Core Psychiatry

This book is dedicated to our families

Commissioning Editor: *Jeremy Bowes*
Development Editor: *Lulu Stader/Ailsa Laing*
Project Manager: *Annie Victor*
Designer: *Stewart Larking*
Illustration Manager: *Bruce Hogarth*

Core Psychiatry

THIRD EDITION

Edited by

Pádraig Wright LRCP&SI LM MB BCh BAO(NUI) MRCPsych MD
Senior Lecturer (Honorary), Institute of Psychiatry, London

Julian Stern BA MB ChB FRCPsych
Consultant Psychiatrist in Psychotherapy, St Mark's Hospital, Harrow

Michael Phelan BSc MB BS FRCPsych
Consultant Psychiatrist, Department of Psychiatry, Charing Cross Hospital, London

SAUNDERS
ELSEVIER

Edinburgh London New York Oxford Philadelphia St Louis Sydney Toronto 2012

SAUNDERS
ELSEVIER

© 2012 Elsevier Ltd. All rights reserved.
© Harcourt Publishers Limited 2000 © 2005, Elsevier Limited.

First edition 2000
Second edition 2005
Third edition 2012
Reprinted 2016

ISBN 9780702033971

British Library Cataloguing in Publication Data
A catalogue record for this book is available from the British Library

Library of Congress Cataloging in Publication Data
A catalog record for this book is available from the Library of Congress

Notices
Knowledge and best practice in this field are constantly changing. As new research and experience
broaden our understanding, changes in research methods, professional practices, or medical treatment may
become necessary.

Practitioners and researchers must always rely on their own experience and knowledge in evaluating
and using any information, methods, compounds, or experiments described herein. In using such
information or methods they should be mindful of their own safety and the safety of others, including
parties for whom they have a professional responsibility.

With respect to any drug or pharmaceutical products identified, readers are advised to check the
most current information provided (i) on procedures featured or (ii) by the manufacturer of each product to
be administered, to verify the recommended dose or formula, the method and duration of administration,
and contraindications. It is the responsibility of practitioners, relying on their own experience and
knowledge of their patients, to make diagnoses, to determine dosages and the best treatment for each
individual patient, and to take all appropriate safety precautions.

To the fullest extent of the law, neither the Publisher nor the authors, contributors, or editors, assume
any liability for any injury and/or damage to persons or property as a matter of products liability,
negligence or otherwise, or from any use or operation of any methods, products, instructions, or ideas
contained in the material herein.

ELSEVIER your source for books,
journals and multimedia
in the health sciences

www.elsevierhealth.com

Working together to grow
libraries in developing countries

www.elsevier.com | www.bookaid.org | www.sabre.org

ELSEVIER | BOOK AID International | Sabre Foundation

The
Publisher's
policy is to use
**paper manufactured
from sustainable forests**

Printed in Great Britain

Core Psychiatry was originally conceived as a single volume postgraduate textbook, primarily for psychiatrists in training, and preparing for the Membership of the Royal College of Psychiatrists.

While our broad intention in preparing the third edition has not changed, the march of time means that we ourselves have changed and can no longer be described as authors who have 'recently attained' Membership of the Royal College of Psychiatrists. The march of time also means that there is much that is new in the sciences that underpin psychiatry and in the practice of clinical psychiatry itself, since the second edition was published. These factors coupled with changes to the curriculum of the Royal College of Psychiatrists have led us to invite several new authors, all experts in their fields, to contribute to this edition. It has also meant that many chapters incorporate much new material and have required extensive revision.

Like the previous editions, this third edition is divided into three parts. Part 1 – The foundations of psychiatry – describes the sciences that underpin the practice of psychiatry. Part 2 – Clinical psychiatry – describes the clinical syndromes with which psychiatrists must be familiar, along with their general treatment and the healthcare settings in which it is delivered. Part 3 – Diagnosis, investigation and treatment – describes the clinical evaluation and clinical investigation of patients and provides a detailed account of our current use of psychotherapeutic, psychopharmacological and neuromodulatory treatments.

Core Psychiatry has become a well regarded textbook since its first publication in 2000, and in 2005 it was 'Highly Commended' in the Mental Health category of the British Medical Association Book Awards.

As with previous editions, many of the authors who have contributed to this edition have been or continue to be associated with the Maudsley Hospital, the Institute of Psychiatry and other leading London teaching hospitals. Other authors have equally illustrious affiliations and we now have chapters written by authors based not only in the UK but also in Australia, Canada, Iceland, Ireland, the Netherlands and the USA. We thank all of them for their excellent contributions.

We hope that this third edition of *Core Psychiatry* will be a useful companion to all students of psychiatry. While originally intended as a postgraduate textbook for psychiatrists, we are pleased that the book is widely used by colleagues in other disciplines, as well as by medical students, nurses, psychologists and other health professionals. We hope that this new edition will also prove useful, informative and enjoyable to a wide readership.

PW, MP, JS 2012

Our intention in producing the first edition of *Core Psychiatry* was to provide a single volume postgraduate textbook for candidates sitting the examinations for Membership of the Royal College of Psychiatrists. We have tried to remain faithful to this intention while preparing this second edition. Thankfully however, we have been thwarted in this intention by the current pace of discovery and development in psychiatry. This is such that every chapter (including the chapter on Clinical Neuro-anatomy) has required considerable revision and the book has grown overall by five chapters.

Like the first edition of *Core Psychiatry*, this second edition is divided into three parts. The first two sections describe the sciences that underpin the practice of psychiatry (*The foundations of psychiatry*) and the clinical syndromes and their treatment, along with the health care settings, with which psychiatrists must be familiar (*Clinical psychiatry*). The final section (*Diagnosis, investigation and treatment*) provides a description of the clinical evaluation and investigation of patients and of current psychotherapeutic, psychopharmacological and other treatments. Again like the first edition, the authors contributing to this second edition are or have been associated with the Maudsley Hospital and Institute of Psychiatry or with other leading London teaching hospitals.

It is our hope that this second edition of *Core Psychiatry* will prove a useful addition to the bookshelves (and better still the desktops and briefcases) of all students of psychiatry, be they trainee or consultant psychiatrists, clinical psychologists, psychiatric nurses or senior medical students.

This book originated from a highly successful revision course for candidates sitting the Parts I and II examinations for Membership of the Royal College of Psychiatrists that two of us (JS, MP) have organized twice yearly in London since 1994 and from the suggestion by one of us (PW) that the knowledge and expertise of the lecturers on this revision course should be collected in a single volume.

Core Psychiatry is divided into three parts. Part I (The Foundations of Psychiatry) describes the historical development of psychiatry and the basic sciences with which all psychiatrists must be familiar, including the rapidly expanding field of psychiatric genetics, and discusses the skills required when reviewing scientific publications. Part II (Clinical Psychiatry) describes the major psychiatric syndromes and disorders, including the sequelae of childhood sexual abuse, and provides a detailed discussion of community psychiatry. Finally, Part III (Diagnosis, Investigation and Treatment) describes how patients should be interviewed and examined and how a diagnosis should be made, provides accounts of contemporary psychotherapeutic, psychopharmacological and other treatments, and discusses contemporary investigational techniques.

All of the authors contributing to *Core Psychiatry* are, or have been, associated with the world-renowned Maudsley Hospital/Institute of Psychiatry or with other London teaching hospitals and most now hold senior clinical or academic appointments in the UK, Ireland or Iceland. They have assumed little previous knowledge of psychiatry and have attempted to provide both introductory and in-depth coverage of their topics.

Thus while *Core Psychiatry* is primarily intended as a postgraduate textbook for candidates sitting the Parts I and II examinations for Membership of the Royal College of Psychiatrists and other similar examinations, it is also a suitable text for postgraduate medical and psychology students, for senior undergraduate medical students and for nursing students. *Core Psychiatry* will also serve as an excellent single volume reference for newly appointed consultant psychiatrists and for other specialists such as neurologists and general practitioners.

PW JS MP 2000

Gwen Adshead MBBS MA PRCPsych
Consultant forensic psychotherapist, West London Mental Health Trust, Broadmoor Hospital, Crowthorne, UK

Stephen Attard MBChB MRCPsych
Locum Consultant Forensic Psychiatrist, The Trevor Gibbens Unit, Hermitage Lane, Maidstone, Kent, UK

Jeremy Berman MBChB MRCP MRCPsych
Consultant Forensic Psychiatrist, The John Howard Centre, London, UK

Sadgun Bhandari MBBS MRCPsych
Consultant Psychiatrist in General Adult and Assertive Outreach Affiliation; Honorary Visiting Fellow, University of Hertfordshire, UK

Rahul Bhattacharya MBBS DPM MRCPsych
Consultant Psychiatrist, East London NHS Foundation Trust, London, UK

Kamaldeep Bhui MBBS MSc MD FRCPsych
Professor of Cultural Psychiatry & Epidemiology, Queen Mary University of London; Honorary Consultant Psychiatrist, East London Foundation Trust, London, UK

Peter Byrne MB MRCPsych
Consultant Liaison Psychiatrist, Department of Psychological Medicine, Newham University Hospital, London; Honorary Senior Lecturer in Social Psychiatry, University College London, London, UK

David J. Castle MB ChB MSc DLSHTM MD FRCPsych FRANZCP
Chair of Psychiatry, St Vincent's Hospital, Melbourne and the University of Melbourne; Consultant Psychiatrist, St Vincent's Hospital, Melbourne, Australia

Heather A. Church MBBCh BAO BA
Senior Registrar in Child & Adolescent Psychiatry, Adolescent Unit, St Patrick's University Hospital, Dublin, Ireland

Anthony Cleare MBBS MRCPsych PhD
Reader in Affective Disorders, Institute of Psychiatry, King's College, London; Consultant Psychiatrist, National Affective Disorders Unit, South London and Maudsley NHS Foundation Trust, London, UK

John Cookson DPhil FRCP FRCPsych
Consultant Psychiatrist, The Royal London Hospital (St Clements), London, UK

John M. Cooney MD MRCPI MRCPsych MD
Consultant in Liaison Psychiatry, St Patrick's Hospital, Dublin, Ireland

Frances Connan MD PhD
Clinical Director and Consultant Psychiatrist in Eating Disorders, Vincent Square Eating Disorder Service, Central North West London NHS Foundation Trust, London, UK

Aiden Corvin MRCPsych
Associate Professor of Psychiatry and Consultant Psychiatrist, Trinity College Dublin and St James' Hospital, Dublin, Ireland

Michael Crawford MD FRCPsych
Reader in Mental Health Services Research, Centre for Mental Health, Imperial College, London, UK

Ross A. Dunne MB MRCPsych HRB
Research Training Fellow, Department of Psychiatry & Trinity College, Institute of Neuroscience, St Patrick's University Hospital, Dublin, Ireland

Abebaw Fekadu MD MSc MRCPsych
Associate Professor, Department of Psychiatry, Faculty of Medicine, College of Health Sciences, Addis Ababa University; Consultant Psychiatrist, Amanuel Specialized Hospital, Addis Ababa, Ethiopia; Honorary Lecturer, Institute of Psychiatry, King's College London, London, UK

Peter Fitzgerald MB MRCPsych
Senior Registrar, Liaison Psychiatry, St James's Hospital, Dublin, Ireland

Stuart Foyle MD
Consultant, The Department of Psychological Therapies and the Department of Liaison Psychiatry, The University Hospital of North Durham, Durham, UK

Michael Gill MD MRCPsych FTCD
Professor of Psychiatry and Consultant Psychiatrist, Trinity College Dublin and St James' Hospital, Dublin, Ireland

Stephen Ginn MRCPsych MChem
General Adult Psychiatry, Tower Hamlets Home, Treatment Team West, Mile End Hospital, London, UK

Nick Goddard BSc MBBS MA MRCPsych
Consultant Child and Adolescent Psychiatrist, De Bascule
(Academic Centre for Child and Adolescent Psychiatry),
Amsterdam, the Netherlands

Claire Henderson MRCPsych PhD
Clinical Senior Lecturer in Psychiatry, Health Service and Population
Research Department, Institute of Psychiatry, King's College,
London; Honorary Consultant Psychiatrist, South London and
Maudsley NHS Foundation Trust, London, UK

Matthew Hotopf MBBS MSc PhD MRCPsych
Professor of General Hospital Psychiatry, King's College, London, UK

Assen V. Jablensky MD DMSc FRCPsych FRANZCP
Professor of Psychiatry School of Psychiatry and Clinical
Neurosciences, The University of Western Australia, Australia

Caroline Jacob MBChB MRCPsych MSc
Consultant Forensic Psychiatrist and Psychotherapist, Calverton Hill
Hospital, Nottingham, UK

Shaloo Jain MBBS MRCPsych
Associate Specialist, West London Mental Health NHS Trust,
Uxbridge Road, Southall, Middlesex, UK

Jelena Jankovic Gavrilovic MD MRCPsych
Clinical Lecturer in General Adult Psychiatry, Barts and the London
School of Medicine, Queen Mary, University of London, London, UK

Mark Jones MBBS MRCPsych FRSA
Consultant Emeritus and Speciality Doctor, The Department of
Psychological Therapies and the Department of Liaison Psychiatry,
The University Hospital of North Durham, Durham, UK

Nicola Kalk MBChB MSc MRCPsych
Clinical Research Fellow, Neuropsychopharmacology Unit, Imperial
College, London, UK

John E. Kraus MD PhD
Director, Medical Sciences, Neurosciences Medicines Development
Center, GlaxoSmithKline, Research Triangle Park, NC; Clinical
Assistant Professor, Department of Psychiatry, University
of North Carolina, Chapel Hill NC, USA

William Lee MBChB MRCPsych
Clinical Research Fellow, Section of General Hospital Psychiatry,
Institute of Psychiatry, King's College, London, UK

Anne Lingford-Hughes PhD BM BCh MRCPsych
Professor of Addiction Biology, Neuropsychopharmacology Unit,
Centre for Pharmacology and Therapeutics, Division of Experimental
Medicine, Imperial College, London, UK

James V. Lucey MD PhD FRCPI FRCPsych
Clinical Professor of Psychiatry, Trinity College Medical School,
Dublin; Medical Director, St Patrick's Hospital, Dublin, Ireland

Paul Mackin MBBS PhD MRCPsych
Senior Lecturer and Honorary Consultant Psychiatrist, Newcastle
University; Academic Psychiatry, Newcastle General Hospital,
Newcastle upon Tyne, UK

Declan M. McLoughlin PhD MRCPI MRCPsych
Research Professor of Psychiatry and Consultant in Old Age
Psychiatry, Department of Psychiatry, Trinity College Institute of
Neuroscience, St Patrick's University Hospital, Dublin, Ireland

Carine Minne MB BCh BAO DRCOG MRCPsych MBPAS
Consultant Psychiatrist in Forensic Psychotherapy, Portman Clinic,
Tavistock & Portman NHS Foundation Trust and Broadmoor Hospital,
West London Mental Health NHS Trust, London; Psychoanalyst,
British Psychoanalytical Society, UK

Joanna Moncrieff MBBS MD MRCPsych
Senior Lecturer/Honorary Consultant Psychiatrist, University College
London and North East London Foundation Trust, London, UK

Stirling Moorey MBBS FRCPsych
Consultant Psychiatrist in Cognitive Behaviour Therapy, Bethlem and
Maudsley NHS Trust, London; Honorary Senior Lecturer, Institute
of Psychiatry, UK

Jean O'Hara MBBS FRCPsych
Consultant Psychiatrist and Clinical Director, Behavioural and
Developmental Psychiatry Clinical Academic Group, South London &
Maudsley NHS Foundation Trust & Institute of Psychiatry, Guy's
Hospital, London, UK

Michael F. O'Neill Phd
Managing Director, Eolas Biosciences Ltd., The Neurosciences
Consultancy; Visiting Fellow, University of Sussex, UK

Oyedeji Oyebode MBBS MPhil MRCPsych
Deputy Medical Director, East London NHS Foundation Trust,
London, UK

Lisa A. Page MRCPsych MSc PhD
Consultant Liaison Psychiatrist, King's College Hospital, London;
Honorary Lecturer, Institute of Psychiatry, London, UK

Catherine Penny MRCPsych LLM
Specialty Registrar in Forensic Psychiatry, The Bracton Centre,
Oxleas NHS Foundation Trust, London, UK

Michael Phelan MBBS FRCPsych
Consultant Psychiatrist, Department of Psychiatry, Charing Cross
Hospital, London, UK

Martin Prince MD MSc FRCPsych
Professor of Epidemiological Psychiatry and Co-Director, Centre for
Global Mental Health, Health Service and Population Research
Department, Institute of Psychiatry, King's College,
London, UK

Lena Rane MBBS MRCPsych
Clinical Researcher, Institute of Psychiatry, King's College London,
London; Honorary Specialty Registrar in Psychiatry, National Affective
Disorders Unit, South London & Maudsley NHS Foundation Trust,
London, UK

Kylie D. Reed MA BMBCh MRCPsych
Honorary SpR and Clinical Research Worker, National Addiction
Centre, Institute of Psychiatry, King's College London,
London, UK

Ajit Shah MB ChB MRCPsych FRCPsych
Professor Emeritus of Ageing, Ethnicity and Mental Health,
International School for Communities, Rights and Inclusion,
University of Central Lancashire, Preston, UK

Thordur Sigmundsson MD MRCPsych
Consultant Psychiatrist, Department of Psychiatry, The University
Hospital (Landspitalinn), Reykjavik, Iceland

Shubuladè Smith MBBS MRCPsych
Consultant Psychiatrist and Clinical Senior Lecturer, Maudsley
Hospital and Institute of Psychiatry, Camberwell, London, UK

Shankarnanarayan Srinath MB MRCPsych
Consultant Psychotherapist, Young People's Service, Psychological
Treatment Services, Addenbrooke's NHS Trust, Cambridge, UK

Julian Stern MB ChB FRCPsych
Consultant Psychiatrist in Psychotherapy, St Mark's Hospital, North
West London NHS Trust, Harrow, UK

Sue Stuart-Smith MBBS PhD MRCPsych TQAP
Consultant Psychiatrist in Psychotherapy, St Albans and Dacorum,
Hertfordshire Partnership NHS Trust; Senior Clinical Lecturer,
Tavistock and Portman NHS Trust, UK

Susannah Whitwell MRCPsych
Consultant Psychiatrist, South London & Maudsley NHS Foundation
Trust, London, UK

Séan Whyte MA BM BCh MRCPsych FHEA LLM
Consultant Forensic Psychiatrist, South-West London Community
Forensic Team, London, UK

Adam Winstock MD MRCP MRCPsych FAChAM
Clinical Senior Lecturer/MSc Programme Leader, National
Addiction Centre, Division of Psychological Medicine & Psychiatry,
London, UK

Pádraig Wright LRCP&SI LM MB BCh BAO(NUI) MRCPsych MD
Honorary Senior Lecturer, Division of Psychological Medicine Institute
of Psychiatry, London, UK

Allan Young MB ChB MPhil PhD FRCPsych FRCPC
Chair of Psychiatry, Imperial College, Centre for Mental Health,
Claybrook Centre, Charing Cross Hospital,
London, UK

Marina Zvartau-Hind MD PhD BC ABPN
Director Neurosciences, GlaxoSmithKline, Uxbridge,
Middlesex, UK

Contents

PART 1

The foundations of psychiatry

A brief history of psychiatry

John Cookson

CHAPTER CONTENTS

Introduction

Many lessons can be learned about the treatment of mental illness from the earlier history of psychiatry. Furthermore, it is useful to consider the use of modern drug treatment and contemporary psychological therapy in the light of the effects of their predecessors. Edward Shorter's *A History of Psychiatry* (1997) and Roy Porter's *The Greatest Benefit to Mankind* (1997) provide excellent comprehensive accounts

by professional historians of much that is discussed in this chapter, which summarizes the history of psychiatry over the last 7000 years.

Ancient and classical times

Neolithic skulls dating from 5000 BC show evidence of trephination, the oldest known form of surgery, which was carried out in ancient times on living patients to release evil spirits or to relieve skull fractures, headaches, convulsions or insanity. The procedure must often have been fatal, but some skulls show bony callus formation, indicative of survival. We know little of what other desperate remedies were attempted by Stone age man, as herbal medicine began its evolution. Archaeological evidence of the use of psychotropic substances in Mexico dates from 8500 BC, with the mescal bean and peyote cactus; samples of peyote containing mescaline from a cave in Texas have been carbon-dated to 5700 years ago (Bruhn et al 2002).

Medicine developed in Mesopotamia and Egypt almost simultaneously and descriptions of epilepsy, dementia and psychotic disorders in the form of spiritual possession are available from both cultures, as indeed they are from the Old Testament of the Bible. Treatment at the time appears to have involved the use of drugs (derived from plants, minerals and animal parts), diets, magical spells and incantations.

Hippocrates (460–377 BC) is regarded as the father of medicine and was among the first to challenge the view that disease was punishment sent from the gods. He especially ridiculed the idea that epilepsy was a 'sacred disease'. Hippocratic texts propounded the notion of four 'humours', of which black bile was associated with melancholia. This broad explanatory scheme (elaborated by Galen, a Greek physician of the first century AD) survived to some extent until the nineteenth century and probably impeded scientific advance.

Mania, melancholia and paranoia were prominent categories in Greek medicine. The writings of Aretaeus (from Cappadocia in Turkey in about AD 150) certainly contain descriptions resembling modern depression and mania. However, it is very difficult to relate ancient accounts of mental illness (or even those from 100 years ago) to their counterparts in modern diagnostic systems.

The Middle Ages

Mentally ill people were the responsibility of their family or community and were often excluded from general society. Mental illness was widely regarded as a spiritual affliction associated with witchcraft or possession by the Devil. This led to the burning of mentally ill people as witches during the Inquisition, to religious institutions becoming responsible for caring for mad people, and to the use of exorcism as a treatment. Thus Bethlem Hospital in London was founded in 1247 to care for the insane and was run by a religious order. 'Shock' was also used in various forms.

The Renaissance and the Reformation

The French philosopher and antipsychiatrist Foucault (1926–1984), has written of the alienation and plight of the insane in these periods, although the historical basis for his statements seems slender (Foucault 1961).

During the Renaissance, at least in literature and painting, the mentally ill were treated with curiosity and fear or even romanticized, but were still excluded from general society and displaced or left to wander.

In the seventeenth century, mental illness began to rank as a problem of the cities. Places of confinement were developed which grouped the poor and the unemployed with criminals and the mentally ill. Workhouses were first established during the Elizabethan era, more from concern about the disruptive social effects of vagrancy than to administer charitable welfare. Houses of correction ('bridewells') existed in England from 1575 for the punishment of vagabonds and relief of the poor. The Poor Law of 1601 made local parishes responsible for electing overseers to provide relief for the sick and work for the able-bodied poor in workhouses. An Act of 1670 gave an increasing sense of a duty of assistance, coupled with the view that work was the cure for idleness and poverty.

In France, a decree of 1656 created establishments (*Hôpital Général*), to which the poor 'in whatever state they may be' could be assigned. One such was the Salpêtrière (previously an arsenal) in Paris. In 1676, an edict of the king required that a *Hôpital Général* be established in each city of France. They were not medical establishments, and the Church was excluded from their administration. Within such places, when the insane became dangerous, their rages were dealt with by mechanical restraint, iron chains, cuffs and bars, leading Foucault to conclude that they were treated as animals, or wild beasts.

The asylum and moral therapy

The history of 'psychiatry' began with the custodial asylum – an institution to confine raging individuals who were dangerous or a nuisance. The discovery that the institution itself could have a therapeutic function led to the birth of psychiatry as a medical speciality. This notion can be traced to clinicians such as William Battie (St Luke's, 1751), Chiarugi (Florence, 1785) and Pinel (Paris, 1795), and lay people such as William Tuke (1796), a Quaker tea merchant who founded the Retreat in York. Such a development was in keeping with the style of thinking of the Age of Enlightenment (that ended with the French Revolution in 1789), with its religious scepticism and its quest for understanding. Pinel (at the Salpêtrière for women and the Bicêtre for men), in particular, anticipated several trends, abolishing the use of restraining chains and recognizing a group of 'curable lunatics' (mainly with melancholia or mania without delusions), for whom a more humanitarian approach in an 'institution morale' seemed to be therapeutic.

The term 'psychiatry' was first used in 1808 by Reil, a professor of medicine in Germany, to describe the evolving discipline, although its practitioners were known as alienists (those who treated mental alienation) until the twentieth century.

During the eighteenth century, there had been a growing trade in lunacy throughout Europe. In Britain, for example, the insane were confined to private madhouses, to which physicians had limited access and input. In 1788, King George III suffered a bout of mental illness for which eventually he received attention from Francis Willis, a 'mad-doctor' renowned for his piercing stare. The constitutional implications were considerable, and parliament subsequently instituted a committee to enquire into this and into the care of the mentally ill in general.

The therapeutic asylums, which sprang up in the nineteenth century, had in common a routine of work and activity and an approach by the staff encompassed in the term 'moral therapy' and variously described as 'a mildness of manner and expression, an attention to their narrative and seeming acquiescence in its truth' (Haslam, Bedlam, 1809), 'the soothing voice of friendship' (Burrows, London, 1828) and 'encouraging esteem . . . conducive to a salutary habit of self-restraint' (Samuel Tuke, York, 1813). Uplifting architecture, as well as access to sunlight and the opportunity to work in the open air, were also valued.

Many of these institutions had charismatic directors and employed attendants who could be trusted not to beat the patients. Reil (1803) described the qualities of a good psychiatrist as having 'perspicacity, a talent for observation, intelligence, goodwill, persistence, patience, experience, an imposing physique and a countenance that commands respect'. These are recognizable ingredients contributing to a placebo effect, and most of the physical treatments at their disposal were largely that: purgatives, enemas, blood letting (advocated, e.g. for mania by Benjamin Rush, the founding father of American psychiatry, 1812) and emetics, aimed to 'draw out' nervous irritants ('catharsis').

During the nineteenth century, the confining of patients to an asylum passed from an unusual procedure born of grave necessity to society's first response when dealing with psychotic illness. Therapeutic asylums were built on a vast scale as politicians responded to the claims of the early enthusiasts. Unfortunately, while the doctors had no effective treatments, the asylums were destined to accumulate more and more incurable patients, leaving the staff overwhelmed, demoralized, and with insufficient time or conviction to sustain their 'moral' approach. The situation was exacerbated by an increase in the numbers of mentally ill people, especially through neurosyphilis and alcoholism, and by the increasing reluctance of families in industrialized society to tolerate their mentally ill relatives.

In 1894, the American neurologist Silas Weir Mitchell told asylum physicians that they had lost contact with the rest of medicine, and that their treatments were 'a sham'. In Britain, apart from the Maudsley Hospital, which opened in 1923 for teaching and research and for the treatment of recently ill patients, asylum psychiatry remained virtually divorced from the rest of medicine until the 1930s.

Academic psychiatry

During the nineteenth century many developments occurred in academic centres in Germany where the new techniques of neuroanatomy (Wernicke), histology (Meynert) and pathology (Alzheimer) were brought to bear. Griesinger wrote an influential textbook (1861) and strove to link psychiatry with general medicine, being of the view that 'psychological diseases are diseases of the brain'. The old humoral theories began to be replaced with new ideas about the connection between mental illness and brain function, and the pursuit of these links was successful for neurosyphilis, cretinism and dementia. By 1900 German academic centres had set a model for psychiatry to be taught alongside medicine.

But despite these developments, the scene was set for a period of therapeutic nihilism, and the rise of the new ideology of psychoanalysis. By the turn of the century, many leading clinicians believed that psychiatric illness was largely incurable, and therefore dedicated themselves to research rather than patient care. Kraepelin (1896) had concluded that mental illness should be defined by its prognosis rather than its cause, and that brain sciences were as yet too nascent to provide an understanding of mental illness. This nullified the premise that enthusiasm for research is a hallmark of better clinical care and failed to recognize that better treatments can be developed without a knowledge of aetiology provided one retains confidence that the illness has a biological basis. Wernicke did attempt to link psychiatric symptoms to brain regions and while successful for aphasia and the speech areas (1874), this approach led to a confusing attempt at classification which Karl Jaspers (1913) later described as 'brain mythology'. Furthermore, the attitude of many clinicians was affected by the doctrine of 'degeneracy' promulgated by Morel in 1857 and the early sexologist, Krafft-Ebing, in 1879, according to which severe mental illness represents the action of hereditary processes progressing over generations, constituting a threat to society. In France the excessive emphasis by Charcot (1825–1893) on 'hysteria' shows us, in retrospect, that illness behaviour may produce the very symptoms that the doctor is keen to treat, through the mechanism of suggestibility.

In the first half of the twentieth century, American psychiatry became dominated by the ideas of Adolf Meyer (Johns Hopkins University) who elevated history-taking, investigations and note-keeping above treatment. Furthermore, academic psychiatrists began to devote more attention to the less severe mental conditions encountered outside the asylum.

A notable voice retaining enthusiasm for developing better treatments was that of Thomas Clouston in Edinburgh, whose textbook (Clouston 1896) described clearly the shortcomings of available physical treatments and the hope for better.

Nervous illness, rest cures and psychoanalysis

By 1900, the public was so frightened of psychiatry that care had often to be delivered under the guise of 'nervous illness', and accurate diagnostic terms had to be avoided. The less severely ill and the better-off sought help in less stigmatizing nerve clinics or 'hydros' (spas offering spring mineral water, showers and baths in pleasant resorts). In 1869, George Beard (New York) invented the term 'neurasthenia' to encompass many non-psychotic or psychosomatic disorders attributed to exhaustion of nerves. In 1875, Weir Mitchell – despite his subsequent debunking of 'sham' treatments – devised a 'rest cure' consisting of seclusion, enforced bedrest, a diet of milk products, electrical treatments and massage. It transpired that the essence of the cure was in fact the physician's authority and the patient's submission to it. Its effectiveness in some cases illustrated the importance of the one-to-one relationship between doctor and patient. This method remained in widespread use by neurologists and psychiatrists until the 1940s.

The introduction of psychoanalysis – with its concepts of transference and countertransference – made doctors more aware of the active nature of the therapeutic relationship. It also helped them to understand the content, though not the form, of mental symptoms, while its depth made psychiatrists rather than neurologists the appropriate specialists to deal with nervous illness. However, its initial promise of hope for the treatment of psychosis and other diagnostic groups proved unjustified, and concepts such as that of the 'schizophrenogenic mother' (a term used by Dr Frieda Fromm-Reichmann, 1935) were dogmatic and misleading.

Plant alkaloids and the first drugs

Dioscorides (AD 57), Nero's surgeon, compiled a list, the 'materia medica', of medicines, including almost 500 derived from plants. Paracelsus (b.1493, Switzerland) is regarded as the grandfather of pharmacology; he taught that each drug (or plant) should be used alone, that chemistry was the science to produce medicines, and that it is only the dose that makes a thing a poison. See Table 1.1 for the history of psychotropic agents.

Plants with medicinal uses affecting the mind include the poppy (opium, morphine) (mentioned in the Ebers papyrus of about 1550 BC Egypt), hellebore (veratrum), *Rauwolfia serpentina* (reserpine), the Solanacea henbane (hyoscine), belladonna (atropine), St John's wort (hypericum alkaloids) and cannabis. Kava root from South Pacific islands has at least 15 chemical ingredients and effects include relaxation and sedation. NB *Gingko biloba* may help dementia. In their natural forms, the medicines derived from plants lacked purity and varied in strength. They were consequently dangerous to administer, with a significant risk of overdose. Chemical techniques of

Table 1.1 The history of psychotropic agents

Year	Comment
1831	Atropine isolated
1857	Bromides synthesized
1869	Chloral as sedative
1880	Hyoscine isolated
1882	Paraldehyde
1903	Barbiturates (Veronal)
1917	Malaria for neurosyphilis
1930	Insulin coma for schizophrenia
1935	Amphetamine (narcolepsy)
1938	Phenytoin introduced; ECT
1942	Antihistamines
1948	Lithium in mania (Cade)
1952	Chlorpromazine (Delay & Deniker)
1954	Lithium (Schou)
1957	Iproniazid, psychic energizer – MAOIs
1958	Haloperidol (Janssen)
	Imipramine (Kuhn): TCAs, MARIs
1961	Chlordiazepoxide: benzodiazepines
1967	Depot antipsychotic injections: Modecate
1968	Lithium prophylaxis
1973	Carbamazepine in mania
1982	Zimelidine: SSRIs
1988	Clozapine (Kane et al)
	Fluoxetine (Prozac) approved
1988	SSRIs in panic disorder
1994	Valproate in mania (Bowden et al 1994)
	Atypical antipsychotics: risperidone, olanzapine
1999	Atypical antipsychotics for bipolar disorder

the nineteenth century enabled the active alkaloid ingredients to be extracted, purified and identified.

Opium had long been used, and morphine was isolated in 1806 and used both orally and by subcutaneous injection as a sedative (after the introduction of the hypodermic syringe by the Scots physician, Alexander Wood, in 1855), until it was realized how addictive it was. Henbane and later hyoscine (isolated in 1880) were used to calm agitated and manic patients, as was atropine. *Rauwolfia serpentina* was used in India more than 2000 years ago for *Oonmaad* (insanity). Reserpine was isolated from it in 1953, and synthesized and introduced as an antipsychotic in 1954; it provided insights into the role of dopamine, noradrenaline (norepinephrine) and serotonin (5HT) in the brain, and the mechanisms of antidepressant drug actions. *Veratrum* was the source of modern calcium antagonists, some of which may have psychotropic properties. St John's wort has now been confirmed to have mild antidepressant activity, and its ingredients share biochemical properties with modern monoamine reuptake inhibitors and serotonin agonists.

Heroin (diacetyl morphine) was synthesized in Bayer laboratories towards the end of the nineteenth century and was initially promoted as a cough remedy. Its name arose because it was said to make factory workers feel 'heroic'. At about the same time, chemists at Bayer were creating aspirin by acetylating salicylic acid, the active ingredient of myrtle, meadowsweet and willow bark; a drug was thus made that was more stable and less bitter. Such was the success of Bayer in making vast sums from healing common ailments that at the Treaty of Versailles, the Allies expropriated the Bayer trademark – and with it aspirin – as part of First World War reparations. Only in the 1970s did Vane discover that aspirin blocked prostaglandin production; work for which he received a Nobel prize, and which led to further uses for aspirin, including stroke prophylaxis.

The French physiologist Claude Bernard (1856) had predicted that certain drugs (such as curare from South American arrow poison) could be used as 'physiological scalpels' to dissect the workings of neurotransmission. This proved prophetic with regard to biochemical theories of depression and schizophrenia, which arose from knowledge of the mechanism of action of antidepressants and antipsychotics, and anticipated the search for drugs with selective actions at particular receptors.

Sedatives, anticonvulsants and bromides

The synthesis by chemists, particularly in Germany, of sedative drugs in the nineteenth century represents the beginning of the modern pharmaceutical industry. Chloral (1832) was synthesized by von Liebig (the founder of organic chemistry), found to be a sedative (1869) and produced by the pharmaceuticals division formed by Bayer (1888). It became widely used in psychiatry, although prone to abuse and addiction, and was the occasional cause of sudden death.

Paraldehyde was introduced into medicine in 1882 and used as an anticonvulsant and sedative, being regarded as relatively safe, albeit unpleasant treatment.

Bromide salts were produced by French chemists in the nineteenth century and found to be sedatives, and in 1857 Locock (London) reported the use of potassium bromide for epilepsy and hysteria. Bromides became popular and remained in use as cheap alternatives to chloral for sedation until the 1940s. In higher doses, they produce bromism, a toxic confusional state. McLeod (1899) used high doses of bromides to induce long periods of deep sleep in patients with mania, with reportedly good results.

Barbituric acid was first synthesized in 1864 but its first useful hypnotic and anticonvulsant derivative, diethyl barbituric acid (Veronal), was only produced much later, in 1904. Sedatives were used to assist catharsis or abreaction in victims of 'shell shock' in the First World War.

Many other barbiturates followed, including phenobarbitone (phenobarbital). These drugs induced sleep and relieved agitation, and paved the way for deep sleep therapy, or prolonged narcosis, in which patients were induced to sleep for 16 hours a day for several days, with drowsy intervals to eat and drink. Although widely used, and much appreciated by hospital personnel, the long-term efficacy of this treatment was never proven in a controlled trial. Prolonged narcosis also carried a significant risk of respiratory and cardiovascular depression, pneumonia and death. The subsequent use of benzodiazepines for prolonged sedation was safer. The first benzodiazepine, chlordiazepoxide, was introduced in 1961, and diazepam, which became the most commonly prescribed drug in the world, followed soon after. The risk of dependence on therapeutic doses of benzodiazepines was not widely recognized until 1981.

Malaria, insulin coma and ECT

The Austrian Julius Wagner-Jauregg had noted in 1883 that a psychotic patient was cured when she developed a streptococcal fever with erysipelas. In 1887, he proposed fever treatment with malaria for psychosis. In 1917, he returned to the subject, treating advanced neurosyphilis patients successfully by injecting blood infected with malaria, which induced a series of fevers that were later terminated by the use of quinine. In 1927, he was awarded a Nobel prize for this. Subsequently, penicillin, discovered by Fleming in 1929 and available clinically from 1944, virtually put an end to neurosyphilis in the developed world. These discoveries provided the first evidence to psychiatrists that a mental illness could be cured, and suggested that heroic methods might be justified.

Insulin was isolated by Banting and Best in 1922. Sakel thought that insulin-induced hypoglycaemic coma could relieve opiate withdrawal problems, and suggested its use in schizophrenia, claiming success in 1934. Insulin units were set up in many hospitals; in some centres, coma was induced with increasing doses of insulin until convulsions occurred. By 1944, insulin coma therapy was the main physical treatment recommended for acute schizophrenia, for instance by Sargent and Slater (1946) in London. However, in 1953, Bourne, a junior psychiatrist, challenged its efficacy; several academic psychiatrists wrote in its defence, but the controlled trial that followed, comparing insulin coma and barbiturate-induced sleep, failed to demonstrate any advantage of insulin coma therapy (Ackner et al 1957). This dangerous treatment gradually fell into disuse and the antipsychotic drugs took its place.

Camphor was used to induce convulsions and claimed to effectively treat melancholia in the eighteenth century (although the convulsions could result in fractured bones). Convulsions induced by the chemical metrazol (Cardiazol), were proposed by von Meduna (1934) to relieve schizophrenia. However, the procedure itself was extremely unpleasant and a more controlled means of inducing convulsions was subsequently devised by Cerletti and Bini (Rome, 1938), using brief electrical currents applied through electrodes on the temples. Electroconvulsive therapy (ECT) was found to alleviate schizophrenia temporarily. The treatment was introduced at St Bartholomew's Hospital in London by Strauss in 1940; Felix Post (1978) described its dramatic impact on the practice of psychiatry at the Bethlem Hospital in relation to depressive psychosis during the 1940s. The subsequent introduction of anaesthetics and muscular relaxants reduced many of the dangers associated with ECT, and its efficacy was established scientifically in double-blind controlled trials in the 1980s.

Diagnostic precision

Accurate diagnosis becomes more important when treatments are discovered which are effective in specific conditions. The description of schizophrenia developed from Kraepelin (1899), through Eugen Bleuler (1911) to Kurt Schneider (1959). The notion of bipolar disorder has developed from Falret's (1794–1870) circular insanity, through Baillarger's (1809–1890) 'folie à double forme' to Kraepelin's manic-depressive insanity (1899), and thence to the refinement by Leonard (1957) into 'bipolar' and 'unipolar' forms.

There is a tendency to overdiagnose conditions for which a new treatment has been discovered, as occurred in the USA with bipolar disorder after the introduction of lithium. When Baldessarini (1970) compared the frequency of affective illness to schizophrenia in patients discharged from hospital before and after the introduction of lithium, a reciprocal pattern was noted, with increasingly frequent diagnosis of bipolar illness and decreasing frequency of schizophrenia. Stoll et al (1993) confirmed this finding in the discharge diagnoses of six psychiatric hospitals from the early 1970s. In the UK, the situation was different. There, affective illness was often diagnosed in patients whom US colleagues regarded as having schizophrenia. This resulted from differences in definition, with a broader concept of schizophrenia in the USA, as shown by the US/UK diagnostic project (Cooper et al 1972). Subsequently, the general acceptance of criteria-based diagnostic systems, particularly the DSM-III in 1982, introduced greater diagnostic reliability. However, the definition of bipolar mood disorder was broadened to include patients with mood-incongruent psychotic features, who would previously have been regarded as having schizoaffective disorder or schizophrenia. Thus, the availability of lithium and the wider use of standard diagnostic systems have led patients to receive a diagnosis of bipolar disorder, who might previously have been diagnosed with schizophrenia, at least in the USA.

Psychotherapies

Sigmund Freud (1856–1939), a Viennese neurologist who studied with Charcot in 1885, abandoned hypnosis in favour of free association and the interpretation of dreams, as a means of attaining 'catharsis' and understanding symptoms. The other ingredients of his 'models', which changed over the years, included the role of the unconscious, infantile sexuality, repression (developed from Pierre Janet) and other 'defence mechanisms' (later listed systematically by his daughter Anna Freud), identification with the lost 'object' in mourning, and the ambivalence of feelings. He also described the dangers and the therapeutic potential of 'transference' – the feelings

Antipsychiatry

It may be no coincidence that following a decade of genuine innovation and progress in treatment in the 1950s, the following decade became known as the era of 'antipsychiatry'. It was also a time of liberal thinking, student socialism, experimentation with mind-altering drugs and the beginning of the widespread abuse of illicit addictive drugs which later expanded into epidemic proportions. Abuse of the new psychopharmacological agents by prescribers was also seen in the almost indiscriminate use of benzodiazepines in general practice, and in the use of inappropriately high doses of antipsychotic drugs in hospitalized patients who seemed resistant to treatment.

The success of psychiatry, which had led to open-door policies and the rundown of psychiatric beds, left the mental hospitals even more vulnerable to criticism. Indeed they were blamed for causing some of the very diseases that patients suffered, such as institutionalization or the deficits of chronic schizophrenia. The influential 'three hospitals' study, by Wing and Brown, appeared in 1961. This seemed to show that patients deteriorated more in a hospital where they were given less individual attention, had fewer personal possessions and were generally treated less well than they would be in a family – the antithesis of moral therapy. This finding in a non-randomized study was often misinterpreted. The terms 'institutionalism' and 'institutionalization' were misapplied as descriptions of, and as an explanation for, the social impoverishment of chronic schizophrenia, even though the same phenomenon could be seen in patients who had little exposure to psychiatric wards, let alone spent years in a mental hospital.

The asylum in its twentieth-century incarnation was rightfully criticized by Goffman (1961) as a total institution that could degrade its inmates. At the same time, however, attacks, regarded by many as sinister and unwarranted, were made upon the very concept of mental illness, and upon the claims of doctors to be able to treat it. Those articulating these ideas included Szasz and Scheff in the USA, R.D. Laing in the UK, and Foucault in France. Gradually, their claims were exposed and discredited by thoughtful argument, based on well-conducted studies of the epidemiology, genetics and psychopharmacological responses of the major mental disorders. Vestiges of these philosophies are still occasionally encountered, usually among those who became acquainted with sociology during the 1960s, but also understandably in those with bad personal experiences of psychiatric services.

Integrating treatment approaches

Accompanying the clinical and financial success of modern drug treatments, there has been a tendency to polarize treatment approaches into the 'organic' or 'biological' and the 'psychological'. The polarization can also be extended to the doctors who favour one or other approach. Such a division may be valid for focusing research interests, but is unhelpful for clinicians. Doctors should avoid becoming identified as solely organic; it may give a sense of knowledge and authority, but it undermines the basis of the doctor–patient relationship, which has been important

for as long as psychiatry, and indeed medicine, has existed. The expanding knowledge base of psychopharmacology places an additional strain upon the therapeutic relationship, which is one that entails a degree of trust. The doctor is expected to be knowledgeable about the treatments being used. Patients may easily acquire detailed information, which can seem to expose gaps in their doctor's knowledge rather than supporting a constructive dialogue. There is also a growing expectation about what the doctor should tell the patient about his/her illness and treatment; again, trust in the doctor can be eroded if the patient feels that he or she has not been given accurate or sufficient information.

The pharmaceutical industry recognizes the value of promoting drugs directly to the public, and uses various means of 'health awareness' to achieve this. Such campaigns became so prevalent, that in 1997, the US Food and Drugs Administration (FDA) made direct-to-consumer advertising of prescription drugs legal. Doctors now have an important role in helping patients to make decisions based on information they may have received from a variety of sources.

Regulatory authorities

Disasters with drugs, such as that associated with thalidomide and fetal malformations in 1961, have led to legislation to regulate the marketing of medicines, for instance the Medicines Act of 1968 in the UK. These agencies, the Food and Drug Administration (FDA) in the USA and the European Medicines Agency (EMA), now set standards for the approval of new drugs and dictate much of the research that is done.

Conclusions

At the start of the twenty-first century, the physical treatments available in psychiatry include an increasing number of highly 'crafted' molecules with selective actions on neurochemical systems. They also include three older treatments that are relatively crude in their mechanism of action: two drugs, lithium and clozapine, which have extensive biological actions and side-effects, and ECT. Although relatively crude, these treatments are still used because they are of proven efficacy. As our understanding of the mechanisms of action of drugs develops, so too does the possibility of developing more sophisticated treatments, with greater efficacy and with fewer side-effects. Psychopharmacology is particularly fascinating because it spans the spectrum of knowledge and understanding from molecules to the mind of the patient.

Experimental techniques play a crucial role in advancing scientific knowledge. The new techniques of structural and functional imaging, combined with isotope-labelled drugs with known sites of action, provide powerful tools with which to explore the brain in health and disease and to expand our understanding of treatments. Together with the new science of molecular genetics, they offer hope that the era of effective treatments in psychiatry will advance much further – and will do so rapidly.

Further reading

Bourne, H., 1953. The insulin myth. Lancet 2, 964–969.

Healy, D., 1996. The psychopharmacologists I and II: Interviews by David Healy. Altman, London.

Healy, D., 1998. The antidepressant era. Harvard University Press, London.

Mitchell, P.B., Hadzi-Pavlovic, D., Manji, H.K. (Eds.), 1999. Fifty years of treatments for bipolar disorder: A celebration of John Cade's discovery. Aust. N. Z. J. Psychiatry 33, S1–S122.

Shepherd, M., 1990. The 'neuroleptics' and the Oedipus effect. J. Psychopharmacol. 4, 131–135.

Part of a special issue on the History of Psychopharmacology, including papers by Carlsson and Kuhn. Discusses the early impact of phenothiazines, and the term 'neuroleptic'.

References

Ackner, B., Harris, A., Oldham, A.J., 1957. Insulin treatment of schizophrenia: a controlled study. Lancet 272, 607–611.

Baldessarini, R.J., 1970. Frequency of diagnoses of schizophrenia versus affective disorders from 1944 to 1968. Am. J. Psychiatry 127, 757–763.

Ballenger, J.C., Post, R.M., 1980. Carbamazepine in manic-depressive illness: a new treatment. Am. J. Psychiatry 137, 782–790.

Bleuler, E., 1911. Dementia Praecox or the Group of Schizophrenias (translated edition 1950). International University Press, New York.

Bowden, C., Brugger, A., Swann, A., et al., 1994. Efficacy of divalproex vs lithium and placebo in the treatment of mania. J. Am. Med. Assoc. 271, 918–924.

Brain, R., 1965. The Second Report of the Interdepartmental Committee on Drug Addiction. HMSO, London.

Bruhn, J.G., De Smeet, P.A., El-Seedi, H.R., et al., 2002. Mescaline use for 5700 years. Lancet 359, 1866.

Carlsson, A., Lindqvist, M., 1963. Effect of chlorpromazine or haloperidol on formation of 3methoxytyramine and normetanephrine in mouse brain. Acta Pharmacol. Toxicol. (Copenh) 20, 140–144.

Cerletti, U., Bini, L., 1938. Un nuovo metodo di shockterapia: 'L'elettroshock' (Riassunto). Communicazione alla Seduta del 28 maggio 1938–XVI. Della Reale Accademia Medica di Roma.

Clouston, T., 1896. Clinical lectures on mental diseases. J. & A. Churchill, London.

Cooper, J.E., Kendell, R.E., Gurland, B., et al., 1972. Psychiatric diagnosis in New York and London: A comparative study of mental hospital admissions. Oxford University Press, New York.

Dale, H.H., Laidlaw, P.P., 1910. The physiological action of beta-iminazolylethylamine. J. Physiol. 41, 318–344.

Delay, J., Deniker, P., 1952. Réactions biologiques observées au cours du traitement par l'chlorhydrate de deméthylaminopropyl-N-chlorophénothiazine. C.R. Congrès. Méd. Alién. Neurol. (France) 50, 514–518.

den Boer, J.A., Westenberg, H.G., 1988. Effect of a serotonin and noradrenaline uptake inhibitor in panic disorder: a double-blind comparative study with fluvoxamine and maprotiline. Int. Clin. Psychopharmacol. 3, 59–74.

Dole Vincent, P., Nyswander, M.E., 1965. A medical treatment for diacetylmorphine (heroin) addiction. A clinical trial with methadone hydrochloride. J. Am. Med. Assoc. 193, 646–650.

Foucault, M., 1961. Madness and civilisation. English translation. Cambridge University Press, Routledge.

Goffman, E., 1961. Asylums. Essays on the social situation of patients and other inmates. Anchor Books, New York.

Kane, J.M., Honigfeld, G., Singer, J., et al., the Clozaril Collaborative Study Group, 1988. Clozapine for the treatment-resistant schizophrenic: a double-blind comparison with chlorpromazine. Arch. Gen. Psychiatry 45, 789–796.

Kuhn, R., 1958. The treatment of depressive states with G 22355 (imipramine hydrochloride). Am. J. Psychiatry 115, 459–464.

Porter, R., 1997. The greatest benefit to mankind: a medical history of humanity from antiquity to the present. Harper Collins, London.

Post, F., 1978. Then and now. Br. J. Psychiatry 133, 83–86.

Sargent, W., Slater, E., 1946. An introduction to physical methods of treatment in psychiatry. Churchill Livingstone, Edinburgh.

Schneider, K., 1959. Clinical psychopathology. Grune and Stratton, New York.

Schou, M., Juel-Nielsen, N., Stromgren, E., 1954. The treatment of manic psychoses by the administration of lithium salts. J. Neurol. Neurosurg. Psychiatry 17, 250–260.

Shorter, E., 1997. A history of psychiatry: from the age of the asylum to the era of Prozac. Wiley, New York.

Stoll, A.L., Tohen, M., Baldessarini, R.J., et al., 1993. Shifts in diagnostic frequencies of schizophrenia and major affective disorders at six North American psychiatric hospitals, 1972–1988. Am. J. Psychiatry 150, 1668–1673.

von Meduna, L., 1934. Arch. Psychiatr. Nervenkr. 102, 333–339.

Wing, J.K., Brown, G.W., 1961. Social treatment of chronic schizophrenia. J. Ment. Sci. 107, 847–861.

Clinical neuroanatomy

2

Anne Lingford-Hughes   Nicola Kalk

CHAPTER CONTENTS

Although not an absolute maxim, apraxia generally results from dysfunction in the dominant hemisphere and agnosia from dysfunction in the non-dominant hemisphere. These terms are more fully described after discussing signs and symptoms associated with dysfunction in specific lobes of the cerebral cortex.

Frontal lobe

The frontal lobe includes the prefrontal cortex, motor and supplementary motor cortices, Broca's area and frontal eye fields. Damage to the frontal lobes generally results in changes in personality, often profound, but in the presence of few other symptoms or signs. Consequently, changes or lesions in the frontal lobe can be 'silent' for a considerable length of time.

Functions of the frontal lobe

The prefrontal cortex (PFC) is divided into the medial and lateral surface and the latter into the ventrolateral, dorsolateral and anterior prefrontal regions. The PFC mediates executive functions of the brain such as focusing attention on relevant information and processes, and inhibiting irrelevant ones, switching focused attention between tasks, planning a sequence to achieve a goal, updating working memory to make sure a plan is 'on-task', as well as coding this information. Tests of frontal lobe function therefore generally include tasks that require attention, switching attention, planning and manipulation of information such as learning new rules, e.g. Wisconsin Card Sort Test.

The prefrontal cortex is also involved in encoding and retrieval of memories. The dorsolateral prefrontal cortex is particularly involved in working memory, i.e. short-lasting memory associated with active maintenance and rehearsal of information to achieve a goal in behaviour, speech or reasoning. The prefrontal cortex is also part of the mesolimbic or mesocorticolimbic system and receives dopaminergic projections from the ventral tegmental area in the brainstem. It is hypothesized that hypofunction in this pathway contributes to the negative features of schizophrenia.

The anterior cingulate cortex is part of the limbic system and is strongly implicated in attention and emotional processing. For example, its activity increases in response to emotionally significant stimuli. Its ventral subdivision appears to be the 'affective' component and impaired function here is strongly implicated in depression. The orbitofrontal cortex (OFC) is also part of the limbic system and is involved in processing the reward value of stimuli and in suppressing motor responses. It therefore plays a key role in decision-making and appropriate responsiveness. OFC dysfunction has been reported in some disorders of impulse control such as obsessive-compulsive disorder and addiction. Patients with OFC dysfunction can show inability to appreciate and avoid possible negative future consequences of their actions.

Personality changes

Damage to the prefrontal cortex results in changes in personality which broadly fit into categories of disturbed mood, poor judgement, and impaired social awareness and motivation (Box 2.3).

The changes seen in mood tend to be those of euphoria rather than depression, but all changes have an 'empty' feeling to them.

Box 2.3

Personality changes associated with frontal lobe dysfunction

- Disinhibition – Reduced social awareness and control
- Loss of finer feelings – Sexual indiscretions
- Errors of judgement – Decreased abstracting ability
- Irritability – Elevated mood (fatuous, childish)
- Lack of concern for others – Lack of drive
- Catastrophic response – Inability to adapt to the unexpected
- Impaired initiation – Impaired concentration and attention

Childishness may be a feature, including making jokes and performing pranks (*Witzelsucht*). Lack of drive and motivation coupled to an inability to plan, impaired judgement and poor social awareness often result in profound disability. Other features include perseveration, both of speech and movements, palilalia or repetition of phrases and sentences and decreased verbal fluency. Basal/medial damage tends to have the most profound effects on personality. Damage to the lateral frontal lobe is associated with decreased motivation referred to as 'pseudodepressive' frontal lobe syndrome.

Motor changes

The primary motor cortex lies in the posterior part of the frontal lobe. The body is represented somatotopically and inverted with areas such as the face taking up more area than the lower limb. If this area is damaged, contralateral hemiparesis will be present. The signs can be subtle but the grasp reflex is invariably elicited. If the frontal lobe superior to the eye is damaged, 'forced utilization' may be seen. Here, when objects are placed in front of the subject, an object will be picked up and used appropriately, even when the subject is told not to do so. Urinary incontinence can also be a sign of frontal lobe dysfunction.

Other changes

If the lesion is in the posterior part of the dominant frontal lobe, apraxia of the face, motor aphasia and motor agraphia may also be present. A lesion of Broca's area, which is in the motor area in the posterior frontal cortex, will result in problems with verbal expression. This is revealed by poor articulation and sparse speech. This is known as expressive or Broca's aphasia.

Clinical examination

The appearance and behaviour of the subject will provide many clues to frontal lobe dysfunction. The following bedside tests are sensitive to frontal lobe dysfunction: verbal fluency; ability to interpret proverbs (abstract thinking); movements requiring coordinated series of actions such as the Luria 3-step test.

Temporal lobe

Damage to the temporal lobe can result in amnesia, personality disturbances and visual field and sensory deficits, depending on the location of the lesion. Typically, lesions involving the dominant lobe result in more symptoms and signs. Components of the temporal lobe, such as the hippocampus and amygdala, play important roles within the limbic system and are more fully described below.

Sensation

The temporal lobe is the final destination for different sensory modalities including auditory, vestibular, gustatory and olfactory senses.

Memory and amnesia

The medial temporal lobe, including the hippocampus, plays a crucial role in mediating declarative memory, i.e. memory of personal events (episodic memory) and factual knowledge (semantic memory). The hippocampus serves as a final common pathway for other structures in the medial temporal cortex, such as the amygdala, parahippocampal and entorhinal cortices. Profound amnesia results from bilateral medial temporal lobe lesions. Causes of such lesions include infections, tumours, epilepsy and bilateral occlusion of the posterior cerebral artery. Subjects with such lesions will have preserved performance at tasks requiring intact immediate memory (e.g. digit span). Both retrograde and anterograde memory, i.e. memory of events before and after the lesion, respectively, will be impaired. Retrograde amnesia may not be as severe as the anterograde amnesia and memory for remote events may be well preserved. Semantic memory remains intact. More specific lesions of the hippocampal formation, if they occur bilaterally, will also result in global amnesia. The deficit resulting from unilateral lesions of the temporal cortex involving the hippocampus will depend on whether the dominant or the non-dominant lobe is affected. Problems with learning new verbal material results from dysfunction of the dominant lobe, with impaired learning of new non-verbal information (e.g. music) resulting from lesions of the non-dominant lobe.

Personality changes

Personality changes include depersonalization, emotional instability, aggression and antisocial behaviour. Psychosis may also be present, as can be seen in temporal lobe epilepsy. Manic psychoses are associated with right-sided lesions.

Visual field deficit

Lesions deep within the temporal lobe which involve the optic radiation result in a contralateral homonymous upper quadrant visual field defect.

Other changes

If lesions are in the dominant lobe, sensory or receptive aphasia will be present. Lesions in the posterior part of the temporal lobe will also result in alexia and agraphia. Hemisomatognosia, prosopagnosia and visuospatial problems may be present after damage to either hemisphere, but more commonly occur with non-dominant hemisphere dysfunction.

Lesions within Wernicke's auditory association area in the dominant superior temporal cortex result in problems of reduced verbal comprehension and reading and writing abilities. Despite their speech being fluent, reduced comprehension means that the speech may be nonsensical or so-called jargon aphasia. This is also referred to as Wernicke's or receptive aphasia.

Klüver–Bucy syndrome

This syndrome results from bilateral ablation of temporal lobes and destruction of the uncus, amygdala and hippocampus. In monkeys, an increase in oral and sexual behaviours, placidity and a loss of fear or anger with apathy and pet-like compliance is seen. A similar syndrome is seen in humans in association with a number of disorders such as Pick disease, Alzheimer dementia, arteriosclerosis, cerebral tumours and herpes simplex encephalitis. The syndrome is also associated with visual agnosia and sometimes prosopagnosia and hypermetamorphosis (patients touch everything).

Parietal lobe

The parietal lobe is involved in a number of complex tasks involving attention, integration of information such as recognition, visuospatial abilities and appreciation of environmental cues and the appropriate connection of sensory input to action. Hence, while patients with parietal lobe impairment are not visually blind to a visual stimulus, they cannot interpret the stimulus, particularly its spatial attributes, or use visual information to guide movements of the body. The parietal lobe syndrome consists of constructional apraxia, visuospatial agnosia, topographical disorientation (getting lost, inability to learn new routes), visual inattention and cortical sensory loss, when objects can be felt but not fully interpreted or discriminated.

Lesions in the dominant lobe result in motor aphasia if the lesion is anterior, or sensory aphasia if the lesion is posterior. Other consequences include agraphia with alexia, motor apraxia and bilateral tactile agnosia. Visual agnosia occurs if the parieto-occipital region is affected.

A specific syndrome, Gerstmann syndrome, is associated with lesions of the dominant parietal lobe. This consists of dyscalculia, agraphia, finger agnosia and right-left disorientation. Lesions in the nondominant hemisphere result in anosognosia, hemisomatognosia, dressing apraxia and prosopagnosia. Balint syndrome is caused by bilateral damage to the posterior parietal lobe and is characterized by optic ataxia, oculomotor apraxia and simultanagnosia.

Occipital lobe

The occipital lobe is involved in processing visual information. Although all of the following can occur with dysfunction of either hemisphere, the more common associations are described. Lesions in the dominant lobe result in alexia without agraphia, colour agnosia and visual object agnosia. Lesions in the non-dominant lobe result in visuospatial agnosia, prosopagnosia, metamorphosia (image distortion) and complex visual hallucinations.

The occipital lobe syndrome consists of contralateral homonymous hemianopia, scotomata and simultagnosia.

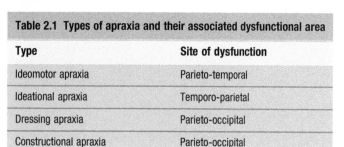

Table 2.1 Types of apraxia and their associated dysfunctional area

Type	Site of dysfunction
Ideomotor apraxia	Parieto-temporal
Ideational apraxia	Temporo-parietal
Dressing apraxia	Parieto-occipital
Constructional apraxia	Parieto-occipital

Table 2.2 Types of agnosia and their associated dysfunctional area

Type	Site of dysfunction
Visuospatial agnosia, e.g. prosopagnosia, simultagnosia	Parietal (especially right-sided lesions result in left-sided neglect)
Visual identification problems, e.g. hemisomatognosia, anosognosia, autotopagnosia	Temporal lesions (especially, right)

Table 2.3 Glossary of apraxias and agnosias

Constructional apraxia/ visuospatial agnosia[a]	Inability to construct or copy figures
Dressing apraxia	Difficulty dressing and undressing
Ideomotor apraxia	Difficulty carrying out requested movements or intended movements
Agraphia	Inability to write
Alexia	Inability to read
Dyscalculia	Inability to calculate
Topographical disorientation	Getting lost, inability to learn new routes
Autotopagnosia	Inability to name, recognize or point to parts of own or someone else's body
Hemisomatognosia	Part of body felt to be absent
Prosopagnosia	Inability to recognize faces
Anosognosia	Failure to recognize a disabled limb
Finger agnosia	Inability to name/number fingers
Simultagnosia	Inability to recognize complex pictures

[a]There is considerable overlap in the signs of these two syndromes.

Specific signs and syndromes seen with cortical lobe dysfunction

Apraxia

Apraxia is the inability to carry out purposeful voluntary movements. This cannot be accounted for by paresis, incoordination, sensory loss or involuntary movements. The same movements can, however, be performed in another context such as part of a reflex. The different types of apraxia and associated site of dysfunction are listed in Table 2.1.

Agnosia

Agnosia is the inability to recognize an object through sensation, however it is presented, e.g. touch, sight, smell. The impairment cannot be attributed to sensory defects, mental deterioration, disorders of consciousness or attention or to non-familiarity with the object. Some different types of agnosia are listed in Table 2.2. Examples of various agnosias and apraxias are described in Table 2.3.

Cerebellum

The cerebellum develops from the metencephalon and lies posteriorly to the pons and medulla. It is concerned with coordination of movement, maintenance of muscle tone and equilibrium. Increasingly, the role of the cerebellum in cognition is being recognized. There are two hemispheres flanking the midline vermis.

Phylogenetically, there are three parts to the cerebellum. The archicerebellum is the inferior portion of vermis and receives efferents from and sends efferents to the vestibular nuclei. Lesions here result in a broad-based gait. The paleocerebellum is the anterior lobe and receives afferents from the anterior and posterior spinocerebellar tracts and sends efferents to vestibular and reticular nuclei. The role of the paleocerebellum is concerned with muscle tone and lesions here affect extensor tone. The neocerebellum consists of the posterior lobe and the tonsil. Afferents come from the pontine nuclei, which is a relay for cortical information. Thus, this part of the cerebellum is concerned with skilled voluntary movements.

Cellular constituents of the cerebellar cortex

The cerebellar cortex is three-layered (Table 2.4). The ascending fibres to the cerebellum all terminate in specific parts of the cortex and send collaterals to one or more of the cerebellar nuclei. They are all excitatory. Mossy fibres are excitatory fibres that are the terminal projections of spinocerebellar, pontocerebellar

Table 2.4 Layers of the cerebellar cortex

	Cell type	Function
Superficial		
Molecular layer	Basket cell, Stellate cell	Inhibitory on Purkinje cell
Purkinje layer	Purkinje cell	Predominant cell type, receives all afferent information and provides only efferent pathway contains GABA
Granular layer	Granule cell; Golgi cell	Axon ascends to molecular layer and bifurcates to run parallel to surface; synapses on dendrites of Purkinje cell
Deep		

and vestibulocerebellar tracts. The fibres terminate in glomeruli, which are synaptic arrangements involving a granule cell, its dendrites and Golgi cells. Climbing fibres provide excitatory input from the olivocerebellum and reticulocerebellum. These fibres terminate on the GABA-containing Purkinje cells, in a 1:1 arrangement, wrapped around their dendrites. Descending fibres from the cerebellum all originate from Purkinje cells and end in cerebellar nuclei where they exert an inhibitory influence. The cerebellar nuclei are the dentate, emboliform, globose and fastigial nuclei.

Connections of the cerebellum

The cerebellar peduncles contain the afferent and efferent tracts of the cerebellum. The inferior cerebellar peduncle contains four afferent tracts (posterior spinocerebellar, vestibulocerebellar, olivocerebellar and reticulocerebellar) and one efferent tract (the cerebellovestibular tract). The middle cerebellar peduncle is the largest and contains only afferent fibres from the pontine nucleus. This pontocerebellar tract provides an important connection between the cerebral cortex and cerebellum and modulates skilled activities of hands and fingers. The superior cerebellar peduncle contains one afferent, anterior cerebellar tract and one efferent tract from the cerebellar nuclei to the red nucleus, thalamus and medulla.

Cerebellar function

The cerebellum receives information from eyes, ears, proprioceptors, brainstem, cerebral cortex and reticular formation, which is integrated and relayed to other centres involved in controlling movement in the brain. The result of this integration is smooth, coordinated motor function. Patients with cerebellar dysfunction may show truncal ataxia and disequilibrium. Muscle tone will be reduced, muscles will tire easily and decreased reflexes will be present. Incoordination of movements will be manifest by poor ability to perform rapid alternating movements (dysdiadochokinesis), past-pointing in finger–nose testing (dysmetria) and intention tremor. Speech may be slurred, jerky, explosive and intermittent. Nystagmus will prevent visual fixation on an object, and gait will be that of a wide-based ataxia.

Until relatively recently, the cerebellum has only been thought of in terms of its key role in motor control. Functional neuroimaging studies have shown that the cerebellum is also involved in working memory, implicit and explicit learning and memory and language. However, there are no clinical tests that specifically probe this aspect of its function.

Diencephalon

The diencephalon is composed of four constituents (see Box 2.4).

> ### Box 2.4
>
> #### Constituents of the diencephalon
> - Thalamus
> - Hypothalamus
> - Epithalamus
> - Subthalamus

Thalamus

The thalamus is a collection of many nuclear groups and hence consists largely of grey matter. It is a relay station for both sensory and motor information. The connections and functions of the nuclei, with particular reference to psychiatry, are described in Table 2.5. Damage to the medio-dorsal nucleus of the thalamus is thought to be important in the pathogenesis of Korsakoff's psychosis.

Hypothalamus

Like the thalamus, the hypothalamus consists of groups of nuclei, involved in endocrine control, neurosecretion, regulation of autonomic function, regulation of body temperature, the biological clock, food and water intake and sexual function. It is also part of the limbic system and is involved in mediating emotion, rage, fear, pleasure and reward.

In addition to being named (Table 2.6), the nuclei of the hypothalamus are also described by their anatomical location within the hypothalamus. Thus the ventromedial nucleus which controls satiety and feeding has a lateral feeding centre and a medial satiety centre. Ablation of the satiety or feeding centres leads to hyperphagia and aphagia, respectively. The control of water intake is similarly located. A major role of the hypothalamus in controlling endocrine function is to release hypothalamic releasing factors which stimulate or inhibit the release of hormones from the anterior pituitary. The hypothalamic releasing factors and their corresponding anterior pituitary hormones are described in Table 2.7.

Connections of the hypothalamus

Many of the connecting pathways of the thalamus are part of a two-way system projecting between the midbrain and limbic lobe (Fig. 2.2).

Afferent pathways

There are a number of pathways that connect the hypothalamus with other components of the limbic system, the medial forebrain bundle, fornix and stria terminalis. The medial forebrain bundle consists of projections from the olfactory part of forebrain and septal nuclei and passes through the hypothalamus, to the tegmentum in the midbrain. Fibres from the medial forebrain bundle project into the lateral hypothalamus.

The fornix arises from the hippocampus and projects to the mammillary bodies, and is more fully described in relation to the hippocampus. The stria terminalis arises in the amygdala, a nuclear complex with a key role in the formation and processing of emotional content. In addition to terminating in the nucleus of stria terminalis, projections terminate in the preoptic, tuberal and anterior nuclei of the hypothalamus.

Other afferent fibres arise in the forebrain, upper brainstem, thalamus and visual pathways.

Efferent pathways

Many of the pathways described above also carry efferent projections from the hypothalamus. The medial forebrain bundle carries fibres from the lateral hypothalamus to the septal nuclei

Amygdala

The amygdaloid complex contains many nuclei involved in both sensory and motor functions. It is an important component of the limbic system. The amygdala plays a key role in emotional processing and associative learning, making emotional memories easier to recall than non-emotional events. Damage to the amygdala can result in impaired emotional processing of stimuli, such as increased threshold, e.g. degree of fear, threat, disgust, anger and impaired emotional learning and deficits in emotional perception and expression. Stimulation of the amygdala produces aggressive behaviour in animals, while ablation causes placidity. Recent neuroanatomical studies have suggested that the amygdala, part of the nucleus accumbens and the stria terminalis represent one functional unit, referred to as the 'extended amygdala'.

Nucleus accumbens

The nucleus accumbens is contained within the ventral striatum in man but is not visible as an anatomically separate division within this part of the striatum. The nucleus accumbens is part of the mesolimbic system and receives dopaminergic projections from the ventral tegmental area (VTA) in the brainstem. Release of dopamine in the nucleus accumbens is critical in mediating positive reinforcement or pleasure for both natural rewards such as food or sex and also substances of abuse such as alcohol and cocaine. Dopamine-dependent processes are involved in recognizing stimuli and in 'labelling' them with appetitive value, predicting and detecting rewards and signal alerting and novel events. More recently, it has been recognized that release of dopamine here also occurs in response to aversive stimuli. An alternative theory that dopaminergic stimulation of the nucleus accumbens determines the salience of stimuli rather than reward per se has subsequently been proposed. Hyperdopaminergic states in the mesolimbic tract may be involved in delusional perception – the attribution of salience to inconsequential events.

Basal ganglia

Components of the basal ganglia

The basal ganglia consist of the corpus striatum, globus pallidus, claustrum and specific nuclei of the amygdaloid complex (Fig. 2.3 and Box 2.6). The corpus striatum comprises the caudate nucleus and putamen. The combination of the putamen laterally and globus pallidus medially is referred to as the lentiform nucleus. The claustrum is the strip of grey matter lateral to the lentiform nucleus.

Connections of the basal ganglia

The caudate and putamen receive afferent fibres from all parts of the cerebral cortex and topographically project onto the globus pallidus. Efferent fibres from the globus pallidus project to

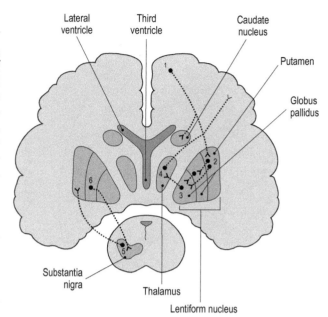

Figure 2.3 • Basal ganglia and its connections: coronal stylized section. Pathway 1→4 is the mechanism by which voluntary movement is modulated. Pathway 5→6 is the nigrostriatal/striatonigral pathway.

Box 2.6

Components of the basal ganglia

- Corpus striatum caudate nucleus putamen
- Lentiform nucleus globus pallidus putamen
- Claustrum
- Amygdala

---

the ventral nuclei of the thalamus and brainstem. The ventral nuclei of the thalamus also project to the premotor cerebral cortex, completing a circuit whereby motor activity arising in the motor cortex can be monitored and modulated by the basal ganglia. The other major reciprocal connection is between the striatum and the substantia nigra, the nigrostriatal and striatonigral pathways (Fig. 2.3).

Functions of the basal ganglia

The basal ganglia are responsible for programming, integration and termination of motor activity. Motor activity controlled by the basal ganglia forms a significant part of the extrapyramidal motor system (see below). However, the traditional view that the basal ganglia are simply involved in the control of movement has been challenged in recent years. Activity in some parts of the basal ganglia is higher during cognitive or sensory functions and circuits exist between the basal ganglia and cognitive areas of the cerebral cortex. The basal ganglia appears to be involved in fundamental aspects of attentional control (often covert), in the guidance of the early stages of learning (especially reinforcement-based learning, but also in encoding strategies in explicit paradigms), and in the associative binding of reward to cue salience and response sequences via dopaminergic mechanisms.

Basal ganglia dysfunction

Dysfunction involving the basal ganglia results in a number of motor disorders. The resulting typical signs and symptoms are described in Table 2.8. The nigrostriatal projection to the globus pallidus and striatum from the substantia nigra contains dopamine. Degeneration of this pathway, due to loss of neurons in the substantia nigra and consequent loss of dopamine, underlies Parkinson disease. The symptoms of Parkinson disease or so-called parkinsonism can be reproduced by blockade of dopamine D_2 receptors in the basal ganglia. This is commonly seen secondary to the use of typical antipsychotic medication.

Other disorders associated with dysfunction of the basal ganglia include Huntington chorea, caused by degeneration of the caudate, and Wilson disease, caused by copper deposition in the basal ganglia and liver. In Huntington chorea, loss of caudate function causes choreiform movements and neuropsychiatric symptoms such as depression, psychosis and dementia. Huntington chorea is an autosomal dominant disease, with the gene on chromosome 4. In addition to dysfunction of the basal

Table 2.8 Basal ganglia dysfunction

Disturbance of muscle tone	Rigidity: cog-wheeling
Loss of automatic associated movement	Swinging arms when walking, facial expression
Unwanted movements, uncontrollable, purposeless, usually distal	Choreiform: 'fidgety' movements Hemiballismus Athetoid: slow, writhing movements of arms and legs Resting tremor

ganglia, the classic sign of Wilson disease is the Kayser–Fleischer ring – a brown coppery ring around the cornea. Wilson disease is due to an inborn error of copper metabolism.

Brainstem

The brainstem ascends from the spinal cord through the medulla, pons and midbrain and into the diencephalon (Box 2.7).

Spinal cord

The spinal cord consists of a number of ascending and descending tracts that convey sensory and motor information between the periphery and the brain (Fig. 2.4).

Ascending tracts

The ascending tracts carry sensory information from the periphery to the central nervous system.

Proprioception, tactile discrimination and vibration sense

The fasciculus gracilis and cuneatus constitute large tracts in the posterior part of the spinal cord. Fibres in these tracts are organized such that those from sacral to cervical spinal nerves lie medial to lateral, respectively. They carry sensory information regarding proprioception, tactile discrimination and vibration sense. The tracts are ipsilateral until they reach the medulla, where they synapse in their respective nuclei. Fibres project from here, cross over, ascend as the medial lemniscus and terminate in the ventral posterior nucleus of thalamus. Fibres project from the thalamus to the somatosensory, parietal cortex, via the internal capsule. The body is mapped somatotopically and inverted with the face most inferior.

Box 2.7

Contents of the brainstem

Medulla

Decussation of pyramids – corticospinal tracts
Rubrospinal, vestibulospinal, tectospinal tracts
Medial longitudinal fasciculus – ascending and descending fibres (involves eye movements – III, IV, VI)
Inferior olivary nucleus – projects to cerebellum
Nucleus gracilis and cuneate
Decussation of medial lemniscus – fibres from gracilis and cuneus to thalamus
Nuclei of cranial nerves XII and spinal root of XI
Spinal root of cranial nerve V
Medial, lateral, superior and inferior vestibular nuclei
Anterior and dorsal cochlear nuclei
Dorsal motor nucleus of cranial nerve X
Solitary nucleus
Nucleus ambiguus – motor – for IX, X, XI
Reticular formation
Fourth ventricle
Inferior cerebellar peduncle

Pons

Corticobulbar, rubrospinal tracts
Medial longitudinal fasciculus
Spinal trigeminal nucleus and tract
Mesencephalic nuclei of V
Nucleus of VI
Nucleus of VII
Trapezoid body
Superior olivary nucleus – auditory
Lateral and superior vestibular nuclei
Reticular formation
Locus coeruleus (noradrenaline)
Floor of fourth ventricle
Middle and superior cerebellar peduncles

Midbrain

Mesencephalic nucleus of V
Nucleus of IV
Oculomotor nucleus (III) (Edinger–Westphal)
Medial longitudinal fasciculus
Reticular formation
Raphe nuclei (serotonin)
Periaqueductal grey matter
Superior cerebellar peduncle
Medial and lateral lemniscus
Crus cerebri
Substantia nigra
Inferior colliculi – auditory
Superior colliculi – visual cerebral cortex and efferents to spinal cord, cranial nuclei
Red nucleus – afferents from cerebellum and cerebral aqueduct

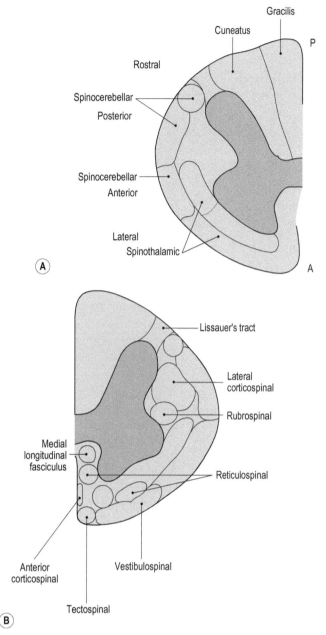

Figure 2.4 • Spinal cord tracts. (A) Ascending tracts. (B) Descending tracts. A, anterior; P, posterior.

Pain and temperature

The lateral spinothalamic tract carries information about pain and temperature. The anterior spinothalamic tract carries sensory information regarding light, poorly localized touch. This information is carried in slow-conducting fibres (Aδ and C fibres) in contrast to the rapidly conducting fibres carrying information about pain and temperature. After joining the spinal cord, the fibres cross after ascending 1–2 segments and synapse in Lissauer's tract. From there, the fibres ascend as the lateral or anterior spinothalamic tract, and terminate in the ventral posterior nucleus of the thalamus. Fibres are also given off to the reticular formation and periaqueductal grey matter. The sensory cerebral cortex receives the final projections as described above.

Since the dorsal columns and spinothalamic tracts contain ipsilateral and contralateral fibres, respectively, transection of one-half of the spinal cord leads to a characteristic pattern of sensory loss. This is known as Brown–Sequard syndrome or sensory dissociation. Below such a lesion, there is loss of two-point discrimination and proprioception ipsilaterally and loss of pain and temperature sensation contralaterally.

Muscle and tendon function

The spinocerebellar tract relays information from muscle spindle or tendon–organ receptors. It is an ipsilateral tract.

Descending tracts

The descending tracts relay information from cortical and subcortical regions and the brainstem to the periphery to initiate and modulate movement.

Corticospinal or pyramidal tracts

The corticospinal tracts mediate voluntary movements and arise from the cerebral cortex as described previously. The lateral corticospinal tract is present throughout the entire length of the spinal cord. The anterior corticospinal tract is different in two respects from the lateral corticospinal tract in that it is ipsilateral and terminates at the level of the thoracic vertebrae.

The extrapyramidal tracts

There are several tracts that constitute the extrapyramidal motor system. The vestibulospinal tract arises from the vestibular nuclei and terminates on the anterior horn cells. Information in this tract facilitates activity in all anti-gravity (extensor) muscles. The rubrospinal tract arises from the red nucleus in the midbrain and terminates on interneurons. This tract terminates in the thoracic part of the spinal cord and controls flexor tone. The tectospinal tract arises from the superior colliculus and terminates on interneurons. This tract relays information to the cervical level about postural reflexes to do with visual and auditory stimuli. The reticulospinal tract arises from brainstem nuclei and also terminates on interneurons.

Mixed ascending and descending tract

The medial longitudinal fasciculus contains both ascending and descending fibres. It relays information regarding visual tracking of a moving object through coordinated movements of eyes, head, neck and trunk. The descending fibres arise from the superior colliculus, motor nucleus of the IIIrd cranial nerve (visual, visual tracking), and pontine and vestibular nuclei (balance). The fibres terminate on anterior horn cells. Ascending fibres arise from vestibular nuclei and terminate in the IIIrd, IVth and VIth cranial nerve nuclei.

Overview of sensory and motor systems

Sensory system

Conscious appreciation of sensation occurs in the post-central gyrus of the parietal lobe, of visual stimuli in the occipital lobe and of auditory stimuli in the temporal lobe. The sensory nerve for all of these modalities arises in the dorsal root ganglion, the processes of which terminate at the peripheral receptor in the tissue and centrally at nuclei specific to the information being carried. A projection then relays the information topographically to the thalamus, from which the final projection to the parietal cortex arises.

Receptors

There are a number of different peripheral receptors. Flower-spray and anulospiral endings in muscle spindle organs and Golgi tendon organs register stretching or movement. Thus they play an important role in proprioception, perception of limb position and control of posture and muscle tone.

Touch, temperature and pain are detected by unencapsulated receptors such as free or Merkel's discs. The encapsulated receptors, the Pacinian and Meissner corpuscles, detect pressure and vibration and two-point discrimination, respectively. Sensory information is carried in myelinated Ad and Ab fibres and in unmyelinated C fibres. Touch is mediated by Ad and Ab, pain by Ad, and temperature by C fibres. Each spinal nerve carries information from a specific dermatome, or area of cutaneous and subcutaneous tissue. The pathways running within the spinal cord to the brainstem and associated with each sensory modality are described above.

Motor system

Voluntary movement is initiated in the primary motor cortex of the frontal lobe. The body is mapped somatotopically and inverted, with the face most inferior on the lateral surface and lower limbs represented on the medial surface of the frontal lobe. The pyramidal cells of this region give rise to fibres that run through the internal capsule, decussate in the midbrain and travel down the spinal cord as the corticospinal tract. The tracts terminate on the anterior horn cells and also on interneurons within the spinal cord.

In addition, collaterals are given off to the basal ganglia – predominantly the putamen – and to the cerebellum. This allows modulation and coordination of voluntary movement. These systems constitute part of the extrapyramidal system (see above).

The corticospinal tract provides an excitatory input to the anterior horn cells, whereas the extrapyramidal system tends to be inhibitory. All projections onto the anterior horn cell are referred to as upper motor neuron, and from the anterior horn cell to the muscle as lower motor neuron. The effects of lesions of lower and upper motor neurons are described in Table 2.9.

Table 2.9 Effects of lower and upper motor neuron lesions

Lower motor neuron	Upper motor neuron
Hypotonia	Hypertonia
Flaccid paralysis	Spastic paralysis
Hyporeflexia	Hyperreflexia
Wasting of muscles with fasciculation, fibrillation	Babinski sign

Autonomic nervous system

The autonomic nervous system (Fig. 2.5) is that part of the peripheral nervous system that innervates and regulates smooth and cardiac muscles and glands. The autonomic system and the central nervous system, including the hypothalamus and limbic system, interact in order to integrate activity appropriately. However, many autonomic responses are at an unconscious level and are governed through reflexes.

The autonomic nervous system comprises sympathetic and parasympathetic systems. These nervous systems tend to have the opposite effect on target organs such that parasympathetic stimulation leads to increased gut motility, for example, while sympathetic stimulation causes reduced motility.

The peripheral target organ is reached through a two-neuron relay in the autonomic system. The preganglionic neuron is located in the spinal cord or brainstem and terminates in a peripheral ganglion. Arising from this ganglion, the postganglionic neuron innervates the target organ. In the sympathetic nervous system, the postganglionic fibres are much longer than the preganglionic fibres. The reverse is true in the parasympathetic system. Thus, the ganglia in the sympathetic system lie close to the central nervous system while the ganglia of the parasympathetic lie close to the target organ. Another difference between these two systems is the neurotransmitter released by the postganglionic fibres. Parasympathetic postganglionic fibres release acetylcholine, while sympathetic fibres release noradrenaline with the exception of those that terminate in sweat glands which release acetylcholine. In both parasympathetic and sympathetic systems, the preganglionic neurons release acetylcholine.

The site of origin of the sympathetic and parasympathetic nervous systems also differ anatomically. The sympathetic nervous system arises from the intermediolateral grey column of thoracolumbar segments T1–T12 and L1–L2 of the spinal cord. The preganglionic cell bodies of the parasympathetic system are located in the brainstem, and in the intermediate grey matter of sacral segments S2–S4 of the spinal cord. Brainstem parasympathetic nuclei include the Edinger–Westphal nucleus (IIIrd cranial nerve), the superior and inferior salivatory nuclei (VIIth and IXth cranial nerves) and the dorsal motor nucleus of the vagus (Xth cranial nerve) (see Cranial nerves, below, and Fig. 2.5).

The vagus (X) nerve supplies a great number of organs over an extensive area, including the heart, lungs, gut and other abdominal organs. The ganglia from which the postganglionic fibres arise are sited usually in the walls of the target organ. Vagal stimulation results in reduced heart and respiratory rate, constriction of bronchi and increased bronchial secretion, and increased gut motility and secretions therein.

The sacral component of the parasympathetic nervous system arises in the neurons of the lateral horn of sacral segments S2–S4 of the spinal cord. The preganglionic fibres are termed the pelvic splanchnic nerves. The target organs include the colon, rectum, urinary bladder and reproductive organs. Stimulation results in emptying of the bladder, increased gut motility and erection of the penis or clitoris. In addition, vaginal secretions are increased in women.

Cranial nerves

There are 12 pairs of cranial nerves. Their exit foramina from the skull are described in Table 2.10. Each cranial nerve is described as to whether it has sensory or motor, or somatic or autonomic components.

Olfactory nerve

The Ist cranial nerve is the olfactory nerve, a sensory nerve arising peripherally in the mucous membrane of the nasal cavity. The nerve passes through the cribriform plate of the ethmoid bone and synapses in the olfactory bulb. The second-order neurons form the olfactory tract and project to the septal area, and from there to the hippocampus and hypothalamus. The primary

(amygdaloid complex and piriform cortex) and secondary (entorhinal cortex) olfactory areas are the final projection areas.

Optic nerve

The retina

This sensory cranial nerve arises from the retinal ganglion cells. The outermost layer of the retina comprises pigmented epithelium under which lie the rods and cones. These are sensitive to light. The rods are more sensitive to light than the cones and hence are responsible for night vision. The cones contain one of three different pigments that are maximally sensitive to light in the blue, green or orange range. They are concentrated in the fovea centralis. Both rods and cones synapse with bipolar cells, cones in a 1:1 relationship while rods may synapse with many bipolar cells. The bipolar cells then synapse with ganglion cells, whose axons form the optic nerve.

The optic nerve and radiation

The medial fibres of the optic nerve, which represent the temporal visual fields, cross in the optic chiasma to join the contralateral optic tract (Fig. 2.6). The lateral fibres of the optic nerve,

Table 2.10 The cranial nerves and the skull foramina through which they exit

Olfactory nerves	I	Cribriform plates of ethmoid bone
Optic nerve	II	Optic canal with ophthalmic artery
Oculomotor nerve	III	Superior orbital fissure
Trochlear nerve	IV	Superior orbital fissure
Ophthalmic (1st) of trigeminal nerve	V	Superior orbital fissure
Maxillary (2nd) of trigeminal nerve	V	Foramen rotundum
Mandibular (3rd) of trigeminal nerve	V	Foramen ovale
Abducens nerve	VI	Superior orbital fissure
Facial nerve	VII	Internal auditory meatus
Vestibulocochlear nerve	VIII	Internal auditory meatus
Glossopharyngeal nerve	IX	Jugular foramen
Vagus nerve	X	Jugular foramen
Both roots of accessory nerve	XI	Jugular foramen
Spinal roots of accessory nerve	XI	Foramen magnum
Hypoglossal nerve	XII	Hypoglossal canal

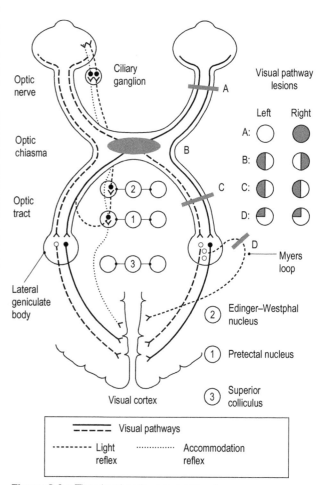

Figure 2.6 • The visual pathway and its reflexes.

representing the nasal visual field, pass through the optic chiasma to the ipsilateral optic tract. The fibres of the optic tract synapse in the lateral geniculate body of the thalamus. From here, the optic radiation runs within the posterior part of the internal capsule. The optic radiation terminates in the visual cortex, which is part of the occipital lobe, with fibres also going to association areas of the parietal cortex. Myer's loop is part of the optic radiation that loops anteriorly from the lateral geniculate ganglion into the temporal lobe before travelling posteriorly to terminate in the occipital cortex. Fibres in Myer's loop carry information from the top half of the visual field. In the occipital cortex, the visual fields are inverted such that the inferior cortex receives information from the upper visual field.

Effects of lesions of the visual pathway

Lesions within the visual pathway produce characteristic visual defects that pinpoint the site of the lesion (Fig. 2.6). A lesion anterior to the optic chiasma results in loss of the visual field to that eye. Any lesion of or posterior to the optic chiasma will result in visual defects in both eyes. A pituitary tumour compressing the optic chiasma and hence the temporal visual field fibres as they cross will result in bitemporal heteronymous hemianopia. Homonymous hemianopia results from loss of the optic tract or radiation on one side. Damage to Myer's loop results in homonymous superior quadrantanopia and may be the first indication of a lesion within the temporal lobe. Papilloedema is characterized by blurring of the optic disc on fundoscopy and can be caused by a number of different conditions (Table 2.11).

Oculomotor nerve

The oculomotor nerve is a motor nerve containing both somatic and parasympathetic components.

Motor somatic

The oculomotor nuclei are within the midbrain, next to the periaqueductal grey matter and superior colliculus, and give rise to a nerve that ascends and passes through the superior orbital

Table 2.11 Common causes of papilloedema

Intracranial mass lesion
Encephalitis
Subarachnoid haemorrhage
Accelerated hypertension
Disc infiltration
Retinal vein obstruction
Optic neuritis (MS)
CO_2 retention
Chronic anoxia
Optic neuropathy

Table 2.12 Movements of the eye and the muscles responsible

Muscle	Nerve	Movement
Medial rectus	III	Horizontally inwards
Inferior rectus	III	In abduction: depresses eye
Superior rectus	III	In abduction: elevates eye
Inferior oblique	III	In adduction: elevates eye
Superior oblique	IV	In adduction: depresses eye
Lateral rectus	VI	Horizontally outwards
Levator palpebrae	III	Lifts eyelids

fissure. The eye muscles innervated by the oculomotor nerve are the inferior rectus, medial rectus, superior rectus, inferior oblique and levator palpebrae. The role of these muscles and their innervation is described in Table 2.12.

The motor nuclei of the IIIrd, IVth and VIth nerves are linked through the medial longitudinal fasciculus, which coordinates movement of the eyes. Fixation to a target or searching the visual fields involves involuntary and voluntary movement of the eyes respectively. The former involves a reflex arc including the occipital association areas. Visual search or saccadic eye movements involves a projection from the occipitoparietal cortex to the frontal eye fields in the frontal lobe.

Motor parasympathetic

The parasympathetic motor nucleus of the third nerve is the Edinger–Westphal nucleus, which sends preganglionic fibres to the ciliary ganglion. The short ciliary nerves comprise the postganglionic fibres and project to the ciliary and sphincter pupillae muscles of the iris. Stimulation results in pupillary constriction and focusing for near vision or accommodation.

Pupillary reflexes

Light reflex

The pupillary light reflex functions to allow the size of the pupil to respond to light conditions by contracting and dilating and also allows both pupils to react together or consensually. The afferent limb consists of the optic nerve, projecting through the optic chiasma and optic tract bilaterally to the pretectal nucleus and the parasympathetic Edinger–Westphal nucleus. The efferent limb consists of parasympathetic preganglionic fibres from the Edinger–Westphal nucleus, which accompany the oculomotor nerve and synapse in the ciliary ganglion. From there, postganglionic fibres innervate the ciliary and constrictor muscles of the iris. The light reflex does not involve the visual cortex (Fig. 2.6).

Accommodation reflex

The accommodation reflex functions to allow the eye to focus on near objects. Projections from the primary visual cortex via the superior colliculus and/or pretectal nucleus terminate in the Edinger–Westphal nucleus. From here, parasympathetic nerves follow the same pathway as for the light reflex and project to the ciliary muscle. On contraction of this muscle, lens convexity increases, facilitating near vision (Fig. 2.6).

Effects of lesions

Lesions of the oculomotor nerve result in ptosis and deviation of the eye downwards and outwards. If parasympathetic innervation is also lost, the pupil will be dilated. Argyll Robertson pupils occur in neurosyphilis and are small, unequal, irregular pupils that do not react to light. The convergence reflex, however, is normal. In Horner syndrome, the pupil is constricted due to the loss of sympathetic innervation. Ptosis, anhydrosis and enophthalmos also occur (Table 2.13).

Trochlear nerve

The trochlear or IVth cranial nerve is a motor nerve that supplies the superior oblique muscle of the eye (Table 2.12).

Abducens nerve

The abducens nerve (VI) is also solely a motor nerve and supplies the lateral rectus muscle of the eye (Table 2.12). This nerve emerges at the cerebellopontine angle and has the longest intracranial course, both of which make this nerve particularly vulnerable to damage. Loss of nerve function results in 'cross-eye'. This nerve is the most commonly affected in ophthalmoplegia associated with Wernicke–Korsakoff syndrome.

Trigeminal nerve

The trigeminal nerve is the largest cranial nerve and contains both motor and sensory, and somatic and autonomic components. It emerges at the cerebellopontine angle, along with cranial nerves VI, VII, VIII and IX.

Motor somatic

The motor nucleus lies close to the sensory nucleus, and fibres run within the mandibular branch. Thus, unlike the other two branches of the trigeminal nerve, the mandibular branch contains both sensory and motor nerve fibres. It supplies the muscles of mastication, which are temporalis, masseter and pterygoids,

and in addition supplies tensor tympani of middle ear, tensor veli palatini of pharynx and digastric muscles of mouth. A lesion involving this nerve results in loss of the jaw jerk.

Sensory somatic

The cell bodies of primary sensory somatic neurons are located in the trigeminal ganglion and give rise to three peripheral divisions or branches:

- The ophthalmic division enters the orbit through the superior orbital fissure with the ophthalmic artery and IIIrd, IVth and VIth cranial nerves. This branch innervates skin on top of the head and scalp and is involved in the corneal reflex, via the nasociliary branch.
- The maxillary branch innervates skin on the cheek area.
- The mandibular branch innervates skin on the lower part of the face, buccal cavity, external ear, lower teeth and lip.
- Centrally, fibres from these sensory nerves convey impulses to three sensory nuclei:
  - The spinal trigeminal nucleus mediates facial touch, temperature and pain via the spinal trigeminal tract.
  - The main sensory nucleus mediates touch, position sense and two-point discrimination.
  - The mesencephalic nucleus of the Vth nerve mediates proprioception of muscles of mastication.

From the spinal trigeminal nucleus and main sensory nucleus, fibres relay information to the sensory cortex of parietal lobe via the ventral posterior nucleus of the thalamus.

Autonomic

While it has no parasympathetic nucleus, as seen with the IIIrd nerve, various branches of the trigeminal nerve include autonomic – both parasympathetic and sympathetic – components.

Facial nerve

The VIIth nerve contains motor somatic and parasympathetic, and sensory somatic and autonomic components. Like the Vth nerve, it emerges at the cerebellopontine angle.

Motor somatic

The motor somatic component supplies the facial muscles. Its course runs through the ear, giving off a branch to the stapedius muscle, and it emerges from the facial canal into the parotid gland. There it divides into the temporal, zygomatic, buccal, mandibular and cervical branches, which supply all the muscles of facial expression. Other muscles innervated include the posterior belly of digastric and the stylohyoid.

There are a number of sites on its course where the facial nerve is particularly vulnerable to damage. These include the internal auditory meatus (by a tumour of the VIIIth nerve), in the facial canal (by infection of the middle ear) or within the parotid gland (by tumour or surgery). Peripheral lesions result in paralysis or weakness ipsilaterally, i.e. Bell's palsy. Central lesions, which are upper motor neuron lesions, result only in the

Table 2.13 Eponymous pupil abnormalities	
Marcus Gunn pupil	Relative afferent pupillary defect
Holmes–Adie pupil	One pupil relatively wide in bright light, relatively constricted in dark
Argyll Robertson pupil	Intact accommodation but abolished light reflex – syphilis
Hutchinson's pupil	Pupil on one side constricts then dilates, followed by the same pattern on the other side. Occurs in rapidly increasing intracranial pressure
Horner syndrome	Ptosis, miosis, anhidrosis

contralateral muscles in the lower part of the face being affected. Since forehead muscles are supplied by crossed and uncrossed fibres, there is seldom any objective paralysis of these muscles.

Motor parasympathetic

The secretomotor parasympathetic nerves arise from the superior salivary nucleus and supply the nasal, palatine, sublingual, submandibular and parotid glands. The parasympathetic nerves run in the greater and lesser petrosal nerves. The lacrimal nucleus supplies the lacrimal gland.

Sensory somatic

The cell bodies of the sensory somatic nerves arise in the geniculate ganglion and terminate in the spinal trigeminal nucleus. Touch, pain and temperature from a small area of skin on the external ear are mediated through these nerves. The spinal trigeminal nucleus subserves these modalities for a number of cranial nerves (V, VII, IX and X).

Sensory autonomic

The cell bodies of the autonomic nerve lie in the nucleus solitarius and convey taste from the anterior two-thirds of the tongue in the greater petrosal nerve. The nucleus solitarius also sends fibres to the IXth and Xth cranial nerves.

Vestibulocochlear nerve

The VIIIth nerve is solely sensory and subserves both hearing and balance. This nerve also emerges at the cerebellopontine angle and is vulnerable to damage.

Cochlea – hearing

Fibres from the cochlea terminate in the superior and inferior cochlear nuclei, situated at the inferior cerebellar peduncle. Fibres then ascend ipsilaterally to the superior olivary nucleus or cross in the trapezoid body to the contralateral superior olivary nucleus in the pons. From here fibres constitute the lateral lemniscus and terminate in the inferior colliculus, where some fibres also cross. The final part of the pathway is via the auditory radiation, which is part of the internal capsule, to the superior temporal or Heschl's gyrus (auditory cortex). Since the fibres cross, lesions within the auditory cortex cause minimal deafness. However, a lesion of the peripheral nerve will cause unilateral deafness.

Vestibular – balance

The vestibular nerve mediates balance and its projections terminate within the cerebellum and nuclei of the oculomotor nerves.

Glossopharyngeal nerve

The IXth nerve is both motor sensory and parasympathetic, and sensory somatic and autonomic. The nerve emerges at the cerebellopontine angle.

Motor somatic

This component supplies stylopharyngeus and superior constrictor muscles of pharynx and hence lesions result in ipsilateral paralysis and difficulty in swallowing. The cell bodies are in the nucleus ambiguus, which also gives rise to motor fibres for the Xth and XIth cranial nerves.

Motor parasympathetic

Cell bodies for the motor parasympathetic division lie in the inferior salivatory nucleus and terminate in the parotid gland. Stimulation results in watery secretions, rich in amylase.

Sensory somatic

The somatic sensory nerve innervates the skin of the external auditory meatus and the back of the ear. Fibres terminate in the spinal trigeminal nucleus.

Sensory autonomic

The autonomic sensory nerve mediates:

- Pain and poorly localized sensation from palate, pharynx, tonsils
- Carotid sinus – pressure receptors at bifurcation of carotid artery
- Carotid body – chemoreceptor for hydrogen ion, CO_2 and O_2
- Taste on the posterior third of the tongue.

All fibres join together in the inferior (petrosal) ganglion and the central processes terminate in the nucleus solitarius. This nucleus also receives fibres from the VIIth and Xth cranial nerves and projects to the ventral posterior nucleus of the thalamus.

Vagus nerve

The Xth nerve is both motor somatic and parasympathetic, and sensory somatic and parasympathetic.

Motor somatic

The motor somatic nerve fibres arise in the nucleus ambiguus and innervate muscles of pharynx and palate. A branch, the recurrent laryngeal nerve, innervates the laryngeal muscles. Unilateral lesion of this nerve results in a partially obstructed airway and dysphonia while a bilateral lesion results in closed vocal cords and a narrowed airway. This nerve is particularly vulnerable to damage in thyroid surgery.

Motor parasympathetic

Postganglionic fibres arise from ganglia in cardiac, pulmonary, gastric and intestinal walls. Stimulation results in contraction of smooth muscle, slowed heart rate and secretomotor activity in all glands including liver, pancreas and gallbladder.

Sensory somatic

This is a small branch that innervates the skin of the external ear and whose fibres terminate in the spinal trigeminal nucleus.

CSF circulates from the lateral to the IIIrd ventricle via the inter-ventricular foramina of Monro, then into the IVth ventricle via the cerebral aqueduct to Sylvius and finally via the foramina of Magendie (midline) and Luschka (two, lateral) into the subarachnoid space where it is reabsorbed passively from the subarachnoid space by arachnoid villi within the dural venous sinuses.

Obstruction of CSF flow in the IIIrd or IVth ventricles or their communicating pathways leads to non-communicating hydrocephalus. Raised intracranial pressure is associated with non-communicating hydrocephalus and the symptoms and signs reflect this: nausea and vomiting, headache made worse on lying down, reduced pulse, raised blood pressure and papilloedema.

Obstruction to CSF flow in the subarachnoid space leads to communicating or normal pressure hydrocephalus. The symptoms associated with this condition are ataxia, urinary incontinence and nystagmus with impaired cognition.

Further reading

Diamond, M.C., Scheibel, A.B., Elson, L.M., 1985. The human brain coloring book. HarperCollins, New York.

Gilam, S., Newman, S.W., 1987. Manter & Gatz's essentials of clinical neuroanatomy and neurophysiology. FA Davis, Philadelphia.

Lishman, W.A., 1998. Organic psychiatry. Blackwell Science, Oxford.

Talley, N., O'Connor, S., 1989. Clinical examination. Blackwell Science, Oxford.

Williams, P.L., 1995. Gray's anatomy, thirty eighth ed. Churchill Livingstone, Edinburgh.

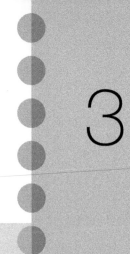

Psychiatric genetics

Aiden Corvin   Michael Gill

3

Introduction

Genetics is the scientific study of the inheritance of physical and behavioural traits. Genes, the units of inheritance, provide an assembly code for the complex molecules that make up life and enable reproduction of living organisms. Genes are located at varying intervals along chromosomes, which are highly compacted linear molecules of deoxyribonucleic acid (DNA) housed in cell nuclei. Within species they pass from generation to generation providing familial resemblance and individual variation, which through evolution, is responsible for the diversity of life. This chapter describes the basic principles of genetics and their relevance to psychiatric practice.

Genetics

The history of genetics

Knowledge of heredity has been exploited in the breeding of animals and plants since prehistoric times. The first recorded reference and response to genetic disease (haemophilia) was recorded 1500 years ago. Although the term 'genetics' was coined in 1906 by the British biologist William Bateson, the science of genetics began 40 years earlier. In 1866 an Austrian monk, Gregor Mendel, described the pattern of inheritance of seven simple, bimodal traits in pea plants including seed shape (round or wrinkled) and colour (yellow or green). Mendel suggested that each parent plant had a pair of units of inheritance for each trait but contributed only one unit from each pair to its offspring. He developed two laws to account for his observations and noted that all possible combinations of the seven traits could occur:

- Mendel's first law (the law of segregation) states that one of an individual's two genes (alleles) at any locus is randomly distributed to each gamete.
- Mendel's second law (of independent assortment) states that the segregation of the alleles for any one trait to a gamete occurs independently of the segregation of the alleles for any other trait to that gamete.

The significance of Mendel's work was only realized at the turn of the twentieth century, and the laws he derived became the foundation of modern genetics. Mendel's research informed the work of Thomas Hunt Morgan, an American geneticist who studied fruit flies. He demonstrated that genes were arranged linearly on chromosomes within cell nuclei, so that, contrary to Mendel's second law, genes on the same chromosomes could be inherited together depending on the physical distance between them and the frequency of recombination (see below) in that region of the chromosome. Genes inherited in this way are said to be linked, and the phenomena of genetic linkage (or departure from Mendel's second law) has enabled genetic maps to be constructed and used to locate genes responsible for diseases. Morgan also demonstrated that linkage is rarely complete and that some traits are sex-linked.

In 1944 Oswald Avery, a Canadian bacteriologist, confirmed that genes were composed of DNA by transferring DNA from one strain of bacteria to another and showing that the second strain acquired traits from the first, and could pass these traits to future generations. Also in the 1940s the American geneticists George Beadle and Edward Tatum discovered that specific genes produced specific polypeptide enzymes. In 1953, geneticists James Watson and Francis Crick, American and British, respectively, discovered that the DNA molecule was composed of two long strands that form a double helix (Watson & Crick 1953). Their deduction of the structure of DNA was made from X-ray photographs taken by a British scientist, Rosalind Franklin, and a New Zealander, Maurice Wilkins. Crick and Watson determined that DNA resembled a long, spiral ladder with a sugar-phosphate backbone and rungs composed of pairs of complementary nucleotide bases. This proposition immediately suggested that genetic information could be transmitted across generations if the two strands of DNA unwound and separated at the nucleotide bases and new complementary nucleotide bases linked to each separated strand. Such a mechanism would result in the production of two identical double helices.

By this time it was known that genes produced proteins and scientists speculated that a genetic code, encrypted in the order of nucleotide bases, must determine the sequence of amino acids in proteins. Only four different nucleotides had been identified in DNA, but at least 20 different amino acids were known to occur in proteins. In 1962, Crick found that the coding sequence was a series of three nucleotide bases and that each amino acid was specified by at least one of these sequences (a codon). Recent developments have made significant contributions to the new science of molecular genetics. The British biochemist Fredrick Sanger developed methods for analysing the molecular structure of proteins and for rapidly determining the nucleotide sequence of nucleic acids. The American

biochemist Kary Mullis in 1983, developed a refinement of the polymerase chain reaction (PCR), which allowed rapid enzymatic synthesis *in vitro* of specific DNA sequences. From these breakthroughs came the Human Genome Project, a 13-year international effort, which completed the sequencing of a human genome of 3 billion bases in 2003, only 50 years after the discovery of the structure of DNA. Sequencing technology has evolved rapidly and large-scale sequencing of thousands of individuals will soon be feasible.

Chromosomes, cell division and genes

The nucleus of a human cell has 23 homologous pairs of chromosomes (46 in all), one member of each pair being inherited from each parent. Each chromosome consists of a single molecule of DNA, and the total DNA complement in a cell is referred to as its genome. The human genome is over 2 m long and contains approximately 3.9×10^9 base-pairs (bp). Only 2–3% of the genome contains the complement of approximately 20 000 genes: the remainder of the genome is not 'junk' and is being discovered to have many functions including regulation of DNA structure, repair and expression.

A gene is a length of DNA that codes for a sequence of amino acids. Each gene is located at a specific site on a chromosome called a locus. Because chromosomes exist in homologous pairs there is a pair of genes at any given locus. The DNA base sequence throughout the genome, including within genes, varies considerably between individuals and between the two copies possessed by an individual. These different forms are called alleles and are often denoted by letters such as A or a, B or b. As stated in Mendel's first law, only one allele for each gene may be inherited from each parent. Individuals who inherit the same allele for a gene from both parents are said to be homozygous (e.g. AA or BB), while those who inherit different alleles for a gene from their parents are termed heterozygous (e.g. Aa or aA). This means that an individual has two genes for every trait. At a locus the alleles of the two genes constitute the individual's genotype. The expression of the trait coded for by the genotype is called the phenotype. If AA and Aa individuals have the same phenotype, the allele A is said to be dominant over allele a (or allele a is recessive to allele A). If the Aa phenotype is intermediate between AA and aa phenotypes, the alleles A and a are termed codominant.

The nucleus of the human cell generally contains 46 chromosomes (23 pairs). This is termed the diploid state and applies to somatic cells, but sex cells (gametes) have only 23 chromosomes and are termed haploid. These differences in chromosome number, on which sexual reproduction depends, arise because somatic cells replicate by mitosis and gametes by meiosis. In mitosis chromosomes are duplicated in the *prophase* stage of the cycle. The duplicated chromosomes join at a constricted chromosomal region called the centromere to form sister chromatids. In *metaphase*, a spindle forms from a centriole at each cell pole to the centromere. During *anaphase* the spindles retract, pulling a chromosome to each pole and distributing the chromosomes equally between two daughter cells identical to the parent cell (*telophase*).

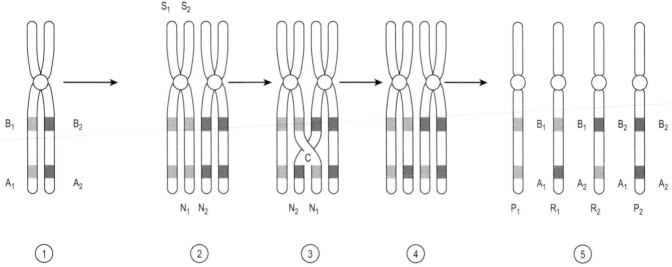

Figure 3.1 • Meiosis and crossing over. (1) Pairing of homologous chromosomes. A_1 and A_2 are different alleles of the same gene A. Similarly, B_1 and B_2 are different alleles of the same gene B. (2) Duplication of homologous chromosomes to form 4 chromatids (referred to as the tetrad). S_1 and S_2 are sister chromatids while N_1 and N_2 are non-sister chromatids. (3) Crossing over of non-sister chromatids N_1 and N_2 at the chiasma, C. (4) For clarity, only one crossing over is illustrated. However, for any pair of non-sister chromatids, crossing over occurs at numerous chiasmata; genes that were originally on the same chromosome are dispersed to separate chromosomes (and vice versa) at each crossing over. (5) Separation of the tetrad to chromatids. R_1 and R_2 are recombinant chromatids while P_1 and P_2 are parental chromatids. The four daughter cells resulting from this meiosis will each contain a chromatid. (From original drawings by Pádraig Wright.)

In contrast, gametes are produced by meiosis in which daughter cells receive only half the number of chromosomes (Fig. 3.1). During the prophase stage of meiosis, each chromosome of each homologous pair duplicates itself, and the resulting sister chromatids are joined at the centromere. Each homologous pair of chromosomes produces a tetrad consisting of four chromatids. Non-sister chromatids pair together, and recombine (cross over) exchanging genetic information. On average, one recombination occurs per chromosomal arm in meiosis. This means that genes originally on different members of a pair of parental (non-recombinant) chromosomes may become located on a single daughter (recombinant) chromosome. The cell now divides into four daughter cells, each haploid and each containing a single chromatid from the tetrad. At fertilization, when gametes fuse, the normal diploid state of 46 chromosomes is restored. These two processes, recombination and random assortment of chromosomes at fertilization, contribute to individual differences and diversity within species.

Human chromosomes can be easily visualized by microscope in cells undergoing mitosis obtained from a stained buccal smear. For chromosomal studies the chromosomes are paired and sorted in roughly decreasing length from 1–22 and called autosomes. The remaining two chromosomes are the sex chromosomes X and Y. Females have two X chromosomes (genotype XX) and males have an X chromosome and a shorter Y chromosome (XY). Early in female development, one of these X chromosomes is inactivated and is known as the Barr body (or sex chromatin); whether the active X chromosome is of maternal or paternal origin is a random event. Healthy females are therefore mosaics of cells with active X chromosomes of either maternal or paternal origin (mosaicism is described more fully below).

Each chromosome is divided by the centromere into two arms, usually of different lengths. The shorter arm is designated the p (for petit) arm and the longer is designated q (because q comes after p in the alphabet). Some chromosomes (e.g. 8–11) are of similar length, and with a homogenous stain it may not be possible to distinguish them. Additional staining procedures produce pale or dark bands of varying thickness specific to each chromosome, allowing individual chromosomes or chromosomal regions to be consistently identified. A standard nomenclature is used when studying chromosomal regions. For example, a locus in the second subdivision of the first band on the p arm of chromosome 8 would be termed 8p1.2. Based on the increasing availability of full human genome sequence information, there is a gradual shift from nomenclature based on cytogenetic bands to one using base-pair location in reference DNA sequences.

Molecular genetics

Molecular genetics is the branch of genetics that investigates the chemical and physical nature of genes and the mechanisms by which genes control development, growth and physiology.

Basic molecular genetics

Each chromosome contains a molecule of DNA composed of a backbone of sugar (deoxyribose) and phosphate, the purine bases adenine (A) and guanine (G), and the pyrimidine bases cytosine (C) and thymine (T). These repeating units of 5-carbon sugar, phosphate and organic bases are called nucleotides. The DNA molecule resembles a spiral ladder, where each side is composed of alternating deoxyribose and phosphate molecules with pairs of bases as rungs. Because bases can only pair by forming hydrogen bonds between T and A, or G and C, the sequence

DNA variation and genetic markers

In any two randomly selected human genomes 99.9% of the DNA sequence is identical. The remaining 0.1% accounts for population diversity and individuality including susceptibility to disease. Molecular genetics seeks to correlate differences between this DNA polymorphism/variation (genetic markers) and phenotypic differences (such as having a disease or trait). Many different types of polymorphisms can be used as genetic 'markers', including small deletions or insertions, variability in small (1–5 bp) repeat sequences (microsatellite markers) or single nucleotide polymorphism (SNPs), the commonest form of polymorphism. To date many thousands of microsatellite markers and more than 20 million reference SNPs have been identified and are publicly available to researchers (www. ncbi.nlm.nih.gov/SNP) seeking to map disease or trait genes.

Mendelian inheritance

The patterns of inheritance described by Mendel are due to the relative effects of complementary genes on both members of a pair of autosomes or the sex chromosomes. Where a mutation interferes with the function of one gene it is likely that the complementary gene will be unaffected and in this case gene expression may occur but at a reduced level that may or may not influence cell function or phenotype. Mendelian inheritance applies to the bimodal traits described by him in pea plants, but also to human diseases caused by single mutations, where the mutation is both necessary and sufficient to cause the disease and is said to have a major gene effect:

- *Autosomal dominant disorders*: these are the most common Mendelian disorders (7 per 1000 live births), apparent in individuals having one (heterozygous) or two (homozygous) mutant genes. Such conditions will, on average, affect half of all individuals in a sibship. If a proband has a dominant disorder one of their parents will also be affected, unless the disorder represents a new mutation. The extent to which a heterozygote shows features of the disorder is described as the penetrance of the condition, e.g. the Huntington's mutation has a penetration of almost 100%.
- *Autosomal recessive disorders*: these are less common (<3 per 1000 live births), partly because the disorder is expressed only in homozygotes. As with dominant disorders, the extent of expression depends on the penetrance of the mutations. If both parents are heterozygous for the mutant gene then, on average, one in four children will be affected. These conditions are rare as it is less likely that both parents will have a copy of the mutant gene unless they are related (e.g. in a geographically or ethnically isolated population) or the mutant is common in the general population (e.g. haemochromatosis or cystic fibrosis in the European population). For this reason, recessive disorders may appear to 'skip' generations.
- *X (or sex)-linked disorders*: these arise from mutations of the sex chromosomes and follow different inheritance patterns because males can only pass on their Y-chromosomes to sons. Most X-linked conditions are recessive. A heterozygotic

mother may pass on the mutant gene to her son and he will be affected, while his heterozygotic sister will be a carrier. Affected males transmit the carrier state to half of their daughters but do not transmit the disease to their sons. Examples include Duchenne muscular dystrophy and haemophilia A and B. In pedigrees with a dominant X-linked disorder, each generation usually has an affected individual, as all daughters of affected males are affected and both sons and daughters of an affected heterozygous female may be affected. Dominant X-linked disorders, such as nephrogenic diabetes insipidus, are extremely rare.
- *Mitochondrial disorders*: rare single gene disorders caused by mutations in a mitochondrial gene. They follow a distinct inheritance pattern because mitochondrial DNA in fertilized embryos is exclusively acquired from the ovum, as sperm do not contain mitochondria. Similarly, Y chromosomes are exclusively inherited through sperm in males. For mitochondrial disorders, the children of an affected woman, but none of the children of an affected man, are affected depending on disease penetrance.

Inheritance of complex genetic disorders

Many common biological traits or behaviours are, in the statistical sense, distributed normally in the general population and are likely to be determined by the interaction between multiple genes of minor effect and the environment rather than single genes of major effect. Within the normal distribution of biological traits, offspring of parents who are at the extremes of a continuously distributed trait (e.g. very tall individuals) tend to be closer to the population mean, a phenomenon called regression to the mean. Genes or locations on the genome that contribute to biological traits or behaviours that display these characteristics are called quantitative trait loci (QTLs). Biometrical analysis and quantitative genetics study the contribution of QTLs and environmental effects to phenotypes that approximate to a continuous normal distribution within the population.

Each minor or risk gene may have an effect independent of all other genes (an additive component), an effect that is dependent on the other allele at that locus (a dominant interaction) or an effect that is influenced by genotype at other loci (epistatic interactions). Overall, the proportion of the total variance of a trait in a population explained by additive genetic effects is called its narrow heritability (h^2). (The genetics of complex disorders is covered in greater detail by Plomin et al 1994.)

To date, where common variants are shown to be involved in a disorder, they collectively account for only a very small proportion of the total genetic variance or heritability. An alternative view, emerging as more data become available on copy-number variants or CNVs (a segment of DNA in which differences in the number of copies of a molecule or copy-number have been found by comparison of two or more genomes) and sequencing studies, is that for some common disorders (e.g. autism and schizophrenia) a proportion of susceptibility may be the consequence of rare risk variants or mutations which have a greater effect on risk in those with the variant, but which each impact on only small numbers of individuals.

Molecular genetics: techniques and terminology

Recombinant DNA technology

Also called molecular cloning, this is an umbrella term for the process of introducing a gene from an organism into a host cell, where it can be replicated and studied. This technology developed from the discovery in the 1970s of restriction enzymes produced by various bacteria that recognize particular short nucleotide sequences (4–8 base-pairs) and cut the DNA molecule specifically at such a location. This enables the bacteria to 'restrict' which foreign DNA could be incorporated into the bacterial genome. Using these enzymes *in vitro*, lengths of DNA could be cut to manageable sizes, and could be ordered into fragments of varying lengths as part of a restriction 'map'. These fragment lengths, called restriction fragment length polymorphisms (RFLPs), could be used to detect DNA polymorphism/variation if, as a consequence of the polymorphism, a restriction site is created or removed.

Vectors and cloning

When two different DNA samples are treated with a specific endonuclease enzyme to produce a staggered cut and then mixed together in the presence of another enzyme (DNA ligase) the two ends anneal forming a new DNA sequence, which can be inserted into a cloning vector, often a plasmid. This vector, when inserted into a host bacterial cell, replicates with the bacteria when cultured, allowing millions of copies of the original DNA sequence to be obtained (cloned). Cloning vectors include extrachromosomal bacterial elements (plasmids), bacterial viruses (bacteriophages), combinations of sequences from both these sources (cosmids) and phage, bacterial or yeast artificial chromosomes (PACs, BACs or YACs).

Polymerase chain reaction – enzymatic DNA amplification

DNA can be caused to unwind when heated to over 90°C; cooling causes the double helix to reform. In polymerase chain reactions (PCR) small pieces of DNA, called oligonucleotide primers, are chemically synthesized to be complementary to the DNA on either side of the sequence to be amplified. Mixing these primers with DNA containing the sequence to be amplified, a supply of individual nucleotides, and a heat-stable DNA polymerase enzyme at a suitable temperature, these primers bind to their complementary sequences on each strand. Next, the individual DNA bases extend along the strand reforming the double helix. Returning to over 90°C the strands separate and the process begins again with twice the number of molecules at the target. This procedure is automated by machines that cycle the reaction mixture through at the different temperatures to produce a very large number (many millions) of copies of the target DNA sequence.

Visualization

Fragments of DNA produced by cloning and/or other methods may be electrophoretically separated in agarose or acrylamide gels according to size, and visualized using dyes or radiolabelling. Further analysis is possible if DNA fragments are transferred and attached to a membrane (Southern blotting). Specific single-stranded DNA molecules can be detected by immobilizing the DNA molecule on a membrane and testing it with a DNA molecule complementary to that sought. This technique (using cDNA to hybridize RNA transcripts) has been extended so that expression levels of thousands of genes can be simultaneously investigated using microarrays of probe sequences immobilized on glass or silicon (Bunney et al 2003).

Genotyping

Newer methods of detecting DNA variation (genotyping), using hybridization with allele-specific probes or single nucleotide primer extension, have superceded the traditional enzyme cleavage RFLP method. These modern methods detect DNA sequence differences using a range of chemistry and detection devices. Such innovations mean that thousands or millions of individual genotypes can now be rapidly produced using automated procedures.

Human genome project

The completed draft of the sequence of the human genome sequence has recently been released. It has already produced insights into the collective history of humans, our shared identity and our individuality. It will also open up exciting possibilities for the understanding, identification, treatment and prevention of disease. Sequencing the genome involved its fragmentation using site-specific restriction endonucleases. Each segment (of approximately 150 bp in length) was inserted and replicated using a bacterial artificial chromosome or BAC vector, and the resulting clones were restricted to produce small fragments called 'fingerprints'. A physical map of overlapping fingerprints was assembled and sequenced using computer technology to assemble the raw sequence. At 3.2 gigabases (Gb), the human genome is 25 times larger than any previously sequenced genome. What is now available is a map of the genome encompassing most of the 'euchromatin' (2.95 Gb of the genome, where most genes are found). The task underway is to annotate the sequence with all its elements including genes, regulatory elements, repeats and duplications. Additional tasks include the comparison between the human sequence and that of other organisms.

As mentioned above, one of the most surprising findings is that the estimated number of genes is much smaller, at 20 000–25 000, than previously predicted. Proteins encoded by these genes can be grouped into families on the basis of their similarity to one another, and it turns out that humans share most of the same protein families with worms, flies and plants. However, humans generally have many more genes in a particular family than other organisms. For example, humans have 765 genes with immunoglobulin subunits, while the fly has 140 and the worm 64. The increased complexity in humans seems to be due to a number of factors, including additional genes within families, more complex regulatory mechanisms and alternative splicing of RNA (see above). Around 60% of human genes have two or more alternatively spliced transcripts, compared, for example, with only 22% in the worm. Humans have twice as many proteins that switch genes on and off as the fly and nearly five times as many as the worm. Another unexpected finding is that the human genome has a substantially higher proportion of segmental duplication (segments of DNA with almost identical sequences and covering ~5% of the euchromatic genome), than in other species. Some of these regions are under positive selection and may be important in evolutionary terms.

Genomics and bioinformatics

Genetics is the study of single genes and their effects. Genomics is the study of the functions and interactions of all the genes in the genome. Genomics as a science has been driven by the increased availability of entire genomes for comparison between species and the application of human genome information to common conditions. Bioinformatics is a new science that has evolved to cope with the growing banks of molecular sequence data. This involves computational methods for retrieval and analysis of data, including algorithms for sequence similarity searches and prediction of the structure and function of genes.

Confirming a genetic contribution to disease: family, twin and adoption research

Family studies

If a disease is genetic it should be familial, i.e. it should be more common in first-degree relatives of an affected proband (who share on average 50% of their DNA) than in second-degree relatives (who share 25% of their DNA) and more common in this group than in the general population. This information can be collected either by taking a detailed family history from affected individuals or their relatives (the family history method), or more rigorously by using a family study approach, where all affected individuals are directly interviewed. Many psychiatric disorders including schizophrenia, bipolar affective disorder and autism cluster in families.

Family studies by themselves are insufficient to define an illness as genetic because families share common environments to a greater extent than unrelated individuals. Shared effects reflect the environmental influences, which make family members similar for a trait. Non-shared influences are the effects that cause members of a family to be different and in psychiatry reflect how different individuals cope with the same stressors.

Two natural forms of biological and social experiment, namely, twin births and adoption, allow some separation of genetic and environmental effects.

Twin studies

Monozygotic (MZ) twins arise from a single fertilized ovum and thus have identical genes; dizygotic (DZ) twins develop from different ova and like any full siblings share an average of 50% of their genes. Twin research assumes that twins share environmental effects equally. If both twins have a disease, they are said to be concordant for that condition, but if only one twin is affected they are described as discordant. Higher concordance of disease in MZ than DZ twins is strong evidence of a genetic contribution to disease.

Early twin studies measured pair-wise concordance, where the total number of concordant twins is divided by the total number of twins studied. However, if twins have been ascertained independently, they may be counted twice and MZ concordant twins will be over-represented. Another method,

proband-wise concordance, is now more common as it avoids this problem by dividing the number of affected co-twins of an affected proband by the total number of co-twins in the study. Ascertainment bias at recruitment is also a potential flaw, but researchers in the USA, UK, Denmark and Sweden have overcome this problem by exploiting national or local twin registers to systematically screen all twin births. Twin studies assume that twins within a family share the same environment. This may not be completely true:

- Environmental factors including prenatal nutrition or birth trauma may differ between twins.
- MZ twins may share a different microenvironment to DZ twins.
- Being a twin, in itself, may contribute to illness.

Despite these caveats, twin studies remain a powerful tool in the elucidation of the genetic component of behavioural and psychiatric phenotypes. Twin studies have also proved valuable by exposing different aspects of gene expression in identical individuals. A study by Gottesman and Bertelsen (1989) of twin pairs discordant for schizophrenia showed that, for MZ twins, offspring had the same increased rate of schizophrenia, whether their parent was the affected co-twin or not. This finding suggested that the genetic risk, although unexpressed in one of the MZ twins, is nonetheless passed on to offspring. Apart from environmental differences, a number of genetic factors have been proposed to account for discordance including DNA methylation, somatic mutations, and imprinting (discussed below).

Adoption studies

These studies examine the effect of being adopted into, or out of, a family with a specific disorder using a variety of designs. In the Danish adoption study of schizophrenia (Kety 1988), adopted children who become ill are ascertained and rates of illness are compared in their adoptive and biological families (the adoptee family method). Adoption can also be studied prospectively, by using the parent as proband. In this adoptee study method, the rates of illness in adopted offspring of affected individuals are compared with rates in adopted offspring of individuals without the disorder. A third method is the cross-fostering design where rates of illness are compared between adoptees of affected biological parents raised by healthy adoptive parents and adoptees of unaffected biological parents raised in a family where an adoptive parent has become affected. As with twin studies, there are caveats:

- A child having affected biological parents may influence potential adoptive parents.
- Adopted children may experience particular intrauterine effects.
- Age at adoption is often overlooked.
- Adoption is a rare event.

Mode of inheritance

Family, twin and adoption studies may each have their limitations, but if independent evidence from all three methods points to a significant genetic component to a disease or trait then it is not unreasonable to assume that one exists. Other methods are required to identify the mode of inheritance involved.

Mode of inheritance can be investigated by examining the recurrence risk of disorder in different classes of relatives and in the general population. A rapid decrease in risk from MZ co-twins to 1st-degree relatives to the general population is inconsistent with a single gene model of inheritance. An alternative method of investigating inheritance patterns is segregation analysis, where the segregation of phenotypes within pedigrees is observed and statistically compared to expected patterns for known models of inheritance. Analyses of many common psychiatric disorder phenotypes including schizophrenia, depression and bipolar affective disorder indicate that the observed patterns of inheritance in many families are not compatible with Mendelian inheritance, at least involving the core phenotype. Ruling out a simple Mendelian model is a much simpler proposition than distinguishing between more complex genetic models. It is becoming apparent that some psychiatric disorders, such as Alzheimer disease, attention deficit hyperactivity disorder (ADHD) and possibly schizophrenia, are oligogenic, where a small number (5–20) genes might account for most of the genetic risk. For other conditions, the genetic risk may be attributable to many genes, each of very small effect. This is the polygenic model which better fits continuous traits, although with the addition of a threshold it may also account for categorical diagnoses. To complicate matters further, different genes may account for illness in different families. This is known as genetic heterogeneity. The most recent genomic data concerning disorders such as schizophrenia and autism is that genetic heterogeneity may be much more extensive than previously considered. The reality is that for a given disorder some or all of the models may apply and may be impossible to distinguish without further genomic information.

Quantitative and mathematical aspects of genetics

Hardy–Weinberg law

The English mathematician Godfrey Harvey and the German obstetrician Wilhelm Weinberg independently formulated this law in 1908. This states that the frequencies of alleles will, in the presence of random mating and in the absence of disturbances including mutation, natural selection, migration, inbreeding or random genetic drift, remain constant from generation to generation. Thus let two alleles 'A' and 'a' exist in a population. If their frequencies of occurrence (expressed in decimals) are 'p' and 'q', respectively, then $p + q = 1$; and if mating between individuals is random, after one generation the frequencies of the three genotypes will be p^2, $2pq$ and q^2. This generation will produce gametes (A and a) with frequencies p and q, similar to the previous generation. A sample of individuals is said to be in Hardy–Weinberg equilibrium if the frequencies of the observed genotypes AA, Aa and aa are not statistically different from the expected frequencies derived from allele frequencies using the above formula.

Recombination fraction

We have already described the process of recombination during meiosis. Genetic markers on separate chromosomes will segregate independently of each other and statistically therefore parental versions of the markers are as likely to transmit together into gametes as not. Even on the same chromosome, many markers will segregate independently. The recombination fraction is defined as the number of recombinant gametes divided by the total number of gametes and for independently segregating markers takes the value 0.5. This means that if the recombination fraction (θ) between two loci is <0.5, they are not independently segregating and instead are linked, meaning in physical terms that they lie close together on the same chromosome.

Genetic distance

Where two loci are linked, the probability of recombination occurring between them (θ) is proportional to the physical distance between them. This fraction is expressed in Morgans (M), where 1 M corresponds to the length of DNA on which one recombination is expected on average (roughly equivalent to 100 million bp), but is usually written as centiMorgans (cM), where 1 cM is the genetic distance corresponding to a recombination fraction of 0.01. This is roughly equivalent to 1 million base-pairs of DNA, but the relationship between genetic and physical distance is imprecise as recombination rates vary across the genome.

Linkage analysis

Linkage studies investigate possible cosegregation of genetic markers and disease in one or more families. This process of genetic tracking or mapping follows the descent of DNA markers down generations in pedigrees and their segregation with illness. Large multiply affected pedigrees or many small families or even multiple pairs of affected siblings may be studied, and each approach has advantages and disadvantages (further details are provided in Lander & Kruglyak 1995). Now that sufficient genetic markers are available, most linkage studies take a genome-wide approach using regularly spaced genetic markers or polymorphisms to locate the disease gene on the map of the genome. Linkage studies have two aims:

- To establish whether two loci (genetic locations, e.g. genes or polymorphic markers) segregate independently during meiosis.
- If there is a departure from independent segregation, to estimate the amount of recombination between the marker and the putative disease gene.

The value of θ is <0.5 when two loci are co-inherited more often than expected by chance and generally means they are physically located close together on the same chromosome. If two loci are physically close, crossing over is unlikely to occur between them during the small number of meioses that might be observed in a family. Linkage analysis estimates θ and tests whether $\theta = 0.5$. The conventional statistical method of doing this is to calculate a log of the odds (LOD) score. This is the common logarithm of the probability that the recombination fraction has some given value, divided by the probability that the value is 0.5. Where the mode of inheritance is known and the phenotype can be clearly defined a LOD score of 3.0 (odds in favour of linkage 1000:1) is accepted as proof of linkage and a score of −2.0 (odds against of 100:1) as proof of exclusion of linkage. However, the LOD score takes Bayesian theory into account, whereby the prior odds that two loci are linked is ~1:50. The observed odds ratio of a LOD score of 3 is 1000:1 leading to a posterior probability of about 20:1, roughly equivalent to a *p* value of 0.05.

Genetic association methods and linkage disequilibrium (LD)

In their simplest form, association studies look for differences in allele frequencies between populations of patients and healthy controls. If the patient population has a specific allele more frequently than the control population that allele is said to be associated with the disorder. It is important to match populations carefully for studies of this type, because different allele frequencies among ethnic groups, called population stratification, can cause false positive results. To avoid this difficulty, many studies use ethnically homogenous populations or a family based approach including the non-transmitted parental allele as the control group (haplotype relative risk or transmission disequilibrium test methods). Association studies may be hypothesis-driven and select potential candidate genes or polymorphisms based on genes associated with known biological systems. An example of a candidate gene is the ApoE gene in late-onset Alzheimer disease (see below).

Evidence of association may also be found where a marker is closely linked to an involved gene. This can occur because of linkage disequilibrium (LD), which is a form of linkage where the 'pedigree' selected is the entire population and the number of generations is unknown. If two genetic variants are in close proximity they are said to be in LD when recombination between them is rare, even over many generations. The extent of LD is variable throughout the genome for many reasons including the local rate of recombination and age of the original mutation. Association/LD studies are a powerful way of identifying even small genes effects, but to date, they have been confined to candidate genes. This is because the likely extent of LD at a local level may be small, meaning a huge number of markers would be required to produce a genome map. Neither the density of markers required nor the variation in LD between populations is fully understood. For this reason, a public collaboration, the International HapMap Project, was formed in 2002 to characterize LD across the human genome.

Clinical and molecular genetics of psychiatric disorders

The importance of diagnosis

Operationalized diagnostic systems such as DSM-IV and ICD-10 have considerably improved the reliability of diagnosis. Using these systems, a more consistent pattern of results has emerged from genetic epidemiology confirming a heritable component to many psychiatric and behavioural phenotypes. Although reliable, the biological validity of psychiatric diagnoses is yet to be established and recent studies are supporting earlier observations of genetic overlap across psychiatric diagnoses.

Single gene/chromosomal abnormalities in psychiatry

Early molecular methodologies have allowed the identification of single gene/chromosomal abnormalities which of themselves are both necessary and sufficient to cause psychiatric morbidity.

For example, many rare single gene disorders are recognized which clinically present with learning disability or neuropsychiatric symptoms. Illustrative examples are velocardiofacial syndrome (VCFS), Prader–Willi syndrome and the heritable dementias. This group of dementias includes familial Alzheimer disease (FAD), Huntington disease (HD), Creutzfeldt–Jakob disease (CJD) and cerebral autosomal dominant arteriopathy with subcortical infarcts and leukoencephalopathy (CADASIL). Information about each specific human genetic disorder is available from a catalogue called Online Mendelian Inheritance in Man (OMIM), available at: www.ncbi.nlm.nih.gov/Omim/. Details about clinical aspects of specific genetic learning disability or dementia phenotypes are discussed elsewhere in this volume.

Velocardiofacial syndrome (VCFS)

VCFS (also known as diGeorge syndrome and 22q11 deletion syndrome) affects 1/4000 live births and is caused by a common chromosomal microdeletion in the q11 band of chromosome 22. The syndrome has a complex phenotypic expression affecting multiple organs. Typical features are facial dysmorphology (long face, narrow palpebral fissures, flattened malar eminences, prominent nose and small mouth); palate abnormalities (cleft palate or hypernasal speech); borderline learning disability; congenital heart disease; and psychiatric disorders. In particular, psychotic disorders are much more common in VCFS populations (affecting ~30% of patients), and VCFS may be over-represented in schizophrenia (Murphy 2002).

Prader–Willi/Angelman syndrome

These learning disability syndromes are discussed here because they exhibit the phenomenon of imprinting. Imprinting, also known as a parent-of-origin effect, is where different phenotypes are associated with paternal and maternal inheritance of a disorder. The changes involved are known as epigenetic phenomena as they are inherited but involve phenotypic but not genotypic change. The mechanism is uncertain but it is assumed that activation or inactivation of genes from one parent occurs in the germline DNA. Prader–Willi syndrome follows an autosomal dominant pattern of inheritance and is caused by deletion of seven paternally inherited genes at 15q11–13. This results in mild or moderate learning disability with short stature, overeating and hypogonadism. In contrast, inactivation of the maternally inherited genes at the same locus results in Angelman syndrome. This disorder is less common, and presents with severe learning disability, lack of speech, epilepsy and ataxia.

Huntington disease (HD)/trinucleotide repeat expansion diseases (TREDs)

HD is a progressive, fatal, neurodegenerative disorder with an incidence of 1 in 100 000. The condition commonly presents between ages 35 and 50 with impaired muscle coordination, choreiform movements, psychiatric symptoms and progressive subcortical dementia. Almost all cases are familial with an autosomal dominant mode of inheritance. The disease is caused by an expansion of a CAG trinucleotide repeat coding for glutamine in exon 1 of the HD gene. Non-HD individuals have <35 CAG repeats, those with 36–39 repeats may have phenotypic expression of HD and those with higher numbers of repeats are more severely affected. Expansions of more than 55 repeats frequently cause a juvenile form of the disease. Unlike other mutations trinucleotide repeats are unstable and vulnerable to dynamic mutation, meaning that longer repeat sequences are more likely to undergo further expansion. This effect, called anticipation, explains why the disease tends to become more severe and have an earlier onset in successive generations of HD families. Since the early 1990s more than 20 trinucleotide expansion diseases have been identified including fragile X syndrome, myotonic dystrophy, juvenile myoclonic epilepsy and Friedrich's ataxia.

Familial Alzheimer disease (FAD)

Most cases of Alzheimer disease develop after the age of 65 (late onset) and are sporadic. Familial Alzheimer disease represents a small subset of all AD cases, and typically several generations of a family will be affected with early onset disease (<55 years). The first gene linked to the disease was the gene coding amyloid precursor protein (APP) on chromosome 21. Although at least five common mutations have been identified they only occur in a small number of families. By contrast, mutations of the presenilin-1 gene on chromosome 14q24.3 account for 40–50% of all early onset familial cases with mutations at the related presenilin-2 gene on chromosome 1 accounting for a further small percentage of early onset cases. Both genes produce membrane proteins that are highly expressed in brain, but only recently has presenilin-1 been linked to our biological understanding of the disorder. It appears to be the secretase enzyme (or a cofactor of the enzyme) involved in APP processing (Xia et al 2000). At present, a DNA diagnosis is possible in ~80% of people with FAD, but in the absence of preventive treatment the take-up for testing is likely to be low, as has been the case for HD. The contribution of genes to general AD risk will be considered below.

Common psychiatric disorders with a genetic contribution

The most important chromosomal loci and susceptibility genes for the major psychiatric disorders are presented in Table 3.1.

Schizophrenia

Schizophrenia affects between 0.5% and 1% of the population at some time in their lives. It has a point prevalence of approximately 4 cases per 1000 and is equally common in males and females, but with a later mean age at onset in females than males. The biggest risk factor for schizophrenia is the sharing of genes with someone who is affected, as evidenced by family, twin and adoption studies. Lifetime risk for schizophrenia in 1st-degree relatives is ~10%; in dizygotic twins 10–15%; in monozygotic twins 50% and in the offspring of two parents with schizophrenia or a related disorder, ~40%. The genetic architecture involved is poorly understood at present but is likely to overlap with other psychiatric disorders, in particular other major

psychotic disorders. For example, 1st-degree relatives of probands with either schizophrenia or bipolar disorder are at increased risk of both of these disorders, which suggests a common genetic contribution to schizophrenia and bipolar disorder (Lichtenstein et al 2009).

Segregation analysis supports a polygenic, complex genetic aetiology in most affected families. As with other complex genetic disorders, traditional linkage and functional candidate

Table 3.1 The most important chromosomal loci and susceptibility genes for the major psychiatric disorders

Disorder	Linked locus	CNV/other structural variant	Gene
Schizophrenia	6p 8p	1q21.1 15q11.2 15q13.3 22q11 DISC1	HLA region ZNF804A TCF4 NRGN
Bipolar affective disorder			CACNA1C ANK3
Recurrent depressive disorder			
Autistic spectrum disorders	2q 7q 15q X	NRXN1 NLGN1 SHANK3	
Attention-deficit hyperactivity disorder			DRD4 DRD5 DAT1
Panic disorder	13q 14q 4q31–34		
Obsessive–compulsive disorder	9p24		SLC1A1
Alzheimer disease	19q13 10p		Apolipoprotein E CLU CR1 PICALM BIN1
Specific language/ reading impairment			FOXP2 CNTNAP2 ATP2C2 CMIP DYX1C1 KIAA0319 DCDC2
Alcohol dependence syndrome	1 4 11		ADH2 ALDH2 GABRA2
Eating disorders	1p 4 10p		5-HT2A BDNF

gene association studies have met with limited success. More than 20 linkage scans of schizophrenia have been performed and a meta-analysis of these studies (n ~2000 affected individuals) provides statistical support for a number of loci including chromosome 6p, 8p and 22q (Lewis et al 2003). Functional candidate gene studies are heavily dependent on an understanding of disease aetiology: our current understanding of schizophrenia is such that few genes can be definitively excluded as candidates and the prior-probability for involvement of any particular gene is low. Emerging most prominently from the genetic association literature, although not definitive, have been genes with additional linkage (NRG1, DTNBP1, DAOA) or cytogenetic evidence (DISC1).

These approaches have been largely superseded by collaborative genome-wide association studies (GWAS) which provide reasonable power to identify common risk variants of moderate effect across the genome. These have provided more robust statistical support for at least eight susceptibility loci including the major histocompatibility complex (MHC) region, the zinc finger protein 804A (ZNF804A), transcription factor 4 (TCF4) and neurogranin (NRGN) genes (International Schizophrenia Consortium 2009; O'Donovan et al 2008; Stefansson et al 2009). Analysis of GWAS data also supports overlapping susceptibility with bipolar disorder and suggests that the number of small, common genetic effects that contribute to this susceptibility may measure in the hundreds, if not more (International Schizophrenia Consortium 2009).

Cytogenetic studies have reported numerous associations between schizophrenia and chromosomal mutations such as translocations, inversions, deletions and trisomies. Because schizophrenia is relatively common, many may have been coincidental; however, recent evidence is that they may play a larger role in causing schizophrenia than had been anticipated. It has been know for some time that chromosome 22q deletions are more common in individuals with schizophrenia and expression of the chromosome 22q deletion phenotype (VCFS) increases risk of psychosis. Strong evidence for linkage has also been reported for a balanced (1;11) (q42.1;q14.3) translocation which segregates with schizophrenia and related psychiatric disorders in a large Scottish pedigree (St Clair et al 1990). This translocation disrupted a previously unknown gene, called disrupted in schizophrenia 1 (DISC1), which is now known to be expressed in the brain and involved in neurodevelopment. Advances in technology have allowed identification of smaller, submicroscopic copy number variants in the human genome and their investigation in human disease. Deletions at an additional four loci, 1q21.1, 15q11.2, 15q13.3 and the gene neurexin-1 (NRXN1), and microduplications at 16p11.2 have all been reported as significantly over-represented in schizophrenia compared with controls. Taken together, the structural variation identified up to the present time may account for <2% of schizophrenia cases, but these rare events have a major effect on risk for individual carriers (e.g. odds ratios for these events are reportedly in the range 3–30) (Sebat et al 2009). An added striking finding is that the same or similar structural variants have also been found in some cases with other phenotypes including learning disability, autism, cardiac anomalies and obesity (Mefford et al 2008). More information on structural variation in the general population, in these patient groups,

and the availability of more refined sequencing methodologies will be required to quantify the total contribution made by this type of variation and to accurately estimate the risk to those affected.

Affective disorders

Recurrent depressive disorder

Evidence from family, twin and adoption studies in European and US community, and clinical samples, support a genetic component to major depressive disorder. There also appears to be genetic overlap between depression and anxiety disorders. The odds ratio for depression in 1st-degree relatives of depressive probands when compared with relatives of unaffected probands is 2.8 and heritability has been estimated to be ~40%. Several studies have suggested that more severe depressive disorder may have a substantially higher heritability (McGuffin et al 1996). A complex aetiology involving both genetic liability and a major environmental component is most likely. Indicators of familial liability include recurrence of depression, early age at onset and more severe functional impairment. Research points to the environmental effects being unique to the individual rather than due to common effects within families (such as poverty or parenting style). It has been suggested that individuals at low genetic risk develop depressive episodes in response to stressful life events, in contrast to individuals at higher genetic risk who are more likely to develop spontaneous depressive episodes (Kendler et al 2001). A number of candidate gene, linkage and GWAS studies have been conducted to date. These have provided little consistent support for individual loci which may reflect underlying heterogeneity of the phenotype but also the limited study power of recent studies compared to the larger collaborative studies available for other neuropsychiatric disorders.

Bipolar affective disorder (BP)

The mean population risk for BP is approximately 0.5% and at least 30 published family studies report an increased risk of BP in the relatives of affected probands. The relative risk to 1st-degree relatives of bipolar probands (measured in odds ratios, OR) is OR = 7 (CI 5–10), equivalent to a population risk of 10–18%. A meta-analysis of six twin studies indicates an average MZ concordance for BP of 50% with an average DZ concordance of 7%. There is also an increased risk of unipolar depression and schizophrenia within the families of bipolar probands, which may represent shared genetic susceptibility (Table 3.2). The lifetime risk is increased for probands with early age of onset, and in families with more affected members, but risk does

Table 3.2 Risk of BP disorder

	Risk of BP (%)	Additional UP risk (%)
MZ co-twin	50	15–25
1st-degree relative	5–10	10–20
Population controls	0.5–1.5	5–10

not seem to be influenced by either the sex or type of affected relative. The only adoption study of sufficient size to provide statistically meaningful results showed a significantly greater risk of affective disorder (bipolar, unipolar and schizoaffective disorder) in the biological parents of bipolar adoptees compared with adoptive parents.

BP linkage studies in the 1980s focused on rare, large pedigrees where the disorder appeared to follow an autosomal dominant pattern. Early promising linkage results were later retracted as key unaffected members of pedigrees became ill and examination of new members reduced linkage evidence. As with other complex diseases, the linkage approach has provided equivocal support for a number of susceptibility loci. A number of potential candidate genes, particularly involved in neurotransmitter function, have been well studied (e.g. the serotonin transporter gene (5-HTT) and a common functional variant (*val108/158met*) of the COMT gene), but none of the findings from candidate gene approaches have met with consistent, unambiguous support.

As has been the case with schizophrenia, promising findings have emerged from early GWAS studies and in particular from large meta-analytic efforts to combine GWAS datasets. Common genetic variants at two genes CACNA1C and ANK3 both meet rigorous threshold criteria for genome-wide significance (Ferreira et al 2008). These early findings strongly implicate ion channel dysfunction in BP susceptibility. CACNA1C encodes the alpha 1C subunit of the L-type voltage-gated calcium channel and ANK3 encodes the ankyrin-G protein), which regulates the assembly of voltage-gated sodium channels. Both genes are also known to be downregulated in mouse brain in response to lithium (McQuillin et al 2007) and are now the subject of intensive investigation. In line with emerging evidence for overlap between disorders, ZNF804A, the schizophrenia susceptibility gene mentioned above may also be involved in bipolar susceptibility.

As evidence emerges for shared common risk variants involved across psychotic disorders an obvious question is whether the same effect is true for rare variation (e.g. CNVs, see above). The evidence for involvement of CNVs in BP susceptibility is more equivocal, but further investigation of rare variation in BP will be required.

Autism/autistic spectrum disorders

Autism is a complex neurodevelopmental disorder characterized by significant disturbances in social, communicative and behavioural functioning. It is one of a group of disorders called pervasive developmental disorders (PDDs), which include Asperger syndrome, Rett syndrome, childhood disintegrative disorder, and 'pervasive developmental disorder not otherwise specified' (PDDNOS). A review of multiple epidemiological surveys estimates the prevalence of autism at ~1 per 1000 children, with the prevalence for all PDDs at ~7 per 1000 (Fombonne 2003).

Autism is considered by many to be the most strongly genetically influenced multifactorial childhood psychiatric disorder. The rate among siblings (called the sibling recurrence risk ratio) is at least 50 times higher than in the general population. Four twin studies have reported increased MZ:DZ twin concordance, averaging 73:7 across studies. Adopted away children have been identified, but formal adoption studies have not been possible because the condition is so rare. From family and twin data heritability has been estimated at ~90%. The mode of inheritance is unknown but likely to be complex and involve either multiple genes of small effect with epistatic interactions, or multiple rare but more highly penetrant mutations, or a combination of both models. Autism appears genetically related to the more common pervasive developmental disorders/autistic spectrum of disorders (ASDs), so both narrow and broad definitions of the disorder have been suggested for use in genetic studies. Both autism and ASDs are more common in males. Data from a large twin study also indicates that some autistic traits may be continuously distributed in the general population.

Genome-wide linkage studies of autism have provided suggestive, but not significant linkage evidence, to loci on chromosomes 2q, 7q, 15q and X. Cytogenetic abnormalities have also been reported in autistic individuals at each of these loci. Analysis of subsets of autistic individuals with (a) delayed speech increased linkage evidence at chromosomes 2 and 7, and (b) insistence on sameness increased evidence at 15q. Overall, however, linkage studies have not provided genome-wide evidence for linkage with only a small number of loci replicated in independent studies (e.g. chromosomes 7q31 and 17q11). Several genome-wide association studies have been reported but with little or no commonality between studies. If common variants of small effect are involved they are of very low penetrance and likely to account for only a small overall proportion of risk. However, using these arrays for an analysis of copy number variation has revealed multiple rare copy number variants, many of which arise *de novo* in the affected individual. In a recent study (Pinto et al 2010) cases were found to carry a higher global burden of rare CNVs than matched controls. The genes identified disrupt function gene sets involved in cellular proliferation, cell projection, cell motility and GTPase/Ras signalling. Genome-wide arrays targeted specifically at CNVs (comparative genomic hybridization) are now identifying rare and likely causative structural genomic variation in an increasingly large proportion of cases.

Speech, language and reading disorders

Specific language impairment (SLI) and dyslexia/specific reading disability (SRD) are frequent childhood disorders which appear to be related. They affect between 5 and 8% of pre-school children and are strongly familial in nature (see Williams 2002, for review). Twin studies estimate the heritability of SLI and SRD as 0.76 and 0.8, respectively.

Substantial progress has been made in our molecular understanding of these disorders. For SLI, the first step was the identification of a mutation in the gene FOXP2 in a monogenic form of speech and language disorder (Lai et al 2001). Although the mutation itself is rare and the resultant language disorder phenotype is not typical of SLI, the finding is likely to be important to our understanding of the biology of language processing. FOXP2 plays a key role in regulation of other genes critical to the development and function of the motor cortex, striatum and cerebellum. Downstream targeting of the molecular networks dependent on FOXP2 identified involvement of CNTNAP2, a neurexin gene in SLI susceptibility. CNTNAP2 and other members of the neurexin gene family interact with neuroligins in cell adhesion between pre- and postsynaptic membranes. Both neurexins and neuroligins have been implicated in autism, which strongly overlaps with SLI. Two other promising candidate genes have been identified, through positional cloning of a chromosome 16q locus identified by linkage. These genes, the calcium-transporting ATPase 2C2 (ATP2C2) and the cMAF inducing protein (CMIP) gene, are both brain-expressed but their involvement in brain function is poorly understood. In SRD there is promising evidence to support the involvement of three genes, DYX1C1, KIAA0319 and DCDC2. All have been implicated in neuronal migration but are also expressed in mature neurons. Further molecular biological research is required to understand both their function and how they relate to the SRD phenotype.

Anxiety and related disorders

There is significant co-morbidity between individual anxiety disorders and between anxiety disorders and depression; this may represent discrete or shared genetic or environmental risk factors. The most robust genetic epidemiological data is in relation to panic disorder (PD). Other anxiety phenotypes, including OCD, social phobia, post-traumatic stress disorder and neuroticism have also been investigated. The processes that underlie anxiety disorders are also substantially heritable. For example, twin research indicates a significant genetic component to the habituation, acquisition and extinction of fear stimuli.

Panic disorder

Numerous worldwide studies indicate that PD is more prevalent in 1st-degree relatives of affected probands ($\sim$8%) than in relatives of controls (1–3%). Twin studies provide evidence for a heritability estimate in the 40–48% range. Linkage studies provide suggestive evidence for loci at chr 13q, 14q and 4q31–34. More than 350 candidate genes have been investigated and the likelihood is that few if any play a significant role in PD risk. Larger GWAS studies are currently underway.

Obsessive–compulsive disorder (OCD)

OCD affects approximately 2% of the population but obsessional traits occur more commonly. Both the disorder and trait are familial and twin data indicate heritability in the 0.25–0.5 range (Clifford et al 1984; Jonnal et al 2000). Three genome-wide linkage studies have been completed to date, with suggestive but not highly significant results. In addition, over 80 candidate gene studies have been published. Most of these studies have focused on genes in the serotonergic and dopaminergic pathways. None have achieved genome-wide significance, and, with the exception of the glutamate transporter gene, none have been replicated. In the brain, the glutamate transporter is crucial in terminating the action of the excitatory neurotransmitter glutamate and in maintaining extracellular glutamate concentrations within a normal range. Two of the genome linkage scans have identified a region of chromosome 9p24 where DNA variants show suggestive linkage to OCD. Three studies have identified evidence of genetic association with DNA variants at the SLC1A1 gene with no negative evidence reported to date (Pauls 2010).

Anxiety and fear behaviour

Few human molecular studies of anxiety/fear have been conducted. Because anxiety/fear is readily reproduced across species and appears to share common neurophysiology, many animal studies have been performed. Artificial selection has been used to create mouse strains with heritable differences in anxiety behaviour. QTL mapping of these mice has identified susceptibility loci for mouse 'anxiety'. This information may prove valuable in identifying candidate loci for molecular studies of human anxiety.

Attention deficit hyperactivity disorder (ADHD)

ADHD is a common condition of childhood affecting 3–6% of school-age children worldwide with males being affected three times more commonly than females. Its clinical features include excessive motor activity, impaired attention and impulsivity. ADHD causes marked educational, social and family difficulties for sufferers and their relatives. The condition is of early onset (usually before age 7) and tends to persist throughout childhood. A substantial genetic element has been implicated by family, twin and adoption studies. The heritability (h^2) of ADHD has been estimated to be between 0.50 and 0.98.

Converging evidence from human and animal studies implicates dysregulation of frontostriatal and frontocerebellar catecholamine circuits in the aetiology of ADHD (Biederman & Faraone 2005). The mainstay of treatment for ADHD is methylphenidate and other psychostimulant medications (dextroamphetamine, pemoline) that are known to inhibit the dopamine transporter. These drugs ameliorate hyperactivity, inattention and impulsivity in ADHD cases. Animal models also support a dopaminergic hypothesis in ADHD. Mice without a functioning dopamine transporter (DAT1 knockout mice) have high extracellular striatal dopamine levels, a doubling of the rate of dopamine synthesis, and a nearly complete loss of functioning of dopamine autoreceptors. They display markedly increased locomotor and stereotypic activity compared to normal (wild-type) mice. Structural brain imaging studies in affected children have shown abnormalities in the frontal lobe and subcortical structures (globus pallidus, caudate, corpus callosum), regions known to be rich in dopamine neurotransmission and important in the control of attention and response to organization. Thus, unlike many other psychiatric disorders, reasonable candidate genes exist.

Many genetic association studies have been conducted and for the dopamine system, the receptors DRD4 and DRD5 and the dopamine transporter (DAT1) have shown strong evidence for association in many but not all samples examined. Meta-analyses of DRD4 studies (Faraone et al 2001; Li et al 2006) show strong support for association with an odds ratio (OR) of 1.4 for family based designs ($p = 0.02$) and a stronger OR of 1.9 for case control studies ($p = 0.08 \times 10^{-6}$). A joint analysis of a DRD5 polymorphism (Lowe et al 2004) showed association with the *DRD5* locus ($p = 0.00\,005$, OR = 1.24, 95% CI 1.12–1.38). Interestingly, this association appears to be confined to the predominantly inattentive and combined clinical subtypes. Meta-analysis of DAT1 variants are mixed, with a stronger effect in cases of European origin than of Asian origin, and there is some evidence that haplotypes made up of several variants are reliably associated (Franke et al 2009). Other dopamine-related candidate genes showing positive but mixed results. Genome-wide studies are being reported but to date have not found variants with genome-wide significance. Larger studies are underway as part of the Psychiatric Genetic Consortium (PGC). One of the most promising findings is for a variant at the cadherin 13 gene, the protein of which is expressed in neurons regulating cell migration and cell–cell adhesion.

Gilles de la Tourette syndrome (TS)

TS is a familial neuropsychiatric disorder of childhood onset characterized by both motor and vocal tics. Individuals with TS and their relatives often have symptoms of OCD that may be an alternative expression of the TS gene (s) in TS families. Some studies of TS have included other tic disorders and OCD as part of the phenotype, although tic disorders may be genetically heterogeneous. Five genome-wide linkage scans of TS have been completed. These have provided suggestive evidence for linkage to several loci, with two studies reporting linkage to chromosome 11q23 and the largest study, conducted by the Tourette Syndrome Association International Consortium for Genetics (TSAICG) showing strong evidence for linkage to DNA variants on chromosome 2p23.2. Most candidate gene studies, including studies of variants under the above linkage region, have reported negative findings to date. No GWAS have been reported to date.

Alzheimer disease

Alzheimer disease (AD) is the commonest form of dementia and is substantially heritable (Hollingworth et al 2010). As previously discussed, the investigation of rare families with early-onset forms identified causative mutations in the genes APP, PSEN-1 and PSEN-2, but taken together these account for <1% of all AD cases and have little effect on susceptibility to late-onset AD. These mutations are of pathophysiological interest, as they alter production of the Aβ peptide, the principal component of senile plaques.

For late-onset AD, early progress was made with linkage being observed between late-onset and chromosome 19q13.2, a region known to include the apolipoprotein E gene (APOE). Extensive linkage and candidate gene analysis failed to yield other confirmed genes. Apolipoprotein E is synthesized primarily in astrocytes and transports cholesterol and triglycerides from cellular debris to neurons where they are used for synaptic membrane formation. The APOE gene is polymorphic for three common alleles, each of which encodes a distinctive isoform: APOEε2, APOEε3 and APOEε4. Candidate gene studies have found significant evidence that the APOEε4 allele is associated not only with normal age-related cognitive change but also with late-onset AD. The association between APOE4 and AD is additive: ε4/ε4 genotype has a greater risk than ε4/ε3. The APOE2 allele has been shown to be protective. The increased risk for AD between those with no ε4 alleles and those with two copies is 12-fold. This is still not predictive of AD as 50% of those homozygous for ε4 who survive to 80 show no evidence of AD. The mechanism by which ApoE increases risk is uncertain, but this may involve a differential effect of different isoforms on Aβ aggregation and clearance (Kim et al 2009).

As of early 2010, 14 GWAS studies, of varying sizes, have been reported. These have confirmed that APOE is the only common risk variant of moderate or large effect. As has proved to be the case with most other common disorders, the effect sizes for most common risk loci are likely to be in the OR range of 1.05–1.5. Efforts to combine GWAS samples have been extremely successful in identifying additional novel susceptibility genes for late-onset AD including the genes CLU, PICALM, CLU, CR1 and BIN1. These are recent discoveries, and much work is still to be done to elucidate the mechanisms involved in AD pathogenesis. Based on what is already known about these genes CLU, like APOE, is a brain apolipoprotein which may be similarly involved in Aβ aggregation and clearance; the PICALM and BIN1 genes are both involved in vesicular formation. A key question is whether these genes contribute to one or more molecular pathways and different aspects of pathophysiology.

Alcohol abuse/dependence

Family, twin and adoption studies indicate that 40–60% of the individual variation in alcohol preference and vulnerability to alcohol dependence syndrome (ADS) is genetic in origin. The largest proportion of this genetic vulnerability is substance-specific although nicotine addiction may be co-inherited. All studies point to a large and complex environmental contribution as the prevalence differs widely between cultures, in the same culture over time (e.g. due to the effect of prohibition in the USA), and between the sexes within the same culture. Indeed the lifetime rates in partners of affected women are similar to rates in male relatives, suggesting that learned behaviour and assortative mating may play an important role.

Polymorphisms of two major enzymes of alcohol metabolism, alcohol dehydrogenase and aldehyde dehydrogenase, are well established as genetic factors for reduced susceptibility to ADS. The alcohol dehydrogenase allele (ADH2 His47) increases metabolism of alcohol to acetaldehyde and the aldehyde dehydrogenase allele (ALDH2 Lys487) decreases the rate of acetaldehyde removal. Both alleles are found in half the population of South-Eastern Asian countries but are rare in Caucasian and African populations. Both lead to an accumulation of acetaldehyde after alcohol intake and a flushing reaction similar to that produced by disulfiram. Even for Japanese people with one ALDH2 Lys487 allele (30–40% of the population), the risk of alcoholism is reduced 5- to 10-fold. Studies of alcoholism in Americans of Asian ancestry imply that the protective effect of both polymorphisms varies across different environmental backgrounds.

Rodent models of alcohol sensitivity are being used to increase our molecular understanding of ADS. For example, differences in GABA$_A$ receptor function appear to be a critical determinant of ethanol sensitivity. QTL mapping in rodents has identified candidate genes and loci for alcohol-related behaviour for further investigation in humans. In such models withdrawal severity is attributable primarily to loci at chromosome 1, 4 and 11; the chromosome 11 locus contains a GABA$_A$ gene cluster that may contribute to this differential alcohol response. Fine mapping of the chr 4 locus has demonstrated replicable association at the GABRA2 gene in ADS.

be selected, and discriminated against as genetically abnormal, or in need of corrective treatment? Selection on the basis of genetic tests might also include prenatal testing, the streaming of children in schools on IQ or aptitude, screening by employers, and the use of genetic information for insurance purposes. Is this type of selection acceptable? Is an individual with a genotype known to be associated with impulsiveness, for example, less responsible for their behaviour? Could this have legal implications? Could the study of normal behavioural traits contribute adversely to their medicalization? If so, the boundaries between normal variation and disorder may shift towards the centre and social tolerance for previously normal traits may be undermined and the role of the environment undervalued. Are there dangers in the widening of diagnostic boundaries?

It is likely that the predictive value of individual genetic tests will be so low as to be of no value for screening purposes, for determining optimal treatment, or for attributing diminished responsibility. However, the potential value of a combination of many genetic tests and environmental information has yet to be determined and will require careful consideration. We are as yet uncertain as to the impact of rare genetic variation, which may have significant relevance to risk for a few, or many individuals with major mental disorders. Currently, public opinion supports the use of legislation to prevent the misuse of genetic information but this may vary between nations and with the proposed use of the information. Legal opinion suggests that tests for traits within the normal range fall outside of the current legal definitions of insanity and diminished responsibility and cannot, therefore, be used as a defence. However, many issues remain to be resolved and new ethical issues will undoubtedly arise in the future. These ethical questions and dilemmas will require debate. It is important that the scientific community takes part in that debate, and provides accurate and unbiased information to help construct reasonable guidelines.

References

Alia-Klein, N., Goldstein, R.Z., Kriplani, A., et al., 2008. Brain monoamine oxidase-A activity predicts trait aggression. J. Neurosci. 28, 5099–5104.

Biederman, J., Faraone, S.V., 2005. Attention-deficit hyperactivity disorder. Lancet 366, 237–248.

Bulik, C.M., Devlin, B., Bacanu, S.A., et al., 2003. Significant linkage on chromosome 10p in families with bulimia nervosa. Am. J. Hum. Genet. 72, 200–207.

Bunney, W.E., Bunney, B.G., Vawter, M.P., et al., 2003. Microarray technology: a review of new strategies to discover candidate vulnerability genes in psychiatric disorders. Am. J. Psychiatry 160, 657–666.

Caspi, A., McClay, J., Moffitt, T.E., et al., 2002. Role of genotype in the cycle of violence in maltreated children. Science 297, 851–854.

Clifford, C.A., Murray, R.M., Fulker, D.W., 1984. Genetic and environmental influences on obsessional traits and symptoms. Psychol. Med. 14, 791–800.

Davis, O.S., Butcher, L.M., Docherty, S.J., et al., 2010. A three-stage genome-wide association study of general cognitive ability: hunting the small effects. Behav. Genet. 40, 759–767.

Eichler, E.E., Nickerson, D.A., Altshuler, D., et al., 2007. Completing the map of human genetic variation. Nature 447, 161–165.

Fairburn, C.G., Harrison, P.J., 2003. Eating disorders. Lancet 1361, 407–416.

Faraone, S.V., Doyle, A.V., Mick, E., et al., 2001. Meta-analysis of the association between the 7-repeat allele of the dopamine D(4) receptor gene and attention deficit hyperactivity disorder. Am. J. Psychiatry 158, 1052–1057.

Ferreira, M.A., O'Donovan, M.C., Meng, Y.A., et al., 2008. Collaborative genome-wide association analysis supports a role for ANK3 and CACNA1C in bipolar disorder. Nat. Genet. 40, 1056–1058.

Fombonne, E., 2003. The prevalence of autism. J. Am. Med. Assoc. 289, 87–89.

Franke, B., Neale, B.M., Faraone, S.V., 2009. Genome-wide association studies in ADHD. Hum. Genet. 126, 13–50.

Goldberg, T.E., Egan, M.F., Gscheidle, T., et al., 2003. Executive subprocesses in working memory: relationship to catechol-O-methyltransferase Val158Met genotype and schizophrenia. Arch. Gen. Psychiatry 60, 889–896.

Gottesman, I.I., Bertelsen, A., 1989. Confirming unexpressed genotypes for schizophrenia. Results in the offspring of Fisher's Danish identical and fraternal twins. Arch. Gen. Psychiatry 46, 867–872.

Grice, D.E., Halmi, K.A., Fichter, M.M., et al., 2002. Evidence for a susceptibility gene for anorexia nervosa on chromosome 1. Am. J. Hum. Genet. 70, 787–792.

Hollingworth, P., Harold, D., Jones, L., et al., 2010. Alzheimer's disease genetics: current knowledge and future challenges. Int. J. Geriatr. Psychiatry Oct 19 [Epub ahead of print].

International Schizophrenia Consortium, 2009. Common polygenic variation contributes to risk of schizophrenia and bipolar disorder. Nature 460, 748–752.

Jonnal, A.H., Gardner, C.O., Prescott, C.A., et al., 2000. Obsessive and compulsive symptoms in a general population sample of female twins. Am. J. Med. Genet. 96, 791–796.

Kendler, K.S., Thornton, L.M., Gardner, C.O., 2001. Genetic risk, number of previous depressive episodes, and stressful life events in predicting onset of major depression. Am. J. Psychiatry 158, 582–586.

Kety, S.S., 1988. Schizophrenic illness in the families of schizophrenic adoptees: findings from the Danish national sample. Schizophr. Bull. 14, 217–222.

Kim, J., Basak, J.M., Holtzman, D.M., 2009. The role of apolipoprotein E in Alzheimer's disease. Neuron 63, 287–303.

Lai, C.S., Fisher, S.E., Hurst, J.A., et al., 2001. A forkhead-domain gene is mutated in a severe speech and language disorder. Nature 413, 519–523.

Lander, E., Kruglyak, L., 1995. Genetic dissection of complex traits: guidelines for interpreting and reporting linkage results. Nat. Genet. 11, 241–247.

Lewis, C.M., Levinson, D.F., Wise, L.H., et al., 2003. Genome scan meta-analysis of schizophrenia and bipolar disorder, part II: schizophrenia. Am. J. Hum. Genet. 73, 34–48.

Li, D., Sham, P., Owen, M.J., et al., 2006. Meta-analysis shows significant association between dopamine system genes and attention deficit hyperactivity disorder (ADHD). Hum. Mol. Genet. 15, 2276–2284.

Lichtenstein, P., Yip, B.H., Bjork, C., et al., 2009. Common genetic determinants of schizophrenia and bipolar disorder in Swedish families: a population-based study. Lancet 373, 234–239.

Lowe, N., Kirley, A., Hawi, Z., et al., 2004. Joint analysis of the DRD5 marker concludes association with attention-deficit/hyperactivity disorder confined to the predominantly inattentive and combined subtypes. Am. J. Hum. Genet. 74, 348–356.

Malhotra, A.K., Lencz, T., Correll, C.U., et al., 2007. Genomics and the future of pharmacotherapy in psychiatry. Int. Rev. Psychiatry 19, 523–530.

McGuffin, P., Katz, R., Watkins, S., et al., 1996. Hospital-based twin register of the heritability of DSM-IV unipolar depression. Arch. Gen. Psychiatry 53, 129–136.

McQuillin, A., Rizig, M., Gurling, H.M., 2007. A microarray gene expression study of the molecular pharmacology of lithium carbonate on mouse brain mRNA to understand the neurobiology of mood stabilization and treatment of bipolar affective disorder. Pharmacogenet. Genom. 17, 605–617.

Mefford, H.C., Sharp, A.J., Baker, C., et al., 2008. Recurrent rearrangements of chromosome 1q21.1 and variable pediatric phenotypes. N. Engl. J. Med. 359, 1685–1699.

Mulle, J.G., Dodd, A.F., McGrath, J.A., et al., 2010. Microdeletions of 3q29 confer high risk for schizophrenia. Am. J. Hum. Genet. 87, 229–236.

Murphy, K.C., 2002. Schizophrenia and velocardiofacial syndrome. Lancet 359, 426–430.

Nuffield Council on Bioethics, 2002. Genetics and human behaviour, the ethical context. Online. Available:www.nuffieldbioethics.org/publications/pp_0000000015.asp (accessed 01.05.04.).

O'Donovan, M.C., Craddock, N., Norton, N., et al., 2008. Identification of loci associated with schizophrenia by genome-wide association and follow up. Nat. Genet. 40, 1053–1055.

Pauls, D.L., 2010. The genetics of obsessive-compulsive disorder: a review. Dialogues Clin. Neurosci. 12, 149–163.

Pinto, D., Pagnamenta, A.T., Klei, L., et al., 2010. Functional impact of global rare copy number variation in autism spectrum disorders. Nature 466, 368–372.

Plomin, R., Owen, M.J., McGuffin, P., 1994. The genetic basis of complex human behaviours. Science 264, 1733–1739.

Sebat, J., Levy, D.L., McCarthy, S.E., 2009. Rare structural variants in schizophrenia: one disorder, multiple mutations; one mutation, multiple disorders. Trends Genet. 25, 528–535.

StClair, D., Blackwood, D., Muir, W., et al., 1990. Association within a family of a balanced autosomal translocation with major mental illness. Lancet 336, 13–16.

Stefansson, H., Ophoff, R.A., Steinberg, S., et al., 2009. Common variants conferring risk of schizophrenia. Nature 460, 744–747.

Treutlein, J., Cichon, S., Ridinger, M., et al., 2009. Genome-wide association study of alcohol dependence. Arch. Gen. Psychiatry 66, 773–784.

Verweij, K.J., Zietsch, B.P., Medland, S.E., et al., 2010. A genome-wide association study of Cloninger's temperament scales: implications for the evolutionary genetics of personality. Biol. Psychol. 85, 306–317.

Watson, J.D., Crick, F.H.C., 1953. Molecular structure of nucleic acids. Nature 171, 737–738.

Williams, J., 2002. Reading and language disorders. In: McGuffin, P., Owen, M.J., Gottesman, I.I. (Eds.), Psychiatric genetics and genomics. Oxford University Press, Oxford, pp. 129–146.

Xia, W., Ray, W.J., Ostaszewski, B.L., et al., 2000. Presenilin complexes with the C-terminal fragments of amyloid precursor protein at the sites of amyloid beta-protein generation. Proc. Natl. Acad. Sci. U.S.A. 97, 9299–9304.

Human personality development

4

Nick Goddard

CHAPTER CONTENTS

Introduction

Development is a complex process, involving physical, cognitive, personality and social changes and adaptations throughout life. Attention is often focused on the early years of life, but development continues throughout life and a lifespan developmental approach will encompass not only the major changes in infants, but also the adjustments made in adolescence, in adult life and in old age, that occur as well as the major events that impact on life, e.g. bereavement, chronic illness.

Human development is clearly a diverse topic, which has given rise to many models and theories. The main areas are covered in this chapter.

Nature vs nurture

Conceptualizing development has led to several polarized approaches and the nature/nurture or genetics/environment debate has a long history.

The nurture argument was perhaps first articulated by John Locke in the seventeenth century. He contended that at birth, children were blank slates (*tabula rasa*) and that what they became was dependent on learning and experience. Therefore, their environment determines their development.

In contrast, Jean Jacques Rousseau supported the nature argument, believing that development was an invariant sequence of Nature's plan and that all a child required was guidance.

This argument has been repeated in various forms, more recently as the environment versus genetics debate. While there has been no clear resolution to the debate, at best it is reductionist. More recent research has focused on the interaction of genes and environment, giving rise to behavioural genetics. Of interest here, is how the genetic developmental plan is dependent on environmental factors (both protective and adverse) for its expression. Genes can also influence the environment through reactive, evocative and proactive interactions.

Cognitive development

Jean Piaget, a Swiss born psychologist, brought a new approach to cognitive development. He moved away from environmental or biological components of development to how a child's naturally developing abilities interact with the environment.

Piaget proposed a 'stage' model in which a child passes through development in an *invariant sequence*, through a process of *assimilation* (taking in new information) and *accommodation* (modifying existing information or *schema*). Such information requires *organization* and the whole process involves active participation (Piaget & Inhelder 1969).

Piaget, through his observations and discussions with children, including his own, proposed the following four-stage process of development:

- **Phase 3 (6 months–3 years):** intense attachment and proximity seeking. Infants become intensely attached, usually to the principal carer, showing distress if left (separation anxiety) and a wariness of strangers (fear of strangers). As mobility increases babies begin to attempt to follow the carer.
- **Phase 4 (3 years–adulthood):** partnership behaviour. The child becomes more aware of the carer's actions, allowing them to leave and working more in partnership.

The main emphasis of Bowlby's work is on early infancy and while there is little on phase 4 or attachments in later life, more recent work is attempting to examine these periods.

Bowlby had a major impact on child-rearing practices. He described that separation leads to a process of *protest*, followed by *despair* and then *detachment*. The adverse effect of such separations was one factor influencing the attitudes of hospitals to parents staying with their children during paediatric admissions.

Attachment work has been furthered by Mary Ainsworth. She was interested in how babies used mothers as a secure base from which to explore. Their reactions were investigated using the *Strange Situation Procedure*. Baby and carer enter an unfamiliar room, containing a one-way viewing screen. A stranger enters and the carer leaves the baby for a predesignated period of time, then returns. The baby's reactions are observed at each stage. From this work, Ainsworth described three patterns of attachment (Ainsworth et al 1978), later adding a fourth:

- **Securely attached:** these infants use mother as a base from which to explore. When mother leaves, their play decreases and they look upset. On mother's return they greet her, remain close and then begin to re-explore. About 60–70% of infants demonstrate this pattern of attachment.
- **Insecure–avoidant:** infants in this category look independent and do not check with mother while exploring. When mother leaves they do not appear upset. As mother returns they seek proximity to her, though avoid her if picked up. This pattern is present in about 20% of infants.
- **Insecure–ambivalent:** infants are clingy and preoccupied with mother, exploring little. They appear upset when left, but are ambivalent on mother's return, reaching out to mother but pushing her away at the same time. Around 10% of infants show this pattern.
- **Disorganized:** this category, added at a later date, describes a subgroup whose behaviour lacked any coherent pattern. Some 10–15% of infants fall into this category.

There is increasing interest in the implications of attachment for adult life. The *Adult Attachment Interview* developed by Mary Main seeks to examine adults' perceptions of their early relationships. Four categories of adult attachment have been described, which in turn have been linked with childhood attachments (Table 4.2).

This is an on-going area of research in development. Research suggests that the pattern of attachment expressed by mothers may determine the attachment of infants. Attachment styles are also being examined in relation to specific mental illnesses, though as yet there are few robust connections.

Table 4.2 Patterns of attachment and their relationships to childhood attachment

Adult attachment	Childhood attachment	
Autonomous	Secure attachment	Typically, such adults are self-reliant, coherent in describing their early experiences, objective and not defensive. They give a history of good supportive relations or have come to terms with their absence
Dismissing	Insecure–avoidant	Adults with this pattern of attachment appear to have few emotional memories of childhood. Caregivers are often idealized and the effect of traumatic experiences are minimized
Preoccupied	Insecure–ambivalent	These adults appear to be still caught up in childhood events, often expressing anger towards the parents
Unresolved	Disorganized	The narrative of adults in this group is characterized by lapses or gaps, particularly around traumatic events

Language development

Language development is a complex phenomenon, acting as a means of developing reasoning, thought and communication. The development of language is a mixture of learning and innate processes.

Learning processes

Imitation plays some role in learning language, but cannot be the only means of developing language. Conditioning may also help the process, but adults do not pay attention to every detail of speech uttered by infants.

Children also appear to learn a set of operating principles, which allows them to generalize certain constructions, e.g. the addition of '-ed' to a verb to form the past tense, e.g. 'walk, walked'. Children learn gradually not to over-generalize, e.g. 'go, goed', and to recognize irregular verbs.

Innate processes

All children, regardless of culture, seem to go through the same sequence of language development, implying an innate knowledge. Language development also has critical periods when it is easier to learn languages, such as the early years of life.

One of the foremost theorists in this area is Noam Chomsky, whose work has spawned a new science of neurolinguistics. He suggests that language development is built in (Chomsky 1972). The theory then becomes very dense, but a summary is shown in Table 4.3.

Table 4.3 Language development

Age	Theory of Chomsky	
0–12 months	Early language	Babies respond to speech. At 1 month they gurgle and coo and by 6 months babble
1 year	One-word utterances	Single, simple words
1–1½ years	Two-word utterances	Connecting words, e.g. 'good boy'
2–3 years	Grammar development	Begin to make noun phrases, e.g. 'I making tea', and over-generalize rules, e.g. 'I runned'
3–6 years	Transformations	Increasingly complex grammar. Form questions using transformations, i.e. changing a sentence around, e.g. 'I can put it where?' → 'Where can I put it?'
5–10 years	Near-adult grammar	Develop more subtle aspects of grammar, e.g. the passive voice

Chomsky has been criticized on the grounds of reading adult meanings into children's speech. He also believes that language should be studied separately from other aspects of development.

Family development

Development is not confined to individuals but also applies to the social units in which individuals live.

Defining the exact nature of what constitutes a family is difficult. One definition is to consider the family to be everyone living in a household, but also to extend this to others important to members of that household, e.g. extended family members, estranged parents.

In Western society, the nuclear family of husband, wife and children has tended to be regarded as normal. This view has been challenged. The following types of family have been defined:

- Nuclear
- Childless couple
- One-parent families – widows/widowers, divorced/separated, non-married
- Adopted – husband, wife, plus adopted children
- Communal – groups of families
- Reconstituted – with eight combinations:
  - **i.** Divorced man – single woman
  - **ii.** Divorced man – widowed woman
  - **iii.** Divorced man – divorced woman
  - **iv.** Single man – widowed woman
  - **v.** Single man – divorced woman
  - **vi.** Widowed man – single woman
  - **vii.** Widowed man – widowed woman
  - **viii.** Widowed man – divorced woman.

Family lifecycle

Development may vary because of the different forms of families. Classically, family development is described in the form of the family lifecycle. McGoldrick and Carter (1982) described six stages:

- **i.** Unattached young adult – between families
- **ii.** Joining of families through cohabitation or marriage
- **iii.** Family with young children – adults become parents
- **iv.** Family with adolescents – child becomes more independent
- **v.** Launching children – children leave and may begin their own family lifecycle, leading to the 'empty nest'
- **vi.** Family in later life – parents become grandparents and acquire new interests.

The above is a simplistic model as many other events can occur, such as death, divorce, illness and other life events. Families may get into trouble at these points of stress or transition. Barnhill and Longo (1978) defined nine 'transition points':

- **i.** Commitment – two people decide to form a relationship
- **ii.** Developing parent role – man/woman becomes father/mother
- **iii.** Accepting new personality – adapting to child's development
- **iv.** Introducing child to institutions outside of family – such as school
- **v.** Accepting adolescence – parents come to terms with adolescent changes
- **vi.** Allowing experimentation with independence – late adolescence
- **vii.** Preparations to launch – as young adult moves into outside world
- **viii.** Letting go – facing each other – father/mother face each other again as partners without child-rearing responsibility
- **ix.** Accepting retirement/old-age.

Family functioning

Families adopt their own styles of getting along together. In working with families a normative model is used based on the characteristics of well-functioning families. Difficulties can arise because of:

- **Discord:** family discord refers to arguments, hostility and criticism in the family setting. Discord often relates to poor and inconsistent discipline in the home. An association has been established between child psychiatric disorders and exposure to family discord.
- **Over-protection:** parents seeking to prevent exposing the child to the stressors of daily life can become over-protective. Overprotection is part of a group of four patterns of family interaction (enmeshment, over-protection, rigidity and lack of conflict resolution) described by Minuchin as characterizing family functioning in families with children presenting with psychosomatic disorders (see Ch. 37).
- **Enmeshment:** families can be considered as systems, where boundaries operate to demarcate one system from

surrounding systems or parts of the system from each other, e.g. parents from children. Enmeshment occurs if boundaries are not clear enough, leading to the functions of child and parent becoming blurred and overlapping. Such a situation can reduce autonomy and lead to difficulties in separation.

Parenting

Parents use a variety of styles in rearing their children. Some may be relaxed and warm, others aloof and cold. *Child-centred* parenting refers to being involved with the child and aware of their needs, while *parent-centred* parents are more preoccupied with their own needs and interests.

Several models of parenting have been described. Maccoby and Martin (1983) divide parenting into two areas: the amount of control exerted and responsiveness. This produces four styles of parenting:

- **Authoritative:** these parents are responsive, warm, accepting and child-centred. They have expectations about behaviour and exert control and authority when required, while also being responsive to the child's needs. Children of such parents tend to be independent, make good peer and parental relationships. Also, they tend to be well motivated.
- **Authoritarian:** parents in this class also exert control but in a parent-centered manner, attempting to control the behaviour of the child without responding to the child's needs. Children from this category can be responsible and contented, but boys may be more aggressive and girls less motivated.
- **Indulgent:** parents are child-centred but make few demands on children, exerting little authority. Children are often positive but can be immature and the lack of authority contributes to increased aggressive behaviour.
- **Neglecting:** this is not used in the abuse sense, but to describe parents who are parent-centred, unresponsive and exert little control. Children may be more likely to be impulsive, with poor concentration and prone to temper outbursts.

While these four parenting styles are convenient, parents do not always fall into one category and may use different styles at different times.

Adolescence and development

The physiological changes marking the onset of puberty also herald a period of social development. Resolution of this period involves:

- Attainment of separation
- Establishment of a sexual identity
- Commitment to work
- Development of a moral system
- Development of the capacity to form lasting relationships
- Establishment of a relationship with parents based on relative equity.

During this time, adolescents often work hard at understanding themselves and shaping further their sense of self.

Identity

One of the fundamental tasks of adolescence is to establish this sense of self or identity. Marcia (1966, 1980) suggests four identity statuses:

- **Identity achievement:** this follows a period of active questioning and self-definition.
- **Foreclosure:** an identity may develop, though often without an active period of questioning. Adolescents may just adopt family values without question.
- **Moratorium:** during this period, adolescents may be actively seeking answers and an identity. At this time, adolescents can be open and sensitive or anxious and self-righteous.
- **Identity diffusion:** the adolescent has no sense of self and is not taking steps to test out ideas.

These are not necessarily distinct stages, although there is some progression to identity achievement with age. It is also possible to be in one status with respect to one set of beliefs, e.g. religious values, and not to have formed any opinion in other areas, e.g. occupational interests.

Adolescent turmoil

The classic picture of adolescent–parent relationships is of highly charged atmospheres and stormy arguments, with adolescents in a state of emotional flux or 'turmoil'. Research suggests that major difficulties are not common and may be more characteristic of the small proportion referred to psychiatric services. Family conflict may be more common, but usually revolves around everyday matters, e.g. housework, homework, curfew times. Resolution occurs by negotiating a new working relationship with parents and the adolescent being granted more autonomy in return for increased responsibility.

'Turmoil' may be slightly more common. Around one-fifth of adolescents report feeling miserable and depressed, although this may be mild and transient. However, adolescence is the time when rates for depression and deliberate self-harm do begin to mirror adult patterns.

Sexual development

Sexual development is also complex, representing an interplay of biological, psychological and social influences. The three main components are:

- **Gender (anatomical) identity:** an awareness of the two different categories, male or female, like father or like mother. By the age of 2, 80% of children can correctly answer the question 'are you a boy or girl?' By age 3, 80% can pick an appropriately sexed doll.
- **Sex-typed behaviour:** refers to activities considered by society to be appropriate. Sex differences in play are evident by the age of 3–4 years, although even 1-year-olds may show toy preferences (girls prefer soft toys and dolls; boys mechanical toys).
- **Sexual orientation:** the direction of emotional/romantic and erotic interests. Typically evident in early adolescence, although probably present at a much earlier age.

Much research is based on 'atypical' development with competing claims for genetic and environmental influences.

Adulthood and development

Physical changes continue through adulthood, e.g. hair loss, slowing of reflexes, etc. and social development also continues. Less work has been done on formalizing patterns of development in adulthood. Levinson et al (1978) suggest the following stages:

- **Early adult life:**
  - 22–28: entering the adult world: a period of stability, developing careers and families
  - 28–33: 'age 30 transition': decisions about where life will go
  - 33–40: settling down: stable and become more autonomous.
- **Middle adulthood:**
  - 40–45: mid-life transition: 'mid-life crisis', re-evaluation of life, which can result in changes of jobs, re-marriage, etc.
  - 45–50: entering mid-adulthood: either develop a more compassionate, wise view of life or stagnate
  - 50–55: transition: similar to 'mid-life crisis' at age 40, if no crisis at earlier stage
  - 55–60: culmination: preparing for late adulthood.
- **Late adulthood:**
  - 60+: retirement and late life.

These stages are not comprehensive and there may be sex differences, but they give a flavour of the changes in adult life.

Late adulthood and development

Late adulthood is a time of great physical change and also of cognitive decline. A reappraisal of life is required with retirement from work. Older people on the whole feel just as satisfied with life, though this is dependent on physical health. Many adjust well but others have difficulties. Those who are more positive are more likely to be financially comfortable, healthy, to have planned their retirement and do not consider work as central to their lives.

Death

Late adulthood inevitably leads to the end of life. Older people's attitudes to death depend more on the degree of control they feel they can exert on the environment, rather than number of years lived.

A 'dying trajectory' has been described, tracing the process of anticipation of death. Kübler-Ross (1969) describes the following stages:

- **Denial and isolation:** the prospect of death is initially denied. The individual may appear calm and carry on with life in the usual manner.
- **Anger and resentment:** angry feelings can surface, directed against others or self.
- **Bargaining:** this may represent partial acceptance, though often immediate problems are denied. Miracle 'cures' can be looked for.
- **Depression:** sadness at understanding that death will occur.
- **Acceptance:** coming to terms with the inevitable.

These phases do not always occur in the same sequence, and some may not be experienced at all. Individuals may move backwards and forwards through the stages depending on their state of health, their personality and the support they receive.

Development is not necessarily a straight pathway. Events can occur along the way that add or change the process, e.g. pregnancy, illness and bereavement. Human development is therefore a lifelong process.

Further reading

Nolen-Hoeksema, S., Frederickson, B.L., Loftus, G.R., et al., 2009. Atkinson and Hilgard's Introduction to psychology, fifteenth ed. Cengage Learning, New York.

Clarke-Stewart, A., Dunn, J. (Eds.), 2006. Families count: effects on child and adolescent development (Jacobs Foundation Series on Adolescence). Cambridge University Press, Cambridge.

Oates, J. (Ed.), 1995. Foundation of child development. Open University, Blackwell, Oxford.

Schlesinger, L.B., 1980. Distinctions between psychopathic, sociopathic and anti-social personality disorders. Psychol. Rep. 47, 15–21.

References

Ainsworth, M.D., Blehar, M., Waters, E., et al., 1978. Patterns of attachment: a psychological study of the strange situation. Lawrence Erlbaum, Hillsdale, NJ.

Bandura, A., 1977. Social learning theory. Prentice Hall, New Jersey.

Barnhill, L.H., Longo, D., 1978. Fixation and regression in the family life cycle. Fam. Process 17, 469–478.

Bowlby, J., 1969/1982. Attachment and loss: attachment. Basic Books, New York.

Chomsky, N., 1972. Language and mind. Harcourt Brace, New York.

Erikson, E., 1963. Childhood and society, second ed. Norton, New York.

Gilligan, C., 1985. In a different voice. Harvard University Press, Cambridge.

Kohlberg, L., 1976. Moral stages and moralisation: the cognitive–developmental approach. In: Lickong, T. (Ed.), Moral development and behaviour. Holt, Rinehart & Winston, New York.

Kübler-Ross, E., 1969. On death and dying. Macmillan, New York.

Levinson, D.J., Darrow, C., Klein, E., et al., 1978. The seasons of a man's life. Knopf, New York.

Maccoby, E.E., Martin, J.A., 1983. Socialisation in the context of the family: parent–child interaction. In: Mussen, P.H. (Ed.), Handbook of child psychology. vol. 4. Wiley, New York.

Marcia, J.E., 1966. Development and validation of egoidentity status. J. Soc. Psychol. 3, 551–558.

Marcia, J.E., 1980. Identity in adolescence. In: Adelson, J. (Ed.), Handbook of adolescent psychology. Wiley, New York.

McGoldrick, M., Carter, E.A., 1982. The family life cycle. In: Walsh, F. (Ed.), Normal family processes. Guildford, New York.

Piaget, J., Inhelder, B., 1969. The psychology of the child. Basic Books, New York.

Introduction

Psychology is the scientific study of behaviour and cognitive processes. The scientific method was first applied to the study of the mind and mental processes at the start of the twentieth century. Early methods of inquiry involved introspection; these were soon replaced by behaviourist theories which focused on only what can be measured or observed. Later, the Gestalt psychologists (mainly interested in perception) became prominent. From the 1950s onwards, cognitive theorists dominated; initially the brain was seen as analogous to a computer: a sequential, serial processor. Today cognitive theorists still dominate the research field in understanding mental processes.

A number of branches of applied psychology exist today: occupational, educational, clinical and counselling being the most prominent. Psychiatrists are most likely to encounter clinical psychologists in their work, based in mental health settings, or educational psychologists who work primarily within the education system. While clinical practice has moved far from the basic theories outlined here, it is these that represent the building blocks of knowledge in psychological treatment approaches such as cognitive therapy, behaviour therapy and broader clinical practice.

Learning theory

Learning is a hypothetical construct representing a relatively permanent change in observable behaviour, which results from prior experience. It is not the result of maturational factors or reversible influences such as hunger or fatigue. There are three main forms of learning:

- **Associative learning:** refers to the behavioural approach and covers classical and operant conditioning.
- **Cognitive learning:** relates to the cognitive processes of perception and language.
- **Social learning:** relates to learning from observations and modelling.

Forms of associative learning

Classical conditioning

Classical conditioning is the pairing of two stimuli, usually a reflex behaviour (e.g. blinking when air hits the eye) with a neutral response. The work of Pavlov, an influential physiologist and behaviourist in the early part of the twentieth century, was extremely valuable in demonstrating this phenomenon. Interested initially in the process of digestion in dogs, he noticed that the dogs would often start salivating (the *unconditioned response*) not only before food was given to them (the *unconditioned stimulus*), but also when they heard the bell that signalled mealtimes (a *conditioned stimulus*). The dogs were pairing a stimulus usually unconnected with a salivatory response (the bell) with another stimulus, which was associated with that response (i.e. food). The three stages of classical conditioning are shown in Figure 5.1.

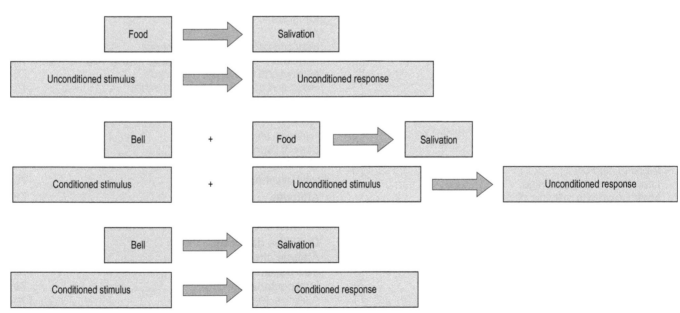

Figure 5.1 • The three stages of classical conditioning.

Pavlov (1927) demonstrated different types of classical conditioning based on relationships between the conditioned and unconditioned stimuli:

- **Delayed/forward conditioning:** the conditioned stimulus (CS) is presented before the unconditioned stimulus (UCS) and remains 'on', while UCS is presented until the unconditioned response (UCR) appears. Strongest learning occurs when the delay is no more than 0.5 seconds. The longer the interval, the poorer the learning.
- **Simultaneous conditioning:** CS and UCS are presented together and conditioning occurs when the CS has produced the CR alone.
- **Trace conditioning:** CS is presented and removed before UCS is presented; only a 'trace memory' of the CS remains to be conditioned. The shorter the interval, the stronger the conditioning. Usually this tends to be a weaker pairing than in delayed or simultaneous conditioning.
- **Backward conditioning:** CS is presented after the UCS. Used widely in advertising, i.e. set the sunny scene, then introduce the drink to be drunk in the sunny scene.
- **Stimulus generalization:** where a similar CS can generate the same CR, e.g. different bells give rise to the CR. The further the stimulus differs from the original CS, the weaker the response. Watson, often referred to as the founder of behaviourism, attempted to apply the work of Pavlov with dogs to humans. He described the case of Little Albert, an 11-month-old infant who developed a generalized fear of white fluffy things after touching a white rabbit that had been paired with a loud scary noise and this is one of the most famous examples of this concept (Watson & Rayner 1920).
- **Higher order conditioning:** CS can be paired with another stimulus (CS^2) to produce a further CR, e.g. once the CR (salivation) had been paired with the bell, the bell could be paired with a light, which then when presented alone elicits the CR. The original CS (the bell) serves as a UCS for the new association, in the same way as did the food originally. Higher order conditioning tends to be fairly weak, as the CS^2 is never actually paired with the UCR. Third and fourth order conditioning are possible, but become weaker with each pairing.
- **Extinction:** when the CS (bell) is continually presented without the UCS (food) the CR (salivation) stops. Through presentation of the CR without CS the response becomes 'unlearned'. If after a time the pairing is repeated, the association appears again and the CR will again bring on the CS. Spontaneous recovery of the response may occur after a period of time but in a weaker form.

Operant/instrumental conditioning

Operant conditioning was clearly demonstrated by Skinner, working a little before Pavlov, through his work with rats in mazes. He was the first behaviourist to make a distinction between respondent behaviour (that which is triggered automatically) and operant behaviour (that which occurs voluntarily). Skinner believed that most animal or human behaviour is not elicited by a specific stimulus, but is a voluntary, active process. He argued that people 'operate' on their environment and that behaviour is 'instrumental' in leading to certain

'consequences', which lead to the behaviour being repeated. Contingent upon the consequences of the action, responses that bring pleasure or satisfaction are likely to be repeated; those that bring discomfort or pain, are not (Skinner 1938).

Thorndike's law of effect

Skinner's work was much influenced by Thorndike, who had carried out experiments with cats in puzzle boxes (Thorndike 1898). These boxes had a latch, which opened a door enabling the cat to get out. The cat's task was to open the latch to escape the box and get to the waiting fish outside. Thorndike found that the more times the cats attempted to get out of the box, the quicker they became at opening the latch. Thorndike explained their quicker responses in terms of trial and error learning, so proposing a link between the stimulus (the puzzle box and latch) and the response (getting out). He called this the *Law of Effect* showing that what happens as a result of a behaviour will affect that behaviour in the future. In classical conditioning, it is what happens before the behaviour that is said to determine the behaviour.

A variety of terms for clarifying behaviours has been developed:

- **Reinforcement:** there are two types of reinforcers:
  - i. Primary reinforcers are those stimuli that meet biological needs, e.g. hunger, thirst, etc.
  - ii. Secondary reinforcers are those which one has to learn the value of. These do not rely on basic needs but tend to be those that we have chosen to value, e.g. self-esteem, money, etc.
- **Consequences of conditioning:** the consequences of operant conditioning may be positive reinforcement, negative reinforcement or punishment:
  - i. Positive reinforcement: refers to the presentation of something pleasant to make the behaviour stronger, in order that the behaviour will be repeated.
  - ii. Negative reinforcement: relates to acting or behaving in order that an aversive stimulus is removed. Both positive and negative reinforcement serve to strengthen behaviour.
  - iii. Punishment: refers to pain or annoyance administered to decrease or weaken behaviour, i.e. electric shocks given to those who respond in an unwanted way to a certain stimulus. Punishment tends not to be as effective in learning situations as positive or negative reinforcers which increase the probability of the desired behaviour.
- **Reinforcement schedules:** how often and how regularly the reinforcement is presented will effect behaviour:
  - ○ Continuous reinforcement: reinforcing every occurrence of the response. Very easily extinguished.
  - ○ Partial reinforcement: reinforcement is given to only some responses.
  - ○ Fixed interval: reinforcement is given regularly, for example every 30 seconds. The response rate will increase, as the next reinforcement becomes available. Extinction achieved fairly easily.
  - ○ Variable interval: reinforcement is given regularly but the interval varies from trial to trial, it is unpredictable. Extinction takes a long time to occur.

○ Fixed ratio: reinforcement given for a fixed number of responses. Extinction occurs fairly easily.

○ Variable ratio: reinforcement given regularly but the number of responses required changes from trial to trial. Extinction is extremely hard to achieve.

Applications of conditioning today are found in basic behavioural management schedules, for example in fears and phobias, in biofeedback and in programmed learning.

Observational learning

This refers to learning by watching rather than by doing and stems from social learning theory. Bandura, a major proponent of these theories, posited that while both classical and operant conditioning are important, they cannot account for novel behaviour (behaviour which has not been displayed before) and therefore that novel behaviour must develop from observational learning (Bandura 1977). Bandura also argued that a variety of cognitive factors mediate the learning process:

• Attention
• Perception
• Memory
• Reproduction of the seen motor activities
• Motivation.

This kind of learning is especially relevant to the development of children with their expanding repertoire of behaviours. Observational learning is discussed in greater depth in Chapter 4.

Insight learning

From this theoretical viewpoint, learning is seen as a purely cognitive process. The Gestalt theorists, of whom Kohler (1947) was a major author, argued that all psychological theory should be treated holistically, looking at the whole rather than only certain relationships. These theorists, best known for their work on perception, saw learning as a process involving the perceptual restructuring of elements that constitute a problem situation, with the addition of a piece of information that was previously missing. Whereas in stimulus–response theories, learning is said to occur by trial and error, in insight learning, cognitive processes are put into play and the situation thought about. Then a solution will suddenly become evident when the missing piece of information becomes 'seen' and therefore available for use in solving the problem. It is the cognitive relationship between the means and the end that is learned, not a specific set of conditioned associations, thus ensuring easier application to similar problems in the future. Kohler did not believe that past experience had an impact on learning processes, and this is one major weakness of the theory.

Linking stimulus–response and cognitive theories: learning sets

Harlow argued that stimulus–response (S–R) learning and insight learning are based along a continuum, where stimulus–response learning dominates early on and cognitive or insight learning appears later (Harlow 1949). He argued for a learning

set, or a way of *learning to learn*; this is a process that occurs somewhere between S–R and insight learning. A set comprises a general rule or skill applicable to a whole class of problems and demonstrates the transfer of learning, in that earlier learning influences later learning. The more sets a person has, the better equipped they are to learn new information.

Motivation

Motivated behaviour is goal-directed, purposeful behaviour. The study of motivation is highly dependent upon one's theoretical approach, whether:

• Psychoanalytic (examining unconscious motives and desires)
• Behaviourist (based on learning and reinforcement schedules)
• Humanist (related to self-actualization, as described above)
• Cognitive (looking for appraisal and attribution)
• Neurobiological (looking at nervous system, endocrine system and other bodily systems).

There are two broad categories of motivational drives – survival or physiological motives and competence or cognitive motives. Social motives are an occasionally used third category.

• **Homeostatic or primary drives:** described by Cannon (1929) are those that are guided by a physiological need, i.e. hunger or thirst. The drive leads to behaviour aimed at reducing a tissue deficiency need, i.e. finding food or something to drink, leading to the restoration of the internal balance of homeostasis. The primary reinforcers for primary drives are food, water and sex.

• **Drive reduction theory:** Hull (1943) relates to his theory of learning and the notion of reinforcement described earlier. Here a physiological need is noted, along with a drive to reduce that need; behaviour is then directed to reduce the drive and this drive reduction reinforces the drive reducing behaviour.

• **Competence or secondary drives:** are those things that people seek out that do not fulfil a physiological need. These are continuous motives, unlike primary motives that come and go. Play is an example of a competence motive. It is now clear that behaviour is much more complex than simple reactions to physiological or even secondary drives. These motives tend to involve the search for stimulation, through curiosity and exploration, without any extrinsic reward.

Perception

An understanding of the sensory processes is important in building a full picture of cognitive learning. Perception is an effortless but active process involving the selection, inference, organization and interpretation of information received by the senses at any one time in conjunction with prior knowledge and memory. It is an immediate discriminatory response of an organism to energy-activating sense organs. By means of perception it is possible to build up a mental representation of the world, a process that occurs from birth. The process of perception encompasses a variety of processing systems, including the physiological systems of each sensory modality and central brain processes.

Visual perception

It has been estimated that about 90% of the information received about the world comes through the eyes. Vision is therefore the most widely researched sensory system.

Given the vast amount of information available to the sensory systems at any one time, it is possible to use only a small percentage of it. The brain has limited capacity to process the information and is able to attend or select some things and not others. At times, the information received is incomplete and the whole picture may not be seen. It is therefore necessary to supplement the incoming information with previous experience and knowledge of the world, in order to infer the whole picture. The notion of *constancy* describes this.

Constancy is the ability to perceive objects as they are, rather than as they may be seen. Constancy can be found in:

- Shape: a cup may appear, due to perspective, as an ellipse but is still known to be round; a tree will be perceived as vertical even when one's head is tilted to the side
- Size: whether an object is 1 or 10 metres away, we are able to judge its approximate breadth and height
- Colour: whatever the availability of light, the colour or hue of an object can be perceived
- Brightness: regardless of the brightness of the light in which it is seen, coal is seen as black
- Location: even if a person spins round, kinaesthetic feedback ensures that the person knows they, rather than the world, are spinning.

Pattern recognition is a key feature of visual perception. It involves assigning meaning to visual input by identifying objects in the visual field. Three main theories exist:

- **Template matching theories:** suggest that pattern recognition involves a comparison between the information held in the sensory register and miniature copies or templates of previously seen information, held in long-term stores. If this theory were true there would have to be an infinite number of templates in the long-term storage facility and the search for a match would take a very long time; it also does not explain how the search would happen.
- **Prototype theories:** suggest that each stimulus belongs to a category, and shares key attributes with the other stimuli in that category, so a smaller number of pieces of information are stored than with template theories. In order to recognize a pattern, the basic elements or features are compared with the stored prototypes. While this theory is better substantiated than template theories, it does not explain how the matching process works.
- **Feature detection theories:** the best-developed theories. They suggest that each stimulus pattern represents a specific organization of certain basic attributes or features. Perception involves extracting these attributes from the

presented stimuli, which are then compared with previously stored information. While these theories are better able to explain the complexities of pattern recognition, and much support has been generated from behavioural and neurological studies, they still have inherent weaknesses.

Set and schema

Allport (1955) described a *set* as a perceptual bias, predisposition or readiness to perceive particular features of a stimulus; a way of selecting some parts of information and ignoring others. A *schema* is a persistent well-organized classificatory system of perceiving, thinking and believing. The set first works as a selector based on the expectations formed by the schema and then as an interpreter, using information from the schema to classify, understand and infer from the information. Set is influenced by both organismic or perceiver variables and situational variables.

Perceptual organization: figure–ground differentiation

Visual information is almost always organized into a way that makes sense of the information presented. Figure–ground differentiation is a clear example of how this organization works, and can make mistakes. Distinct parts of a visual field are said to stand out from other parts; this has been called the figure–ground relationship. A classic example of this is the Rubin vase, where some part of a stimulus always stands out at any one time. The vase also demonstrates how the part that stands out can change (Fig. 5.2).

Figure–ground organization appears to be an automatic process, and Gestalt psychologists have argued that it reflects an important part of the innate organizational ability of the visual system. Other organizational principles relate to proximity

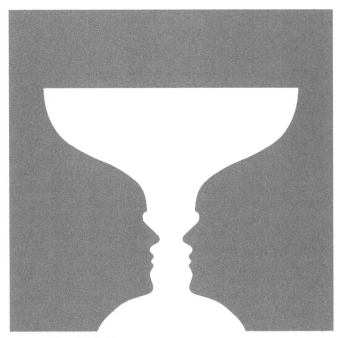

Figure 5.2 • The Rubin vase.

held in STM for longer than 30 seconds by using techniques of auditory rehearsal or repetition, which 'refresh' the memory trace. Coding in the STM tends to be acoustic, whether information was primarily visual or verbal.

Forgetting and short-term memory

There has been much debate as to whether information held in STM disappears due to trace decay (i.e. the memory trace disintegrates and is lost from the memory system) or interference/displacement of old information by new information entering the system. As might be expected, short-term forgetting seems to be a combination of the two, the trace weakens over time and becomes harder to be retrieved or be discriminated from other competing traces.

Working memory

Alan Baddely and colleagues proposed that STM should be replaced with working memory (Baddely & Hitch 1974), a system which could hold and manipulate information and that was vital in performing a range of cognitive tasks comprising three parts:

- **Central executive:** has a limited capacity and is used when dealing with cognitively demanding tasks. It closely resembles attention.
- **Articulatory or phonological loop:** temporally and serially, encodes phonemic information. It is used to supplement the storage capacity of the central executive in verbal tasks.
- **Visuospatial scratch pad:** less well understood, but appears to manipulate visuospatial images, managing visual information, again feeding into the central executive. It seems to be useful in tasks involving visuospatial manipulation.

The early model has been expanded, now comprising a central executive controlling the articulatory loop, visuospatial scratch pad and primary acoustic store (Salame & Baddely 1982).

Long-term memory storage

Long-term memory (LTM) is thought to have an unlimited capacity, in which memories can last from a few minutes to many years. The LTM store is highly organized around a central store. Information tends to be stored semantically (i.e. verbal meaning is encoded) or visually (i.e. in pictures). There also appears to be an episodic memory store, demonstrated by patients who have suffered brain damage, who may forget personal information (episodic memory) but do not forget their native language (semantic memory).

Mnemonics: one example of long-term memory organization

Mnemonics are rules of learning that aid recall by providing a fast way of learning new information with the help of existing memory structures. A common example would be trying to visualize a new piece of information displayed in every room of a familiar house. As one visualizes the rooms of the house, the new information is recalled as well.

Retrieval from the long-term memory

Retrieval of information relies of information being stored in a logical, rational order. There are several forms of remembering:

- **Recognition:** involves being able to recognize but not spontaneously recall an answer to a question, e.g. when presented with a multiple choice of answers to a problem, it is easy to pick out the correct one, whereas it would not have been possible to spontaneously generate the correct response.
- **Recall:** involves actively searching the memory stores and reproducing something that was learned. Retrieval clues are sparse here.
- **Relearning:** involves learning something which been learned and then forgotten. It takes less time the second time around, as the existing memory, although inaccessible, is likely to have left some trace.
- **Reconstructive memory:** the type of remembering involved in the passing on of information from one person to another, often involving distortion of the information received. It is this kind of memory that is implicated in eye witness testimony, described in Chapter 31.
- **Confabulation:** a memory error often made at times of high arousal, where if a full memory cannot be found, pieces are added to make the story seem more appropriate. Confabulation is frequently found in patients with Korsakoff syndrome.
- **Redintegration:** recollection of past experiences based on certain cues, e.g. a perfume, an unusual sound. A small amount of the memory is triggered and then a systematic search of memory stores gives rise to the whole memory.

Context and memory storage

Context and state-dependent memory are concerned with:

- The state of the person (e.g. under the influence of alcohol)
- The place in which the memory was initially encoded for the retrieval of information.

Retrieval of information is generally better given similar rather than different contextual cues.

Motivational and emotional factors

These are also likely to affect recall and forgetting. Freud argued that painful or emotionally salient memories can be repressed and placed out of conscious access as a protective mechanism. Clinically, this may be seen in amnesia in patients following severe emotional trauma. Motivated forgetting is, however, hard to assess empirically. Some research suggests that high levels of arousal may lead to enhanced recall under certain circumstances, due to the positive effect of arousal on memory trace consolidation.

Mood and retrieval

A person in a gloomy mood is more likely to recall gloomy information, a person in a happy mood is more likely to remember cheerful information. Patients with clinical depression have been found to recall more negatively focused information than nondepressed controls. However, stress and anxiety states may distort the attentional processes rather than the memory processes and hence may lead to distorted encoding of a stimulus due to heightened attention to salient aspects of a traumatic scene.

Forgetting in long-term memory

It is impossible to say that information can be forgotten from LTM, rather that it is not accessible or available at the present time.

- **Passive decay theory:** as time goes by, memory traces may decay unless maintained. It has been suggested that this may in part be due to metabolic processes or neural decay, although there is little evidence for this (Solso 1995).
- **Systematic distortion of the memory trace:** the longer the memory is stored, the more subject to distortions it becomes. Evidence now suggests that distortions may occur at all points of the memory system.
- **Interference theories:** the greater the similarity between two things, the more likely they are to interfere with the memory trace. Thus, as more is learned over time, forgetting is more likely to occur due to increasing competition between similar memories. What is learned will be influenced by proactive (prior learning) and retroactive (future learning) interference.

A full understanding of the memory system has not as yet been reached and further exciting work is continuing, especially with regard to understanding the development of memory in children.

Intelligence

Intelligence represents one of the most widely studied and controversial areas in psychology today. Many theories have been developed to try and explain it. Many methods for measuring intelligence have been developed, the most influential being the psychometric approaches, which rely on factor analysis. Definitions of intelligence refer to it as: a biological construct (related to adaptation to the environment), a psychological construct (related to the measurement of individual differences), or an operational construct (intelligence defined as what intelligence tests measure). In general, it is seen as a multidimensional cognitive ability, comprising an individual's capacity to understand, reason and problem solve.

Factor analytic approaches

These approaches are based on the analysis of large amounts of data from individuals using factor analysis.

Spearman's two-factor theory: Spearman carried out a factor analysis of the results of children's performance on a number of tests, and found many positive correlations between the tests. From this he concluded that all tests measured both a common factor of general intelligence (g) and a specific factor (s). He believed that individual differences were due to differences in g. His theory of g, although nowadays held to be inaccurate, was extremely influential.

Cyril Burt: a student of Spearman, expanded the two-factor model and developed the Hierarchical model, where g is what all tests measure. He and a colleague, Vernon, proposed that between g and s were major and minor group factors. The major group factors (divided into verbal–educational ability and spatial–mechanical ability) were what all tests measure; the minor group what particular tests measure. They then saw specific factors as what particular tests measured on specific occasions (Vernon 1960).

Guilford: rejected the notion of g and classified cognitive tasks along three dimensions (Guilford 1967):

- Content (what is the problem?)
- Operations (how does the subject need to approach the task?)
- Products (what kind of answer is needed?).

From the different kinds of operations needed in each of these dimensions he calculated at least 120 mental abilities. Results on tests designed using this model often correlated well, suggesting far fewer distinct mental abilities (Brody & Brody 1976).

It is now widely accepted that intelligence is a combination of general mental and specific mental ability. Theorists relying on factor analytic studies to define intelligence have proposed very different theories. This is in part because they used differing subject pools, of different ages with different factor analytic techniques and different tests. A further danger with factor analytic methods is that the factor described (e.g. verbal ability) becomes a reality (the process of reification) rather than simply a statistic.

Other models of intelligence

Fluid and crystallized intelligence

Cattell and Horn (Cattell 1965; Horn & Cattell, 1967), using factor analysis again, proposed that g should be divided into two parts:

- **Fluid intelligence:** relates to untaught abilities, relatively free of cultural bias, e.g. abstract problem-solving abilities. It was argued that this ability peaked during adolescence, then plateaued and decreased after young adulthood, although recent research has not demonstrated this decline.
- **Crystallized intelligence:** relates to cumulative learning experiences and is based on acquired knowledge and skills from school and life experiences. It is said to increase throughout the life span and there is some evidence to support this claim.

Measurement of intelligence

The intelligence quotient

Intelligence quotient (IQ) refers to mental age (MA) expressed as a ratio of chronological age (CA) multiplied by 100. For IQ to remain stable, MA must increase with CA over time. This is true until around 18 years, when intellectual abilities are usually fully developed. As stated above, it was erroneously thought that intellectual ability started to decline after young adulthood.

It now appears that although fluid intelligence may start to decrease, crystallized intelligence continues to develop throughout the lifespan. Intelligence is said to be normally distributed with a slight 'bump' at the lower end of the normal distribution curve, representing those with severe learning difficulties.

Testing intelligence

It is now said that intelligence tests assess a range of cognitive abilities, rather than the more abstract concept of intelligence. Intelligence tests are said to measure the level of performance upon specific tests. While it is then suggested that, due to the fact that the test are standardized, reliable and valid, they measure IQ, the debate continues as to whether this is so and indeed whether tests of intelligence are useful (Kaufman 1994).

The Stanford–Binet test

Generally held to be the first intelligence test, Binet and Simon (1905) developed a measure to identify those school children who would not benefit from mainstream education due to low levels of cognitive ability. The test was modified by an American, Terman, who was working at Stanford University. It then became known as the Stanford–Binet test. It has been revised many times but is not now widely used.

The Wechsler scales

The most widely used tests of intelligence are the Wechsler scales, initially developed for adults in the 1940s and revised many times for different ages and cultural groups. The most commonly used versions in the UK are (Wechsler 1991, 1999a,b, 2003):

- Wechsler Adult Intelligence Scale-R (WAIS-R), for people of 16 years and over
- Wechsler Intelligence Scales for Children-III-UK (WISC-III-UK), for 7- to 16-year-olds
- Wechsler Pre-school and Primary Scales of Intelligence (WPPSI-III-UK) for 3–7.3-year-olds.

The raw scores obtained from all Wechsler subtests are converted into scale scores. Scale scores range from 1 to 19, the average range being 8–12.

The Wechsler tests all contain a variety of subtests, which are divided into two domains of verbal and performance abilities (verbal IQ and performance IQ). The combined standardized scores of the subtests on these two domains give an overall intelligence quotient (IQ). WISC-III-UK scores are also commonly organized into factor indexes, of verbal comprehension, perceptual organization, processing speed and freedom from distractibility (Kaufman 1994). For the IQ and index scores the mean is 100, with 15 points representing 1 standard deviation (SD). So 68% of the population will score between 85 and 115, 14% between 70 and 84, or 116 and 130 and 2% <70 or >130.

The Wechsler Abbreviated Scale of Intelligence (Wechsler 1999b) has also been introduced to screen a wide age-range using 2–4 subtests. This measure is primarily used in research rather than in clinical practice.

Differences between subtest scores provide important diagnostic information: for example, children with attention deficit hyperactivity disorder may perform better on verbal than performance subtests and children with autism may do better on specific performance subtests compared with verbal subtests. While much clinical information can be obtained from an analysis of the cognitive profile, it is rare that an IQ test on its own will yield sufficient information to make recommendations about the care of a person who has demonstrated either global or specific difficulties. Further testing using a variety of attainment and neuropsychological measures is usually indicated.

Other tests such as the British Ability Scales (BAS-II) are also widely used by educational and clinical psychologists. This measure comprises 24 subscales that measure 24 distinct aspects of cognitive abilities in 2.1- to 17-year-olds and gives standardized scores in order that the results can be compared between measures.

Raven's progressive matrices

In order to overcome cultural biases prevalent in intelligence tests, i.e. biased in favour of white, middle-class children and adults, tests like the Raven's progressive matrices were developed (Raven et al 1983). This test comprises a series of non-verbal pattern-matching exercises. The object of the test is evident without much understanding of language. However, the test is still considered to be culture-dependent as the skill of pattern matching is more commonly used in some cultures than in others.

Cultural and racial factors

Jensen, an American psychologist, argued that there were intellectual differences between different races (Jensen 1980). His research has been shown to be biased and it is now clear that there are not actual differences in the intellectual abilities of different racial or cultural groups but that environmental factors, test bias and genetic differences all play a part in any individual's performance.

Factors affecting test performance

A test result is meaningless unless it is evaluated together with all other relevant information about the person (social and medical history, school or work reports, information from family and significant others) including the following variables:

- **Arousal and anxiety:** can impinge on a person's ability to perform as well as they otherwise might on these tests. People with depression tend to perform more poorly due to motor and thought slowing.
- **Ability to plan and organize one's approach to test materials:** these factors can affect the speed with which a person can complete a task and give clues as to how they may approach tasks in everyday life.
- **Lack of motivation:** may reduce the overall score.
- **Changes in neurological functioning:** may be responsible for decreases in functioning, as might changes in psychiatric status.

- **Physical difficulties:** such as motor difficulties, visual field deficits, may impair performance, especially on timed tests.
- **Linguistic and cultural background:** if English is not fluent, the person may not be able to demonstrate their true ability. As stated above, different stimuli may be applicable to different cultural groups.
- **Familiarity with the test material:** if a test is repeated frequently, practice effects will occur and the person will be seen to improve. The Wechsler tests should not be repeated within less than 6 months, in order to avoid this.

Indications for testing

The testing of cognitive ability has a variety of uses in clinical practice and should be carried out only when the result is likely to influence clinical practice, for example:

- In the assessment and diagnosis of specific and global learning difficulties
- In examining the effect of a brain injury or systemic illness upon a person's functioning
- To aid in rehabilitation planning following a brain injury.

Emotion

Emotions

There have been many attempts to classify emotions; Plutchik (1980) proposed the existence of eight primary emotions, composed of four pairs of opposites. These are arranged in a wheel and are surrounded by eight complex emotions (Fig. 5.3).

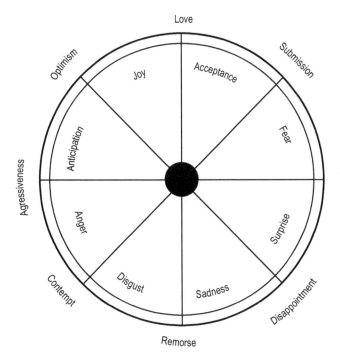

Figure 5.3 • Plutchik's wheel.

Plutchik argues that the primary emotions are biologically and subjectively distinct.

However the spectrum of emotions interrelate, it is argued that there are three components to every emotional response:

- Subjective experience: the experience of joy, sadness, anger, etc.
- Physiological changes: changes in the autonomic nervous system and endocrine system, over which the individual has little control, such as sweating
- Behavioural associations: specific patterns associated with specific emotions such as smiling when happy.

Theories of emotion

Initial theories of emotion focused purely on physiological reactions, later theories include the importance of cognitive aspects into the understanding of emotional experience.

The James–Lange theory: (originally described by James in 1890) viewed the emotional response to a situation as the result of physiological reactions, i.e. we feel frightened because we are running away from something, not because something makes us scared. It is the notion of feedback from bodily changes that is key to this theory. The theory suggests that each emotion results from a different physiological state. Critics of the theory argue that as emotion is felt instantly (without time for physiological responses to begin), physiological arousal might not even be necessary for the experience of emotion. Furthermore, they point out that similar physiological reactions can occur when no emotion is felt, e.g. exercise may bring about the same physiological changes as those experienced in fear.

The Cannon–Baird theory: (Cannon 1929) suggested that the autonomic nervous system responds in the same way to all emotional stimuli, so emotional experience must be more than basic physiological arousal. The thalamus was seen as central in emotional regulation, in sending impulses to the sympathetic nervous system and to the cerebral cortex. While this theory also has weaknesses, it is clear that physiological factors play a large, interdependent role in emotional experience.

The two-factor theory of emotion: Schachter (1964) argues that an emotional reaction involves initial peripheral physiological changes, such as heart rate and blood pressure and the interpretation or appraisal of those changes. Emotional specificity is therefore based on what the arousal is attributed to, i.e. the cognitive appraisal of the arousal.

More recently, there has been much work on the role of cognition in the experience of emotion, especially by Lazarus and Folkman (1984).

Emotion and performance

An important relationship between the level of emotional arousal and performance is demonstrated by the Yerkes–Dodson curve (Yerkes & Dodson 1908; Fig. 5.4). The theory suggests that there is an inverted U-shaped relationship between arousal (or motivation) and performance level. As the level of emotional arousal increases, so does performance efficiency, to an optimal level. As emotional arousal increases above this point, performance

These are not dimensions that could be applied to all people. These individual traits take three forms:

i. Cardinal traits – all pervading, directing most of an individual's behaviour

ii. Central traits – blocks that make up the core personality

iii. Secondary traits – refer to tastes, preferences, political views, etc.

It has been argued that Allport's idiographic methods are basically nomothetic theories applied to individuals.

Kelly and personal construct theory

Kelly (1955) described the person in terms of their own experiences and view of the world (the phenomenological approach). He proposed that an individual has their own concepts or ideas which are used to understand the world, and make predictions about future events. He defined the way in which one sees the world through constructs (each person's construct system being hierarchically organized; based on broad (superordinate) and narrow (subordinate) constructs).

The Repertory Grid Technique, devised to test construct systems, involves choosing elements (e.g. the most important figures in the person's life) and describing in what way these elements are alike or different from a third element. These differences or similarities (the constructs) are then applied to all other elements. This process is reproduced until the person has produced all the constructs they can. The information is presented in a grid, which can be analysed statistically to enable a person to gain a clearer sense of the way they see the world. Kelly (1955) and Bannister and Fransella (1980) produced a thorough review of Personal Construct Theory, which is helpful in understanding the complexities of the theory.

Rogers and client-centred therapy

Rogers (1951) (who, along with Maslow, was one of the most influential humanistic psychologists), saw people as rational, whole beings who know about their feelings and reactions. He argued that self-knowledge is the basis of personality and that it develops from interactions with the world. It aims for consistency but can change as a result of its interactions. The basic need for positive regard is one of Rogers' key arguments. Difficulties arise if there is a discrepancy between an individual's self-concept and their experiences.

The Q-Sort Technique, developed from this theory, involves a person sorting cards with statements on them, into piles. They may be asked to sort the cards into piles indicating how they think of themselves presently, or indeed how they would like to be. The task can then be repeated over the course of therapy in order to monitor the person's changing views of themselves.

Maslow and the hierarchy of needs

Maslow's approach was also phenomenological in that he was concerned with individuals' experiences of their world. He postulated a hierarchy of needs (Fig. 5.5), factors that need to be fulfilled in order that one can become 'self-actualized', the highest form of personal growth. In order to reach the higher levels, the lower levels (involving basic survival needs) must be satisfied (Maslow 1943). Maslow's hierarchy of needs is in essence more about needs and motivation so is not a 'pure' theory of personality, such as that of Eysenck or Cattell.

Freud and psychoanalytic approaches

Freud construed personality as having three main components:

- **Id:** responds directly to impulses and biologically based needs, e.g. food, warmth, shelter
- **Ego:** that part of the id that has been modified by the direct influence of the external world through the medium of conscious perception
- **Superego:** this develops once a person has absorbed moral values which determine the acceptability of behaviour, representing the moral or judicial part of the personality.

These concepts are covered in depth in Chapter 37.

It is now generally accepted that attempting to explain all behaviour in terms of personality is unwise: behaviour in any one situation is a reflection of both person and situation variables and even these situational variables have to do with the psychological meaning of the situation to the person.

Consciousness

Freud described the 'topographical model', in which the mind was divided into the conscious, preconscious and the unconscious, with only limited access to those thoughts held in the unconscious and preconscious systems. Psychologists tend to see the unconscious more as a continuum from being fully conscious to being totally unconscious. Different amounts of thoughts, feelings, memories can be accessed, often referred to as the subjective awareness of actions and of the world around us (Rubin & McNeil 1983). Consciousness also has links with attention, and is often described as what we pay attention to.

Arousal

Arousal relates to the level of alertness of the individual and refers to a continuum of possible behavioural and physiological states. Levels of arousal are influenced by circadian rhythms (the 24-hour patterns of biological change). Sleep represents the common, daily change in levels of arousal, and is described further in Chapter 35.

Hypnosis and suggestibility

Hypnosis has been described as an altered state of consciousness, where the hypnotized subject can be influenced to behave and to experience things differently than he or she would have in the ordinary waking state (Rubin & McNeil 1983). Others would argue that it is not an altered state of arousal. It was first demonstrated by Mesmer, who showed that when hypnotized, a patient could be instructed to change their behaviour when the hypnotic session was finished. The Stanford Hypnotic Susceptibility Scale can measure suggestibility, relating to how readily hypnotizable the subject is (Weitzenhoffer & Hilgard 1959). Suggestibility is highest in children, reaching a peak at around age 10 and declining with age.

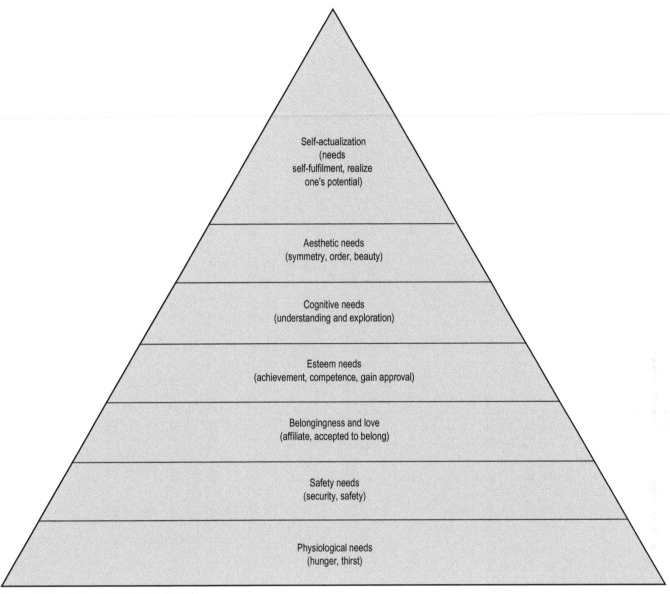

Figure 5.5 • Maslow's hierarchy of needs.

Uses of hypnosis

Hypnosis is commonly used to help people overcome habits such as smoking, and in the treatment of pain. The subject is hypnotized and then receives instructions that the quality or intensity of the pain they are experiencing is altered, turned down or transferred in location. A typical experiment to demonstrate the efficacy of hypnosis is the cold pressor response, where a patient is asked to immerse their arm in a bucket of cold water. Patients who have been hypnotized will report less pain or discomfort than those who have not (Hilgard 1978). Hilgard also refers to the hidden observer phenomenon: when the hypnotized person is asked about the pain or discomfort, they report low levels, but when the 'hidden observer' (i.e. another part of the person's consciousness) is asked, levels almost the same as a non-hypnotized subject are reported. This is referred to as Hilgard's neo-dissociation theory.

The debate as to whether hypnosis is a real state of altered consciousness continues and studies abound trying to prove or disprove its existence and its mechanisms (Wagstaff 1995).

Meditation and trances

Meditation refers to a technique of clearing the mind through focused thought. It represents a way of trying to alter consciousness to achieve inner calm. There are two main forms of meditation:

• *Concentrate meditation* as practised by some Hindus, which seeks an alteration of consciousness through detachment from the external environment and from internal thought processes, by concentrating on a mandala (a visual image on which all attention is focused) or a mantra (a single word, repeated silently to oneself).

- *Mindfulness meditation*, as practised by Zen Buddhists, where all mental attention is directed at the thoughts that pass through the mind, the object of the exercise being to observe these things in a detached manner rather than challenge them or direct the mind in any way. Mindfulness has been incorporated with cognitive behaviour therapy (mindfulness-based cognitive therapy – MBCT) as a treatment for depression and dialectical behaviour therapy (DBT) for the treatment of borderline personality disorder (see Chapter 38).

Through meditation, thought to be mainly a right-hemisphere activity, people have been able to control their bodily processes, slow down heart rate and reduce the amount of oxygen capacity used, akin to the aims of biofeedback.

Social psychology

Social psychology is the study of how people perceive, think and feel about the social world and how we interact and influence one another. Behaviour is then determined according to the power of the situation and a person's interpretation of the situation.

Attitudes

Attitudes are a set of beliefs (favourable and unfavourable evaluations) that predispose an individual to particular behaviours. There are three components:

- **Cognitive:** beliefs based on information, e.g. exercise is good for your health
- **Affective:** (often very hard to change), e.g. 'I love long-distance running'
- **Behavioural:** e.g. 'I run every day'.

In general, people hold similar attitudes on a range of subjects.

Measurement of attitudes

There are several ways of measuring attitudes, e.g. projective tests such as Rorschach inkblots, physiological tests, e.g. galvanic skin response, and questionnaires. The following are the three main forms of questionnaire:

- **Likert scales:** agree/disagree on a 5-point scale. Such scales are relatively sensitive and simple to design, though similar scores can be obtained with different answers.
- **Thurstone scales:** a range of statements is presented and you pick those you agree with. These scales are less sensitive than Likert scales and can have value-laden biases.
- **Semantic-differential:** a visual analogue scale with polarized adjectives separated by a line. Subjects mark their attitude between the two. These are easy to complete and reliable but may be subject to positional response bias.

Social effects may also impact on measurements of behaviour:

- *Response set*: tendency to always agree/disagree to a set of questions
- *Bias to middle*: avoidance of extreme responses
- *Halo effect*: the observer allows preconceptions to influence responses

- *Hawthorn effect*: positive social interactions between experimenter and subject affects response.

Attitudes and behaviour

A major reason for studying attitudes is expectation that they will predict a person's behaviour. Attitudes predict behaviour best if they are:

- Strong and consistent
- Based on experience
- Related to the behaviour being predicted.

Behaviour may also determine attitudes as expressed in cognitive dissonance theory.

Cognitive dissonance theory (Festinger 1957)

Individuals strive for consistency in their attitudes with discomfort or dissonance arising if two cognitions are held that are inconsistent.

This was demonstrated in an experiment where subjects were recruited for a very dull task and paid $20 or $1. They were then asked to tell others how interesting and fun the task was. Those paid $1 did change attitudes and said the task was fun, while the $20 group were less enthusiastic. Cognitive dissonance theory implies that $20 was sufficient reason to take part, while receiving $1 and doing a boring task was harder to justify leading to the subjects decreasing dissonance by changing attitudes.

Dissonance is increased if there is:

- Low pressure to comply
- Increased choice of options
- Awareness of responsibility for consequences
- Expected unpleasant consequences of behaviour to others.

Dissonance is decreased by:

- Changing behaviour
- Dismissing information/cognitions
- Adding new cognitions.

The theory has little predictive power as to what course of action will be chosen. Other psychologists have argued that dissonance is linked to self-concept or as a way of protecting a public self-image.

Attitude change

Advertising attempts to change/influence attitudes using new information (cognitive), appealing to emotions and offering rewards (behaviour). Similar processes are used in persuasive communication. There are three main areas to consider:

1. **Communicator factors.** More persuasive if:
   - Expert or leader of opinions
   - Motivation clear (no vested interest)
   - Attractive/likeable
   - Uses non-verbal cues – attention paid to body language, etc.

2. Recipient factors. These are influenced by:
- ○ Self-esteem – increased cooperation if simple message in low self-esteem
- ○ Intelligence – though relationship not simple.

3. Message
- ○ An interactive personalized discussion – with a two-sided discussion to a neutral audience and a more one-sided discussion to an already favourable audience
- ○ Fear – excess fear may be counter-productive but also depends on anxiety levels. Low anxiety requires a higher fear content, with medium fear in highly anxious states.

Self-psychology

Self-concept refers to a set of attitudes that an individual holds about themselves, e.g. 'I am popular', 'I am thin'.

Self-esteem is a sense of contentment and self-acceptance arising from a process of appraisal of one's own worth, significance, attractiveness, etc. and one's ability to satisfy aspirations. Increased self-esteem is associated with social activity, fulfilling relationships, etc. Decreased self-esteem is associated with mental illness, a vulnerability to depression and some physical illnesses.

Self-image is a descriptive view of self, derived from experiences of success and the content of social interactions.

Self-perception theory (Bem 1972) proposes that we make judgements about ourselves using the same inferential processes and errors that we use for making judgements of others (see below). Specifically, individuals form their attitudes by inferring them from the observation of their behaviours and situations. If internal cues are weak, then we rely on external cues. Fundamental attribution errors (see below) also mean that self-perception is affected by the tendency to give too much weight to personal characteristics rather than situations, e.g. in a conversation someone who selects topics for discussion will feel and be seen as more knowledgeable than others who follow the conversation flow.

Self-concept is influenced differently by various characteristics, e.g. gender, age:
- Gender:
  - **a.** Males – predominance of activity, dominance
  - **b.** Females – affection, sensitivity.
- Age:
  - **a.** Childhood – physical characteristics, kindness
  - **b.** Adolescents – interests
  - **c.** Adults – occupation, family role.

Interpersonal psychology

Of all attitudes, one of the most interesting is the attitudes of others and factors that influence interpersonal attraction. Attraction is mediated by:
- **Physical attractiveness:** while individuals do not rate this as important, research suggests it does play a major part. People are rated more favourably if with an attractive partner,

and photos of attractive people are rated as being more popular.
- **Proximity:** research suggests that one of the best predictors is how close people live to each other. Being in close proximity to someone is likely to promote friendship.
- **Familiarity:** proximity also promotes familiarity and familiarity also increases liking for something or someone.
- **Similarity:** couples tend to have similar interests or outlooks, similar psychological characteristics, e.g. intelligence and physical attributes – *assortative mating*.

Social exchange theory

This theory suggests that people like their partner more according to the rewards received compared to those given. Relationships can be divided into 'exchange' relationships (rewards exchanged predominantly) and 'communal' relationships (rewards given out of concern for other). 'Exchange' relationships are characterized by insecurity and dissatisfaction.

Stereotypes

A limited amount of information about an individual will result in them being fitted into a specific group and other behavioural characteristics will be ascribed to that individual even with no evidence to support them, e.g. age. In general, the first information received has the greatest effect on the overall impression: the *primacy effect* or *first impressions count*!

Stereotypes persist, even if data do not confirm them, and cause us to interact with people we have stereotyped in ways that cause self-fulfilling stereotypes.

Attribution theory

Attribution theory (Heider 1958) suggests that we develop attitudes based on what we observe. If we infer something based on a belief that it is due to that individual's characteristics, then this is an internal or *dispositional* attribution. If we conclude that an external cause is responsible, e.g. money, then this is a *situational* attribution.

The *fundamental attributional error* suggests a bias towards dispositional attributions, e.g. in a debate. If people are randomly allocated to each side of the debate, people will still estimate the debater's own personal attitudes to be close to the position argued, despite clear evidence that the situation was responsible.

Social interaction and influence

Interacting with others helps determine our actions and beliefs, while the influence of others attempts to change these for positive or negative reasons. Such influence can be direct or indirect and unintentional. Social norms (implicit rules) also influence behaviour, e.g. standing face forward in a lift.

Wagstaff, G.F., 1995. Hypnosis. In: Colman, A.M. (Ed.), Controversies in psychology. Longman, London.

Watson, J.B., Rayner, R., 1920. Conditioned emotional reactions. J. Exp. Psychol. 3, 1–14.

Wechsler, D., 1991. Wechsler Intelligence Scale for Children, third UK ed. Psychological Corporation, London.

Wechsler, D., 1999a. Wechsler Adult Intelligence Scale. Psychological Corporation, London.

Wechsler, D., 1999b. Wechsler Abbreviated Scale of Intelligence. Psychological Corporation, London.

Wechsler, D., 2003. Wechsler Pre-School and Primary Scales of Intelligence, third UK ed. Psychological Corporation, London.

Weitzenhoffer, A.M., Hilgard, E.R., 1959. Stanford Hypnotic Susceptibility Scale, Forms A and B. Consulting Psychologists' Press, Palo Alto.

Yerkes, R.M., Dodson, J.D., 1908. The relation of strength of stimulus to rapidity of habit formation. J. Comp. Neurol. Psychol. 18, 459–482.

Descriptive psychopathology

Sadgun Bhandari

Introduction

Descriptive psychopathology is the method of precisely describing and categorizing abnormal experiences as recounted by psychiatric patients and observed in their behaviour. It eschews explanations and is atheoretical. The uses of descriptive psychopathology are adapted from Sims (1991):

- **Diagnostic:** facilitates communication of the clinical features to other professionals
- **Scientific:** allows precise observations and deductions to be made
- **Therapeutic:** facilitates the establishment of an empathic relationship
- **Forensic:** medico-legal evaluation of the patient is largely based upon psychopathology.

According to Jaspers (1959), phenomenology is the description of the actual experiences of the patient without reference to the sources of these experiences, the emergence of one psychic phenomenon rather than another, or to theories of underlying cause. Psychic phenomena should be elicited empathically in an attempt to render the patient's experience understandable.

Schneider (1959) commented that clinical diagnosis often precedes enquiry and that symptoms tend to be subsequently evaluated in the light of the diagnosis. Ideally, unbiased observation and description of symptoms should precede diagnosis.

The principal symptoms encountered in clinical psychiatry occur in the realm of perception, thinking, affect, motor activity, consciousness, sense of self and memory. Disorders of consciousness and memory will be discussed later in this volume.

Disorders of perception

Disorders of perception are classically divided into sensory distortions, in which real objects are perceived as altered in some way, and false perceptions, in which non-existent objects are perceived (Table 6.1).

Sensory distortions

In sensory distortion, a real perceptual object is perceived as distorted. The intensity of a perception can become heightened or diminished and qualitative changes can occur. This commonly affects the visual modality when toxicity from certain drugs alters colour vision (e.g. santonin causing violet or yellow vision). Quantitative changes include micropsia, macropsia or dysmegalopsia, in which objects are seen as smaller or larger than they really are, or as altered in shape, respectively. Such phenomena may be due to end organ disease or to acute organic disorders and epilepsy.

False perceptions

Illusions are thought to occur when stimuli from a perceived object are combined with mental images to produce a false perception. Illusions are associated with inattention when external sensory stimuli are meagre or when attention is impaired due to delirium. Illusions are also associated with prevailing affect, thus shadows may appear like human figures to a frightened individual. Illusions almost always disappear when sensory stimuli increase or when attention improves.

Pareidolia is a type of illusion that occurs when imagination is used to create images and is the misperception of vague or obscure stimuli being perceived as something clear and distinct. It is a normal phenomenon (especially in children) that does not disappear when attention is focused, and the images are recognized as unreal by the individual.

Hallucinations are the most clinically significant false perceptions. Hallucinations are not distortions of real perceptions but arise *de novo* and occur alongside real perceptions (Jaspers 1959). Hallucinations are not experienced in inner subjective space, but occur in the individual's external

environment. They have the substantiality of a normal perception and are not under voluntary control (Box 6.1).

Hallucinations may occur due to disorders of peripheral sense organs, sensory deprivation and while falling asleep or awakening (these are referred to as hypnagogic hallucinations or hypnopompic hallucinations, respectively). Hallucinations should be differentiated from illusions, pseudohallucinations, hypnagogic and hypnopompic images and from vivid imagery.

Pathologically significant hallucinations occur most commonly in patients with organic psychoses, schizophrenia or affective disorders (Table 6.2).

Auditory hallucinations

Auditory hallucinations may range from elementary noises to fully formed voices. Voices may be single or multiple and may talk to or about the person. When eliciting auditory hallucinations, the interviewer should ensure that the patient is not stating that he hears actual voices. Furthermore, auditory hallucinations need to be clearly distinguished from the patient's own thoughts.

Diagnostic significance
Auditory hallucinations are one of the most important symptoms for the diagnosis of psychosis, especially schizophrenia. Schneider (1959) included three particular types of auditory hallucinations as symptoms of the first rank for the diagnosis of schizophrenia. These particular hallucinations are part of the diagnostic criteria for schizophrenia in both the ICD-10 and DSM-IV. The three types are thought echo (which is also known as Gedankenlautwerden and écho de la pensée), running commentary hallucinations, and third person hallucinations of two or more voices arguing about or discussing the patient. Other types of auditory hallucinations can also occur in

Table 6.1 Disorders of perception

Sensory distortions	False perceptions
Altered intensity of perception	Illusions and pareidolia
Qualitative alteration of perception	Hallucinations
Quantitative alteration of perception	

Table 6.2 Classification of hallucinations

Modality specific	Special types
Auditory	Functional
Visual	Reflex
Bodily senses	Extracampine
Gustatory	Autoscopic
Olfactory	

schizophrenia, including voices commanding the patient and voices talking directly to him. Paraphrenia may also present with prominent auditory hallucinations.

Auditory hallucinations occur in affective disorder, in which case the content often reflects the underlying mood; these hallucinations are referred to as mood congruent hallucinations.

Alcoholic hallucinosis is characterized predominantly by auditory hallucinations with a derogatory or persecutory content. Delirium due to any cause is also associated with auditory hallucinations, as is cerebral dysfunction, even when consciousness is not impaired.

Visual hallucinations

Visual hallucinations can range from elementary flashes of light through fully formed visions of animals, objects and persons, to complex scenes. It is sometimes difficult to distinguish between internal images, illusions and clear visual hallucinations.

Diagnostic significance

Visual hallucinations characteristically occur in delirium of any cause, but dementia due to Alzheimer disease, Pick disease and Lewy bodies is also associated with visual hallucinations. Intoxication with hallucinogenic drugs, such as lysergic-acid-diethylamide (LSD) is a relatively common cause of visual hallucinations. Visual hallucinations are very uncommon in patients with schizophrenia and affective disorders (Sims 1995) and if present, suggest an organic disorder (Box 6.2).

Bodily senses

These hallucinations include those affecting the skin, muscle and joint sense and inner organs (Sims 1995), and can include sensations of heat or cold, electric shocks, sexual experiences and visceral sensations. The term tactile hallucination is used commonly to describe hallucinations affecting the skin (another term commonly used, haptic hallucination, refers to hallucinations of touch). Tactile hallucinations are unique, in that they are invariably delusionally elaborated; the commonest delusions are those of being controlled. This is somatic passivity, which is a first rank symptom. Possibly deriving from this, the term

Box 6.2

Charles Bonnet syndrome

The Charles Bonnet syndrome is a condition of the elderly, in which individuals, mostly female, experience extremely vivid visual hallucinations. These occur persistently and repetitively without any delusions or hallucinations in any other modality, and without disturbance of consciousness. Insight is preserved. Age-related macular degeneration (ARMD) with secondary decline in central vision is the most common ocular disease in which CBS occurs (Vukicevic & Fitzmaurice 2008). It is believed that the hallucinations represent release phenomena due to de-afferentation of the visual association areas of the cerebral cortex (Manford & Andermann 1998).

A similar phenomenon has been described in impaired hearing and presents as musical hallucinations (Ali 2002).

somatic hallucination is also used to describe hallucinations of bodily senses.

Diagnostic significance

Hallucinations of bodily senses along with the delusional elaboration occur in schizophrenia. In certain acute organic psychoses and cocaine intoxication, tactile hallucinations occur in the form of formication, which is the sensation of animals crawling all over the body. This differs from Ekbom syndrome.

Gustatory hallucinations

Gustatory hallucinations refer to false perceptions of taste and are often difficult to diagnose. They may sometimes present with changes in taste, which may be persistent.

Diagnostic significance

Gustatory hallucinations may occur in schizophrenia where they may be delusionally elaborated, for example a change in taste may be elaborated as a delusion of being poisoned. They may also present as a feature of a temporal lobe epileptic attack (see Ch. 27).

Olfactory hallucinations

Olfactory hallucinations are not common and may range from the experience of something smelling to the patients complaining that they themselves smell unpleasantly. This needs to be distinguished from the rare olfactory reference syndrome where a person is preoccupied with emitting foul odour (Stein et al 1998).

Diagnostic significance

Olfactory hallucinations are a feature of temporal lobe epilepsy. They have also been described in schizophrenia and depression, and in the latter they may reflect the underlying mood.

Functional hallucinations

In functional hallucination, the hallucination is provoked by a stimulus and occurs in the same sensory modality as the stimulus. Both the stimulus and the hallucination are perceived simultaneously and are also perceived as being distinct. Thus, a patient may hear a voice only when a tap is turned on and then hears both the sound of running water and the sound of the voice.

Reflex hallucinations

In reflex hallucinations, a stimulus in one sensory modality provokes a hallucination in another modality. This is thought to be a morbid form of synaesthesia. Synaesthesia is a normal phenomenon, in which stimulation of one sense triggers anomalous perceptual experiences. Experiencing letters and numbers with colours or textures is an especially prevalent form that affects at least 1% of the population. This is known as 'grapheme-colour' synaesthesia (Eagleman 2010).

Hypochondriacal delusions

These are also referred to as delusions of ill-health. They range from the belief that something vague and generalized is wrong, to beliefs in the presence of specific diseases. Delusions of infestation are also included under the category of hypochondriacal delusions.

Diagnostic significance
Hypochondriacal delusions can present as single systematized delusions in delusional disorders or as symptoms of depression and schizophrenia.

Delusions of love, delusions of infidelity, nihilistic delusions, the delusion of doubles, delusions of infestation and shared delusions are discussed in Chapter 23.

Overvalued ideas

Overvalued ideas are isolated, preoccupying beliefs, accompanied by a strong affective response which manifests as anxiety and anger when there is a threat to the loss of their goal or object of the belief. In addition an overvalued idea is an isolated sustained belief which:

* Is held strongly, with less than delusional intensity
* Is ego-syntonic compared to most obsessions
* Often develops in an abnormal personality
* Is usually comprehensible with knowledge of the individual's past experience and personality
* The content is usually regarded as abnormal compared to the general population (but not bizarre as some delusions)
* Causes disturbed functioning or distress to the patient and others.

Compared to many delusions, overvalued ideas are more likely to lead to repeated action which is considered justified (McKenna 1984; Veale 2002).

The DSM-IV-TR defines overvalued ideas solely on the strength of the belief in that it is held with less than delusional intensity and also considers that the belief is abnormal compared to other members of the patient's culture.

Diagnostic significance
Disorders which are characterized by overvalued ideas include the querulous paranoid state, morbid jealousy, hypochondriasis, dysmorphophobia, parasitophobia, anorexia nervosa, pseudocyesis and apotemnophilia (McKenna 1984; Veale 2002). Apotemnophilia is a rare disorder in which a person feels that one or more limbs do not seem to belong to them. Overvalued ideas may also be features of an emerging psychosis or an organic disorder.

Dysmorphophobia

The term 'body dysmorphic disorder' is used in the DSM-IV-TR and this describes the development of an excessive concern with the imagined unsightly appearance of a single, often facial, feature (Hay 1970). The DSM-IV-TR also describes a delusional subtype. The commonest features affected are nose, hair and complexion. The disfigurement is believed to be noticeable to other people but the actual appearance lies within the normal

limits. Patients more often consult plastic surgeons than psychiatrists. Usually, dysmorphophobia is the only complaint, although personality disorders may coexist, or the complaint may be an early symptom of schizophrenia or, less often, depression (McKenna 1984).

Disorders of control of thinking

Normally, a person is in control or possession of his thinking but some symptoms are characterized by a dysfunction of this control. The two main phenomena discussed here are obsessions and thought alienation (passivity of thought).

Obsessions

Obsessions are recurrent ideas, thoughts, impulses or images that are experienced as being intrusive and senseless but are recognized as the person's own thoughts. The experience is distressing and attempts to resist its content or form are not successful.

Compulsions include actions or cognitions such as praying or counting and are also referred to as rituals.

Thought alienation

Thought alienation is characterized by the experience of one's thoughts being alien, not emanating from one's own mind, and not being under voluntary control. Three forms of this passivity phenomenon in relation to thinking were described by Schneider (1959) and included as symptoms of first rank for the diagnosis of schizophrenia. These are thought broadcasting (diffusion of thought), thought insertion and thought withdrawal (interruption of thought). Thought withdrawal may be responsible for thought blocking. In both thought blocking and thought withdrawal the patient describes his thoughts as being controlled or influenced by an external agency, therefore these experiences are delusions of control, and are also ego-alien.

Other passivity experiences described by Schneider (1959) are those in which feelings, impulses and will are believed to be the product of others or to be under the direct control of others and are referred to as 'made' phenomena. The term made action has been used interchangeably with made impulse. These experiences represent disturbances of the sense of identity and are delusions of control. Schneider (1959) considered these to be symptoms of first rank for schizophrenia. Somatic passivity is also a first rank symptom. It consists of somatic hallucinations associated with the belief that outside influences are responsible. Thus again, a hallucination is accompanied by a delusion of control and is considered to be a passivity experience. Clinically, it is essential to ensure that the patient is not using a figure of speech, for example 'as though' arms feel electrified. First rank symptoms are important diagnostic criteria for schizophrenia in both ICD-10 and DSM-IV and are summarized in Box 6.4.

First rank symptoms were described by Schneider (1959) who suggested that in the absence of any organic symptoms, the presence of a first rank symptom suggests a diagnosis of schizophrenia. Further studies have suggested that they are not exclusive to schizophrenia, but there is evidence that when

Box 6.4

First rank symptoms
- Thought echo (Gedenkenlautwerden and écho de la pensée)
- Running commentary hallucinations
- Voices discussing the patient in the third person (voices arguing)
- Delusional perception
- Thought broadcast
- Thought insertion
- Thought withdrawal
- Made feeling (emotion)
- Made impulse
- Made volition (action)
- Somatic passivity

narrower definitions are used they are exclusive to schizophrenia. They lack predictive value with regard to the prognosis and are not inherited. One of their major advantages is their reliability, which has been demonstrated by studies such as the International Pilot Study of Schizophrenia (IPSS) (Sartorius 1974), which used the Present State Examination which relies on the first rank symptoms.

Disorders of the flow of thought

These include flight of ideas, retardation, thought blocking, perseveration and circumstantiality.

Flight of ideas

Flight of ideas occurs when thoughts follow each other rapidly, the connections between successive thoughts are understandable and clang associations, alliterations and other similar phenomena occur. Flight of ideas often occurs in the context of pressure of speech.

Diagnostic significance
Flight of ideas is typical of mania. It can also occasionally occur in schizophrenia and in some organic disorders, especially those resulting from lesions of the hypothalamus (Fish 1967).

Retardation

In retardation, thinking is slowed down and the number of ideas entering consciousness is decreased. This is experienced as difficulty making decisions, loss of concentration and lack of clarity of thinking.

Diagnostic significance
Retardation of thinking is typical of depression.

Thought blocking

This refers to the complete interruption of speech before a thought or an idea has been completely expressed. Occasional loss of the train of thought may be due to poor concentration or distractibility. Thought blocking should only be accepted as present when the patient voluntarily describes it or when on questioning it is clear that a pause in speech is due to the experience of thoughts breaking off or ceasing.

Diagnostic significance
Thought blocking occurs in schizophrenia. It may occur in the context of thought withdrawal.

Perseveration

Perseveration refers to the adherence of an individual to the same concepts and words beyond the point at which they are relevant.

Diagnostic significance
It is characteristically an organic symptom and occurs when consciousness is impaired as in acute organic disorders as well as chronic organic disorders such as dementia.

Circumstantiality

In circumstantiality speech is very indirect and delayed in reaching its goal due to the inclusion of tedious details.

Diagnostic significance
It is a feature of obsessional personality disorder and probably of temporal lobe epilepsy. Milder forms may be encountered in the absence of any psychiatric or organic disorder.

Formal thought disorder

The term 'formal thought disorder' refers to abnormalities of thought expressed in language, most commonly in speech but also in writing. A review found 68 terms used to describe disordered thinking and concluded that there was significant redundancy in these terms (i.e. more terms than significantly different concepts described) and also different sources gave different definitions for the same terms (Rule 2005). Some of the terms used historically to describe formal thought disorder are presented in Table 6.5, along with their originators (see also Box 6.5).

The concept of thought disorder is problematic. Thought disorder is inferred on the basis of disordered speech, that is, an assumption is made that speech directly mirrors thought, but language is self-contained and has a structure independent of thought. Andreasen (1979) has suggested that formal thought disorder is not a homogenous entity but is a multilevel

Table 6.5 Historical terms used to describe formal thought disorder, and their originators

Kraeplin (1919)	Acataphasia
Bleuler (1911)	Loosening of associations, condensation, displacement, misuse of symbols
Cameron (1939)	Asyndesis, metonyms, overinclusion
Carl Schneider (1930)	Derailment, substitution, omission, fusion, drivelling
Other terms	'Knight's move thinking', paraphasia, neologisms, tangentiality, circumstantiality

Box 6.5

Commonly used terms describing formal thought disorder

- **Derailment (loose associations, flight of ideas):** a pattern of spontaneous speech in which ideas slip from one track to another that is clearly but obliquely related or to one that is completely unrelated
- **Incoherence (word salad, jargon aphasia, paragrammatism):** a pattern of speech which is essentially incomprehensible at times due to several different mechanisms. The difference between derailment and incoherence is based on the abnormality in derailment occurring within the level of sentences and clauses
- **Neologism:** a completely new word or phrase whose derivation cannot be understood
- **Tangentiality:** involves replying to a question in an oblique, tangential or irrelevant manner
- **Poverty of speech:** a restriction in the amount of spontaneous speech so that replies to questions tend to be brief, concrete and unelaborated
- **Poverty of content of speech:** occurs when speech is adequate in amount but tends to convey little information. Language tends to be vague, over-abstract, repetitive and stereotyped.

Adapted from Andreasen 1994. *Note:* some terms are included in parenthesis to highlight the overlap in the definitions.

disturbance involving abnormalities of thinking, language and social cognition. She has therefore proposed the use of the term 'communication disorders'.

Explanations for thought disorder

- Derive from association psychology (Bleuler 1911)
- Overinclusive thinking (Cameron 1939), which may be studied using object sorting tests
- Concrete thinking (Goldstein 1944) which may be studied with proverb tests
- Personal construct theory (Bannister 1963).

Recent research into positive thought disorder has found consistent evidence for association with impaired executive functioning and impaired processing of semantic information (Kerns & Berenbaum 2002).

Diagnostic significance
Historically formal thought disorder has been always associated with the diagnosis of schizophrenia and this is reflected in the ICD-10 and the DSM-IV. However, thought disorder is not exclusive to schizophrenia (Andreasen 1979) and frequently occurs in mania. It is not a common feature of depression. Thought disorder tends to persist in schizophrenia and patients tend to exhibit negative thought disorders such as poverty of speech in addition to positive thought disorders such as derailment (Andreasen 1994).

Disorders of motor activity

Abnormal motor behaviour is a feature of many psychiatric illnesses, either as a disorder of movement intrinsic to the illness or more commonly, as side-effects of commonly prescribed drugs. In addition, several neurological disorders, with prominent motor symptoms (Huntington's chorea, Parkinson disease) also present with psychiatric symptoms.

Psychiatric motor disorders include increased or decreased motor activity and catatonic symptoms.

Increased motor activity

This manifests as hyperactivity and agitation. In hyperactivity the increased motor activity is goal-directed and is associated with pressured speech and distractibility usually in the context of mania.

In agitation, the increased activity is non-goal-directed and the subject is distressed. Agitation occurs in depression, schizophrenia, organic disorders and anxiety states. In cases where antipsychotic medication has been commenced, agitation should be distinguished from akathisia.

The term excitement is also used to describe increased motor activity. Excitement occurs in a variety of disorders but catatonic excitement occurs predominantly in schizophrenia and consists of senseless and purposeless overactivity (Fish 1967).

Decreased motor activity

This manifests as retardation or stupor and is usually a symptom of depression with melancholic symptoms (endogenous depression) and organic disorders. The term psychomotor retardation implies a slowing down of both psychic and motor activity. Stupor is a state of extreme motor retardation characterized by akinesis and mutism in a setting of preserved consciousness. Tumours of the third ventricle also cause stupor or akinetic mutism.

Stupor can occur in schizophrenia, affective disorders (usually depression but occasionally manic) and hysteria. Stupor, also referred to as 'catatonic stupor', always merits careful investigation.

Catatonia is a motor dysregulation syndrome with patients unable to move normally, despite full physical capacity. Movements cannot be initiated or stopped and become repetitive; posture is frozen or oddly positioned and actions become contrary to intent. The principal features of catatonia are listed in Table 6.6.

Diagnostic significance
Catatonia has always been associated with the diagnosis of schizophrenia. However, catatonic presentations may occur with focal neurological lesions, intoxications, metabolic disturbances and in affective disorders particularly bipolar disorder (Fien & McGrath 1990; Fink & Taylor 2009). Catatonia is a major clinical feature of anti-NMDA-receptor encephalitis (Dalmau et al 2008).

Disorders of emotion

Describing mood and feelings and eliciting their associated symptoms is one of the most important skills of clinical examination because mood disorders are extremely common.

The terms used to describe this aspect of psychopathology are often employed interchangeably and overlap with everyday

Table 6.6 Principal features of catatonia

Spontaneous movement disorders

Posturing or catalepsy	The maintenance of strange and uncomfortable postures for long periods of time includes *psychological pillow* and *Schnauz-krampf* (an exaggerated pucker)
Stereotypies	Unusual repetitive, non-goal directed movements
Mannerisms	Unusual, repetitive, goal directed movements (both stereotypies and mannerisms can affect speech too)

Induced movement disorders

Waxy flexibility (flexibilitas cerea)	After an initial resistance the patient may be placed in strange uncomfortable positions, and will maintain them for a minute or more
Automatic obedience	The patient carries out every command in a literal concrete fashion despite instructions to the contrary. Automatic obedience includes *mitmachen and mitgehen*. In mitmachen (cooperation), only a light pressure is needed to move the patient's body into new positions. Mitgehen (extreme cooperation): is an extreme form of mitmachen
Echolalia/echopraxia	The patient repeats the actions or speech of the examiner
Negativism	The patient actively resists all attempts to make contact during the examination. Negativism includes gegenhalten where the patient opposes all passive movements with the same degree of force as that applied by examiner
Ambitendency	The patient alternates between resistance to and cooperation with the examiner's instructions

words (e.g. 'feeling', which has multiple meanings). Definitions of these terms vary, and sometimes they are differentiated on the basis of duration and intensity.

Definitions:

- *Feeling* describes a positive or negative subjective reaction to an experience.
- *Affect* is used to describe the overall emotional state, inferred objectively.
- *Mood* is a prolonged emotional state.

In practice, the terms are often used interchangeably.

Abnormal moods (Table 6.7)

Depression

Depression of mood is common and subjective experience may include feeling sad, despondent, dejected, despairing, hopeless, apathetic or indifferent. Anxiety is a common concomitant symptom. Depressed mood may be accompanied by slowing of thoughts and actions (psychomotor retardation), occasionally stupor, and by agitation and restlessness. Concentration and decision making are impaired. Feelings of guilt hopelessness, helplessness and unworthiness occur, and suicidal thoughts are common. Depression is also associated with anhedonia, the loss of ability to experience pleasure.

Table 6.7 Abnormal moods

Depression	Apathy
Elation	Affective blunting/flattening
Emotional lability	Anxiety
Euphoria	Irritability
Ecstasy	

Elation

Elation of mood, the subjective experience of feeling happy and cheerful, is often accompanied by overactivity, rapid thoughts, distractibility, pressure of speech and flight of ideas. It is a classic feature of mania. Elation may turn to irritability if attempts are made to curtail the patient's overactivity. Elation may occur in schizophrenia and organic disorders and is distinguished from mania on the basis of the lack of communicability of the mood and the absence of associated features such as flight of ideas or grandiosity.

Emotional lability

This is characterized by rapid changes of mood from one extreme to the other. Lability of affect occurs in personality disorders, in the manic phase of bipolar affective disorder and in mixed affective states.

Affective incontinence is characterized by a complete loss of control over emotions, the patient crying or laughing for long periods of time with no provocation. It occurs in multi-infarct dementia, pseudobulbar palsy and multiple sclerosis.

Euphoria

This is a state of excessive, unreasonable cheerfulness. It can be a normal phenomenon but more often occurs in mania and organic conditions such as multiple sclerosis and general paresis of the insane. In frontal lobe syndrome, a silly euphoria with lack of foresight and general indifference may occur. This is called moria or Witzelsucht.

Ecstasy

This is a state of extreme wellbeing associated with a feeling of bliss and grace. It can occur in healthy individuals and during religious experiences, but more often occurs in schizophrenia and organic states, especially temporal lobe epilepsy.

Social psychiatry and sociology

7

Claire Henderson   Stephen Ginn

CHAPTER CONTENTS

Introduction

Social psychiatry is the study of: (1) social factors associated with the onset, course and outcome of psychiatric disorders; (2) social influences on the nature and availability of treatment; (3) the social implications of mental illness for patients, their carers and their families. All of these areas are discussed in this chapter, along with the sociological theories and concepts that underpin social psychiatry.

Social factors associated with the onset, course and outcome of psychiatric disorders

Epidemiology is the main tool used for examining the influence of social and demographic factors on psychiatric disorder. Data from large populations can provide evidence for possible aetiological theories and guide rational service planning. This section summarizes the research findings on rates of psychiatric morbidity within the general population and highlights the populations most at risk. Some of the aetiological theories explaining these findings are considered and specific psychosocial factors, such as life events and expressed emotion are discussed. Epidemiological methodology is described in Chapter 9.

Social and demographic factors associated with mental disorder

Social class

Definition and measurement

Social class has traditionally been defined in the UK on the basis of occupation using the Registrar General's classification introduced in 1911 (Box 7.1). People who do not work full time are

Box 7.1

Registrar General's classification of social class

I   Professional, landowners and higher managerial
II Intermediate
III Skilled workers
IV Semi-skilled workers
V   Unskilled workers
O   Students, retired

hard to classify using this system, and some job titles, for example 'engineer', may be applied to a wide range of occupations, with very different levels of qualifications and pay. The broader concept of socioeconomic status (SES) is increasingly used, which combines measures of education and income, and sometimes of occupation and area of residence.

Sociologists are moving away from hierarchical models of social class to models involving a core and peripheries. The core is composed of full-time employees; moving away from the centre are part-time, temporary and self-employed workers, and beyond them are the short- and long-term unemployed. Outside this is the 'underclass', including homeless people and refugees. Related to this concept is that of 'social exclusion'. Unlike 'poverty', the term does not simply concern economic hardship but is multidimensional, referring, for example, to disadvantages in employment, political engagement, social participation and the ability to access services.

Despite the problems inherent in defining and measuring social class, there are clear and consistent social class gradients in morbidity and mortality for all ages and for nearly all diseases. Thus, individuals classified as social class V are twice as likely to die before retirement and have twice the neonatal mortality compared with those in social class I.

Social class and mental illness

In Britain, a survey by the Office of National Statistics (Singleton et al 2000) demonstrated that rates of non-psychotic disorders are highest among people in social classes IV and V, and that functional psychotic disorders and drug and alcohol dependence are commonest in social class V (Box 7.2). When the individual components of social class were examined, having no educational qualifications increased the risk of a depressive episode, while being economically inactive or unemployed increased the risk of most disorders (see below). Similarly, in the USA, the Epidemiological Catchment Area (ECA) study demonstrated that the

Box 7.2

Summary of sociodemographic factors associated with psychiatric morbidity rates

Strong research evidence	Reasonable research evidence
Economic inactivity	Inner city residence
Social class	High residential mobility
Sex	
Ethnic group	
Marital status	

association between SES and mental disorder is strongest for schizophrenia, intermediate for alcohol abuse and dependence, and weakest for depression (Holzer et al 1986). Studies on the true prevalence and treated incidence of schizophrenia, suggest that low class confers a relative risk of 2–3. Other studies, which have included less developed countries, have not replicated these findings consistently (WHO 1979).

Two hypotheses have been proposed to explain the differing rates of schizophrenia in industrialized countries. The social causation theory suggests that exposure to social stressors induces the onset or relapse of schizophrenia. The selection/drift model, in contrast, proposes that schizophrenia itself causes a reduction in social status compared to the parental generation, and a progressive deterioration in the patient's socioeconomic status. These processes are not mutually exclusive, and the relative importance of each may vary over time and place. Social selection is most visible before any process of social drift has started. However, the onset of social drift relative both to the parental status and to expectations based on early academic performance may begin very early, often before admission to hospital (Goldberg & Morrison 1963). After many years during which the drift theory held sway, it is now being challenged by the suggestion that social deprivation and city life (e.g. Mortensen et al 1999) are mainly responsible for the social class gradient (see Ch. 19).

Age

Psychiatric disorders common to children and adolescents show the same patterns for risk by social class and geographical location as those in adults (Rutter 1989). The group at highest overall risk of mental illness includes children and adolescents in care.

In elderly people, depression is not more common, but is more severe and more likely to require hospital admission. Admission is related not only to severity but to the higher rates of living alone (50% over the age of 75 years), coexistence of physical disorder and risk of suicide. Among the elderly, those at greatest risk of depression are those in residential homes and medical wards, where the rate of depression, at 20–30%, is two or three times higher than that of the background population.

Sex

In the UK, the survey by the Office of National Statistics (Singleton et al 2000) showed a 1-week prevalence for neurotic disorders of 19.4% in women, compared with 13.5% in men. Men had higher rates of alcohol and drug dependence. While there were no sex differences in the overall rates of psychoses, service use appears to be higher in men with schizophrenia; the onset of illness is earlier; and the course, outcome and treatment response are less favourable when compared to women.

Marital status

For both sexes, the prevalence of non-psychotic disorders is lowest for married individuals and highest for those who are divorced or separated (Singleton et al 2000). A similar pattern exists for schizophrenia, although people with psychoses are more likely to be unmarried.

Ethnic group

In countries with large immigrant populations, some ethnic groups have similar rates of mental illness as exist in the general population (e.g. people from South Asia in Britain), whereas other groups have higher rates. In Britain, for example, particular attention has been paid to African Caribbeans, who are 3–5 times as likely to be admitted to hospital with schizophrenia, compared with the native population (London 1986). A study in Nottingham found that rates of hospitalization for schizophrenia may be even higher among second-generation African Caribbeans (Harrison 1988). More recent research has highlighted the contribution of social disadvantage and isolation to these findings (Morgan et al 2008).

Employment status

Unemployment can impair physical and mental health and increase the risk of suicide and deliberate self-harm. Unsatisfactory and insecure employment may have a similar impact. The extent to which this is due to the resulting impoverishment versus the non-financial benefits of working may vary with individual circumstances.

Geographic variation

Area level factors

In recent years, there has been a resurgence of research into the effects of residential environments on the risk of mental disorder and suicide for all or certain groups of residents, regardless of their individual characteristics. The hypothesis is that contextual features of residential environments, usually referred to as area level factors, may be related to health outcomes even after individual factors are taken into account. This adjustment for individual level factors represents a refinement of the ecological study where only area level factors are studied (see Ch. 9), as well as an improvement on surveys of individuals, which ignore their context. The influence of context may be exerted, for example, through chronic stressors related to neighbourhood characteristics or aspects of neighbourhoods that affect social support and access to goods and services; at a wider level public policies may exert an effect. The geographic areas investigated have ranged from large regions of countries with populations of several million to neighbourhoods of a few thousand people.

One example of an area level effect is that of group density. This has been studied most extensively for ethnic density; it is suggested that, for people from a specific ethnic group, rates of mental disorder decrease if the proportion of people from the same ethnic group increases in the local population (Halpern 1993). A similar protective effect has also been described for density of occupation and religious affiliation. The effect is thought to be mediated through increased levels of social support and reduced levels of stress (Whitley et al 2006), and has been shown for: common mental disorder (anxiety and depression) (Halpern & Nazroo 1999); rates of psychiatric hospitalization (e.g. Faris & Dunham 1939); treated rates of psychoses (Boydell et al 2001); suicide (Neeleman & Wessely 1999); and non-fatal self-harm (Neeleman et al 2001).

For ethnic minorities, the protective relationship of ethnic density on mental health found by these authors remained after adjustment for language fluency, and was strengthened by adjusting for economic hardship.

Intra-urban patterns

For 70 years, ecological studies have shown higher rates of admission for schizophrenia in inner city populations, when compared with populations from suburban areas (e.g. Faris & Dunham 1939). These patterns are stable over time and to some degree independent of the ethnicity, housing status or age composition of the local population.

Urban–rural differences

Dohrenwend (1975) reported that overall prevalence rates of psychosis showed little rural–urban difference, but that the prevalence of schizophrenia appeared higher and manic-depressive psychosis lower, in cities. More recent work has demonstrated that being born in a city is associated with a higher risk of developing schizophrenia, indicating that social drift cannot explain this variation entirely (Marcelis et al 1999). For non-psychotic disorders, the ONS survey (Singleton et al 2000) discovered higher rates of neurotic disorders in urban compared to semi-rural and rural populations.

Residential mobility

Higher rates of schizophrenia in areas of high residential mobility were suggested by the work of Faris and Dunham in Chicago (1939) and reinforced by further research in Los Angeles (Dear & Wolch 1987).

Homelessness

Homeless individuals are a heterogeneous group, found in a variety of accommodation settings:

- 'Roofless' (e.g. sleeping in parks)
- Hostels for the homeless
- Emergency accommodation
- Precariously housed (e.g. squatting, staying with friends)
- Institutional (e.g. prisons, hospitals).

People who are street homeless (roofless) are the visible minority of the overall homeless population. It is difficult to count the homeless, and routine indicators of psychopathology such as social withdrawal, suspiciousness and poor personal hygiene may erroneously suggest the presence of mental illness in a population in whom these features may be the norm. Estimating the rate of mental disorder among homeless people is therefore difficult. But while estimates vary, they are universally high when this population is compared to the general population, along with rates of suicides and childhood adversity (Shelton et al 2009).

Closure of large mental hospitals does not appear to have increased the number of homeless mentally ill people directly, because few patients discharged after long-stay hospitalization ('the old long stay') become homeless. However, 'new long stay' patients (defined as those in acute hospital beds for over 6 months) accumulate in hospitals because of the difficulty in finding them suitable accommodation. About 10% of patients

Nature of care

Mental health services have to cater for a diverse population. Diversity is a concept that refers to the presence of differences between people; it is most often applied to, but not limited to, historically marginalized groups such as women, homosexuals, and racial and ethnic minorities. The psychology of diversity examines why these differences are important, how the resulting social categories are used for viewing and evaluating other people and how this can lead to interpersonal and intergroup tensions. With respect to service provision, there are particular problems in relation to individuals from ethnic minority groups. Black patients in Britain are not only over-represented among hospitalized patients and less satisfied with mental health services than other patients (Parkman et al 1997), but are also more likely to be detained under the Mental Health Act (Bhui et al 2003), to be admitted to psychiatric intensive care facilities and to have been imprisoned. In one study, the proportion of African Caribbeans with poor outcome at 1 year was 2.5 times that of white individuals with schizophrenia (Bhugra et al 1997). Behind these findings lies the problem that black patients find statutory service provision unacceptable and thus are less likely to seek help. The development of voluntary sector services supported by the statutory sector may be an appropriate alternative, particularly since the numbers of black patients in a given area will usually not warrant the provision of an entire sectorized mental health team.

An important subgroup of patients requiring care in certain areas of most countries is refugees and asylum seekers. People who have been forced to migrate, especially those who have been subjected to organized violence or torture, have a particularly high prevalence of mental disorder, but local mental health services are often ill-equipped to identify and manage psychiatric problems in this context. Linguistic and cultural differences can further impede access to care and, additionally, individuals who are detained while their refugee status is investigated are often suspicious of government agencies and may therefore be unwilling to seek or accept help (see Ch. 8).

Social impact of mental illness

Stigma

Stigma is the attribution of prejudicial characteristics to a whole class of people. Those with chronic mental illness are viewed with distaste and fear (e.g. Thornicroft 2006), which has a profound impact upon them. Stigma operates both through discrimination by others and through 'self-stigmatization', resulting in loss of self-esteem and confidence to participate in activities that might facilitate recovery. Mechanic et al (1994) demonstrated that patients who do not attribute their problems to mental illness (and thus reject the label 'mentally ill') have a higher measured quality of life, lower sense of stigma and higher self-esteem, than those who perceive themselves as mentally ill. Furthermore, the consequences of stigmatization, such as loss of social support and unemployment, are themselves powerful risk factors for mental illness (see above).

Stigma also impacts on families who have to cope with 'stigma by association' (for a more detailed discussion see Ch. 12). Mental health professionals might be expected to have less negative attitudes than others, but while they endorse treatment and community care, they tend to be pessimistic about clinical outcomes and have concerns about dangerousness similar to the general public (Schulze 2007). Large scale programmes to reduce mental health related stigma and discrimination have been launched in several countries in recent years, including *Like Minds Like Mine* in New Zealand, *See Me* in Scotland, *Time To Change* in England and *Opening Minds* in Canada.

Impact of mental illness on social roles

The direct impact of mental illness and its associated stigma will often reduce the number of social roles (e.g. mother, housewife, employee, friend) undertaken by an individual. However, Greenberg et al (1994) have highlighted the positive roles played by many patients with a mental illness within their families, particularly in the provision of companionship and help around the house.

The 'sick role' was first described by Parsons (1951). When ill, an individual is relieved of occupational and domestic obligations and becomes entitled to care and sympathy. At the same time, such an individual is expected to demonstrate a desire to recover, for example by accepting the doctor's diagnosis and complying with treatment. The 'sick role' concept is less applicable in the context of rehabilitation for chronic illness during which the patient is encouraged to resume his or her normal duties to as great an extent as possible. It is also less applicable to illness that is regarded as self-induced (such as addictions), and illness that is stigmatized and thus does not attract care and sympathy. Furthermore, disagreements between patients and psychiatrists about the cause and meaning of their symptoms or behaviour are frequent, and may lead to patients being described as without insight or non-compliant with treatment. The resolution of such difficulties by reattribution therapy has become an important part of treatment for individuals with psychogenic physical symptoms.

Throughout medicine the shared decision-making model of chronic illness care is increasingly aspired to as a replacement for the paternalism implied in Parson's model. Shared decision-making requires information exchange so that a way forward based on the patient's values and preferences as well as medical expertise can be agreed on, although this might not be the most preferred choice of either party (Charles et al 1997).

For many patients, mental health professionals and fellow patients may be the only people who do not automatically reject them. This can lead to an understandable unwillingness on the part of patients to reduce contact with services when deemed appropriate by professionals. This may on occasion lead to a worsening of symptoms or to problematic behaviours. This may frustrate professionals, and may result in rejection or pejorative labelling. However, this sequence of events has also been described in a more constructive manner in terms of attachment theory by Adshead (1998), who has considered mental health professionals as attachment figures.

The rejection or acceptance of a psychiatric diagnosis and treatment may be described as facets of 'illness behaviour', a term introduced by Mechanic (1968) to describe people's responses to illness (or at least to what many regard as illness). This commences with the perception of a problem on the part of the sufferer (or those close to him or her), followed by decisions as to whether this problem represents illness or not, and if so, future decisions about advice and treatment (usually from family or friends initially). Different patterns of consulting with doctors, e.g. a higher frequency among women when compared with men, has been suggested to result from differences in illness behaviour rather than in actual morbidity. In addition to sociodemographic factors, prior experience of health services is also likely to play a role in deciding whether or not to seek help from the same source again.

Receipt of treatment is no longer the only relationship people with mental illness can have with mental health services. Service user groups are beginning to play a part in the selection of mental health professionals and the training of students and junior psychiatrists. Services users are increasingly involved in research that is either collaborative or user-led, and are employed in some Trusts as peer support workers. They also campaign for improvements in mental health services and against stigma and discrimination through service user and survivor groups and mental health charities.

Sociology of residential institutions

The specific social roles of people with mental illness within the context of the mental health care system have been described by sociologists and anthropologists such as Goffman (1961). Goffman wrote of the potentially dehumanizing effects on patients of 'total institutions', such as prisons or psychiatric hospitals where there are rigid hierarchies. Now that the majority of the psychiatric asylums of which Goffman wrote have closed the applicability of his work to modern acute wards is uncertain. Some more recent work suggests that the inpatient psychiatric experience remains difficult (Quirk & Lelliot 2001). Organizational pressures, such as a high turnover of staff and patients, can have a negative impact on the quality of care, with reduced nurse–patient contact, and patients are critical of ward conditions, viewing life there as boring and unsafe. A number of initiatives, such as the 'Star Wards' programme, have been started to improve both the physical environment and the treatment provided on inpatient units, and many units have succeeded in reducing levels of violence, coerced treatment and staff turnover while increasing satisfaction of services users and staff.

Social networks

Social networks are formed by the connections between people who frequently communicate with each other. Such communication involves the exchange of emotional, physical, economic and informational support and involves family members, colleagues, friends and neighbours. Beyond the emotional and practical support that social networks provide, they also give a sense of belonging to individuals, in turn promoting self-esteem, self-worth and self-confidence (Greenblatt et al 1982).

The quality and quantity of social networks experienced by people with severe long-term mental illness differ from those experienced by members of the general population. Healthy individuals can usually list around 22–25 people who are important to them, with five or six in each of the categories of family, other relatives, friends and neighbours, and social and work associates. By contrast, people with chronic psychiatric disorders can only list around half this number, of whom about two-thirds are relatives. Thus, such individuals have few links to other social groups. This finding has led to the emphasis on enlarging and strengthening a patient's social network as part of a treatment plan. This can be undertaken within institutions and with outpatient populations, and may utilize social skills training and other group activities. The increasing use of hostels in the community facilitates social contacts, and family work such as psycho-education may be useful in strengthening pre-existing connections. The social networks of carers also become diminished over time, often as a result of giving up work or other activities in order to look after an ill relative, but also because of 'stigma by association'. Communication between carers through relatives' support groups and other organizations may allow new contacts to be made and these may provide particularly salient emotional and informational support.

Carers

Unlike the families of patients with other chronic illnesses, the families of those suffering chronic mental illnesses have in the past been seen as having a causal role (Tsiegel et al 1991). This was particularly the case with respect to mothers of patients with schizophrenia. In 1948, Fromm-Reichmann published a theory that hostile and rejecting feelings expressed by mothers were responsible for schizophrenia in the child. Bateson et al (1956) described the 'schizophrenogenic mother' who, by behaving in a rejecting manner while verbalizing affection, placed the infant in a 'double-blind'. Lidz et al (1965) broadened the aetiology to marital partners, using the terms 'marital skew' and 'marital schism' to describe pathogenetic relationships thought to cause schizophrenia (see Ch. 19).

These ideas have are now widely discredited, as they were based on uncontrolled and subjective studies. However, there is sound evidence that some forms of family interaction may precipitate relapse in people with schizophrenia (see below). It is also true that there is greater than average psychopathology in the relations of people with schizophrenia, probably due both to the strain of caring and to genetic loading (Schulz et al 1990).

The concept of 'burden' (Tsiegel et al 1991) is used to encompass the broad effects on a family of caring for a sick relative. These include effects on income and employment, social and leisure activities, domestic routine, caring for children at home, health of household members and relationships with neighbours. Many standardized instruments exist to measure burden, but these have been criticized for not being based on an explicit theory of care-giving, for using predominantly white, middle-class respondents and for being beset by the difficulty of measuring burden objectively (Szmukler et al 1996). The study of care-giving, more established in the relatives of patients with dementia and the concept of 'stress-appraisal-coping' that has been widely used in this field, is now being applied to carers of people with major mental illness. The most common problems experienced by carers are:

- Difficult behaviours exhibited by patient
- Negative symptoms exhibited by patient
- Inaccessible services
- Bereavement
- Patient dependency
- Impact on other family members
- Stigma.

Expressed emotion

The observation that patients with schizophrenia discharged from hospital to live with parents or spouse appeared to relapse more often than those discharged to live with other relatives or non-relatives prompted an examination of various factors correlated with relapse. This led to the concept of *expressed emotion* (EE) (Brown et al 1972), a composite variable with high and low values, that may be determined by the semi-structured Camberwell Family Interview. This rates the number of critical comments, hostility and emotional over-involvement on the part of patient's relatives. These factors each predict the liability for relapse, and give the interview its validity. A number of studies have demonstrated the overall impact of EE, the importance of the amount of time that patients spend in contact with 'high EE' relatives, and the partial role of medication in mitigating these effects.

On the basis of studies on EE and relapse, a number of intervention packages have been designed to reduce the level of EE and, where relevant, the amount of face-to-face contact with relatives. Treatment involves family psycho-education addressing the symptoms, course and treatment of schizophrenia, and the development of alternative coping strategies for dealing with problem behaviours (which may be based on the strategies adapted by low EE families). Interventions have involved meetings with individual families and/or the formation of relatives' groups, as well as the formation of multiple family groups who meet with two therapists but also learn coping strategies from one another (Jewell et al 2009). A meta-analysis of family interventions (Mari & Streiner 1994) showed that changes in EE status between experimental and control groups combining 9-month and 1-year follow-ups were marginally significant, in favour of the experimental group. In addition, the experimental group showed a significant increase in compliance with pharmacotherapy and a reduction in hospitalization during the period studied. The authors calculate that between two and five patients must be treated to avert one episode of relapse during a 9-month treatment period.

Conclusions

This chapter has outlined the significant interplay between social factors and mental illness, and emphasized the importance of considering social factors in the management of patients. As our understanding of the biology of our patients grows, we must never forget their sociology – patients will always be influenced by others, and will always themselves influence others.

References

Adshead, G., 1998. Psychiatric staff as attachment figures: understanding management problems in psychiatric services in the light of attachment theory. Br. J. Psychiatry 172, 64–69.

Bateson, G., Jackson, D.D., Haley, J., et al., 1956. Toward a theory of schizophrenia. Behav. Sci. 1, 251–264.

Bhugra, D., Leff, J., Mallett, G., 1997. Incidence and outcome of schizophrenia in whites, African Caribbeans and Asians in London. Psychol. Med. 27, 791–798.

Bhui, K., Stansfeld, S., Hull, S., et al., 2003. Ethnic variations in pathways to and use of specialist mental health services in the UK Systematic review. Br. J. Psychiatry 182, 105–116.

Boydell, J., van Os, J., McKenzie, K., et al., 2001. Incidence of schizophrenia in ethnic minorities in London: ecological study into interactions with environment. Br. Med. J. 323, 1336–1338.

Brown, G.W., Birley, J.L., Wing, J.K., 1972. Influence of family life on the course of schizophrenic disorder, a replication. Br. J. Psychiatry 121, 241–258.

Brown, G.W., Harris, T., 1978. Social origins of depression. Free Press, New York.

Brown, G.W., Prudo, R., 1981. Psychiatric disorder in a rural and an urban population:

I. Aetiology of depression. Psychol. Med. 11, 581–599.

Charles, C., Gafni, A., Whelan, T., 1997. Shared decision-making in the medical encounter: what does it mean? (or it takes at least two to tango). Soc. Sci. Med. 44, 681–692.

Commander, M.J., Sashi Dharan, S.P., Odell, S.M., et al., 1997. Access to mental health care in an inner city health district. II: Association with demographic factors. Br. J. Psychiatry 170, 317–320.

Dear, M., Wolch, J., 1987. Landscapes of despair. Polity, Oxford.

Dohrenwend, B., 1975. Socio-cultural and social-psychological factors in the genesis of mental disorders. J. Health Soc. Behav. 16, 365–392.

Dunham, W., 1965. Community and schizophrenia. Wayne State University Press, Detroit.

Faris, R., Dunham, H., 1939. Mental disorders in urban areas. University of Chicago Press, Chicago.

Goffman, E., 1961. Asylums. Doubleday Anchor, New York.

Goldberg, D., Huxley, P., 1980. Mental illness in the community. Tavistock, London.

Goldberg, E., Morrison, S., 1963. Schizophrenia and social class. Br. J. Psychiatry 109, 785–802.

Greenberg, K.S., Greenley, J.R., Benedict, P., 1994. Contributions of persons with serious mental illness to their families. Hosp. Community Psychiatry 45, 475–480.

Greenblatt, M., Becera, R.M., Serafetinides, E.A., 1982. Social networks and mental health: an overview. Am. J. Psychiatry 139, 977–984.

Halpern, D., 1993. Minorities and mental health. Soc. Sci. Med. 36, 597–697.

Halpern, D., Nazroo, J., 1999. The ethnic density effect: results from a national community survey of England and Wales. Int. J. Soc. Psychiatry 46, 34–46.

Hare, E., 1956. Mental illness and social conditions in Bristol. J. Ment. Sci. 102, 349–357.

Harrison, G., 1988. A prospective study of severe mental disorder in Afro-Caribbean patients. Psychol. Med. 18, 643–657.

Holzer, C.E., Brent, M.S., Swanson, J.W., et al., 1986. The increased risk for specific psychiatric disorders among persons of low socioeconomic status. Am. J. Soc. Psychiatry 5, 259–271.

Jewell, T.C., Downing, D., McFarlane, W.R., 2009. Partnering with families: multiple family group psychoeducation for schizophrenia. J. Clin. Psychol. 65, 868–878.

Koppel, S., McGuffin, P., 1999. Socio-economic factors that predict psychiatric admissions at a local level. Psychol. Med. 29, 1235–1241.

Lidz, T., Fleck, S., Corneilson, A.R., 1965. Schizophrenia and the family. International Universities Press, New York.

London, M., 1986. Mental illness among immigrant minorities in the United Kingdom. Br. J. Psychiatry 149, 265–273.

Marcelis, M., Takei, N., Van Os, J., 1999. Urbanization and risk for schizophrenia: does the effect operate before or around the time of illness onset? Psychol. Med. 29, 1197–1203.

Mari, J.J., Streiner, D.L., 1994. An overview of family interventions and relapse on schizophrenia: meta-analysis of research findings. Psychol. Med. 24, 565–578.

Mechanic, D., 1968. Medical sociology: a selective view. Free Press, New York.

Mechanic, D., McAlpine, D., Rosenfield, S., et al., 1994. Effects of illness attribution and depression on the quality of life among persons with serious mental illness. Soc. Sci. Med. 39, 155–164.

Morgan, C., Fisher, H., 2007. Environment and schizophrenia: environmental factors in schizophrenia: childhood trauma – a critical review. Schizophr. Bull. 33, 3–10.

Morgan, C., Kirkbride, J., Hutchinson, G., et al., 2008. Cumulative social disadvantage, ethnicity and first-episode psychosis: a case-control study. Psychol. Med. 38, 1701–1715.

Mortensen, P.B., Pedersen, C.B., Westergaard, T., et al., 1999. Effects of family history and place and season of birth on risk of schizophrenia. N. Engl. J. Med. 340, 603–608.

Neeleman, J., Wessely, S., 1999. Ethnic minority suicide: a small group are study in South London. Psychol. Med. 29, 429–436.

Neeleman, J., Wilson-Jones, C., Wessely, S., 2001. Ethnic density and deliberate self harm; a small area study in south east London. J. Epidemiol. Community Health 55, 85–90.

Norman, R.M., Malla, A.K., 1993. Stressful life events and schizophrenia. I: A review of the research. Br. J. Psychiatry 162, 161–166.

Parkman, S., Davies, S., Leese, M., et al., 1997. Ethnic differences in satisfaction with mental health services among representative people with psychosis in South London. Br. J. Psychiatry 171, 260–264.

Parsons, T., 1951. The social system. Free Press, Glencoe, IL.

Quirk, A., Lelliott, P., 2001. What do we know about life on acute psychiatric wards in the UK? A review of the research evidence. Soc. Sci. Med. 53, 1565–1574.

Rogler, L., 1996. Increasing socioeconomic inequalities and the mental health of the poor. J. Nerv. Ment. Dis. 184, 719–722.

Ross, C., 2000. Neighborhood disadvantage and adult depression. J. Health Soc. Behav. 41, 177–187.

Rutter, M., 1989. Isle of Wight revisited: twenty-five years of child psychiatric epidemiology. J. Am. Acad. Child Adolesc. Psychiatry 28, 633–653.

Saxena, S., Thornicroft, G., Knapp, M., et al., 2007. Resources for mental health: scarcity, inequity, and inefficiency. Lancet 370, 878–889.

Schulz, R., Visintainer, P., Williamson, G.M., 1990. Psychiatric and physical morbidity effects of caregiving. J. Gerontol. 5, 181–191.

Schulze, B., 2007. Stigma and mental health professionals: a review of the evidence on an intricate relationship. Int. Rev. Psychiatry 19, 137–155.

Shapiro, S., Skinner, E., Kessler, L., et al., 1984. Utilization of health and mental health services. Three epidemiologic catchment area sites. Arch. Gen. Psychiatry 41, 971–978.

Shelton, K.H., Taylor, P.J., Bonner, A., et al., 2009. Risk factors for homelessness: evidence from a population-based study. Psychiatr. Serv. 60, 465–472.

Singleton, N., Bumpstead, R., O'Brien, M., et al., 2000. Psychiatric morbidity among adults living in private households. Office for National Statistics, London.

Szmukler, G.I., Burgess, P., Herrman, H., et al., 1996. Caring for relatives with serious mental illness: the development of the Experience of Caregiving Inventory. Soc. Psychiatry Psychiatr. Epidemiol. 31, 137–148.

Thornicroft, G., 2006. Shunned: discrimination against people with mental illness. Oxford University Press, Oxford.

Tsiegel, D.E., Salls, E., Schulz, R., 1991. Caregiving in chronic mental illness. In: Family caregiving in chronic illness. Sage, Newbury Park, pp. 164–198.

Wang, P.S., Aguilar-Gaxiola, S., Alonso, J., et al., 2007. Use of mental health services for anxiety, mood, and substance disorders in 17 countries in the WHO world mental health surveys. Lancet 370, 841–850.

Whitley, R., Prince, M., McKenzie, K., et al., 2006. Exploring the ethnic density effect: a qualitative study of a London electoral ward. Int. J. Soc. Psychiatry 52, 376–391.

WHO, 1979. Schizophrenia: an international follow-up study. World Health Organization. Wiley, Chichester.

Wilkinson, R.G., Pickett, K.E., 2007. The problems of relative deprivation: why some societies do better than others. Soc. Sci. Med. 65, 1965–1978.

Box 8.1

Skills of the culturally capable psychiatrist

- Ability to recognize one's own lack of cultural knowledge necessary to deliver effective psychiatric care
- Motivation to learn about cultural factors influencing presentation on their patients – from patients themselves, patient's friends and family (with consent), historical data sources, other colleagues, etc.
- To use interpreters effectively and consider the translations in a cultural and psychopathological context (e.g. avoiding friends or family members as interpreters, booking longer appointments, explaining practical arrangements to a patient; briefing the interpreter about practical arrangements before the session, for example, direct interpreting in the first person, sitting just behind the patient at an angle if patient agrees, always addressing patient in a second person, use simple direct sentences, observe non-verbal interaction between patient and interpreter)
- To ask sensitively about cultural identity and explanatory models, and explore these
- To complete a cultural formulation, taking full account of the transference and counter-transference issues related to race, ethnicity and culture
- To work with families, couples or groups when gathering information or delivering psychiatric interventions and reviewing progress
- To consider cultural variations of psychopathology, pharmacokinetics and pharmacodynamics
- To work effectively with voluntary and independent services which offer specialist care to black and minority ethnic groups
- To be active in research and audit of areas of practice identified locally to be poorly understood and undermine effective treatments.

Box 8.2

Definitions

Ethnic group

- A community whose heritage offers important characteristics in common between members, and which makes them distinct from other communities. The boundary between us and them is recognized by people on both sides of the boundary (Peach 1996)
- A social group characterized by distinctive social and cultural tradition, maintained within the group from generation to generation, a common history and origin, and a sense of identification with the group. Members of the group have distinctive features in their way of life, shared experiences and often a common genetic heritage (Last 1995).

Culture

- Culture is that complex whole which includes knowledge, belief, art, morale, law, customs and other capabilities and habits acquired by man as a member of society (Tylor 1871).
- A set of guidelines which individuals inherit as members of a particular society, and which tells them how to view the world, how to experience it emotionally, and how to behave in it in relation to other people, supernatural forces or gods, and to the natural environment (Helman 1990).

psychiatry has not emerged in a vacuum. 'Cultural studies' assert that our understanding is always unstable and influenced by context; one main aim of cultural studies is to explore power relationships and their expression in modern society. The academic discipline of cultural psychiatry draws on sociology, anthropology, epidemiology, statistics, philosophy, psychoanalysis and health services research to unravel the relationship between culture and mental health. Cultural studies generally, and cultural psychiatry specifically, examines power relationships, and how they are manifest in therapeutic encounters. It does not restrict itself to one discipline or one approach but deploys any method or model to better understand the relationship between culture and mental healthcare. Any study of cultures has to be focused on understanding the limitations of our knowledge and skills, while questioning our assumptions (this approach is more common in social sciences); it contrasts with making positive scientific statement (the approach most often pursued in medicine and epidemiology). This tension between discovering scientific data and recognizing and accepting uncertainty and the limitations of our knowledge has been one of the main sources of controversy and debate among psychiatrists studying culture and mental disorders (Box 8.2).

Culture, society and mental health

Culture determines which social behaviours and institutions are sanctioned and which are prohibited. Through living in a culture, we are informed about how to live, and more specifically, how to react to experiences of dysfunction or disability or distress. Culture influences, and is the substance of, beliefs, attitudes, behaviours and the social and family systems within which we live. Illness behaviour – the way individuals experience, appraise and respond to an episode of illness – is both shaped by culture and constitutes culture. Thus help-seeking patterns, as well as the ascriptions of normality are all defined by cultural norms. These norms are, on the whole, implicit rules for living, experiencing and seeing the world. Each culture has 'rites of reversal' (Helman 1990) when these rules are temporarily flouted, e.g. carnivals, Christmas celebrations, attending football matches in large crowds, being possessed by spirits during a Zar possession in Ethiopia, or speaking in tongues during religious ceremonies. Each of these is normal, even though the rituals and behaviours may seem abnormal to an outsider. However, they are normal only if the behaviours adhere to cultural rules and codes. If speaking in tongues continued for too long, or happened too frequently, or not in a church at all, the peer group that is familiar with these rituals would recognize this as abnormal.

People from different cultural groups will have different norms of behaviour, dress and attitudes towards family, sexuality, relationships, education, religion, state and society. Cultures are characterized by distinct family and kinship patterns, marriage ceremonies and other ritualized social activities. Tseng (2003) summarizes the evidence showing how child development also varies across cultures, and indeed, specific personality types have been ascribed to particular nations. National language films, and books, for example, capture these

are highly prevalent in the world's largest cities, sometimes being the majority.

Cultural psychiatry challenges the assumptions of established 'good clinical practice', and raises some philosophical, theoretical and technical dilemmas for practitioners. Cultural national stereotypes (Bhugra 2003) and can be used to teach cultural psychiatry, although it is recognized that these stereotypes are representations of real but subtle differences in national and cultural characteristics.

Culture can be said to consist of personality dispositions, collective and individual beliefs, knowledge, attitudes and values, and the impact of these on interpersonal relationships, social organizations, and relationships with ancestors, spirits and supernatural forces. Specific cultural knowledge implicitly determines how people appraise their experiences of distress and ill-health and, ultimately, from whom they seek help. The carer they seek out then further informs them how to relieve their suffering or misfortune. Kleinman (1980) considers that the majority of mental distress (60–70%) is remedied within the folk and popular sectors of healthcare, rather than by formal healthcare services. In the popular and folk arena, healing can take place within families, informal groups such as prayer groups, social clubs and shared interest groups. Within such gatherings, individuals seek out opinion and advice, and explain the measures they have taken to remedy their distress. They may not consider or experience their difficulties as being 'mental' in nature, or that they reflect a 'health' problem.

Somatic complaints may reflect true physical illness or co-morbid mental distress that takes a physical-symptom form. The physical complaint may be an idiom of distress, or a metaphorical means of communicating distress, or distress may actually be truly experienced subjectively as having physical origins. Kirmayer (2001) argues that, contrary to the claim that non-Westerners are prone to somatize their distress, somatization is ubiquitous. Somatic symptoms serve as cultural idioms of distress in many ethnocultural groups and, if misinterpreted by the clinician, may lead to unnecessary diagnostic procedures or inappropriate treatment. Clinicians must learn to decode the meaning of somatic and dissociative symptoms, which are not simply indices of disease or disorder but part of a language of distress with interpersonal and wider social meanings. Such distinct ways of experiencing and responding to distress can be better understood using theories about 'explanatory models'.

Key points

- Culture determines our everyday behaviours and attitudes towards each other, and towards the supernatural world.
- Specific cultural knowledge implicitly determines how people appraise their experiences of distress and ill-health and, ultimately, from whom they seek help, i.e. from health services, families and informal groups, healers, etc.

Explanatory models

An explanatory model sets out the patient's own way of naming their problem, describes the patient's explanation of causation, cure and prognosis, as well as who is equipped to help. Explanatory models (EMs) are not fixed cognitive representations or maps of how to behave (Bhui & Bhugra 2002). They are unstable and fluctuate, and are context dependant. They are assessed using a process of mini-ethnography, whereby the practitioner discovers cultural narratives and discourses around health, illness and their mental distress. However, any one individual's set of interrelated EMs constitute their total approach and ways of relating to distress and healers. EMs are operationalized as a set of beliefs about the 'identity' of the problem, and the causes of their distress, as well as what they should do to remedy their difficulties. Thus, some EMs include 'misfortune, breaking a taboo, black magic, karma' and 'an act of God' as forms of 'identity'. More familiar models to the west include: 'cold' and 'damp weather'; 'stress'; 'working too hard'; 'depression'. Causal explanations are patterned by culture, e.g. stormy love affairs and the break up of relationships; loss of status by a job loss; complaints of discrimination; food poisoning; a weak constitution. The veracity of the causal explanation is, in cultural terms, not essential, if the explanation serves a purpose of giving an individual some meaning and also influences their behaviour. A complication to this way of understanding culture is that in more medicalized societies, medical models of health and dysfunction are more likely to penetrate the social imagination and lay explanations for problems. Therefore, 'ME, stress, blood pressure, headache, back pain, a virus' might all be more readily used as explanations for dysfunction in the West. Whereas in the East, e.g. South Asia, explanations may include ghosts, spirits, Gods or the natural elements (e.g. a woman suffering from non-epileptic seizures may believe that it is caused by being possessed by spirits). Lay understandings about how the body works, and how dysfunction arises, include 'blockages, wearing out of parts, or tensions or nerves'. Some societies steeped in religious and strong cultural traditions sustain alternative explanatory frameworks for: misfortune, unexpected events and health problems. There is a danger of labelling patients as 'lacking insight' if their own explanation of their problems is different from those of the health professionals. It is often much more helpful to ask in detail about explanatory models, as it can improve the therapeutic alliance, develop an understanding of patients' experiences and offer possible ideas about appropriate treatment.

Box 8.3 gives an account of an in-depth research interview in which a woman's explanatory model for her depression was explored. This woman was not psychotic and, although depressed, she remained relatively functional in the nursing home where she lived after having to leave her family home, as her children were not prepared to live in an extended family and continue to support her in the way she expected.

Acculturation and cultural identity

Acculturation happens when groups of individuals from different cultures come into continuous first hand contact with subsequent changes in the original cultural patterns of either or both groups. Acculturation is the term given to the changes in everyday practices, attitudes and beliefs that take place when two relatively isolated cultures come into contact. This is a complex process (Box 8.4). Cultural adaptations are seen in language dominance, dress preference, food and leisure pursuits, topics of conversation, attitudes to religious worship, marriage partner selection, child rearing and the balance between work, home

Box 8.3

Case history

Mrs H. is a Muslim woman (Agha Khan group of Muslims). She speaks Hindi, Gujarati and Urdu. She is approximately 70–75 years of age, and has hemiplegia due to a stroke. She needed a translator.

When asked about worry and depression, she said she was depressed due to her family. 'When the family becomes your enemy you inevitably become depressed.' She related family problems as the primary cause of worry and depression. On further questioning, she added that there were also money shortages alongside the difficulties with her family.

When asked, 'Why do people become depressed or develop worry?', she replied that her daughter-in-law had used 'Taveez' against her and had practised magic. God, she said, had intervened and thus she was therefore OK. When asked more about this, she said that her daughter-in-law had used magic water and that one daughter-in-law had asked the second to place it in her curry. Since then, she had not been well. However, they also had suffered and had had major financial worries. Anyone who ate the curry would be affected and she was worried as her name 'was written on the water' and thus, if anyone else was affected by it, it would be her fault in some way.

She did not see doctors as having any role to play as it was a 'family problem' and as such, it had to be resolved within the family. She said that the doctor cannot change things to do with the family and indeed 'family problems' were not shared. 'Doctors give medication only.' She proceeded to explain how the doctor could help identify causes of physical problems and give medication but she did not see that the doctor had a role to play in her financial or family problems, whether they caused her terrible worry or not.

Box 8.4

Psychopathology and culture

- Patho*plastic*: shaping the content of symptoms or the overall picture. For example, a sinking heart as a metaphor for depression and social isolation and interpersonal distress among Punjabi Asians. Also the content of delusions, hallucinations, etc. can vary.

- Patho*selective*: personality and psychological make-up can also recruit specific styles of expressing distress. Deliberate self-harm and anorexia were seen as typical of a Western expression of distress. Personality dispositions influence how people select specific behaviours as expressions of distress.

- Patho*genic* distress can be generated by cultures, e.g. by demands for role fulfilment, or prohibitions on certain behaviours.

- Patho*facilitative*: this suggests that culture does not generate or determine specific psychopathology, but facilitates or makes more likely specific expressions of distress. Thus, the frequency of certain disorders varies across societies, depending upon availability of means and social sanctions for specific expressions of distress.

- Patho*elaborative*: the exaggeration of certain behaviours in specific societies. Latah in the Far East, e.g., is an exaggerated startle reaction as is manifest posturing and taking up instances, after unexpected prodding or startle

- Patho*reactive*: culture influences how people react to illness. The meaning of the symptoms may be interpreted, or there may be stigma or fear about specific manifestations of distress

- Patho*discriminative*: this indicates which behaviours a culture identifies as normal or abnormal.

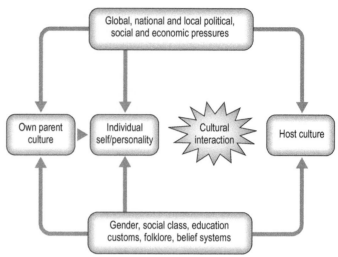

Figure 8.1 • Acculturation as a function of group identity, national and social policy as well as individual demographics.

and family life may all change. Use of health services and attitudes to illness and mental health may also change. This can lead to tensions between the individual and their immediate family, social group and society.

The identity of an individual is in part determined by their culture of origin, but also by their identification with different social groups: older people, women, black people, Nigerian speakers, etc. Focusing only on ethnic identity can be misleading, as people usually relate to more than one cultural group. Identification with either the host or the original culture were once seen as mutually exclusive processes. However, recently, more sophisticated models of identity development suggest people can have multiple identifications, and can be identified with host and original culture on independent domains (Berry 1980). That is, they can be: (1) 'bi-culturally proficient' by synthesizing two cultures; (2) 'traditional' by only identifying with the culture of origin; (3) 'assimilated' by giving up the original culture and adopting the host culture; (4) 'marginalized' by giving up the culture of origin and not adopting the new culture (Fig. 8.1).

The identities that an individual adopts carry with them explanatory models, expectations of healthcare, specific metaphors for describing distress, stigma about mental illness and experiences of mental healthcare. Berry (1980) argues that bi-culturally proficient identities are the most healthy, with the marginalized group being least healthy. However, a great deal of empirical work on cultural identity and acculturation experiences shows this to be a methodologically complex field, with too many value laden assumptions about what constitutes culture, and how to remedy ill health, which is seen to be either generated by immigrant or foreign culture or exacerbated by it.

The cultural formulation

The American Psychiatric Association recommends that all psychiatrists assess cultural identity and explanatory models of their patients (Griffith 2002). This should take place alongside an assessment of the impact on the therapeutic relationship of culture of the professional and/or patient. Cultural factors related to the sociocultural environment (discrimination, unemployment, asylum laws) should also be considered as factors that impact on mental health. Finally, there should be an overall statement outlining any culturally relevant aspects of diagnosis and treatment. Professionals should take particular care to ensure that the rationale for the treatment is understood, and be vigilant about the possibility of breaking cultural taboos or undermining cherished cultural beliefs, as this may lead to potential non-compliance. Most importantly, any further investigations to improve an understanding of the cultural aspects of presentation should be stated explicitly. For example, talking to family or friends of a patient enables the professional to consider their views about psychopathology and ensures that cultural phenomena are not considered as pathology due to a lack of familiarity with the cultural norms of patients. Although the Royal College of Psychiatrists in the UK has not formulated any specific recommendation, there are now capability indicators for trainees reflecting the multicultural nature of the population (Moodley 2002).

Key point

- Always explore the patient's cultural identity and explanatory model (i.e. their own way of naming the problem, their explanation of causation, cure and prognosis, as well as who they believe is equipped to help).

Psychopathology and culture

It is known that first rank symptoms are not specific to schizophrenia and are not uncommon in mania. They are also present to varying degrees in different cultural groups and do not always carry the same diagnostic significance across cultures (Bhugra & Bhui 2001). Breaching individual ego boundaries is not as pathologically regarded as it is in Western societies. In societies with a more sociocentric or diffuse sense of self, where connectedness, dependency and shared communications are not considered immature, incursions from ancestors or family members into the personal space (social or body or mind) of a person are common. For example, in India, spirit possession and exorcisms are not automatically considered abnormal or to need a psychiatrist for treatment. Helman (1990) suggests that all societies allow temporary abnormally behaviours if they obey culturally coded rules. If the rules are broken, then they may be seen as pathology. For example, spirit possession or talking in tongues can be normal experiences, but if they persist or are associated with experiences that people from the reference group consider atypical, then they may be indicators of abnormality. Tseng (2003) has summarized the many ways in which culture affects mental health (Box 8.4).

All of these make the mental state assessment more difficult to interpret in terms of normal or abnormal phenomena. Although psychotic phenomena are often considered to be due to the same universal neurochemical changes in brain which influence perceptions, the same phenomena cannot be assumed to have the same trigger factors, aetiology or meaning for the patient. Furthermore, susceptibility to hallucinations is determined by the relative significance of hallucinations as ordinary events in societies. van Os et al (2000) found that 17.5% of a population sample experienced hallucinations and only 4.5% of these subjects had a diagnosed mental disorder. This presence of a non-clinically-significant psychotic symptom may explain cultural variations if psychotic symptoms can exist in response to social and psychological events compounded by general distress and preparedness to express distress through psychosis. Although visual hallucinations are considered to be rare in schizophrenia, they are not rare in presentations of schizophrenia in some Asian and African countries. A recent study by Suhail and Cochrane (2002) explored the content of psychotic symptoms among Pakistanis in Pakistan, Pakistanis in Britain and white British patients. They found greater differences in phenomenology between Pakistani Pakistanis and British Pakistanis than between British white and British Pakistani patients. This suggests that immediate environment also influences the expression of distress and the content of psychosis.

Can culture influence the form of psychosis? Suhail and Cochrane (2002) also reported that visual hallucinations are more common in Pakistani Pakistanis where religious doctrine encourages 'visions'. They also assert more grandiose symptoms among Pakistani Pakistanis where there is marked poverty and a greater gap between rich and poor. The rates of self-harm among South Asian women in the UK are much higher than among their white counterparts and it has been argued that specific cultural factors, such as level of acculturation, cultural conflicts, stigma and interpersonal relationships, were important factors associated with distress and resilience in this group (Ahmed et al 2007).

These studies challenge a universalistic application of knowledge to all cultural groups, and argue that cultural relativism is necessary and real. There is an active debate about the cultural universality of diagnostic categories. Psychiatric epidemiological studies generate diagnoses using structured interview schedules, so diagnoses are certainly reliably made. Are they as valid? It appears that psychiatric disorders occur around the world, but their recognition as illness varies, and the expectation that doctors can intervene also varies. The more biological the aetiology of specific mental disorders, the more likely it is that these disorders take the same core form in different societies. Thus, common mental disorders such as depression and anxiety are more subject to cultural variation. Any phenomena that psychiatrists label as abnormal (delusions, hallucinations, aggression and paranoia) occur to varying extents in different societies, and many not always be thought of as a mental illness. Such symptoms must be understood in the context of the patient's dominant cultural frame of reference and belief system (Bhugra & Bhui 2001) and prevalence and changes in function associated with these phenomena.

Key point

- Ostensibly 'abnormal' psychopathological phenomena (easily described as delusions, hallucinations, aggression and paranoia) occur to varying extents in different societies, and may not always be thought of as a mental illness. Such symptoms must be understood in the context of the patient's dominant cultural frame of reference and belief system.

Mental health policy

Two policy frameworks have been launched: Inside/Outside and Delivery Race Equality: A Framework for Action (DoH 2003a,b). These documents emerged from extensive discussion with community groups and working parties exploring how to eradicate ethnic inequalities in service users' experiences of services and clinical outcomes.

Key further reading on contemporary debates in cultural psychiatry

Sharpley, M., Hutchinson, G., McKenzie, K., et al., 2001. Understanding the excess of psychosis among the African-Caribbean population in England. Review of current hypotheses. Br. J. Psychiatry 40, S60–S68. *Why do black Caribbean people more often suffer with schizophrenia?*

Bhui, K., Shashidharan, S.P., 2003. Should there be separate psychiatric services for ethnic minority groups? Br. J. Psychiatry 182, 10–12.

Should we have specialist mental health services for specific ethnic minority groups?

Chakraborty, A., McKenzie, K., 2002. Racial discrimination cause mental illness? Br. J. Psychiatry 180, 475–477.

Does racism cause mental disorder?

Bhui, K., Stansfeld, S., Hull, S., et al., 2003. Ethnic variations in pathways to and use of specialist mental health services in the UK.

Systematic review. Br. J. Psychiatry 182, 105–116.

What do we know about ethnic variations in access to mental healthcare?

Minnis, H., McMillan, A., Gillies, M., et al., 2001. Stereotyping: survey of psychiatrists in the United Kingdom. Br. Med. J. 323, 905–906.

Are mental health practitioners racist?

Further reading

Bhugra, D., Bhui, K., 2001. Cross cultural psychiatry: a practical guide. Arnold, London.

Bhugra, D., Bhui, K., 2008. A textbook of cultural psychiatry. Cambridge University Press, Cambridge.

Bhui, K. (Ed.), 2002. Racism and mental health. Jessica Kingsley, London.

Bhui, K., Bhugra, S., 2008. Culture and mental health: a comprehensive textbook. Hodder, London.

Helman, C., 2000. Culture, health and illness, fourth revised ed. Hodder Arnold, London.

Tseng, W.S., 2003. Clinician's guide to cultural psychiatry. Academic Press, San Diego.

References

Ahmed, K., Mohan, R.A., Bhugra, D., 2007. Self harm in South Asian woman: a literature review informed approach to assessment and formulation. Am. J. Psychother. 61, 71–81.

Berry, W., 1980. Acculturation as varieties of adaptation in acculturation: theory, models and some new findings. In: Padilla, A. (Ed.), Acculturation: theory, models and findings. Westview, Boulder.

Bhugra, D., 2003. Using film and literature for cultural competence training. Psychiatry Bulletin 27, 427–428.

Bhugra, D., Bhui, K., 2001. Cross cultural psychiatry: a practical guide. Arnold, London.

Bhui, K., Bhugra, D., 2002. Explanatory models for mental distress: implications for clinical practice and research. Br. J. Psychiatry 181, 6–7.

Bhui, K., Bhugra, D., Goldberg, D., et al., 2001. Cultural influences on the prevalence of common mental disorder, general practitioners' assessments and help-seeking among Punjabi and English people visiting their general practitioner. Psychol. Med. 31, 815–825.

Bhui, K., Brown, P., Hardie, T., et al., 1998. African-Caribbean men remanded to Brixton prison. Psychiatric and forensic characteristics and outcome of final court appearance. Br. J. Psychiatry 172, 337–344.

Bhui, K., Christie, Y., Bhugra, D., 1995. The essential elements of culturally sensitive psychiatric services. Int. J. Soc. Psychiatry 41, 242–256.

Bhui, K., Stansfeld, S., Hull, S., et al., 2003. Ethnic variations in pathways to and use of specialist mental health services in the UK. Systematic review. Br. J. Psychiatry 182, 105–116.

Coid, J., Kahtan, N., Gault, S., et al., 2000. Ethnic differences in admissions to secure forensic psychiatry services. Br. J. Psychiatry 177, 241–247.

Coid, J., Petruckevitch, A., Bebbington, P., et al., 2002a. Ethnic differences in prisoners. 1: Criminality and psychiatric morbidity. Br. J. Psychiatry 181, 473–480.

Coid, J., Petruckevitch, A., Bebbington, P., et al., 2002b. Ethnic differences in prisoners. 2: Risk factors and psychiatric service use. Br. J. Psychiatry 181, 481–487.

Cole, E., Leavey, G., King, M., et al., 1995. Pathways to care for patients with a first episode of psychosis. A comparison of ethnic groups. Br. J. Psychiatry 167, 770–776.

Cooper-Patrick, L., Gallo, J.J., Gonzales, J.J., et al., 1999. Race, gender, and partnership in the patient-physician relationship. J. Am. Med. Assoc. 282, 583–589.

DoH, 2003a. Inside/outside. Department of Health, London.

DoH, 2003b. Delivering race equality: a framework for action. Department of Health, London.

Falkowski, J., Watts, V., Falkowski, W., et al., 1990. Patients leaving hospital without the knowledge or permission of staff – absconding. Br. J. Psychiatry 156, 488–490.

Fearon, P., Kirkbride, J.B., Morgan, C., et al., 2006. Incidence of schizophrenia and other psychoses in ethnic minority groups: results from the MRC AESOP Study. Psychol. Med. 36, 1541–1550.

Frank, J.D., 1993. Persuasion and healing: a comparative study of psychotherapy. Johns Hopkins University Press, Baltimore.

Griffith, E., Committee on Cultural Psychiatry of the Group for the Advancement of Psychiatry, 2002. Cultural assessment in clinical psychiatry. American Psychiatric Publishing, Washington DC.

Gupta, S., 1991. Psychosis in migrants from the Indian subcontinent and English-born controls. A preliminary study on the use of psychiatric services. Br. J. Psychiatry 159, 222–225.

Harrison, G., Owens, D., Holton, A., et al., 1988. A prospective study of severe mental disorder in Afro-Caribbean patients. Psychol. Med. 18, 643–657.

Helman, C., 1990. Culture, health and illness: an introduction for health professionals, second revised ed. Butterworth-Heinemann, Oxford.

Hickling, F.W., McKenzie, K., Mullen, R., et al., 1999. A Jamaican psychiatrist evaluates diagnoses at a London psychiatric hospital. Br. J. Psychiatry 175, 283–285.

Hutchinson, G., Takei, N., Sham, P., et al., 1999. Factor analysis of symptoms in schizophrenia: differences between white and Caribbean patients in Camberwell. Psychol. Med. 29, 607–612.

King, M., Coker, E., Leavey, G., et al., 1994. Incidence of psychotic illness in London: comparison of ethnic groups. Br. Med. J. 309, 1115–1119.

Kirkbride, J.B., Fearon, P., Morgan, C., et al., 2006. Heterogeneity in incidence rates of schizophrenia and other psychotic syndromes: findings from the 3-center AESOP study. Arch. Gen. Psychiatry 63, 250–258.

Kirmayer, L., 2001. Cultural variations in the clinical presentation of anxiety and depression: implications for diagnosis and treatment. J. Clin. Psychiatry 62, 22–28.

Kirov, G., Murray, R.M., 1999. Ethnic differences in the presentation of bipolar affective disorder. Eur. Psychiatry 14, 199–204.

Kleinman, A., 1980. Patients and their healers in the context of culture. University of California Press, Berkeley.

Last, J.M., 1995. A dictionary of epidemiology, third ed. Oxford University Press, Oxford.

Lelliott, P., Audini, B., Duffett, R., 2001. Survey of patients from an inner-London health authority in medium secure psychiatric care. Br. J. Psychiatry 178, 62–66.

Lin, K.M., Anderson, D., Poland, R.E., 1995. Ethnicity and psychopharmacology. Bridging the gap. Psychiatr. Clin. North Am. 18, 635–647.

Mclean, C., Campbell, C., Cornish, F., 2003. African-Caribbean interactions with mental health services in the UK: experiences and expectations of exclusion as (re)productive of health inequalities. Soc. Sci. Med. 56, 657–669.

Moodley, P., 2002. Building a culturally capable workforce-an educational approach to delivering equitable mental health services. Psychiatric Bulletin 26, 63–65.

Myin-Germeys, I., van Os, J., Schwartz, J.E., et al., 2001. Emotional reactivity to daily life stress in psychosis. Arch. Gen. Psychiatry 58, 1137–1144.

Odell, S.M., Surtees, P.G., Wainwright, N.W., et al., 1997. Determinants of general practitioner recognition of psychological problems in a multi-ethnic inner-city health district. Br. J. Psychiatry 171, 537–541.

Parkman, S., Davies, S., Leese, M., et al., 1997. Ethnic differences in satisfaction with mental health services among representative people with psychosis in south London: PRiSM study 4. Br. J. Psychiatry 171, 260–264.

Peach, C., 1996. Introduction to: ethnicity in the 1991 Census, vol 2: The ethnic minority populations of Great Britain, ONS. HMSO, London.

Pote, H.L., Orrell, M.W., 2002. Perceptions of schizophrenia in multi-cultural Britain. Ethn. Health 7, 7–20.

Sainsbury Centre for Mental Health, 2002. Breaking the circles of fear. Sainsbury Centre for Mental Health, London.

Sharpley, M., Hutchinson, G., McKenzie, K., et al., 2001. Understanding the excess of psychosis among the African-Caribbean population in England. Review of current hypotheses. Br. J. Psychiatry 40, S60–S68.

Snowden, L.R., 2003. Bias in mental health assessment and intervention: theory and evidence. Am. J. Public Health 93, 239–243.

Suhail, K., Cochrane, R., 2002. Effect of culture and environment on the phenomenology of delusions and hallucinations. Int. J. Soc. Psychiatry 48, 126–138.

Tseng, W.S., 2003. Clinician's guide to cultural psychiatry. Academic Press, San Diego.

Tylor, E.B., 1871. Primitive culture. Research into the development of mythology, philosophy, religion, art and customs. John Murray, London.

US DoH, HS, 2001. Mental health, culture, race and ethnicity: a supplement to mental health: a report of the Surgeon General. US Department of Health and Human Services, Washington.

van Os, J., Hanssen, M., Bijl, R.V., et al., 2000. Strauss (1969) revisited: a psychosis continuum in the general population? Schizophr. Res. 45, 11–20.

van Ryn, M., Fu, S.S., 2003. Paved with good intentions: do public health and human service providers contribute to racial/ethnic disparities in health? Am. J. Public Health 93, 248–255.

Wessely, S., 1998. The Camberwell Study of Crime and Schizophrenia. Soc. Psychiatry Psychiatr. Epidemiol. 33, S24–S28.

Epidemiology

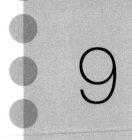

Martin Prince

Introduction and overview

What is epidemiology?

Last's (2001) *Dictionary of Epidemiology* defines epidemiology as:

> The study of the distribution and determinants of health-related states or events in specified populations, and the application of this study to the control of health problems.

What is the purpose of epidemiology?

Epidemiology is concerned with the health states of populations, communities and groups. The health states of individuals is the concern of clinical medicine. Epidemiology may simply describe the distribution of health states (extent, type, severity) within a population. This is *descriptive epidemiology*. Alternatively, it may try to explain the distribution of health states. This is *analytical epidemiology*. The basic strategy is to compare the distribution of disease between groups or between populations, looking for *associations* between hypothesized *risk factors* (genes, behaviours, lifestyles, environmental exposures) and *health states*. These associations may or may not indicate that the hypothesized risk factor has caused the disease (Fig. 9.1).

patient depressed? Does he need treatment? Should he be admitted? Does he have insight? Is he a danger to himself? As Pickering commented (when arguing that hypertension was better understood as a dimensional rather than a dichotomous disorder), 'doctors can count to one but not beyond'. It is important to recognize that a dimensional concept need not contradict a categorical view of a disorder. As with the relativity of the concept of 'a case', it may be useful under some circumstances to think categorically and in others dimensionally. There is, for instance, a positive correlation between the number of symptoms of depression experienced by a person and:

* The impairment of their quality of life
* The frequency with which they use GP services
* The number of days they take off work in a month.

Thus, a dimensional perspective, even more so than broadly based diagnostic criteria, can offer useful insights into the way in which the consequences of mental disorder are very widely distributed in the community (Das-Munshi et al 2008).

From a technical point of view, continuous measures of dimensional traits such as depression, anxiety, neuroticism and cognitive function offer some advantages over their dichotomous equivalents, depressive episode, generalized anxiety disorder and dementia. These diagnoses tend to be rather rare; collapsing a continuous trait into a dichotomous diagnosis may mean that the investigators are in effect throwing away informative data; the net effect may be loss of statistical power to demonstrate an important association with a risk factor, or a real benefit of a treatment.

Validity

Content validity

This refers to the extent to which the construct that the measure seeks to address is real and coherent, and then also to the relevance of the measure to that construct. Content validity cannot be demonstrated empirically, but evidence can be sought to support it. For example, the scope and content of the construct can be identified through systematic reviews of the literature, and open-ended interviews and focus group discussions with experts or key informants. These same informants can review the proposed measure and comment on the appropriateness of the items (face validity).

Construct validity

Construct validity, as first defined by Cronbach and Meehl (1955), referred to a situation in which 'the tester has no definite criterion measure of the quality with which he is concerned, and must use indirect measures. Here, the [elucidation of the] trait or quality underlying the test is of central importance' (Cronbach & Meehl 1955). The answers to these questions would be derived from quantitative research, essentially through a series of hypothesis-driven investigations aimed at identifying the 'nomological net' or theoretical framework consisting of other more or less closely related constructs, which can then be used to help to define it. The investigation of a measure's construct validity is a process that is more or less

comparable to that for developing and confirming theories in observational research. As with a hypothesis in observational research, the construct that is intended to be measured, and the measure itself, can be refined on the basis of findings. This process of testing for associations with related constructs is sometimes termed concurrent validity – convergent when a positive association is hypothesized; divergent when constructs are hypothesized to be unrelated. This, in a validation of the Self Reporting Questionnaire (SRQ 20) as a measure of maternal depression in Ethiopia, SRQ scores, as hypothesized, were associated in a dose-dependent fashion with a range of relevant psychosocial factors (Hanlon et al 2008). The internal measurement properties of a scale can also be explored using factor analysis. Thus, for example, confirmatory factor analysis has been used to validate the Parental Bonding Interview across European centres participating in the World Mental Health Survey, providing strong evidence for the invariance of a three factor solution (care, overprotection and authoritarianism) suggested by exploratory factor analysis, across six countries, both sexes and all age groups (Heider et al 2005).

Known group validity can also be assessed where no established gold standard external criterion exists. Thus, a new questionnaire measuring the amount of time parents spend in positive joint activities with their children could be applied to two groups of parents, identified by their health visitors or teachers as having contrasting levels of involvement with their children (Kumari et al 2000).

Criterion validity

Testing of criterion validity requires a 'gold standard', technically the very thing that one is setting out to measure. In psychiatry there are generally no biologically based criterion measures as, for example, bronchoscopy and biopsy for carcinoma of the bronchus. Much research is currently orientated to the identification of such 'biomarkers'. The first measures developed for psychiatric research were compared with the criterion or 'gold standard' of a competent psychiatrist's clinical diagnosis. Currently, the most commonly used paradigm in psychiatric research is the clinician semi-structured interview, generally the Schedules for Clinical Assessment in Neuropsychiatry (SCAN) or the Structured Clinical Interview for DSM Disorders (SCID), applying ICD-10 or DSM-IV diagnoses. There are several problems that are implicit in this process (Kessler et al 2004). First, the reliability of clinician semi-structured interviews is by no means perfect, particularly in community-based research, and this random error will set an upper limit on the validity coefficients that are likely to be observed. Second, repetition of comprehensive mental state assessments has been shown to be associated with systematic underreporting of symptoms on the second interview compared with the first, again tending towards an underestimate of true validity. Third, the DSM and ICD diagnostic criteria themselves are not fully operationalized, and differing judgments made in the algorithms accompanying the test assessment and gold standard research interviews may be another source of discrepancy. Fourth, Cohen's kappa varies with the prevalence of the disorder even when specificity and sensitivity are constant, limiting the utility of this validity coefficient in comparing the validity of a measure across different populations.

Predictive validity

This assesses the extent to which a new measure can predict future outcomes. Thus, a diagnosis of dementia, if valid, should predict future cognitive and functional decline, and mortality, while stability or recovery would cast doubt upon the diagnosis (Jotheeswaran et al 2010).

Measuring validity

Concurrent validity of a continuous measure against another continuous measure as criterion is measured with a Pearson's (parametric) or Spearman's (non-parametric) correlation coefficient. Criterion validity against a dichotomous criterion is usually expressed in terms of the validity coefficients, *sensitivity*, *specificity* and *positive* and *negative predictive value*. When the same subjects have been assessed using the new measure and the 'gold standard' criterion measure, the results can be summarized in a 2 × 2 table (Table 9.1).

The *sensitivity* of the new measure is the proportion of true cases correctly identified:

$$\text{Sensitivity} = a/a + c.$$

The *specificity* of the new measure is the proportion of non-cases correctly identified:

$$\text{Specificity} = d/b + d.$$

The *positive predictive value* (*PPV*) of the new measure is the proportion of respondents it identifies as cases that actually are cases according to the 'gold standard':

$$\text{PPV} = a/a + b.$$

The *negative predictive value* (*NPV*) of the new measure is the proportion of respondents it identifies as non-cases that actually are non-cases according to the 'gold standard':

$$\text{NPV} = d/c + d.$$

Likelihood ratios

The overall predictiveness of a given test result can be conveniently summarized as the *likelihood* ratio. The likelihood ratio is easily calculated:

LR = Probability of a given test result in diseased persons/
Probability of that test result in non-diseased persons

Using Bayes' theorem, we can calculate the post-test probability of disease given knowledge of the pre-test probability (in this case disease prevalence) and the likelihood ratio (LR) associated with different test results.

Table 9.2 The association of the apolipoprotein E e4 genotype with Alzheimer disease

	Controls	AD cases
Homozygous (two ε4 alleles)	3%	13%
Heterozygous (one ε4 allele)	19%	50%
No ε4 alleles	78%	37%

For example, the apolipoprotein E ε4 genotype is strongly associated with risk for Alzheimer disease (AD). A typical finding for the association is given in Table 9.2. Use of these prevalence rates, and the presence of any ApoE ε4 allele as the test criterion, suggests a test with 78% specificity and 63% sensitivity for a diagnosis of AD.

The LRs derived from the ApoE ε4 frequencies given in Table 9.2 are:

- Homozygous (two ε4 alleles) = 0.13/0.03 = 4.3
- Heterozygous (one ε4 allele) = 0.50/0.19 = 2.5
- No ε4 alleles = 0.37/0.78 = 0.48.

The likelihood ratio for a positive test result (e.g. one or two ε4 alleles) is sometimes known as a likelihood ratio positive and that for a negative test result (e.g. no ε4 alleles) as a likelihood ratio negative.

The LR for a given test result is related to the pre-test and post-test probability of disease, for:

Pre-test odds of disease × LR = post-test odds of disease

If the pre-test probability of Alzheimer disease is 0.10 (a generous estimate for the eventual lifetime prevalence for those who have already survived into their 60s), then the pre-test odds are 0.1/(1 − 0.10) = 0.11. If a person is then found to be homozygous for apoE ε4, their post-test odds, given this additional information, become 0.11 × 4.3 = 0.47. This translates into a post-test probability of disease (positive predictive value for the test) of: 0.47/(1 + 0.47) = 0.32. The post-test probabilities for heterozygosity and for no apoE ε4 allele are 0.22 and 0.05, respectively. The positive predictive values (0.32 and 0.22) therefore encompass too much uncertainty to be of use to screened patients and their clinicians. One reason for this shortcoming is the low prevalence of AD. For a test with given predictive power, the post-test probability of disease is crucially dependent on the pre-test probability. Rarely can a single test be used as an early indicator of a disease with as low a population prevalence as AD. This demonstrates in another way the impact of disease prevalence upon PPV mentioned above. It can be shown that a test with a given LR will provide a maximum 'gain' of post-test diagnostic probability when the pre-test probability is in the region of 0.4–0.6. One solution then might be to apply the test to a target population with a known high lifetime prevalence of the disease; in the case of apoE ε4 and AD, for instance, the test might work satisfactorily in those with a strong family history of AD. Alternatively, Bayes' theorem can be used to combine a number of moderately predictive tests into a more effective package. Given the assumption of conditional independence (that is,

Table 9.1 Validity assessment: a 2 × 2 table

New measure	Gold standard	
	Case	Non-case
Case	a	b
Non-case	c	d

that the results of the second test do not depend on the results of the first) then:

$$\text{Pre-test odds} \times \text{LR}(\text{test 1}) \times \text{LR}(\text{test 2})$$
$$= \text{post-test odds (tests 1 and 2).}$$

Reliability

Test–re-test reliability (intra-measurement reliability)

Intra-measurement reliability tests the stability of a measure over time. The measure is administered to a respondent, and then after an interval of time is administered again to the same person, under the same conditions (e.g. by the same interviewer). The selection of the time interval is a matter of judgement. Too short and the respondent may simply recall and repeat their response from the first testing. Too long, and the trait that the measure was measuring may have changed, e.g. the respondent may have recovered from their depression.

Inter-observer reliability

Inter-observer reliability tests the stability of the measure when administered or rated by different investigators. Administering the measure to the same respondent under the same conditions by first one and then the other interviewer tests inter-interviewer reliability. Having the same interview rated by two or more investigators tests inter-rater reliability.

Measuring reliability

Intra-measurement and interobserver reliability are assessed using measures of agreement. For a continuous scale measure the appropriate statistic would be the intra-class correlation. For a categorical measure the appropriate statistic is Cohen's kappa; this takes into account the agreement expected by chance, and is independent of the prevalence of the condition in the test population.

The internal consistency of a measure indicates the extent to which its component parts, in the case of a scale the individual items, address a common underlying construct. This is conventionally considered a component of reliability. For a scale it is usually measured using Cronbach's coefficient alpha, which varies between 0 and 1. Coefficient alpha of 0.6–0.8 is moderate but satisfactory, above 0.8 indicates a highly internally consistent scale. Another measure of internal consistency is the split-half reliability, a measure of agreement between subscales derived from two randomly selected halves of the scale.

Epidemiological study designs

As with the plots of Hollywood movies, there have only ever been a limited number of epidemiological designs in general use. However, the details of the study designs, and the conduct and analysis of these studies has become increasingly refined and sophisticated. Studies may be experimental or non-experimental (observational). Observational studies may use observations made on individuals, or aggregated data from groups or populations. They may be descriptive or analytic in purpose and design. Figure 9.2 summarizes the main types of study design. On the following pages, the essentials of these basic types of study design are illustrated with reference to their application to the epidemiology of schizophrenia.

Descriptive studies

The cross-sectional (prevalence) survey

In epidemiological research, a cross-sectional prevalence survey provides an estimate of the proportion of individuals within a defined population that have a health condition. The proportion, usually expressed as a percentage, is called the prevalence. Prevalence always refers to a defined time period; point prevalence (prevalence at the instant of the survey), 1-year prevalence (prevalence at any time over the month before the study) and so on. The 1-year prevalence for schizophrenia has been reported generally to lie between 0.3 and 0.8% (Jenkins et al 1997b). Prevalence studies therefore provide a snapshot of the health status of the community at the time that the survey is conducted; for chronic conditions, such as schizophrenia, this will include those who have recently developed the condition (incident cases) and those that have lived with the condition for some time (prevalent cases). The prevalence is therefore the product of the incidence rate and the average length of survival with the illness.

Every survey is of a defined 'base population'. This may be a large population, such as a city or country, in which case a sample is selected, at random, to be representative of the population as whole. Sampling frames for population-based surveys require an accurate register (such as an electoral roll). However, these may not be available to researchers and may be inaccurate. Often, therefore, household surveys are conducted using random samples of addresses and then selecting one individual at

Non-experimental					Experimental
Descriptive		Analytic			
1. Population prevalence/ incidence (a) geographic variation (b) temporal ('secular') variation	2. Ecological correlation	3. Cross-sectional survey	4. Case–control study	5. Cohort study	6. Randomized controlled trial

Figure 9.2 • Types of study design.

random from all eligible household members. In a 'catchment area' survey, all eligible residents of a defined district are assessed, after 'door-knocking' to identify them. The larger the sample, the greater the precision of the estimate of prevalence. Strictly speaking, the prevalence only refers to the base population for the survey, but it may be 'generalizable' to other communities with similar characteristics. In addition to the main health conditions under study, information is typically collected about age, sex and living circumstances (sociodemographic data), as well as information about other health conditions, possible risk factors, use of health and social services, and informal care arrangements. Prevalence is typically reported by age group and sometimes by sex.

There are some special considerations relating to mental health surveys. Some disorders, notably schizophrenia and other psychoses, are relatively rare. Two phase surveys are commonly used, in which all participants are screened in the first phase, and all those meeting screening criteria and a random sample of screen negatives then complete a detailed clinical diagnostic assessment. 'Weighting back' (by the inverse of the probability of selection for the second phase) is required to generate an estimate of prevalence and its confidence intervals (Dunn et al 1999). However, these approaches may be less efficient than they seem, and large samples are still required in order to achieve reasonable precision (Prince 2003). Furthermore, cases will be overrepresented in inpatient facilities, in hostels, in prison populations and among the homeless. These populations may be difficult to access by standard community survey techniques. Unless special attempts are made to sample these subpopulations there is a clear risk of under ascertainment (Jenkins et al 1997a).

Prevalence surveys may be used:

1. To give an accurate assessment of the numbers of cases within a region or country, allowing governments, and health and welfare services to plan adequate services
2. To identify variations in prevalence, allowing epidemiologists to develop and test theories about possible risk factors for the disease; these may be:
   a. Ecological variation: making comparisons with other populations or regions (in a series of comparable surveys conducted in different populations)
   b. Secular variation: charting trends over time (in a series of comparable surveys of the same population)
3. To describe the living circumstances, and care arrangements of people with mental health conditions, identifying met and unmet needs including informal care (by family members) and access to and use of health and social services
4. To describe the impact of mental disorders at the population level including the economic costs
5. To raise awareness, drawing public and political attention to the extent of a mental health problem within a community.

Cross-sectional studies can also be used to compare the characteristics of those in the population with and without the disorder, thus identifying cross-sectional associations with potential risk factors for the disorder. The main drawback of cross-sectional surveys for analytical as opposed to descriptive epidemiology, is that they can only give clues about aetiology. Because exposure (potential risk factor) and outcome (disease or health condition) are measured simultaneously, one can never be sure, in the presence of an association, which led to which. The technical term is 'direction of causality'. Information bias is also a problem. The EURODEP consortium, studying late-life depression across Europe, identified strong and consistent associations between disability (more than physical health conditions) and depression (Braam et al 2005). Patel and Kleinman, reviewing 11 cross-sectional studies of common mental disorder from six low- and middle-income countries, reported consistent associations with low levels of education, rather than with income levels which were less consistently associated (Patel & Kleinman 2003).

Nationally representative surveys of mental health have now been conducted in many countries and regions worldwide, including the Great Britain National Psychiatric Morbidity Survey (Jenkins et al 1997a); the US National Comorbidity Survey (Kessler et al 1994, 2005); the Australian National Survey of Mental Health and Wellbeing (Slade et al 2009); the New Zealand Mental Health Survey (Wells et al 2006) and the European Study of the Epidemiology of Mental Disorders (ESEMeD) (Alonso et al 2004). Several of these studies have participated in a wider venture, the World Mental Health Survey (Demyttenaere et al 2004), using a common methodology, including structured DSM-IV diagnoses derived using the World Health Organization's Composite International Diagnostic Interview (CIDI 3.0).

The incidence study

Incidence studies start with a group of people who do not have the disease, and follow them up over time to measure the incidence rates (the rate at which new cases develop in the population). Incidence risk is defined as the probability of occurrence of disease in a disease free population (population at risk) during a specified time period. There is now a wealth of data on the incidence of schizophrenia. A recent meta-analysis of over 100 studies from 33 countries indicated a wide variation in rates with a median of 15.2/100 000 person years, with a 10th centile of 7.7 and a 90th centile of 43.0 per 100 000 years (McGrath et al 2004). Incidence was generally higher in males compared to females. Studies conducted in urban catchment areas generated higher rates, and the distribution of rates in migrants was significantly higher compared to native-born.

Note that the 1-year prevalence of schizophrenia is approximately 30–40 times greater than the annual incidence risk. Prevalence (P) is approximately equal to the product of incidence (I) and disease duration (T): $P = I \times T$. Disease is terminated either by death or recovery. For conditions with high short-term mortality rates (lung cancer) or short-term recovery rates (common cold), prevalence and incidence rates are similar. Schizophrenia is evidently a chronic condition.

Studying geographic variation

Early studies of schizophrenia have reported clusters of strikingly low prevalence (e.g. among the Hutterite Anabaptist sect in the USA) (Nimgaonkar et al 2000) and an unusually high prevalence (e.g. in Croatia) (Cooper & Eagles 1994). Such findings can be used to generate hypotheses about aetiology, to the extent to

Table 9.5 Case–control and cohort studies: characteristics, advantages and disadvantages

	Case–control	Cohort
Subjects selected according to:	Caseness	Exposure
Perspective	Retrospective (subjects recall exposure)	Prospective (usually) (observers attend outcome)
Sources of bias	Selection Information (recall and observer)	Information (observer only) Non-response
Resources	Quick Relatively cheap	Lengthy Relatively expensive
Useful for	Rare outcomes Single exposures Multiple exposures	Rare exposures Single exposures Multiple outcomes
Measure of effect	Odds ratio	Relative risk

Experimental studies

Randomized controlled trials

Randomized controlled trials are experimental studies. Given the tightly controlled experimental conditions, it may be possible to make direct causal inferences from effects observed to be associated with a particular treatment condition. The ability to make these inferences relies on two essential conditions for a well-conducted trial: blinding and randomized allocation.

A trial is double-blind if neither the participant nor the investigator knows the treatment condition to which the subject has been randomized; it is single blind if the investigator knows but the participant does not. Blinding is an essential condition for a rigorous trial. Information bias may otherwise be a problem. Participants who believe themselves to be receiving an effective treatment may report a falsely positive outcome, and investigators may also bias their assessment of outcome if they know the treatment condition. The adequacy of blinding can be assessed by asking participant or investigator, as appropriate, to guess the participant's random allocation. Blinding the participant can be difficult, or impossible where psychological rather than pharmacological therapies are being trialled. Blinding the investigator should still be feasible.

Assuming that randomization is carried out properly and that the trial is large, then all potential confounding factors, anticipated and unanticipated, should be evenly distributed between the different treatment conditions. Any difference in outcome between the groups should then be attributable to the treatment alone. Confounding should not be a problem unless randomization procedures have failed. This may occur through chance alone, particularly if the trial is small, or through non-random interference with the allocation procedure. The advantages of randomization can also be lost if the data analysis is restricted to those participants who complete the trial. An *intention to treat analysis* analyses all on the basis of their initial randomized allocation, regardless of whether they initiated, complied with or completed the intervention as planned.

The practice of clinical psychiatry is increasingly evidence-based. In the field of treatment and care for people with schizophrenia, the Cochrane Collaboration aims to encourage and disseminate evidence-based practice by sponsoring meticulous and comprehensive reviews and judicious meta-analyses of accumulated data. As the evidence-base develops, then so, increasingly, trials compare one drug with other older treatments rather than placebo (Hunter et al 2003). This can sometimes mean that the evidence for core efficacy is often not as well-established as one would like, and rather reliant on industry sponsored trials (Rattehalli et al 2010). Increasingly, trials are also being conducted into the delivery of care, illustrating, for example, the superiority of intensive case management over other models of provision (Dieterich et al 2010). However, other popular innovations, for example early intervention, are not currently supported by clear evidence of effectiveness (Marshall & Rathbone 2006). Clearly, there is a continuing need for such experimental evidence to guide improvement in care, and cost-effectiveness in service delivery.

Inference

Inference is the 'process of passing from observations to generalizations'. As such, this is a key activity in epidemiological investigation. We have seen already that the observation of an association need not signify that the risk factor *causes* the outcome with which it is associated. The role of chance, bias, confounding and reverse causality first needs to assessed. Only if these competing explanations can be confidently excluded may a causal attribution be considered.

Chance

Statistical inference involves generalizing from sample data to the wider population from which the sample was drawn. Inferences are made by calculating the probability that, given the size of the sample, chance alone might have accounted for a given observation.

Sampling error and sampling distributions

Chance operates through sampling error. If we wanted to know the average height of boys aged 16 in the UK, we would not go to the trouble of measuring the height of every male of that age. We would instead draw a representative sample from a population register. Random selection of participants should ensure representativeness. However, if the sample was relatively small, say 100 boys, then it is quite likely that, by chance, we would happen to sample those who were on average slightly taller or slightly shorter than 16-year-olds in general. If we repeat the study over and over again, drawing each time a sample of 100 boys, and measuring the mean height on each occasion,

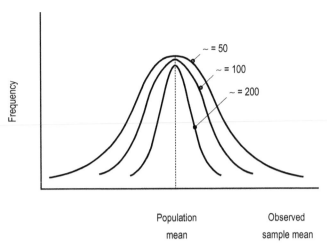

Figure 9.3 • Sampling distribution for different sample sizes.

we would end up with a *sampling distribution* as in Figure 9.3. The observed means from repeated sampling are normally distributed. This tends to be true even if the trait itself is not normally distributed in the population (the proof is referred to as the central limit theorem). The mean (and median and mode) of the sampling distribution are equal to the population mean; sample estimates for the mean that deviate considerably from the true population mean are observed much less commonly, and are represented in the tails of the distribution. Note that if the size of the samples is increased, then the variance of the means obtained through repeated sampling decreases. This is because larger samples tend to give more precise estimates.

Standard errors and confidence intervals

The standard deviation for the sampling distribution is known as the standard error of the mean, and has the property that 95% of sample means obtained by repeated sampling lie ± 2 (actually 1.96) standard errors above or below the population mean. This information can therefore be used to construct limits of uncertainty around an observed sample mean, giving the range of likely values for the population mean. These limits of uncertainty are referred to as 95% confidence intervals. The standard error of the mean is the standard deviation of the population (usually estimated as the standard deviation of the sample) divided by the square root of the sample size. Thus, the observed mean height of the sample of 100 boys might be 160 cm with a standard deviation of 40 cm. The standard error of the mean would then be: $40/\sqrt{100} = 4$ cm. The 95% confidence intervals would then be $160 \text{ cm} \pm 4 \times 1.96$, or 152–168 cm. This would signify that given the sample size and the variance of heights in the sample, there would be a 95% probability that the true mean height of the whole population of 16-year-olds would lie between 152 cm and 168 cm, with only a 5% probability that it lay outside. In descriptive studies, statistical inference therefore allows us to estimate the precision of sample estimates of measures, such as mean anxiety score or prevalence of depression.

In analytical epidemiology, however, we test hypotheses; for example, that those exposed to obstetric complications are more likely to go on to develop schizophrenia than those not so exposed. Statistical inference still works in much the same way as with descriptive studies. Now we are using a *sample* of a certain size to estimate the real relative risk for the association between obstetric complications and schizophrenia *in the general population*. Sampling error may lead us to observe a relative risk (RR) that is lower or higher than the real population effect. We can calculate the standard error of the RR, and use it to construct 95% confidence intervals around our observed value. Again, there will be a 95% probability that the true RR lies within these confidence intervals, and a 5% probability that it lies outside. Thus, in the study of OCs and schizophrenia, an observed RR of 2.0 with 95% confidence intervals of 1.4–2.6 would suggest that a true RR <1.4 or >2.6 would be extremely unlikely (<2.5% probability in each case).

Statistical tests and *p* values

Statistical tests test whether a hypothesis about the distribution of one or more variables should be accepted or rejected. In the case of a hypothesized association between a risk factor and a disease, we can estimate the probability (*p*) of the observed or an even greater degree of association being observed if the null hypothesis were true, i.e. accounted for by chance alone, there being no association. Conventionally, the threshold for statistical significance is taken to be 0.05. This means that, for a population in which two factors were *not* associated, if the same study with the same sample size were to be repeated 100 times, then on average an association of at least the size observed might be recorded five times. It is important to remember that there is nothing magical about the $p = 0.05$ threshold. It represents nothing more than a generally agreed acceptable level of risk of making what is known as a Type I error, i.e. falsely rejecting a null hypothesis when it is true. The probability of rejecting the null hypothesis when it is indeed false (i.e. detecting a true association) is the study's statistical power. The converse scenario, accepting a null hypothesis when it should have been rejected (i.e. failing to detect a true association), is referred to as a Type II error, and the probability of committing this error is clearly (1 – power) (Table 9.6).

Table 9.6 Type I and Type II errors

Null hypothesis	True	False
Accepted	No association Null hypothesis correctly accepted	True association, but null hypothesis mistakenly accepted Type II error Probability = 1 – power
Rejected	No association, but chance observation mistakenly leads to rejection of null hypothesis Type I error Probability = significance	True association, correctly identified Probability = power

The relationship between *p* values and confidence intervals

If we return to the example of the study assessing the association between obstetric complications and schizophrenia, we can see that confidence intervals (CI) convey all of the information given by *p* values, and more besides. The 95% CI for the RR 1.4–2.6, tell us immediately that the null hypothesis RR of 1.0 is implausible given the observed value of 2.0, and thus that the null hypothesis can be rejected with reasonable confidence. The probability of a true RR of 1.0 is certainly <5% and thus the association is 'statistically significant' at $p<0.05$. However, the confidence intervals also give us a range of plausible values, both upper and lower, for the true RR.

Bias

Bias is a special type of error. Most error is random, arising either from sampling error or simple lack of precision in measurement. Such error is equally likely to result in higher or lower estimates. Bias, however, is a non-random or systematic error. In the case of simple descriptive measurements, bias may arise because, for example, a doctor taking blood pressure rounds up every measurement to the next 5 mmHg mark. The estimate of the mean blood pressure level for the population will clearly be biased upwards. In the case of estimating associations, bias occurs where error operates differentially with respect to both exposure and outcome. Thus, in a case–control study addressing the hypothesis that depressed people had low blood pressure, the doctor taking the blood pressure measurements might round up the blood pressure levels of controls but round *down* the blood pressure levels of depressed cases. This bias would overestimate the strength of any true association, or perhaps produce a wholly spurious association between depression and low blood pressure.

Bias is an entirely undesirable feature that cannot be adjusted for once data have been gathered (contrast with confounding below). The epidemiologist's only hope is to limit the scope for bias in the way in which the study has been designed. There are several different types of bias. The most common are:

- Selection bias
- Non-response bias
- Information bias, including:
  - Recall bias
  - Observer bias.

Selection bias

Selection bias is a potential problem wherever individuals are selected for inclusion in a study because of the presence or absence of certain characteristics. This is particularly an issue in case–control studies, where controls are selected to be as similar as possible to the cases who are included in the study, except that they do not have the disease. The golden rule in designing case–control studies is that a control should be eligible to be included as a case, should they develop the disease, and a case should be eligible to be a control if they did not have the disease. A case–control study seeking to identify risk factors for Alzheimer disease, found that arthritis was more common among controls than among cases (Broe et al 1990). This finding might have been taken to suggest that arthritis was in some way protective against AD. However, this case–control study recruited its cases from among new cases of AD recently referred to specialist dementia clinics. Its age and sex-matched controls were selected at random from among patients *attending* primary care surgeries. The flaw in this selection procedure, as the authors of the study acknowledged, was that the controls needed some reason to visit their doctor. One of the most common reasons in this age group was arthritic aches and pains. Had the dementia cases not developed Alzheimer disease, they might not have been eligible to be controls, because they may not have needed to visit their doctor. The cases, simply because of the different selection procedures for cases and controls, were less likely than the controls to have had to have a history of arthritis. This is selection bias. Selection bias can be minimized by following the 'golden rule' cited above. Selection of cases and controls is a critical component of case–control studies. It needs to be attended to very carefully, and inclusion and exclusion criteria described in detail in published papers.

Non-response bias

Non-response bias can occur when subjects who refuse to take part in a study, or who drop out before the study can be completed, are systematically different from those who participate. In simple descriptive epidemiology, for example, the prevalence of depression in a community may be underestimated if those with depression are less likely to participate in the cross-sectional survey than those without depression. An association between lack of social support and depression may be overestimated either if those with good social support are less likely to take part if they are depressed or if those with poor social support are less likely to take part if they are not depressed. Again, note that when an association between an exposure and a disease is being estimated, bias will only occur if the error operates differentially with respect *to both*.

Non-response bias can be minimized by minimizing non-response. Non-response becomes a critical issue when response rates fall below 70%, but significant non-response bias can still occur even at these levels of participation. The likelihood of non-response bias having occurred can be assessed (although not quantified) by comparing the characteristics of responders and non-responders. Usually, some basic sociodemographic information such as age and sex is available from the register or database from which the subjects have been recruited. Similarity of responders and non-responders in terms at least of these basic characteristics is reassuring but does not exclude the possibility that bias has occurred.

Information bias

Recall bias occurs when participants in a study are systematically more or less likely to recall and relate information on exposure depending on their outcome status, or to recall information regarding their outcome dependent on their exposure. This form of bias can be a particular problem in case–control studies. Thus, cases with multiple episodes of major depression as an adult may be more likely to recall and report childhood abuse than controls with no history of mental health problems. Often, the experience of having the disease that is being studied encourages an 'effort after meaning', whereby the person who is a case has already gone over his/her life history in an attempt to understand why he/she had become ill. This clearly predisposes to recall bias.

Observer bias is another form of information bias caused by an investigator incorrectly ascertaining or recording data from a participant in a study. Again, for bias to be a problem, the error must be systematic with respect to both exposure and outcome. The example given above of the investigator selectively rounding up and rounding down blood pressure measurements is an example of observer bias. Alternatively, an investigator who believes that child sexual abuse does cause major depression in adulthood might put extra effort into obtaining disclosure of abuse from subjects whom they knew to be in the depression case group.

Information bias can be reduced in case–control studies by keeping participants and observers blind to the hypotheses under investigation. This can be difficult, and some would argue may challenge the ethical principal of informed consent. However, biased research results are wrong, misleading and a waste of subjects' time. Blinding can be encouraged by making the title of the study non-specific, and by including irrelevant questions in the risk factor questionnaire to distract subjects from the central hypothesis under investigation. Information bias will be less of a problem in cohort studies because neither exposed nor unexposed participants or the investigators know who will go on to develop the disease that is being studied, when their exposure status is ascertained at the beginning of the study.

Confounding

The term confounding derives from the Latin *confundere*, meaning to mix up. Confounding describes a situation in which a measure of the effect of an exposure is distorted because of the association of that exposure with other factors that influence the disease or outcome under study. A confounding variable can cause or prevent the outcome of interest, is not an intermediate variable and is independently associated with the exposure under investigation.

The concept of confounding is best illustrated with an example. Clearly, there is an association between grey hair and the risk of dying. Some imaginary but plausible data are given in Table 9.7. While there is an association between grey hair and

risk for dying, this association is a spurious one, accounted for entirely by the confounding effect of a third variable, age. Thus older people are more likely to have grey hair, and independently (i.e. for reasons entirely unconnected with the grey hair) are at greater risk of dying (Fig. 9.4). When we carry out a *stratified analysis*, we find that the strong association between grey hair and dying is no longer apparent in each of the different age strata. This example illustrates some of the ways in which we may control for confounding in both the design and the analysis of our studies.

In the design, if we had *matched* our grey-haired and non-grey-haired subjects for the suspected confounding variable (age), then we would have been able to make a fair comparison of the death rates of the two groups. Matching could have been carried out on a one-to-one basis, i.e. for every grey-haired person recruited, we recruit a non-grey-haired person of a similar age, or by restriction matching, i.e. we only recruit those aged 40–60. Randomization is the ultimate technique for control of confounding. Where an intervention can be randomly assigned then *all* other factors should be evenly distributed between the intervention group and the control group. Any difference between the two groups can be reasonably confidently attributed to the intervention. The virtue of the randomized design is that all potential confounders, measured and unmeasured, suspected and unsuspected, are automatically controlled for in the design. Of course, ethically, we can only randomize interventions that we believe may benefit, but where no strong evidence exists one way or the other.

In the analysis of the data, where matching has not been carried out, a stratified analysis of the kind seen in Table 9.7 clearly demonstrates the presence or absence of confounding. There are also more complicated forms of statistical analysis, collectively

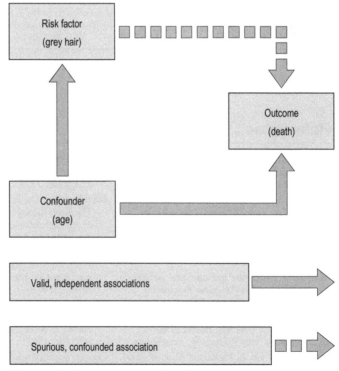

Figure 9.4 • An example of confounding.

Table 9.7 An imaginary example of confounding

	Annual mortality rate		
	Grey hair	No grey hair	RR
All ages	20/1000	5/1000	4.0
20–40 years	1/1000	1/1000	1.0
40–60	10/1000	10/1000	1.0
60+ years	40/1000	40/1000	1.0

Critical appraisal

Reviewing scientific evidence and reading academic papers

10

William Lee   Matthew Hotopf

CHAPTER CONTENTS

Introduction

The duty of the clinician is to use medical knowledge to help patients through correct diagnosis and appropriate treatments. Such medical knowledge, initially acquired in training, is updated as new discoveries are made, but its rate of creation is very great and continues to increase. Much is contradictory, so textbooks such as this exist to distil the literature into that which might reasonably be thought of as 'fact'. Textbooks take time to create, so they can never reflect the most up-to-date knowledge. Further, there is necessarily much simplification, and the choice of material may not be representative, so the knowledge clinicians acquire may be old or distorted, leading to compromised care.

Evidence-based medicine

An approach named 'Evidence-based medicine' (EBM) arose in the 1990s and intended to address these problems. Medical activity informed by evidence was not new (an early clinical trial – on treatments for scurvy – was carried out by James Lind in 1747), but EBM recognized the continuous development of medical knowledge and made it explicit that clinicians should have the skills to assess the scientific literature, rather than absorbing fully formed 'facts' from experts. It has been defined as 'the conscientious and judicious use of current best evidence from clinical care research in the management of individual patients' (Sackett et al 1996). It is an effort to help the clinician be closer to the literature.

There are parts of EBM relevant to clinical directors, health care managers and clinicians, but this chapter will concentrate on evaluating published literature on a particular topic.

Scientific papers and journals

The unit of scientific activity is the 'paper': an article describing some new scientific work written by the team who carried it out. Papers are collected and published in scientific journals. The conventional structure of a paper is an introduction setting the scene, providing a rationale and the explicit aims of the work, followed by a description of what was done (the *Methods*), what was found (the *Results*) and an explanation of what it means (the *Discussion*). There are usually many references throughout, and it is important that an individual paper, which describes particular work in which particular choices were made, is not considered in isolation from the wider literature.

The first scientific journals were published in 1665 in France and England. It is difficult to overstate the importance of their development. Before this, individuals risked losing recognition for their discoveries if they made them public, so they tended to work in isolation until they had a complete process. Once there were scientific journals, a person could 'stake a claim' to recognition for intellectual developments, reducing the need for secrecy. Ideas could build on each other, greatly speeding the process of discovery.

Since the first journals were founded, there has been an enormous and continuously accelerating growth in their number and the total output they publish. According to the website Psychwatch.Com, in December 2009 there were 994 journals concerning psychiatry alone. This number is likely to continue to increase.

Reading the literature

As noted above, the literature is vast: no-one can read all of the published work in even a tiny area of study, and a busy clinician could never reasonably be expected to read the whole of the output of even one psychiatric journal, let alone do justice to the hundreds of others. The problem may seem overwhelming. How can clinical decisions be informed by academic work when to keep abreast of the published work, a clinician could never see any patients?

Fortunately, some papers are more deserving of attention than others. Reading can be concentrated on only those papers on subjects which are particularly relevant and of the best methodological quality available.

Defining a clinical problem

It is common in clinical practice to come across a situation where the correct course of action is uncertain. It is here that EBM practices can improve outcomes for patients and make the job of the clinician more satisfying. Some time spent formulating the question and searching the literature for the answer can be expected to improve outcomes for not only this patient, but future similar patients too. A recent development of an experienced medical librarian attending weekly clinical multidisciplinary meetings, collecting clinical questions and reporting back with the state of the literature is gaining acceptance (Gorring et al 2010). For example, an elderly man is in the general hospital suffering with pneumonia but has developed delirium with psychotic symptoms. Is an antipsychotic medication likely to reduce his symptoms?

Grades of evidence

There are numerous similar 'hierarchy of evidence' schemes, which are used in many different ways, including the creation of the local or regional guidances, which are now widespread. The one published by the Oxford Centre for Evidence Based Medicine (2009) is shown in Table 10.1.

Studies of different designs are differentially vulnerable to the various errors which may affect findings. At the top of these schemes are systematic reviews, followed by randomized-controlled trials, cohort studies, case–control studies, cross-sectional studies, case series, case reports and lastly, expert opinion. Clinical decisions should be informed by the highest level of evidence available.

Therefore, the first type of publication which should be sought is a systematic review, which also includes the various rigorously-created evidence-based guidances from organizations such as the National Institute of health and Clinical Excellence (NICE), as well as reviews published by the Cochrane Collaboration, which may not always appear in peer-reviewed journals (although they are peer-reviewed). Only if there is no reasonably up-to-date systematic review should a search of primary literature be undertaken.

Technology is moving at such a rate that we are loath to advise on internet search techniques, but the search string: 'Cochrane review delirium antipsychotics' typed into Google in December 2009 yielded a link to the abstract of the Cochrane Review, 'Antipsychotics for delirium' by Lonergan et al (2007), which has a three-line summary delivering the take-home message in simple language. This may seem similar to using a textbook, but there are important differences. First, connecting a review directly to a clinician misses out the time-consuming process of textbook writing. Second, no textbook could ever contain the enormous quantity of information which was searched to deliver that page of information. Third, and most importantly, the authors of the review described exactly how they carried out their own search of the literature and which studies they examined, which allows this review itself to be critically appraised, compared with other published reviews for quality and, vitally, the relevance to the clinical situation can be accurately gauged. For example, the studies incorporated into that systematic review may have recruited only young people or people suffering with particular co-morbidities. See Box 10.1 for details of how to read systematic reviews.

Had there been no suitable systematic review or guidance, then Google Scholar, PUBMED or other tools can be used to search the primary literature for randomized controlled trials and other study designs which may be pertinent to the issue. If the reader commences on this course of action, he or she is setting out to produce a systematic review of the available literature on the topic of interest of his or her own. This need not mean ploughing through hundreds or thousands of papers. If the clinical problem is tightly defined it is not rare to find oneself examining only one or two papers. The remainder of this chapter contains guidance on how to read and evaluate individual papers and some worked examples of particular problems.

Reading a paper

When thinking about reading a paper, it is important to consider the academic process as a whole. Researchers carry out the work and write it up. They send the manuscript to a journal and the editor selects a number of reviewers (experts in the field – the authors' peers) who then (usually) anonymously 'peer-review' the manuscript. The reviewers will closely scrutinize the manuscript and judge whether it should be accepted for publication, rejected, or returned to the authors for more detail or explanation to be included. This process means that whoever the intended final audience of a paper, the people for whom it is actually written are the reviewers, so the level of detail and complexity may be too much for someone reading with a clinical problem in mind. This does not mean that the detail is

Table 10.1 Oxford Centre for Evidence-based Medicine Levels of Evidence (May 2001)

Level	Therapy prevention, aetiology/harm	Prognosis	Diagnosis	Differential diagnosis/symptom prevalence study	Economic and decision analyses
1a	SR (with homogeneity) of RCTs	SR (with homogeneity) of inception cohort studies; CDR validated in different populations	SR (with homogeneity) of Level 1 diagnostic studies; CDR with 1b studies from different clinical centres	SR (with homogeneity) of prospective cohort studies	SR (with homogeneity) of Level 1 economic studies
1b	Individual RCT (with narrow confidence interval)	Individual inception cohort study with > 80% follow-up; CDR validated in a single population	Validating cohort study with good reference standards; or CDR tested within one clinical centre	Prospective cohort study with good follow-up	Analysis based on clinically sensible costs or alternatives; systematic review(s) of the evidence; and including multi-way sensitivity analyses
1c	All or none	All or none case series	Absolute SpPins and SnNouts	All or none case series	Absolute better-value or worse-value analyses
2a	SR (with homogeneity) of cohort studies	SR (with homogeneity) of either retrospective cohort studies or untreated control groups in RCTs	SR (with homogeneity) of Level >2 diagnostic studies	SR (with homogeneity) of 2b and better studies	SR (with homogeneity) of Level >2 economic studies
2b	Individual cohort study (including low quality RCT; e.g. <80% follow-up)	Retrospective cohort study or follow-up of untreated control patients in an RCT; Derivation of CDR or validated on split-sample only	Exploratory cohort study with good reference standards; CDR after derivation, or validated only on split-sample or databases	Retrospective cohort study, or poor follow-up	Analysis based on clinically sensible costs or alternatives; limited review(s) of the evidence, or single studies; and including multi-way sensitivity analyses
2c	'Outcomes' research; ecological studies	'Outcomes' research		Ecological studies	Audit or outcomes research
3a	SR (with homogeneity) of case–control studies		SR (with homogeneity) of 3b and better studies	SR (with homogeneity) of 3b and better studies	SR (with homogeneity) of 3b and better studies
3b	Individual case–control study		Non-consecutive study; or without consistently applied reference standards	Non-consecutive cohort study, or very limited population	Analysis based on limited alternatives or costs, poor quality estimates of data, but including sensitivity analyses incorporating clinically sensible variations
4	Case series (and poor quality cohort and case–control studies)	Case series (and poor quality prognostic cohort studies)	Case–control study, poor or non-independent reference standard	Case series or superseded reference standards	Analysis with no sensitivity analysis
5	Expert opinion without explicit critical appraisal, or based on physiology, bench research or 'first principles'	Expert opinion without explicit critical appraisal, or based on physiology, bench research or 'first principles'	Expert opinion without explicit critical appraisal, or based on physiology, bench research or 'first principles'	Expert opinion without explicit critical appraisal, or based on physiology, bench research or 'first principles'	Expert opinion without explicit critical appraisal, or based on economic theory or 'first principles'

Produced by Bob Phillips, Chris Ball, Dave Sackett, Doug Badenoch, Sharon Straus, Brian Haynes, Martin Dawes, November 1998.

completely unimportant; this is how the reader judges the methodological quality and relevance of the work. While the peer-review process exists to increase the quality and reliability of published research, it is far from perfect, so publication in a peer-reviewed journal alone should not be considered a mark of good methodology and research practice. Below are outlined a series of questions which a reader with a clinical question to answer will probably want to address. Of course, there are numerous reasons to read a paper, from mild passing interest to the creation of a new research grant proposal, but here we are concentrating on the clinician attempting to use scientific evidence to answer a clinical question.

Box 10.2

Randomized controlled trials

Participants in a multicentre randomized controlled trial were recruited from primary care and were randomly assigned to receive either five weekly sessions of problem solving or the tricyclic antidepressant amitriptyline. The outcome is assessed by the general practitioner using the Hamilton Rating Scale for Depression at 6 weeks.

Questions and answers

What problems could occur with the randomization and what descriptions would you like to see covered? The main point about this study is that both the doctor and patient are obviously aware that the patient has been prescribed an antidepressant or been enrolled into problem-solving. This is in contrast with the usual 'blinded' (sometimes known as 'masked') drug trials, where not only are patients randomly assigned to receive one of two or more identical tablets, so the patients do not know which they are getting, but also the doctor does not know either. This is known as a *double-blind* trial. Non-blinding has an impact on the randomization, the treatment, and the assessment of the outcome. The problem in randomizing in this trial is that the doctor may have a view about who would and who would not benefit from problem-solving or antidepressants. If the doctor was also delivering the problem-solving intervention, they might only want the most cooperative patients to be allocated into this group. The randomization must *conceal allocation* adequately, such that it is impossible for the doctor to *predict* which patient would go into which group. For example, in some *quasi-randomized* designs, patients would get one treatment if randomized on an odd day of the month, or another treatment if randomized on the even days. It is thus easy to put the randomization off one day, and give the patient the treatment

the investigator thinks will be best for them. In the above example there is also an opportunity to cheat. If the doctor was randomizing patients him- or herself, and the patient was randomized to what he/she saw as the 'wrong' group, the doctor might 'forget' that the patient had been randomized, and try again, hoping that this time they would go into the 'right' group! Such fraudulent practice has happened, and therefore clinical trialists spend much time and energy making sure cheating cannot occur. Good randomized trials will report exactly how the randomization was performed.

It is worth noting that the adequacy of randomization reporting is related to whether 'positive' findings are reported. Trials that use inadequate methods of randomization are far more likely to report 'positive' findings than those that do not, indicating that cheating the randomization may impact upon the research findings (Schulz et al 1995). Improper randomization is akin to selection bias: there is a systematic bias whereby one group is likely to have a worse outcome than the other group.

What problems might arise with the assessment of the outcome? The danger of using the assessment as described is that it could introduce observer bias. The Hamilton Rating Scale for Depression is unstructured: it gives the clinician guidelines on how to assess the severity of depression based on their clinical interview. When the researcher is not blinded to the treatment group to which the patients have been allocated, there is considerable room for observer bias.

Which techniques could reduce such observer bias? There are two main techniques. One would be to blind the rater to the treatment group. The other would be to use a written questionnaire so the doctor is not involved in assessing the outcomes at all.

 Box 10.3

Cohort studies

A study examined the effect of depression as a risk factor for myocardial infarction. Patients with a history of depression were recruited from a psychiatric service and compared with non-depressed individuals identified from general practice lists. The two cohorts were then followed for 10 years, at the end of which those who had died were identified from death certificates. The remaining sample were sent questionnaires in the post, asking whether they had suffered a heart attack or stroke in the past 10 years.

A total of 75% of the survivors with depression responded, whereas 60% of the non-depressed survivors responded. The study found that the rate of non-fatal myocardial infarction was twice as high in the depressed group compared to the non-depressed.

Questions and answers

Could the result have arisen from reverse causality? This is possible, even though a cohort design was used. Cohort studies normally exclude people with the outcome of interest (i.e. heart disease) at the outset. However, there is no evidence that this happened from the above description. Some cohort studies in this area have taken *retrospective* samples of people with depression. This means they may not have been thoroughly assessed at the start of the study. Because heart disease (e.g. angina) is associated with depression, the depressed group may have started off with higher rates of heart disease than the non-depressed, and the result could simply reflect this relationship.

Why might the response rate have differed for the depressed versus the non-depressed? As in the discussion of cross-sectional studies, people with psychiatric disorders may be more or less likely to participate in research. In this case, the people with depression were more likely to be followed-up. This may reflect less mobility among the depressed group (in other words they remained at the same address and were therefore easier to contact at follow-up) or greater interest in participating in research due to their experience of illness.

Could the differential response rate have caused a problem? It certainly is a potential problem. The overall follow-up rate is not especially good. If the non-depressed non-responders had a systematically higher rate of myocardial infarction than the depressed non-responders, this would suggest the reported association is exaggerated.

Are there any additional explanations for the association? Apart from chance, the other possibilities are recall bias, observer bias and confounding. Recall bias could occur if subjects with depression may be more likely to experience chest pain of non-cardiac origin, and to interpret this as a heart attack. Confounding could occur if those with depression had more risk factors for heart attack (smoking, high serum cholesterol or demographic risk factors such as coming from more deprived backgrounds). Observer bias could occur if either group were more assiduously investigated for heart disease.

Box 10.4

Case–control studies

A group of virologists were interested to know whether a particular viral infection was a risk factor for chronic fatigue syndrome (CFS). They ran a clinical service that had attracted patients with debilitating fatigue for some years, and had previously published an influential paper suggesting this hypothesis. They decided to perform a case–control study comparing patients with post-viral fatigue syndrome and healthy controls. They devised a clinical diagnosis of post-viral fatigue syndrome that included debilitating fatigue lasting at least 6 months and a history of viral infection preceding the onset of fatigue.

They decided to measure exposure by estimating viral antibodies (IgG). The healthy control group was identified by asking cases to identify a friend or neighbour who was not fatigued. The research group found that 50% of those with post-viral fatigue had IgG to the infection, whereas only 15% of those without fatigue had antibodies.

Questions and answers

How might the case definition used affect the prevalence of viral antibodies in the cases? The case definition of those affected is not independent of exposure. In other words, in order to be a case, you have to have reported the exposure under study (i.e. viral infection). This is called *ascertainment bias* – the way in which the study population is ascertained has biased the results of the study. Note the circularity; in order to be a case, you have to have recalled exposure to a viral infection. It is therefore no surprise that the cases have higher rates of antibodies.

Could the selection of patients into the clinic have affected the results? The clinic was run by a team who were keen on a certain hypothesis. Local GPs may have been especially keen to refer patients who reported fatigue, and who they also knew had a history of the infection. In other words, there could have been *selection bias* too. It is probably unusual to refer patients to see virologists if there is no history of viral infection.

Could the selection of healthy controls have affected the results? The patients may have selected controls who they knew had not been exposed to a recent viral infection. It is improbable that the patients would have chosen someone just recovering from influenza, hence the controls are not random members of the population. Thus, there could have been a selection bias operating to reduce the chances of exposure among controls.

Selection bias is a common and serious problem in case–control studies. Selection bias is likely to occur in tertiary referral centres, which may represent very unusual populations and where a suitable control group may be difficult to identify. The purpose of the control group is to represent the prevalence of the exposure in the general population *from which the case group is drawn*, and taking into account the various barriers to care, it is difficult to think of, still less recruit, an ideal control group.

Case–control studies are best when they are 'nested' in cross-sectional or cohort studies or where the means of sampling cases is based on some population-based register. In selecting controls, ask: 'If the control had developed the disorder, could he or she have been in the study as a case?' In the example demonstrated above, a control who had chronic fatigue but who had not had a history of viral infection may well not have been included.

Box 10.5

Cross-sectional studies

A cross-sectional study aims to estimate the prevalence of dementia in a community sample of adults aged 65 years or over. The investigators used a database of addresses available from a phone company providing landlines in order to identify their sampling frame. They then sent a letter to a random sample of 1000 adults over 65, inviting them to participate. Those who agreed were seen by a researcher. Those who did not reply were sent a second letter, and later visited by the research team. In the final report, the response rate was reported to be 56%. The estimated prevalence of dementia was 5%.

Questions and answers

How might the sampling procedure have biased the estimate of prevalence? Cross-sectional studies aim to measure prevalence. They therefore need to be representative of the population under study. The sampling frame chosen in this example may not have been representative because:

- *Not everyone has a land-line.* This sampling procedure would not have identified people who did not have a telephone. If people with dementia are less likely to have a telephone, this method would have underestimated dementia prevalence.

- *Many people with dementia will be in long-term residential care.* If the homes they live in did not have individual telephones for each resident, it is again likely that the prevalence of dementia was underestimated.

- *The information from the telephone company may not be typical.* If the company was a relatively new one, people with dementia may have been less likely to have changed company, or vice versa.

These sorts of concerns are especially important in psychiatric disorders where, for many reasons, those affected may be less likely to live at a private residential address. Similar points could be made about surveys of prevalence of schizophrenia that do not consider the homeless population.

Is the response rate likely to have affected the estimated prevalence of dementia? The reported response rate was low – just over half of those eligible were interviewed. It is not hard to see how this sort of survey could get the estimate of prevalence very wrong, if those having the disorder under study were more or less likely to participate. In this example, dementia is likely to affect the ability of sufferers to agree to participate. Those with dementia may be unable to understand the letter or answer it. This sort of problem is common for many psychiatric disorders, including depression and psychotic illness.

Which techniques can be used to assess the impact of non-responders on surveys? Any cross-sectional study should give details of the characteristics of non-responders. For instance, in the example given above of prevalence of dementia, it would be worth knowing whether the non-responders were older than the responders. Age is an important risk factor for dementia, thus if those contacted were, on average 5 years younger than those not contacted, we would be even more concerned about the effects of response bias.

Another useful technique is to guess how far the prevalence estimate could be out by. In the example given above, the estimate could vary enormously. If *all* the non-responders had dementia, the prevalence would rise to 46.8%. Of course it is very unlikely that all non-responders had dementia. However, it is not inconceivable that the rate of dementia was increased three-fold in the non-responders, in which case the total population prevalence would rise to 9.4%. This example illustrates how essential response rates are for cross-sectional studies.

Biological research which, for example, applies a new technology (imaging, neuroendocrine challenge tests, etc.) to a series of patients and compares the results with a control group, often does not name the study design. This sort of research is an example of case–control study design, and is susceptible to the serious flaws inherent to that design. For example, a study that uses functional magnetic resonance imaging on 20 patients with schizophrenia and compares the results with 20 healthy controls can suffer from selection bias (see Box 10.4) which can often overwhelm the true effect, especially if the researcher has used highly educated colleagues or juniors to act as controls. This practice is now discouraged (for both ethical and scientific reasons) but still continues, especially in investigations of more 'biological' exposures where it may seem to some that the exact process by which controls are recruited does not matter (Lee et al 2007).

A useful test of the adequacy of a paper's *Methods* section is whether another researcher would have a chance of replicating the study on the information provided. Would they know how the participants were recruited, what questions they were asked or treatments they received? Inadequacy in this regard is common (Lee et al 2007) and this observation is not new (Altman 1994). This is poor practice. Efforts to improve reporting (and methodology) have included various checklists and guides for authors to use. The most widespread of these is the CONSORT (CONsolidated Standards Of Reporting Trials) statement which tightly specifies the reporting and methodology of randomized controlled trials (Moher et al 2001; Altman et al 2001), but there are others, including the STROBE Statement for observational studies (von Elm et al 2007) and the MOOSE guidelines for reviews of observational studies (Stroup et al 2000). These may not be mentioned by name in a paper, but a little familiarization with these short texts will help the reader judge the quality of the reporting of the primary research.

What are the main results?

The next step is to examine the main results of the paper. These are usually to be found in the *Abstract*, in the *Results* section, including the tables, and at the start of the *Discussion* section. Results can be presented in many different ways depending on the study design, outcomes and statistical techniques used.

Good research should always give the reader a feel for the data. You should expect to see a table where the data are described in a simple way, without complicated statistics. For example, in a cohort study, it is reasonable to see how those exposed to the risk factor compare to those not exposed to it. Are they similar in terms of their main sociodemographic characteristics? Be suspicious if the only results you see are the results of sophisticated statistical models. Data presentation should be transparent.

Ways of describing a finding

Another consideration in digesting the results is the exact form they take. Consider a hypothetical case–control study of obstetric complications in schizophrenia. The paper found that 20% of cases (with schizophrenia) and only 10% of controls (without

schizophrenia) had a history of obstetric complications. Leaving aside alternative explanations for this association (which are discussed below), then each of the following statements could describe these results:

'Individuals with schizophrenia were more likely to report obstetric complications than were controls.'

'Individuals with schizophrenia had a statistically significant (<0.05) higher level of reported obstetric complications than controls.'

'Some 20% of our participants with schizophrenia had obstetric complications as opposed to 10% of controls.'

'Schizophrenia was associated with more reported obstetric complications (odds ratio 2.0; 95% confidence interval 1.1–3.5).'

'Schizophrenia was associated with more reported obstetric complications (odds ratio 2.0; 95% confidence interval 1.1–3.5). Given a population rate of obstetric complications of 10% the population attributable fraction was 9.1%.'

Each statement is describing the same result, but with increasing sophistication. There are five components to these results:

1. The simple result: schizophrenia is associated with obstetric complications
2. The level of statistical significance (described as a *p* value)
3. The effect size (i.e. the fact that 20% of those with schizophrenia vs 10% of those without it had obstetric complications. The odds ratio is also an expression of effect size)
4. The precision of the estimate of effect size (described as the confidence intervals around the odds ratio)
5. The population impact of the exposure. This is the population attributable fraction, which is described in the previous chapter, and is the proportion of cases of schizophrenia that would be avoided if obstetric complications were directly causal and could be eradicated.

Note that the effect size is much more interesting than the level of statistical significance. In older studies, it is very common to see results presented almost solely as *p* values, but it is difficult to understand what this means. With a sufficiently large sample size, it is possible for even very small effect sizes (e.g. an odds ratio of 1.1) to become highly statistically significant. However, it is the effect size combined with the level of significance, rather than the level of significance alone that should determine how much faith the reader will have in the result. As a rule of thumb for observational studies (cross-sectional, case-control and cohort), an odds ratio (OR) or relative risk of <2 is easily produced as a result of bias or confounding. Unless the study is large and well conducted, this sort of effect size should be interpreted with caution. Randomized controlled trials are by no means immune to bias and confounding, but are less susceptible, and therefore smaller effect sizes can be given more credence.

Similarly, a large effect size with very great statistical significance with a miniscule population-attributable fraction may be interesting and important for further research but is unlikely to be of interest to clinicians or (rational) policy-makers. An example of this would be the lethality of a direct meteor strike. If, by some process, this risk could be removed then a highly lethal event could be prevented, but it is so rare that this large expense would have a negligible benefit to the population (see 'A boy claims he was hit by a meteorite' 2009).

What alternative explanations are there?

Good papers point their readers to potential flaws in the research, usually in the *Discussion* section. In some journals, authors are now required to describe the shortcomings for their paper (*British Journal of Psychiatry* 2009). Usually the main shortcomings may be addressed by thinking of the list of alternative explanations of reported associations. These were covered in the previous chapter and are chance, bias, confounding and reverse causality.

Whenever one examines a research finding, it is important to consider each of the possible alternative explanations before giving the straightforward idea of the exposure giving the outcome much credence. It is important for the reader to do this dispassionately because the researchers may have chosen to downplay certain possibilities. Ultimately, human judgement enters the analysis and writing up of results, and no matter how eminent the researchers or peer-reviewers, it is not uncommon for alternative explanations still to be at play.

Chance

Type I and Type II error

Most studies aim to describe reality by taking a sample of the total population and making an *inference* about the population from the sample. However, the sample will not exactly describe the true underlying population distribution; there is always a degree of *sampling error*. This is akin to tossing 10 coins several times and counting different combinations of heads and tails each time. We know *a priori* to expect an unbiased coin to fall with equal probability on heads or tails. Therefore with 10 tosses, the most probable result would be five heads and five tails (which happens about a quarter of the time), but of course any combination of heads and tails is possible. More extreme results (e.g. all tails or all heads) become less probable with increasing numbers of tosses of the coin. In other words, increasing the sample size increases the precision with which the underlying 'true' situation (describing all fair coins) can be estimated. In the example of schizophrenia and obstetric complications described above, we assume that the study is representing reality. Nevertheless, if 10 identical studies were performed, they would produce a variety of results. The size of the difference would depend upon the size of the sample in each study.

Studies that report a 'positive' finding (e.g. they find an association between obstetric complications and schizophrenia) may either be describing the true underlying situation, or (by chance) be reporting a Type I error. Type I error occurs where an association is detected in the sample by chance, but is absent from the population. This is assessed by statistical testing. By convention, the Type I error rate is usually set at $p<0.05$, in other words the probability of the association being false is 1 in 20. It is more probable that a study will detect a true association if that association is a very powerful one. In other words, it is considerably easier to detect the 10-fold increase in lung cancer among smokers than it is to detect the 1.1-fold increase in schizophrenia among those born in winter months.

Studies that report a negative finding (i.e. find no association between obstetric complications and schizophrenia) may either be describing the true underlying situation, or by chance be

Table 10.2 The relationship between the results of a study and 'true life'

		'True life'	
		Association exists	No association exists
Study	Association found	No error	Type I error
	Association not found	Type II error	No error

Most studies set the Type I error rate at ≤ 0.05 or less, and the Type II error rate at 0.1–0.2. The power of a study is 1 minus the Type II error rate (80–90%).

reporting a Type II error. Type II error is a genuine association being missed by chance. A Type II error is assessed in the design of the study by performing a power calculation. This usually sets the Type II error rate at 10–20%. In other words, most studies that perform a power calculation accept that there is a 10–20% chance that they will fail to detect a true difference. The Type II error rate is usually presented as the statistical power (100 minus the Type II error rate – usually set at 80–90%). Statistical power is increased with larger sample sizes. Type I and Type II errors are shown in tabular form in Table 10.2.

Points to consider if a study reports one or more positive associations

It could still be chance. There is no p value that can 'prove' an association, but by convention we often take 'statistical significance' to mean $p<0.05$. This means that one time in 20 we expect to detect the difference by chance, and there is no way of knowing whether the study we are reading is that one instance. This is why cautious researchers will often make comments such as 'our findings require replication'. It may be that the finding was simply a fluke, even with 'statistically significant' results.

Multiple statistical testing. The more hypotheses tested, the greater the likelihood of finding a significant association. If researchers performed a case–control study of risk factors for dementia, and collected data on 40 possible risk factors, they might expect two such risk factors to be associated at $p<0.05$ just by chance. This leaves researchers and their readers with genuine problems. On the one hand, it seems wasteful not to report all possible associations. On the other, it would be misleading to pretend that some of the results reported could not have occurred by chance.

The best way to overcome this dilemma is for the researcher to set out with one or two main hypotheses to be tested. These would form the centre of the research proposal, and the sample sizes would be determined on these hypotheses. All additional findings can be labelled 'secondary analyses', and be seen as a useful by-product of the main research. This consideration is especially important in randomized trials of new treatments as the results of the research may have direct impact on patients. Of course it is up to the reader to decide whether the '*a priori*' hypotheses described by the researchers really were proposed before the results were analysed. Publishing protocols to research projects in advance transforms the credence given to positive findings because the reader could be sure that the positive finding reported is not the product of an extensive 'fishing expedition' for a positive association.

Publication bias is another problem that may lead to chance positive findings being more evident than a true underlying negative relationship. It occurs when the likelihood of research being published is influenced by the results of that research. Journals may prefer to publish results which back up an association, rather than those that report a negative finding. This is discussed further in the section on systematic reviews.

Subgroup analyses are when the researcher breaks down the statistical analysis according to certain characteristics of the subjects. For example, imagine that a randomized trial of a drug and placebo in the treatment of obsessive compulsive disorder finds no overall difference. What many researchers go on to do is find a difference in special groups and end-up making statements like: 'While our findings indicated the drug was no better than placebo for the majority of patients with OCD, it does appear to have a useful effect in females over the age of 55 with a family history of the disorder'. This statement implies that they have made a number of different comparisons and ended up squeezing the data to detect a significant result in this small group. Subgroup analyses are common and deceptive because they are really an example of multiple statistical testing (Assmann et al 2000).

Points to consider if the study reports a 'negative finding'

Imagine an antidepressant drug trial assessing two antidepressants in the treatment of depression. The investigators choose a reference compound and compare it with a new drug. They recruit 50 patients with depression and compare the treatment effects of the two drugs on the change in the Hamilton Depression Rating Scale scores. In presenting their results they state: 'We detected no difference between the two compounds in terms of changes in the Hamilton scores. This indicates that the two drugs are similarly potent and effective.' This sort of study is extremely common (Hotopf et al 1997) and frequently comes to this sort of conclusion.

In this example, the investigators pit two drugs against one another, both of which may be effective in depression. If a true difference exists between the two treatments, it is likely to be a small one. Note that placebo-controlled trials of antidepressants indicate that one-third of people treated with a placebo will be better at 6 weeks. Two-thirds of people treated with most antidepressants get better. Now imagine that people treated with the new drug experience an efficacy rate somewhere between that of most antidepressants and placebo – say a 50% recovery rate. Table 10.3 shows the numbers of people who would have to be randomized to detect these differences setting power at 80% and confidence at 95%.

Table 10.3 indicates that it is not really surprising that the study failed to show a difference between the two treatments. If the investigators had performed a power calculation before embarking on their study, it would have shown that they needed at least 320 subjects to show 50% of people recovering on the drug. These sorts of small trials are common in psychiatry and the rest of medicine. The main thing to be aware of is

Table 10.3 Effect size and power: note how ever-increasing numbers are required as the effect size gets smaller

Recovery rate on Hypexine (%) (compared with 66% improvement on imipramine)	Number required to be randomized
33	82
40	128
50	320
55	654
60	2096

the interpretation of the results: an underpowered study that demonstrates no difference between two treatments does not indicate that the treatments have similar efficacy!

Bias

Bias is a result of study design, and takes two main forms: *selection bias* and *information bias*.

Selection bias

Selection bias is a particular problem of case–control studies and is most likely to occur in situations where cases are derived from highly specialized clinical settings. An example of the role of selection bias is given in the worked example of case–control studies.

Information bias

Information bias occurs in two main ways: *recall bias* and *observer bias*. In recall bias, the disease status of subjects affects their likelihood of reporting the exposure. For example, a patient with cancer may be more likely to recall being a smoker. In schizophrenia research, the disease status may reduce the likelihood that the sufferer will recall an exposure. Recall bias is best avoided either by using cohort studies or by gaining information from alternative sources (such as hospital records).

Observer bias occurs where the disease status or treatment of the subject leads the researcher to ask questions or assess the subject differently. This is the main reason why double blinding of clinical trials is so important, especially when subjective symptoms (e.g. depression) are used as an endpoint.

Confounding

Confounding was described in Chapter 9. The difference between confounding and bias is that confounding is a property of 'real life' situations, whereas bias is an error the researcher introduces into the design of the study. Confounding occurs where an *additional* factor causes the outcome of interest and is associated with the exposure under study. For example, if a study found that alcohol consumption was associated with lung cancer, the obvious confounder would be smoking, because heavy drinkers are more likely to be heavy smokers.

In reading a paper, it is worth considering first: 'Could any confounder have accounted for the association reported?' and second: 'Have the researchers controlled for any of the confounders that I have thought of?'

In the example of alcohol and lung cancer, you will already have identified smoking as an important potential confounder. The researchers could have dealt with this in a number of ways:

Restriction: they could have only included people who had *never smoked* into the study. In other words, they deal with the confounder by removing any variation in exposure to it in the study sample.

Matching: in a case–control study, they may have matched those with lung cancer and those without according to how much they reported smoking, and then assessed alcohol consumption between groups.

Stratifying: they may have collected the data and then broken down the sample into several *strata* according to how much they reported smoking. The association between alcohol and lung cancer could then be examined in never smokers, past smokers, light smokers and heavy smokers.

Statistical modelling: a number of statistical approaches exist whereby confounders are added into a regression equation to determine whether accounting for them reduces the association between the exposure and the disease.

If you can think of a potential confounder and the researchers have not dealt with it using one of these methods, it may be the reason for the apparent association. There is an additional complication known as *residual confounding*, where an attempt has been made to correct for the effect of a potential confounder, but the measure of that factor is too coarse. An example would be to correct for age by stratifying the sample into those under the age of 40 and those of that age and over. Clearly, age could still be an active confounder even within those strata, so the factor would not have been fully corrected.

Reverse causality

Reverse causality occurs when the exposure is caused by the disorder rather than the disorder being caused by the exposure. In the life event literature, one possibility would be that patients with depression are more likely to suffer life events. Their depression may lead to an under-performance at work that may cause them to lose their job. Much of the research on life events has sought to address these concerns.

Sometimes, reverse causality may be quite subtle. For example, obstetric complications are associated with schizophrenia. The usual assumption is that this is because obstetric complications lead to subtle brain damage which predisposes to schizophrenia. An alternative view, however, is that individuals who later develop schizophrenia already have developmental brain abnormalities *in utero* that make them more prone to difficult deliveries, since childbirth requires the active participation of the fetus as well as the mother.

Having satisfied yourself that the reported association was not due to chance, bias, confounding or reverse causality, you are then in a position to take the association at face value – to give credence to the idea of the exposure in the study really being the cause of the outcome.

How does it fit in with the rest of the literature?

In any literature, differences in findings between studies are inevitable. This should not be seen as a problem, or even necessarily requiring explanation beyond the issues of Type 1 and Type 2 errors described above. It is expected and normal for well-conducted studies with the same aims and methodologies to both miss true findings and detect false ones. In this case, one would expect to see the estimates of effect the studies produce to be grouped around a single 'best guess' value.

In reality, however, one is often faced with studies with different sample sizes and methodologies in different settings. If the body of the literature is pointing in the same direction, then the message can be clear, but if studies disagree, then sense needs to be made of it. First, the powerful biases in case–control studies can produce spurious results (Mayes et al 1988) and the results of only the very best conducted case–control study should be considered of equivalent value to a cohort study. Further, no single example of observational research should be considered when compared to a well-conducted randomized controlled trial.

Summary

This chapter has aimed to provide the reader with a grounding in one of the basic skills of evidence based medicine: critical appraisal of the academic literature pertaining to a particular clinical question. This has included describing some of the common flaws in research designs in psychiatry of which readers of academic papers need to be aware.

In critical appraisal it is important to strike a balance between credulity and cynicism. Most research has some flaws and could be wrong. Good critical appraisal involves recognizing those flaws, and pitting them against the main findings of the research the details of the methodology, and examining the literature as a whole. Good evidence-based care is about using the most applicable evidence to inform clinical decisions.

Useful websites

Cochrane Collaboration, www.cochrane.org.
   The Cochrane Collaboration is a non-profit making international organization that aims to assist researchers perform systematic reviews and disseminate their results. It is named after the British epidemiologist Archie Cochrane, who noted the failure of medicine to systematically gather data regarding the efficacy of medical treatments.

National Institute for health and Clinical Excellence (NICE), wwwnice.org.uk.
   This is the UK independent organization responsible for providing evidence-based healthcare guidance.

Oxford Centre for Evidence-Based Medicine, wwwcebm.net.
   Aims to develop, teach and promote evidence-based healthcare and provide support and resources to doctors and healthcare professionals.

NHS Evidence, wwwevidence.nhs.uk.
   Evidence-based medicine tool for healthcare providers on the ground.

Further reading

Crombie, I., 1996. The pocket guide to critical appraisal. BMJ Publishing, London.
This is a short, clearly written book with a useful one-page checklist for each study design.

Greenhalgh, T, 1997. How to read a paper. BMJ Publishing, London.
This is the 'industry standard' text, more detailed than the above.

Prince, M, Stewart, R., Hotopf, M., 2003. Practical psychiatric epidemiology. Oxford University Press, Oxford.
This text has more detail on issues specific to psychiatry.

References

A boy claims he was hit by a meteorite. Available: http://blogs.discovermagazine.com/badastronomy/2009/06/12/a-boy-claims-he-was-hit-by-a-meteorite.

Altman, D.G., 1994. The scandal of poor medical research. Br. Med. J. 308, 283–284.

Altman, D.G., Schulz, K.F., Moher, D., et al., 2001. The revised CONSORT statement for reporting randomized trials: explanation and elaboration. Ann. Intern. Med. 134, 663–694.

Assmann, S.F., Pocock, S.J., Enos, L.E., et al., 2000. Subgroup analysis and other (mis)uses of baseline data in clinical trials. Lancet 355, 1064–1069.

British Journal of Psychiatry, 2009. Instructions for authors. Available: http://bjp.rcpsych.org/misc/ifora.dtl.

Gorring, H., Turner, E., Day, E., et al., 2010. A clinical librarian pilot project in psychiatry. The Psychiatrist 34, 65–68.

Harbord, R.M., Egger, M., Sterne, J.A., 2006. A modified test for small-study effects in meta-analyses of controlled trials with binary endpoints. Stat. Med. 25, 3443–3457.

Higgins, J.P., Thompson, S.G., Deeks, J.J., et al., 2003. Measuring inconsistency in meta-analyses. Br. Med. J. 327, 557–560.

Hotopf, M., Lewis, G., Normand, C., 1997. Putting trials on trial – the costs and consequences of small trials in depression: a systematic review of methodology. J. Epidemiol. Community Health 51, 354–358.

Lee, W., Bindman, J., Ford, T., et al., 2007. Bias in psychiatric case-control studies: literature survey. Br. J. Psychiatry 190, 204–209.

Lonergan, E., Britton, A.M., Luxenberg, J., et al., 2007. Antipsychotics for delirium. Cochrane Database Syst. Rev. (2): CD005594.

Mayes, L.C., Horwitz, R.I., Feinstein, A.R., 1988. A collection of 56 topics with contradictory results in case-control research. Int. J. Epidemiol. 17, 680–685.

Moher, D., Schulz, K.F., Altman, D.G., 2001. The CONSORT statement: revised recommendations for improving the quality of reports of parallel group randomized trials. BMC Med. Res. Methodol. 1, 2.

Oxford Centre for Evidence Based Medicine – Levels of Evidence, 2009. Available: www.cebm.net/index.aspx?o=4590 accessed 05.02.10.).

Sackett, D.L., Rosenberg, W.M., Gray, J.A., et al., 1996. Evidence based medicine: what it is and what it isn't. Br. Med. J. 312, 71–72.

Schulz, K.F., Chalmers, I., Hayes, R.J., et al., 1995. Empirical evidence of bias. Dimensions of methodological quality associated with estimates of treatment effects in controlled trials. J. Am. Med. Assoc. 273, 408–412.

Sterne, J.A., Egger, M., Smith, G.D., 2001. Systematic reviews in health care: investigating and dealing with publication and other biases in meta-analysis. Br. Med. J. 323, 101–105.

Stroup, D.F., Berlin, J.A., Morton, S.C., et al., 2000. Meta-analysis of observational studies in epidemiology: a proposal for reporting. Meta-analysis Of Observational Studies in Epidemiology (MOOSE) group. J. Am. Med. Assoc. 283, 2008–2012.

Turner, E.H., Matthews, A., Linardatos, M., et al., 2008. Selective publication of antidepressant trials and its influence on apparent efficacy. N. Engl. J. Med. 358, 252–260.

von Elm, E., Altman, D.G., Egger, M., et al., 2007. The Strengthening the Reporting of Observational Studies in Epidemiology (STROBE) statement: guidelines for reporting observational studies. PLoS Med. 4, e296.

Ethics and the law in psychiatry

11

Seán Whyte   Catherine Penny

CHAPTER CONTENTS

Introduction

A variety of rules are used in medicine, most of which are there to help put ethical considerations into practice. To a greater extent than doctors in other specialties, the rules psychiatrists work within are complex, overlapping and occasionally contradictory. At times, they can seem supportive: for instance, giving a person treatment against their wishes is made much easier by knowing that this is widely accepted – in specific circumstances – as being in the person's best interests, and that you are following a proper legal procedure which is there to protect the person and you. At other times, these same rules can seem restrictive, as for example when a patient detained with a restriction order cannot be allowed leave to visit a relative until the Ministry of Justice, as well as the multidisciplinary team, have approved it. Some of the sources of the rules applicable to psychiatrists are shown in Box 11.1. The importance of an understanding of ethics and law to psychiatrists is reflected in the Royal College of Psychiatrists' training curriculum and Membership exams (Box 11.2.).

Ethics in psychiatry

Why are ethics – that is, personal or professional moral codes – relevant in psychiatry? Is not psychiatry, and the rest of medicine, essentially a science, where an objective assessment is made of the patient's signs and symptoms, a diagnosis is reached, and treatment is prescribed by reference to a body of scientific knowledge about disease? Even if one regards 'science' itself as being independent of moral and value judgements (and many scientists and philosophers do not; see, e.g. Fulford et al 1994), the processes of diagnosis and treatment in practice inevitably introduce moral questions. What is the 'norm' of speech or behaviour to which to compare this person's speech or behaviour? How do you decide whether a person's relationships count as 'unstable' (part of the definition of borderline personality disorder)? Which of the patients who might benefit from currently expensive or

Box 11.1

Some of the sources of rules affecting psychiatrists

Legal
- Mental Health Act 1983
- Mental Capacity Act 2005.

Quasi-legal
- Care Programme Approach (CPA) guidance
- 'Working Together to Safeguard Children' guidance.

Ethical
- Hippocratic oath
- World Medical and Psychiatric Associations
- General Medical Council
- Royal College of Psychiatrists.

scarce treatments such as acetylcholinesterase inhibitor medication, cognitive–analytic therapy or inpatient alcohol detoxification should be given them? Add to this mix the fact that psychiatrists are expected to judge who is capable of making their own decisions and who is not, and that most psychiatrists are licensed to detain people in hospital against their will, and it then becomes clear that many of the decisions psychiatrists make have a significant ethical component.

Ethical frameworks

The first, and perhaps most famous, statement of ethical principles relating to medicine was that of the ancient Greek physician, Hippocrates. An abridged version of Hippocrates' oath is shown in Box 11.3.; many of the principles he formulated are still considered relevant today. The World Medical Association has produced more detailed and contemporary statements, including the International Code of Medical Ethics for all doctors (World Medical Association 2006) and the Declaration of Helsinki, which covers research on human subjects (World Medical Association 2008). The World Psychiatric Association's Declaration of Madrid applies specifically to psychiatrists (World Psychiatric Association 2005). In the UK, the General Medical Council has produced its own list of doctors' duties, some of which are shown in Box 11.4.; the Royal College of Psychiatrists has endorsed this and produced a companion manual applying these duties in detail to psychiatric practice (Royal College of Psychiatrists 2009).

There are many such codes of professional ethics, mostly embodying the same general values, but differing in detail. With such a profusion of detailed guidance, it can be difficult to see the underlying ethical principles. A useful conventional way of summarizing these ethical codes is provided by Beauchamp and Childress' four principles (2008).

Box 11.2

Royal College of Psychiatrists curriculum and membership exams

The core and general module of the College's competency-based curriculum for specialist training in psychiatry is structured around the domains of good medical practice, the General Medical Council's ethical guidance for doctors. Ethical and legal considerations underpin many of the areas tested in the Membership exams. In addition, the College advises that Paper 1 includes questions on ethics and the philosophy of psychiatry, and that the Clinical Assessment of Skills and Competencies (CASC) may test the assessment of capacity.

Example: Best-of-five Multiple Choice Question (MCQ) (as used in Paper 1)

Ethics and Philosophy – Principles

Select the option that lists all of Beauchamp and Childress' four principles:
A. Non-maleficence, Beneficence, Autonomy and Justice
B. Good will, Duty, Confidentiality and Consent
C. Autonomy, Beneficence, Justice and Fairness
D. Autonomy, Justice, Confidentiality and Beneficence
E. Respect, Justice, Rights and Choice.

Example: Extended Matching Item (EMI) (as used in Paper 1)

Options:
a. The Royal College of Psychiatrists
b. The Common Law 'Bolam' test
c. The World Medical Association
d. The Greek physician, Hippocrates
e. The General Medical Council

f. The Mental Health Act 1959
g. The World Psychiatric Association
h. The Egyptian King, Tutankhamun.

Lead in: Which of the above was/is responsible for the following? Each option might be used once, more than once, or not at all.
1. The Declaration of Madrid
2. The principle that a medical practice is not negligent if it is accepted as proper by a responsible body of doctors skilled in that particular art
3. Providing guidance for UK doctors regarding 'the principles and values that underpin good medical practice'
4. The first surviving statement of ethical principles relating to medicine.

Example: CASC scenario – individual station (7 min, 1 min preparation)

While on call, you are asked to see a 23-year-old man, Mr Brown, who has come to A&E after falling off a ladder and breaking his wrist, while attaching silver foil to the inside of a window. Mr James, his surgeon, is concerned that he says he does not want the operation on his wrist that Mr James recommends. Instead he wants 'more X-rays'. Mr James is also concerned that Mr Brown appears irritable and agitated. He thinks he may have a mental disorder.
- Assess Mr Brown's capacity to refuse treatment
- You do not need to perform a full mental state examination.

MCQ and EMI answers and CASC instructions for role player and examiner's construct are given in the Appendix to this chapter, below.

Box 11.3

The Hippocratic Oath (abridged)

I swear by Apollo Physician and Asclepius and Hygieia and Panaceia and all the gods and goddesses . . . that I will fulfil according to my ability and judgment this oath and this covenant:

. . . I will apply dietetic measures for the benefit of the sick according to my ability and judgment; I will keep them from harm and injustice.

I will neither give a deadly drug to anybody if asked for it, nor will I make any suggestion to this effect.

. . . Whatever houses I may visit, I will come for the benefit of the sick, remaining free of all intentional injustice, of all mischief and in particular of sexual relations with both female and male persons, be they free or slaves.

What I may see or hear in the course of the treatment . . . which on no account one must spread abroad, I will keep to myself . . .

If I fulfil this oath and do not violate it, may it be granted to me to enjoy life . . .; if I transgress and swear falsely, may the opposite . . . be my lot.

Abridged, after Temkin & Temkin 1967.

Box 11.4

The duties of a doctor (abridged)

You must:
- Make the care of your patient your first concern
- Protect and promote the health of patients and the public
- Respect patients' dignity and right to confidentiality
- Work with colleagues in the ways that best serve patients' interests
- Listen to patients and respond to their concerns and preferences
- Keep your professional knowledge and skills up-to-date
- Recognize the limits of your professional competence
- Be honest and act with integrity
- Never abuse patients' trust in you or the public's trust in the profession.

Abridged, after the General Medical Council 2006.

The four principles

These are general principles that are widely thought to underlie guidelines in medical ethics. They are independent of any particular moral system or theory (such as Kantianism, utilitarianism, virtue ethics or casuistry), but they provide a framework for looking at different approaches to ethics. A discussion of these principles, and their relationship with moral systems and with codes of psychiatric ethics, can be found in Bloch et al (1999). The four principles are:

- **Non-maleficence:** often stated as 'first do no harm', this principle states that the doctor should avoid doing anything that would harm the patient.
- **Beneficence:** this principle states that the doctor should promote the welfare of patients. A balance should be sought

which maximizes benefits to the patient (health, disease prevention, etc.) and minimizes harms (pain, disability, side-effects, etc.).

- **Autonomy:** doctors should respect the autonomy of patients, which means both respecting their right to make decisions for themselves (provided that they have the capacity to do so) and promoting their ability to make decisions, such as by providing useful information.
- **Justice:** doctors should treat patients according to what is fair. Among other things, this implies that benefits (such as specific treatments) should be distributed fairly among all those in need of them. This is perhaps the most controversial principle, as there is so much room for disagreement over what is 'fair' and who is 'in need'.

Codes and Laws

The codes of ethics described above are not directly enforced: that is, they are intended to guide practice, rather than representing rules which must be followed to the letter. In contrast, the law provides enforceable rules governing what powers doctors have and when they should be punished for their actions. In this chapter, the focus is on the law in England and Wales, but in many cases broadly similar provisions apply in the rest of the UK and elsewhere.

The law of negligence

This is a very broad area of law, covering situations where a doctor, in their professional capacity, has done something they should not have done (negligence by commission) or not done something they should have done (negligence by omission). Negligence is not a crime, so doctors found to be negligent cannot be imprisoned or otherwise punished. It is a civil wrong or 'tort', and if the doctor (the defendant) is found to be negligent, he or she must pay damages to the person making the complaint (the claimant). The idea is that the damages restore the claimant to the financial position they would have been in had the negligence not occurred – for instance by replacing certain lost earnings from work while in hospital – and compensate the claimant for non-financial hardships such as pain and suffering.

A person claiming that a doctor (or any other person) has been negligent must demonstrate three things: that the defendant owed them a *duty of care*; that the defendant has *breached* that duty; and that this breach led directly to the claimant suffering *damage*. These points are illustrated by the case vignettes in Box 11.5.

In general, doctors owe a duty of care to all their patients; they probably owe a duty of care to people they offer medical treatment to in 'good Samaritan' acts; and they may sometimes owe a duty of care to their patient's carers when they have had dealings with them. However, there is no duty of care to others with whom the doctor has no special or 'proximate' relationship, such as the patient's employer in case 1.

Not all damage suffered by the claimant will be compensated for: the damage suffered must not be too remote from the breach of the duty of care. The usual test for remoteness applied

the patient's best interests, the doctor must take certain steps, as listed in Box 11.7.

The role of independent mental capacity advocates (IMCAs) is to support people who lack capacity and represent their views and interests to decision-makers. They have the right to information about an individual and can see relevant healthcare records.

Advance decisions

A person who does not want a particular treatment, or any treatment at all, if they lose capacity in the future can make a formal record of this in an advance decision. Such a decision, if it meets the requirements set out in Box 11.8, has the same force as a

Box 11.7

Deciding the best interests of a person lacking capacity (MCA Code of Practice 2007)

Consider whether the person is likely to regain capacity and if so whether the decision can wait.

Involve the person as fully as possible in the decision.

Consider the person's past and present wishes and feelings (in particular if they have been written down), any relevant beliefs and values (e.g. religious, cultural or moral), and any other factors that the person would be likely to consider if they were able to do so.

Avoid discrimination, or assumptions about wishes and feelings based on the person's age, appearance, condition or behaviour; in particular, avoid assumptions about the person's quality of life that might lead to a decision not to give life-sustaining treatment.

Consult other people where appropriate, especially anyone previously named by the person as someone to be consulted, anyone caring for or interested in the person's welfare, any attorney appointed under a lasting power of attorney, and any deputy appointed by the Court of Protection.

For decisions about major medical treatment or where the person should live, where there is no one appropriate to consult other than paid staff, instruct an independent mental capacity advocate.

Where more than one option (including no action) seems reasonable in the person's best interests, choose the option that will least restrict the person's future choices.

Box 11.8

Advance decisions (ADs)

ADs are binding only if valid and applicable at the time of the proposed treatment.

To be valid, an advance decision must:
- Not have been withdrawn (while having capacity)
- Not have been superseded by a relevant lasting power of attorney
- Not have been rendered invalid by doing 'anything else clearly inconsistent' with it remaining a 'fixed decision'.

To be applicable, it must be the case that:
- The patient lacks capacity
- The proposed treatment is specified in the AD
- The current situation is envisaged by the AD
- There are no 'reasonable grounds for believing' that the patient would not have made the decision in the AD in the current situation.

ADs do not apply to 'life-sustaining' treatment unless they contain an explicit written, signed and witnessed statement that they do.

contemporaneous decision to refuse treatment, and can only be overridden by detention and treatment under the Mental Health Act.

There is an important legal distinction between a written statement expressing treatment preferences, which a doctor must take into account when making a best interests decision, and a valid and applicable advance decision to refuse treatment, which a doctor must follow. Note that a doctor would not have to follow a written request if they thought that a particular treatment would be clinically unnecessary and therefore not in the person's best interests.

Lasting power of attorney

A person aged 18 or over can appoint an 'attorney' (who can be any person they nominate) to make their health, welfare and financial decisions if they lose the capacity to make such decisions in the future. The LPA may specify limits to the attorney's authority, and can only cover life-sustaining treatment if they include a specific statement to this effect. Attorneys must make decisions in the best interests of the person lacking capacity, having followed the steps in Box 11.7. Doctors directly involved in the care of a person lacking capacity should not generally agree to act as their attorney.

The Court of Protection and court-appointed deputies

If a person lacks capacity to make a decision relating to their welfare or financial affairs, then the Court of Protection can make an order making a decision on their behalf. Alternatively, the Court of Protection can appoint a deputy to make such decisions. Both the court and any deputy, as with attorneys, must make decisions in the person's best interests. The process is complicated and bureaucratic; the costs are paid from the person's estate.

Deprivation of liberty

Making choices on behalf of a person who lacks capacity inevitably restricts the options available to them in the future, and therefore restricts their liberty (e.g. by choosing to use their money to buy them the new clothes that they need, you prevent them using that money to buy something else). However, if the restriction on liberty goes so far as to amount to a *deprivation* of liberty, then additional legal safeguards apply. Whether arrangements for a person's care amount to a 'restriction on' or a 'deprivation of' liberty is a 'difference of degree or intensity, not one of nature or substance' according to the European Court of Human Rights (*HL v UK* 2004). Factors that suggest a deprivation of liberty include the use of restraint and the control of social contacts, residence or movement for a significant period.

Care that deprives a person of their liberty is lawful only if the person is detained under the Mental Health Act, or (if that Act does not apply) if the care provider, such as a nursing home or hospital, has sought approval from the relevant supervisory body, usually the Local Authority or Primary Care Trust. The supervisory body must then take into account the person's age, mental capacity and mental health, any advance decisions or LPAs, and the person's best interests in deciding whether to approve the deprivation of liberty. The person concerned or those acting on their behalf can appeal against such an approval to the Court of Protection.

Research

The Mental Capacity Act imposes additional rules on researchers wishing to include people who lack capacity in their research. The research must have a chance of benefiting the participant individually, and the 'burden' of participation (e.g. the time involved, risk of discomfort or side-effects, etc.) must be reasonable when balanced against the possibility of benefit; or, if there is no chance of personal benefit, the research must aim to increase knowledge about the person's condition or a related condition, the procedures involved must not be intrusive, the risk of harm to the participant must be negligible, and there must be no significant interference with their liberty or privacy.

Ill treatment

Ill treatment or wilful neglect of someone lacking capacity by someone responsible for their care or with decision-making powers is an offence.

Fluctuating capacity

Capacity is not static: a patient can have capacity to make one decision but not another, and even with respect to a single decision, they may have capacity at one time but not at another. Capacity may be temporarily affected by confusion, panic, pain, medication, drugs or alcohol. Mental disorder often contributes to fluctuating capacity; for instance, this is common in the early stages of Alzheimer's dementia where there are periods of lucidity, and in bipolar affective disorder, where the patient may lack capacity during manic episodes but not at other times. In these situations, it may be possible to increase the chance that a patient can make their own decisions: in the case of the patient with Alzheimer's dementia, for example, this might mean interviewing them at a time of day when they are their most alert, conducting the interview in a comfortable, quiet and familiar environment, and ensuring a trusted relative or friend is present. In some cases, it may be possible to put off the decision in the hope that the patient will regain capacity.

When a patient loses capacity, it is permissible to continue to rely on consent given when they had capacity; it is preferable to have recorded the consent, and the fact of their having capacity at the time, in writing (General Medical Council 2008). If the patient regains capacity, their consent should be reviewed with them before treatment continues. It is good practice to establish, while a person has capacity, their views about any clinical intervention that may be necessary during a period of anticipated incapacity, and to record these views. The person may wish to make an advanced decision to refuse treatment or a statement of their preferences and wishes.

Emergency situations

The law governing emergency situations is the same as that described in the sections above. However, in an emergency, it may not be possible to assess a patient's capacity or best interests or whether there is a valid and applicable advance decision, or to give the information that would be required to make an informed decision. In such an emergency, a doctor can provide treatment 'immediately necessary to save their life or to prevent a serious deterioration of their condition' (General Medical Council 2008). Patients who have attempted suicide and are unconscious should be given emergency treatment if any doubt exists as to either their intentions or their capacity when they took the decision to attempt suicide. During such treatment, the patient should be told what is happening, so far as possible. As soon as a patient regains capacity and there is time to give more information, they must be told what has been done and, again, their consent must be sought for any further treatment.

Incapacity for other reasons

The Mental Capacity Act only applies where a person lacks capacity because of an impairment or disturbance of the functioning of the mind or brain. Occasionally, a person with no such impairment or disturbance might lack capacity for other reasons, particularly if they are young – for instance, because they are emotionally overwhelmed by the implications of the decision. In this situation, although the Act does not apply, if they are unable to understand, retain or use relevant information because of this other reason, older common law rules on incapacity apply, and it is lawful to act in their best interests to assist them.

Children

Unlike adults, children under the age of 16 are not presumed by the law to have capacity, and the Mental Capacity Act does not apply to them; the default situation is that a person with parental responsibility must give or refuse consent on their behalf. However, children under 16 can give consent if they have 'sufficient understanding and intelligence to . . . understand fully what is proposed' (Gillick 1986). The courts have not clarified what this means, stating that it is up to the doctor to decide whether a child is 'Gillick-competent' or not; it is suggested that the criteria in the 'capacity' section above should be used to make this decision. A Gillick-competent child can consent to treatment even if their parents refuse, and competent children can be given advice and treatment without their parents' knowledge or consent (R v Secretary of State 2006); however, a parent's consent can override a child's refusal of consent even if that child is Gillick-competent (Re R (A minor) 1991); and even if both child and parents refuse, the doctor can still apply to the High Court for permission to proceed in the child's best interests (something which is not a possibility when the patient is an adult). Emergency treatment of a child is also permissible if consent by the child, a parent or a court is not available or if it is unclear whether a parent's refusal of consent is in the child's best interests.

To complicate matters further, the situation is different for young people aged 16 or 17. The Family Law Reform Act 1969 states that 16- and 17-year-olds are, like adults, presumed to have capacity unless they are shown not to, and allows them to consent to treatment (but not research or non-therapeutic procedures such as organ donation). The Mental Capacity Act applies to 16- and 17-year-olds, although they cannot make advance decisions or LPAs until they turn 18.

At the time of writing, the common law and the Children Act 1989 allows a parent to override their child's refusal of consent, including if the child is 16 or 17. However, this may no longer be lawful under the Human Rights Act 1998 and it would be prudent to obtain a court decision before treating someone in this situation.

Where there is doubt about whether a parent is acting in the interest of a child or young person, for example if a child alleges abuse and the parent supports psychiatric treatment for the child, the Government provides guidance in *Working Together to Safeguard Children* on factors to consider when deciding whether to rely on the parent's consent.

The Mental Health Act

Independently of the powers described above, the Mental Health Act 1983 empowers psychiatrists to detain patients with a mental disorder for assessment and treatment, and to give them treatment for mental disorder without their consent. A breakdown of the main parts and sections of the Act, as amended by the Mental Health Act 2007, is shown in Box 11.9.; for a comprehensive guide to the Act, refer to the Act's Code of Practice (2008) or Jones (2008).

Box 11.9

Principal sections of the Mental Health Act 1983 (as amended)

Part II – Compulsory admission to hospital and guardianship

Section 2: Admission for assessment

Section 3: Admission for treatment

Section 4: Emergency admission for assessment

Section 5: Detention of an informal inpatient

Section 7: Guardianship

Section 12: Approval of doctors to use the Act

Section 17: Leave of absence from hospital

Section 17A: Community treatment order.

Part III – Patients concerned with criminal proceedings

This part provides for patients to be sent to mental hospital from court and from prison (see Ch. 31).

Part IV – Consent to treatment

Section 57: Treatments requiring consent and a second opinion (e.g. psychosurgery)

Sections 58 & 58A: Treatments requiring consent or a second opinion (e.g. ECT, long-term antipsychotic treatment)

Section 62: Urgent treatment

Sections 64A–64H: Treatment under a community treatment order.

Part V – Mental health first-tier tribunals

This part provides for a system to allow patients to appeal against their detention.

Part X – miscellaneous

Section 135: Warrant to search for and remove patients

Section 136: Mentally disordered persons found in public places.

Principles: the basis for detention

As explained above, in most situations, choices can generally only be made for a patient without their consent if they lack capacity. However, the basis for detention under the Act largely ignores capacity. The criteria for detention for treatment under section 3 of the Act are shown in Box 11.10; the specific criteria vary slightly for other sections, but the principles are the same.

The basis for detention is an uneasy compromise between patients' individual needs (as assessed by the professionals – not as seen by patients themselves) and society's desire to stop patients harming themselves or others. Some have suggested there should be one Act to merge the Mental Health Act and the Mental Capacity Act, creating a single regime, based purely on capacity (i.e. the patient's individual needs) that applies to all treatments with no distinction between mental and physical illness (e.g. Zigmond 2009).

Key provisions

The following sections of the Act listed in Box 11.9. will be commonly encountered.

● **Section 2:** allows a person meeting the criteria in Box 11.10. to be detained for up to 28 days for assessment and initial treatment of their condition. They must appear to have a mental disorder: a person with delirium (a physical disorder) or who is intoxicated or dependent on alcohol or drugs cannot be detained for this reason alone, although they may be if there is diagnostic confusion.

● **Section 3:** allows a person meeting the criteria in Box 11.10. to be detained for up to 6 months for treatment. Unlike section 2, it can be renewed. 'Appropriate medical treatment' for the patient must be available; a patient's refusal of consent does not make an available treatment inappropriate.

Box 11.10

Chief criteria for detention under section 3 of the Mental Health Act

● The patient must have a mental disorder ('any disorder or disability of mind')

● The disorder must be severe enough ('of a nature or degree') to need treatment in hospital

● Voluntary treatment is not appropriate (usually because the patient is refusing admission)

● Detention in hospital is necessary in the interests of:
  ● the patient's health, and/or
  ● the patient's safety (e.g. to stop them committing suicide), and/or
  ● other people's safety (e.g. if the patient is violent)

● Two appropriate doctors (usually a psychiatrist approved under the Act and another doctor who knows the patient) and an approved mental health practitioner (usually a social worker) agree on using the section.

- **Section 4:** provides for an emergency procedure when only one doctor is available and the admission cannot be delayed. The patient must still meet the other criteria in Box 11.10. It only authorizes detention for up to 72 h, but can be extended to 28 days if a second doctor later recommends this.

- **Section 5:** is a similar emergency procedure for use when the patient has already been admitted to hospital (i.e. is on a ward – being in A&E does not count as having been admitted). Section 5(4) allows a senior nurse to detain the patient for up to 6 h for assessment; section 5(2) allows a nominated person, usually a doctor, to detain the patient for up to 72 h so that an assessment for section 2 or 3 can take place.

- **Section 7:** guardianship allows for an outpatient to be monitored by a community supervisor (usually a community psychiatric nurse or social worker). The supervisor has the power to require the patient to live in a particular place, to go to other places for medical treatment, education or occupation and to let the supervisor in to see them. Note that the supervisor does not have the power to make the patient accept treatment – just to take them to the place of treatment.

- **Section 17A:** a patient who has been detained in hospital for treatment can be made subject to a community treatment order (CTO), whereby they can be recalled to hospital if they break specified conditions, such as living in a particular place or seeing the professionals involved in their care. It does not allow compulsory treatment in the community but can allow recall to hospital if treatment is not adhered to. Recall to hospital is for up to 72 h, during which treatment can be given without consent if a valid second opinion certificate is in force. If, after assessment during this time, they meet the criteria in Box 11.10, the CTO is revoked and they are detained under section 3; otherwise, they must be allowed to return to the community.

- **Sections 57, 58, 58A, 62 and 64A–H:** these sections deal with treatment. For up to 3 months, doctors can give patients treatments for mental disorder (not for other conditions) without consent; after 3 months, if the patient still refuses consent, treatment can only continue if an independent doctor agrees that the treatment is necessary. However, some treatments are exceptions to this, and from the start, can only be given if the patient consents or if they are incapable of consenting and there is a second opinion in favour (e.g. ECT); other treatments require both consent and a second opinion (e.g. psychosurgery). However, section 62 allows such treatments to begin immediately if they are urgently needed to save the patient's life or prevent serious deterioration. Treatment for patients on CTOs is only authorized where the patient consents (or, if lacking capacity, does not object) and there is a valid second opinion certificate.

- **Sections 135 and 136:** give the police powers to take people whom they suspect are mentally unwell to a place of safety (usually A&E or a psychiatric assessment unit, sometimes the police station). The latter covers people found in a public place; the former allows the police, acting with a doctor and a social worker who has obtained a magistrate's order, to break into private property to remove a person suspected of being mentally unwell.

The Care Programme Approach (CPA)

This is a set of policies introduced by the Department of Health in 1991, made more extensive and binding in 1999 (Department of Health 1999), and further developed in 2008 (Department of Health 2008). The key features of the CPA are shown in Box 11.11 (also see Ch. 30).

Other Acts relevant to psychiatry

Mentally disordered people are sometimes prevented from taking part in activities or are made subject to special conditions.

Appointeeship

If it is decided that a person claiming benefits is unable to act for themselves, the Benefits Agency has the power to appoint somebody who is in regular contact with the claimant and is acceptable to them, to manage their benefits on their behalf.

Driving

The Driver and Vehicle Licensing Agency (DVLA) requires all drivers to inform it of any medical condition that might affect fitness to drive. The rules are complicated; they can be found on the DVLA website (Driver and Vehicle Licensing Agency 2009). For example, a person who is currently psychotic cannot drive; a person with bipolar disorder who has had more than three episodes in the last year cannot drive until they have been well for more than 6 months and the DVLA has given permission; and a person with an anxiety disorder can drive without the DVLA needing to be informed. The duty to inform the DVLA rests with the patient concerned; patients are often understandably reluctant to reveal their illness to the DVLA, as they know (or fear) that they will be told they are not allowed to drive. This can put their GP or psychiatrist in a difficult position. Guidance from the General Medical Council states that the doctor should explain to any patient with a relevant condition their legal duty to inform the DVLA, and if the patient cannot be persuaded to do this, or if the doctor has evidence that they are continuing to

Box 11.11

The main elements of the Care Programme Approach (CPA)

- Systematic arrangements for assessing the health and social needs of people with severe mental illness
- The formation of a care plan which identifies the health and social care required from a variety of providers
- The appointment of a care coordinator to keep in close touch with the service user and to monitor and coordinate care
- Regular review and, where necessary, agreed changes to the care plan.

Research Involving Human Subjects. Online. Available: www.wma.net/e/policy/b3.htm (accessed 29.08.09).

World Psychiatric Association, 2005. Madrid Declaration on Ethical Standards for Psychiatric Practice. Online. Available: www.wpanet.org/content/madrid-ethic-engish.shtml (accessed 29.08.09).

Zigmond, A.S., 2009. Mental illness and legal discrimination. International Psychiatry 6, 79–80.

Cases

Bolam v Friern Hospital Management Committee [1957] 2 All ER 118.

Bolitho v City & Hackney Health Authority [1997] 4 All ER 771.

Bournewood (1998) In Re L (by his next friend GE) [1999] 1 A.C. 458.

Blyth v Birmingham Waterworks [1856] 156 ER 1047.

Chester v Afshar [2004] UKHL 41.

Clarke v Malpas [1862] 45 ER 1238.

Gillick v West Norfolk and Wisbech Area Health Authority [1986] AC 112, HL(E).

HL v United Kingdom [2004] 40 EHRR 761.

Imperial Loan Co v Stone [1892] 1 QB 599.

Re F (Mental Patient: Sterilization) [1990] 2 AC 1 at 75H.

Re R (A minor) (Wardship: Medical Treatment) [1991] 4 All ER 177.

Re W (A minor) (Wardship: Medical Treatment) [1993] Fam 64.

R v Adomako [1994] 5 Med LR 277.

R (Axon) v Secretary of State for Health [2006] EWHC 37 (Admin).

Wagon Mound No.1: Overseas Tankship (UK) Ltd v Morts Dock & Engineering Co [1961] AC 388.

Challenges to psychiatry

Antipsychiatry, the user movement and stigma

12

Joanna Moncrieff   Peter Byrne   Michael Crawford

The antipsychiatry movement

Introduction

Antipsychiatry is usually taken to refer to ideas expressed by some philosophers, sociologists and psychiatrists that first became widely recognized during the 1960s. Although there had been criticism of psychiatry before this, the ideas of antipsychiatry were new in the sense that they presented a fundamental critique of psychiatry from a philosophical and political perspective (Crossley 1998). They became popular and influential and converged with many of the wider changes in social attitudes and behaviour that occurred during the 1960s. Although there are differences between the ideas of individual antipsychiatrists, certain themes emerged as central to a common theory of what psychiatry was really concerned with.

The myth of mental illness

'Mental illness is a myth, whose function it is to disguise and render more palatable the bitter pill of moral conflict in human relations.'

(Szasz 1970: 24)

In his many publications, the psychiatrist Thomas Szasz has argued that the concept of mental illness is a myth, or a 'metaphor'. By this he means that mental illnesses are not the same as physical diseases, and only resemble them by virtue of the fact that 'we call people physically ill when their body functioning violates certain physiological and anatomical norms: similarly we call people mentally ill when their personal conduct violates certain ethical, political and social norms' (Szasz 1970: 23). The brain can be diseased, for example in neurological disorders, such as epilepsy, brain tumours and degenerative brain diseases, but the mind cannot. Diagnosis of physical disorders is quite different from the way in which mental disorders are characterized. In physical diseases there are characteristic pathological findings or objective signs. In contrast, mental illnesses are ascribed on the basis of behaviours that deviate from social norms. Diagnosis of mental disorder is therefore an inherently subjective process, involving normative judgements that will vary depending upon the particular social and cultural context.

Szasz' challenge includes biological models that assume that mental illnesses are actually types of neurological or brain disorder, differing from most other neurological conditions only in the fact that their unique neuropathology has not yet been firmly identified. He argues that regardless of findings of some minor pathological deviations, major mental illnesses such as schizophrenia are still diagnosed on the basis of behavioural criterion, and hence are still defined by deviation from social and ethical norms. If specific and consistent neuropathology is uncovered, then the condition would cease to be a 'mental illness' and would become a neurological condition instead.

Szasz prefers to describe the behaviours that are labelled as mental illnesses as 'problems in living'. They arise from conflict between the individual concerned and the demands of society or the social network around him or her. Psychiatry is thus a 'moral and social enterprise', dealing with 'problems of human conduct' (Szasz 1970: 47). The conflicts may concern low level antisocial behaviour, which may fail to reach the threshold of criminal activity. But often the conflict is about dependency. In a later work, Szasz describes how psychiatry has arisen to provide a solution to the problem of adult dependency: 'the business of psychiatry is distributing poor relief (concealed as medical care) to adult dependents' (Szasz 1994: 149).

R.D. Laing, a Scottish psychiatrist, described the problems labelled as mental illness in slightly different, although not contradictory terms. Laing's main concern was to render the symptoms and behaviours associated with mental illness as meaningful experiences, not merely as the products of pathological processes. His first book, *The Divided Self* (Laing 1960), is a detailed examination of how the 'symptoms' of long-term institutionalized patients could be understood with reference to their lives and histories. His later work is a celebration of the experience of psychosis and its possibilities for expanding consciousness and transcending the alienation of everyday life. These ideas have been much criticized for minimizing the suffering of people with psychotic illnesses, but it should be seen as the product of its time. The late 1960s was a time when experimenting with drug-induced altered forms of consciousness was much valued by the large counter-cultural movement. Some modern accounts of the experience of mental illness also attempt to reclaim the notion that there is positive value in psychotic and other extreme mental states.

Psychiatry and social control

'... psychiatry is a moral practice overlaid by the myths of positivism ...'

(Foucault 1965: 276)

Michel Foucault was a French philosopher, associated with the ideas of post-modernism. His first published book was about the evolution of society's response to madness from the Middle Ages through to the nineteenth century. Foucault's thesis is that up to the medieval period, madness was public and recognized as something to be feared and respected. In contrast, from the enlightenment onwards, madness came to be seen simply as an absence of reason or rationality that needed correcting. First attempts to achieve this involved confinement and discipline, but later a medical approach was adopted which disguised the fact that the management of the mad remained an essentially moral and political enterprise. These developments came about because of social changes wrought by the bourgeois and industrial revolutions that problematized idleness and demanded a strong work ethic and strict discipline. Hence, psychiatry is seen as an institution that helps the modern state to create and maintain a disciplined workforce by controlling behaviour that threatens that discipline. Foucault describes early psychiatric institutions

as 'instruments of moral conformity and social denunciation' (Foucault 1965: 259).

Foucault's work on madness and psychiatry was part of his wider endeavour to uncover the development of methods of control and authority in modern societies. Over the last two centuries, there has grown a belief that social problems and conflicts could be effectively dealt with by experts exercising technical solutions. Handing over these problems to experts or professionals has allowed modern governments to shed some of their thorniest problems and to present themselves as more liberal than they might otherwise appear. For example, in England, it was the government who took the leading role in medicalizing the issue of psychiatric confinement over the twentieth century (Moncrieff 2003).

Szasz also takes up this theme extensively. He has argued that 'The mandate for contemporary psychiatry ... is precisely to obscure, indeed to deny, the ethical dilemmas of life and to transform these into medicalized and technicalized problems susceptible to "professional" solutions' (Szasz 1970: 11). Szasz is a long-time passionate advocate of the complete abolition of involuntary psychiatric hospitalization and treatment. He argues that psychiatric coercion is equivalent to imprisonment without trial. If someone is not breaking the law, they should remain free. He challenges the paternalism that is the basis for much psychiatric intervention. Paternalism is the assumption that others, usually professionals, are in a better position to judge someone's best interests than they are themselves. Szasz argues that paternalism subverts democracy and the rule of law, which rest on the assumption that human beings are autonomous agents that can make their own decisions. It is also easily abused, as people are apt to define others' interests in ways that are actually expressions of their own interests.

Protests and alternatives

The antipsychiatry movement was not just intellectual, however. In the 1970s, protest groups sprang up in parts of Europe and North America, which foreshadowed the more recent rise of the psychiatric users' movement (see below). In the USA and the Netherlands, large demonstrations were held against ECT and biological psychiatry.

Projects offering alternative forms of management of the mentally disordered were also established. In 1965, R.D. Laing and associates David Cooper and Aaron Esterson set up the Philadelphia Association, a charitable Trust that ran a number of therapeutic communities, the first being Kingsley Hall in London. The principle of these communities was that people with psychosis should be encouraged to live through their psychotic episode with the hope that this would lead to an enlightened recovery. There was also an emphasis on breaking down distinctions between staff and patients.

Franco Basaglia, an Italian psychiatrist, established an organization called *Psichiatria Democratica*. This group successfully campaigned for the passing of a law that shut down all psychiatric hospitals in Italy. The benefits or otherwise of this action have been hotly disputed since.

Loren Mosher, an American psychiatrist, set up the Soteria project in the 1970s, which was designed to treat people with severe psychotic illnesses in a small therapeutic environment with no or minimal psychotropic drugs. He conducted a randomized controlled trial of the project comparing it to routine care in a hospital ward. The original project survives to this day, and other similar projects have been developed in the USA and Europe.

Influence of antipsychiatry

The 'antipsychiatrists' have been criticized from many different perspectives and their popularity and influence has declined since their heyday of the 1960s and 1970s. Philosophers and psychiatrists have defended the notion of mental illness, sometimes by pointing to the difficulties of defining physical illness. Others have accused the antipsychiatrists of giving fuel to right wing political imperatives to cut spending on mental healthcare. However, the ideas of antipsychiatry were influential in several respects.

The development of diagnostic criteria, with which we are now so familiar, started in the 1970s, partly in response to the challenge posed by antipsychiatry. The Rosenhan (1973) experiment, in which normal volunteers were diagnosed as having schizophrenia, created a furore and seemed to confirm the idea that psychiatric diagnosis had no objective validity. International research at this time also highlighted big discrepancies in rates of diagnosis of schizophrenia between different countries. Since the publication of DSM III in 1980, diagnosis has become an increasingly detailed, quantitative and apparently objective exercise, although there are still those who doubt its reliability and validity (Kutchins & Kirk 1997).

Psychiatric legislation is another area where the ideas of antipsychiatry can be seen to have had some influence. In England and Wales, the 1959 Mental Health Act had given doctors more powers than any previous piece of legislation. This Act was drafted and passed in an atmosphere of great optimism about the potential of psychiatry to solve all the problems posed by mental illness. However, antipsychiatric ideas suggested this optimism was misplaced and gave fuel to the civil rights movement's arguments that there should, at the very least, be more restrictions on the powers of doctors to admit and forcibly treat mental patients. The 1983 Mental Health Act reflected these concerns. By narrowing definitions of certain categories of mental disorder, shortening periods of maximum detention and placing restrictions on circumstances in which compulsory treatment can and cannot be given, it limited medical power and increased patients' rights.

The ideas of antipsychiatry were influential far beyond psychiatry and were taken up by the media, the arts and the political and social sciences (Crossley 1998). Within psychiatry, they were rarely addressed directly, but their influence and popularity elsewhere presented a challenge to the psychiatric establishment. It has been suggested that the shift towards a more biologically based psychiatry that has occurred over the last three decades represents a tactical response to this challenge (Wilson 1993). Groups and ideas that challenge orthodox views of psychiatry still exist, both within and outside of organized psychiatry and have inherited to greater or lesser degrees the ideas of antipsychiatry. The Critical Psychiatry Network is a group of psychiatrists in the UK, who have united around issues such as questioning some of the assumptions of biological psychiatry, opposition to the introduction of increased coercion in psychiatric legislation and opposing the influence of the pharmaceutical industry. In the United States the Institute for the Study of Psychiatry and Psychology started by the psychiatrist Peter Breggin unites radical professionals, carers and service users against the over-use of psychiatric drugs and other physical treatments. Current ideas such as critical psychiatry, post psychiatry and the limits of psychiatry have all inherited much from their antipsychiatry predecessors.

The user movement

Introduction

Over the last 50 years, people on the receiving end of psychiatric services have played a central role in the debate about the nature of, and appropriate response to, mental distress. While the word 'patient' continues to be the preferred term for many during contact with mental health services, it has generally been rejected by those seeking to challenge the passive role that traditional doctor–patient relationships have assigned to patients. The term 'service user' provides a less value-laden term for describing this role. Others favour terms such as 'service survivor' to indicate the damaging effect they feel psychiatric services have had on their health. More recently, user groups such as 'Mad Pride' in the UK have started to reclaim the language of others as a sign of re-found self-belief in the face of widespread discrimination.

While the term used to describe people who have experienced mental distress may at first seem unimportant, it has been argued that by choosing a term that best describes one's experiences, a person can take an important step towards regaining some of the confidence that mental distress and its treatment may have eroded (Campbell 1998).

Origins of the user movement

Notable examples of user involvement in development of mental health services have occurred ever since the development of institutional responses to mental illness. Protests by inmates of mental institutions occurred in Britain during the seventeenth and eighteenth centuries, and in 1845 the Alleged Lunatics Friends Society was set up in support of those treated in asylums (Barnes & Bowl 2001). The development of a large-scale user movement did not occur until the 1970s and 80s. This movement, which came to the fore in North America and Western Europe, grew in parallel with other social movements of the age that championed the rights of women, ethnic minorities, lesbians and gay men and other groups. In Britain, groups such as the Federation of Mental Patients Union campaigned against compulsory treatment and the overuse of psychiatric drugs.

During this period, service users worked with others in mental health charities such as MIND in the UK and the National Mental Health Association in the USA, to campaign for

Table 12.1 The five components of the stigma process

Components from Link & Phelan (2001)	Examples of other stigma	The stigma of mental illness
1. Labelling differences	A: Physical deformity B: Different ethnic origin	Excess sedation or Parkinsonian symptoms (medication) Person seen leaving a psychiatric hospital or clinic
2. Association with negative attributes	A: Less attractive B: Racist stereotypes	Beliefs that people with MI are weak, self-indulgent Perceptions that people with schizophrenia are violent
3. Separation of 'us' from 'them'	A: Physical barriers B: Racial segregation	Locking people up, or 'asylum in the community' Loss of social networks after diagnosis/admission
4. Status loss and discrimination	A & B: Barriers to employment, tenancy and education	See Table 12.2 for full list of stigma-discrimination: only 17% of people with severe mental illness are in (full or part-time) employment
5. Power differential between stigmatizer (member of dominant in-group) and stigmatized (out-group member)	Dominant culture is A. of different ethnic origin and B. able-bodied, etc.	Potential stigmatizers: health professionals (including psychiatrists), social services, educationalists, police and judiciary, landlords

Table 12.2 The clinical impact of the stigma of severe mental illness

	Presentation	Course	Outcome
Person	Denial of symptoms Other explanations sought Self-medication (alcohol/drugs) Declines referral to psychiatric clinic	Rejection of diagnosis Self-stigmatization Incomplete disclosure of symptoms Non-adherence to treatments ↑ Involuntary admissions	Lack of insight Poor therapeutic relationships Intermittent medication use Loss to follow-up Isolation: loss of relationships, unemployment, homelessness, ?suicide
Family/carers	Denial of symptoms Other explanations: 'lazy' Divisions within families Blaming, scapegoating	Denial of diagnosis: doctor shopping Minimization of symptoms Ambivalence to medications Loss of earnings	Poor relations with professionals 'All or nothing' consultations Chronic illness of family member Economic consequences
Neighbours	Unaware that person is becoming ill	Isolation of individual who is ill Exclusion of family of ill person See only the illness, not the person: 'them and us' reinforced ↑ Calls to police if notice problems	Blame person and family Abuse/bullying of ill person Aversive prejudice/NIMBYism Poor opinions of mental health services: 'only act in extreme emergencies, need to be prodded into action'
Health and social services	(↑ Untreated mental illness in the community) Late presentation of illness ↑ Duration of untreated psychosis ↓ Possibilities for early intervention	'Difficult to engage' patients Social factors more difficult to control if job/supports lost Frustrations at non-compliance ↑ Ratio of involuntary to voluntary inpatients (↑ people on Sections, ?↑ ward violence)	Cycle of low morale and recruitment, loss of trained staff, lack of resources, perception of being undervalued, and reacting only to emergencies and serious incidents: 'take it or leave it' psychiatry Combination of work pressures, ↑ losses to follow-up and isolation make (rare) violence more likely

How does stigma-discrimination operate?

Link and Phelan (2001) conclude by asking four questions of potential stigmatizers: (1) do they have the power to ensure that the human difference they recognize is broadly identified in the culture? (2) Do they have the power to make sure the dominant culture accepts the stereotypes they connect to labelled differences? (3) Do they have the power to separate us from them, and to make the designation stick? (4) Do they control access to education, employment, healthcare and housing? If the answers here are Yes, we can expect stigma to result. If No, 'what we generally mean by stigma would not exist' (Link & Phelan 2001). Put simply, for any act of stigma-discrimination against any group (people with mental or physical disabilities, or of minority ethnic status), a powerful dominant culture needs to identify (label) and act (discriminate). Discrimination can occur at a structural level (think of institutional racism), a group level (residents objecting to a group home in their locality) or an individual level (bullying, verbal and physical abuse).

Stigma and the media

Another approach to understanding stigma is through the media. For some, the media are *the* cause of mental illness stigma, yet this is impossible to prove: various media produce snapshots of stigma, and these are an interesting way to reveal aspects of stigma (Byrne 2000). Characters with mental illness are common in television fiction, and far more frequently violent (than in reality) to capture the ratings. Their currency is the stereotype, at its most extreme in media representations of the psychokiller. The movies of the psychokiller, with (usually) *his* roots in Victorian horror and melodrama, is both mad and bad, and frequently returns to familiar surroundings to effect a terrible revenge for real or imagined wrongs (Byrne 1998). Porter (1991) describes how, in 1793, Philippe Pinel 'struck off the chains from his charges' at Salpêtrière and Bicêtre asylums in Paris, preceding even the enlightened *York Retreat* of Samuel Tuke. Yet it was Pinel who defined madness in stark black and white terms:

> 'Of all the afflictions to which human nature is subject, the loss of reason is at once the most calamitous and interesting. Deprived of this faculty, by which a man is principally distinguished from the beasts that perish, the human form is frequently the most remarkable attribute that he retains of his proud distinction. His character, as an individual of the species is always perverted, sometimes annihilated. His thoughts and actions are diverted from their usual and natural course. The chain which connected his ideas in just series and mutual subserviency is dissevered. His feelings for himself and others are new and uncommon. His attachments are converted into aversions, his love into hatred.'

(Pinel 1806)

Although undoubtedly progressive for its time, Pinel demonstrates the common habit to divide the world into good/evil, sane/insane, human/inhuman, moral/immoral, love/hate, etc. It is this division, crystallized by Robert Louis Stevenson when he wrote *The Strange Case of Dr Jekyll and Mr Hyde* in 1885, which drives the psychokiller stereotype (Byrne 1998). There are parallels between stereotypes of mental illness and ethnic stereotypes. By definition, stereotypes are one-dimensional caricatures that manage limited information efficiently. It is also important to note that recognition of a stereotype (ethnic, racist, ageist, sexist, etc.) is often a neutral finding, in that recognition does not imply agreement with the stereotype. Banner headlines and movie psychokillers do not in themselves prove that there is a stigma of mental illness: they prove that the writer/producer is at least aware that society recognizes the motifs and, on occasions, endorses them as having some basis in reality. Three other stereotypes of mental illness are the pathetic mad, the comedic and the weak. Glasson (1996) makes the point that current media excesses should be seen in the context of wider public concerns about community care. Along with other commentators, she identifies many failures of community care, and cites poor liaison between health and social services, closure of hospitals before development of community facilities, and inadequate community support as important additional considerations (Glasson 1996). In other words, 'don't shoot the messenger'.

Sociological theories

Erving Goffman (1963) first articulated the theoretical concept of stigma from a sociological perspective. It is important to note that stigma is a theoretical concept: Goffman (1963) did not discover stigma, rather he invented it. For Goffman, a stigmatized person:

> 'is disqualified from full social acceptance'

(1963: 9)

> 'is a blemished person, ritually polluted, to be avoided especially in public places'

(1963: 11)

> 'has a discrepancy (stigma) between his actual social identity and his virtual social identity ... that virtual social identity is formed by certain expectations and normative expectations (by others about the stranger)'

(1963: 12)

> 'has a character blemish ... (and) we construct an ideology to explain difference using language'

(1963: 15)

From the perspective of the 'in-group', we do not wish to define ourselves as prejudiced: we idealize our responses ('some of my best friends have mental illness') and seek to minimize acts of discrimination and omissions ('I'd like to hire someone with schizophrenia, but the job would be too stressful for him'). For people with mental illness stigma, shame and secrecy maintain equilibrium until (for some) it can no longer be denied. Equally, the coping mechanisms listed by Goffman (denial, displacement, projection and search for sympathetic others) all make stigma harder to find and to quantify. Such reactions to mental illness by people who become ill, are exactly the same as those found in general public samples (who do not), namely denial, isolation and insulation of mental illness. Although Goffman had considerable expertise about the plight of people with mental illness (an earlier book, *Asylums*, described the experience of being mentally ill with great precision), his work on stigma was intended to cover all possible stigmas within a unified theory.

Thomas Scheff

A second influential sociologist, Thomas Scheff, wrote specifically about people with mental illness: for Scheff, the process of deviance and its labelling overrode other concerns (Scheff 1966). Scheff rejected the psychiatric 'slogan' that mental disorders were an illness like any other, arguing that none of the four components of the medical model (cause, lesion, symptoms and outcome) applied to psychiatry (Scheff 1975). Scheff's Labelling Theory assumed societal conceptions of mental illness would cause deviant behaviour to be so labelled; others' reactions to the behaviour were based on these conceptions; and the person then adopted the 'role of mental illness'. Scheff (1966) believed that 'labelled deviants may be rewarded for playing the stereotyped role ... and are punished when they attempt to return to conventional roles'. He concluded: 'when the individual internalizes this role, incorporating it as a central identity, chronic mental illness is the consequence' (Scheff 1966). Scheff's Labelling Theory has often been cited as implying that there is no mental illness, but he later argued that he did not wish the theory to replace psychiatry, and regretted stating that societal reaction was the *most important single cause* (of mental illness), but perhaps accounted for 5–10%; of cases (Scheff 1975). He continued to disagree that 'stigma may be more profitably viewed as a consequence than a cause of career deviance' (Scheff 1975).

Modified Labelling Theory (MLT) proposed an alteration to the intermediate stage in Scheff's Labelling Theory: it was not the response of others, but rather the response of the labelled individual which predicted consequences for future vulnerability to relapse and self-esteem (Link et al 1989). MLT allowed for multiple relapses in severe mental illness where the person was unaware of the label (insightless about the diagnosis) and it accepted circumstances where psychopathology alone led to negative outcomes.

Social psychology

Social psychology recognizes that all behaviour takes place within a social context, and that even when alone, our actions and inaction are influenced by others. Gross (2000) defines prejudice as an extreme attitude with cognitive, affective and behavioural components, though the third part may not be manifested. Because stigma is a social construct, we must first distinguish between interpersonal and intergroup processes: there are similarities, but the two processes need to be studied within separate frameworks. Crocker et al (1998) produced a comprehensive review of social stigma, of which mental illness is one example. While there are aspects of the stigmatization of people with mental health problems unique to these labels and processes, they provide a useful conceptualization of the power of situations to shape experiences and esteem. One aspect, stereotype threat, occurs where a stigmatized person is aware both of the negative stereotypes (about their status/condition) and that their behaviour will be judged on these grounds. They also conclude that for stigmatizers, 'stigma is about sustaining the belief that I am and we are good (or at least better than they are), maintaining our belief that we are just, fair and deserving' (Crocker et al 1998).

The psychiatric literature

It is worth noting, that stigma became a major subject in psychiatric journals only in the last decade, as a direct result of anti-stigma campaigns. Current diagnostic manuals for mental disorders do not include provision for the effects of any kind of stigma or discrimination in the course of someone's illness. Textbooks of general or social psychiatry have only recently included references, let alone sections, to stigma-discrimination. In these respects, the medical model has failed to address stigma.

It has been argued that institutional psychiatry has contributed to *increasing* the stigma attached to mental illness (Porter 1991; Byrne 2000; Sayce 2000). There is also evidence that psychiatrists are not good at highlighting or understanding the effects of stigma. For example, during the asylum era, patient characteristics that we now recognize as the effects of *institutionalization* were then described as part of the syndrome of schizophrenia (Byrne 2000). One would expect that recently, the profession would have heightened awareness of stigma in severe mental illness, namely schizophrenia. Yet, an extensive review based on meta-analysis (152 references) in a major journal (*Acta Psychiatrica Scandinavica*) failed to consider *any* role for stigma-discrimination in the 'differential diagnosis' of low mood in people with schizophrenia (Hausmann & Fleischhacker 2002). They concluded that depressed mood unrelated to medication, substance misuse, organic pathology, negative symptoms or active psychosis, could be explained by either primary process

schizophrenia (prodrome/postpsychotic depression), schizoaffective disorder or *demoralization*. 'Chronic demoralization should be considered when patients present with a chronic and persistent state of hopelessness and existentialist distress in the absence of somatic features of depression' (Hausmann & Fleischhacker 2002). The concept of demoralization, in contrast to stigma or discrimination, implies that the problem is located within the individual and fails to highlight the role of wider social processes.

What about discrimination?

Service users' surveys measure discrimination by asking people directly about their experiences (Read & Baker 1996; Mental Health Foundation 2000) but have had low response rates (17% and 13%, respectively), and are therefore open to the charge of over-reporting acts of discrimination by a self-selected group. That said, the findings are not easy to ignore. Read and Baker (1996) reported 47% had been abused or harassed in public, 26% had moved home because of harassment, with physical assault in 14%. Other sources of discrimination were the workplace (47%), seeking employment (37%), from friends (26%) and access to housing (10%) (Mental Health Foundation 2000). Of course a major focus on any work should be to measure the consequences of stigma (Table 12.2), and one cannot study stigma without studying discrimination, but addressing discrimination alone will not answer the Why? and How? questions, or uncover hidden (indirect) discriminations. Put another way, discrimination is the behavioural consequence of prejudice and stigma, but limiting studies to discrimination alone is problematic in underestimating the totality of stigma-discrimination.

Stigma includes indirect discrimination

Examination of all aspects of stigma-discrimination is especially important in Western societies where anti-discrimination legislation has unintended consequences in driving discrimination underground. Taking just two examples of this, the workplace and health services, we can identify several aspects of stigma: indirect discrimination, value judgements, prejudice and social exclusion. Goldberg and Steury (2001) identify employers' misconceptions about effective treatments for depression, untreated depression as a workplace disability, and its economic consequences including lower wages, different insurance supports, and a discriminatory workers' compensation system. Levenson and Olbrisch (1993) have measured medical staff opinions as to the suitability of people with schizophrenia for organ transplantation, given the rationing and high costs of these procedures. They report that 'active schizophrenia' (*sic*) is an *absolute* contraindication to transplant in 92% cardiac, 67% liver and 73% renal units; when the condition is described as 'controlled schizophrenia', staff believe this to be either an absolute or relative contraindication: 85%, 80% and 68%, respectively. Phipps (1997) has described 11 years of cardiac transplantation (*n*=706) in Canada: 28 people were denied transplants on 'psychiatric grounds'. These included drug and alcohol misuse (7); non-compliance (3); multiple suicide attempts (2); unrealistic expectations (2); and borderline personality disorder (2) (Phipps 1997). In doctors' daily practice, there are more subtle ways (short of denying life) in which we discriminate against psychiatric patients.

Solutions at the individual level/clinic-based

One of the unique benefits of detailed psychosocial assessment is the ability to understand the meanings of symptoms and events for *that patient* at this time. We can therefore note the interaction of reduced social networks and stigma experiences on service users. It is no more 'dangerous' to enquire about stigma/victimization events than it is to enquire about suicidal ideation. Without assigning blame onto the service user, are there ways in which the outward signs of mental illness can be better disguised? Each day, reflect on the mental health service you provide, and ask yourself: 'is this how I, or a member of my family, would like to be treated?' Mind your language: describing someone as 'a schizophrenic' gives little information to his or her situation or humanity. Better again is the growing practice of increasing service user participation at every stage of service delivery, teaching and research. More than any other intervention, direct contact with service users in a context of equality (not across the clinic table) will reduce the 'them and us' of Table 12.1 There is also a growing evidence base for a cognitive-behavioural approach to stigma, with an emphasis on the problems which can be solved. Equally, everyone who has been or could be stigmatized could do a 'cost benefit analysis' of the benefits and risks of disclosing the secret of mental illness to others including family, employers and landlords.

Solutions at the group-based and structural levels

At every level of society, discrimination against the two *broad* groups – disability and race – is negatively sanctioned. There are laws (Disability and Race Relations Acts) to prevent overt discrimination, verbal abuse and exclusion. Many governments practice positive discrimination: in Italy, firms of a certain size are legally bound to employ people with disabilities (physical or mental) as 15%; of the workforce. Companies who fail to do this pay fines into a social fund. It is also true that people with disabilities and from ethnic minorities are well represented by government and non-governmental agencies, and that as (historical) out-groups, they have united in the common cause. It works against mental illness that, unlike physical disability and race, it can be concealed: secrecy may work as a strategy for the stigmatized individual, but makes collegiality more difficult. In the UK, our culture has changed to such a degree that words such as 'cripple, spastic, nigger, wog, etc.' have been driven underground. By contrast, the media continue to use terms such as 'loony, bonkers, maniac, psycho, etc.', which dehumanize people and make a complex problem even more of a turn off for the public. In their desire to sell newspapers and fill airtime, the (rare) homicides where mental illness is a factor are sensationalized. The challenge is to engage with the media and explain the context even of those instances which could be characterized as psychiatry's failures. Recent successes with target groups such as police, doctors, teachers and schoolchildren, have made anti-stigma research one of the most exciting areas of mental health.

References

Andresen, R., Caputi, P., Oades, L., 2003. The experience of recovery from schizophrenia: towards an empirically validated stage model. Aust. N.Z. J. Psychiatry 37, 586–594.

Barnes, M., Bowl, R., 2001. Taking over the asylum: empowerment and mental health. Palgrave, Basingstoke.

Blackwell, B., Shepherd, M., 1968. Prophylactic lithium: another therapeutic myth? An examination of the evidence to date. Lancet 1, 968–971.

Byrne, P., 1998. The fall and rise of the movie psychokiller. Psychiatric Bulletin 21, 173–175.

Byrne, P., 2000. The stigma of mental illness and ways of diminishing it. Advances in Psychiatric Treatment 6, 65–72.

Campbell, P., 1998. The service user/survivor movement. In: Newnes, C., Holmes, G., Dunn, C. (Eds.), This is madness. PCCS Books, Ross-on-Wye.

Crawford, M.J., Aldridge, T., Bhui, K., et al., 2003. User involvement in the planning and delivery of mental health services: a cross-sectional survey of service users and providers. Acta Psychiatr. Scand. 107, 410–414.

Crocker, J., Major, B., Steele, C., 1998. Social stigma. In: Gilbert, D., Fiske, S., Lindzey, G. (Eds.), Handbook of social psychology, Vol. II. McGraw-Hill, New York, pp. 504–553.

Crossley, N., 1998. R. D. Laing and the British anti-psychiatry movement: a socio-historical analysis. Soc. Sci. Med. 47, 877–889.

Davidson, L., O'Connell, M., Tondora, J., et al., 2006. The top ten concerns about recovery encountered in mental health system transformation. Psychiatr. Serv. 57, 640–645.

Deegan, P.E., Drake, R.E., 2006. Shared decision making and medication management in the recovery process. Psychiatr. Serv. 57, 1636–1639.

Department of Health, 1999. A national service framework for mental health. Department of Health, London.

Foucault, M., 1965. Madness and civilization. Tavistock, London.

Glasson, J., 1996. The public image of the mentally ill and community care. Br. J. Nurs. 5, 615–617.

Goffman, E., 1963. Stigma: notes on the management of spoiled identity. Prentice-Hall, Engelwood Cliffs, New Jersey.

Goldberg, R.J., Steury, S., 2001. Depression in the workplace: costs and barriers to treatment. Psychiatr. Serv. 52, 1639–1643.

Gross, R. (Ed.), 2000. Prejudice and discrimination. In: Psychology. Hodder and Stoughton, London.

Hausmann, A., Fleischhacker, W.W., 2002. Differential diagnosis of depressed mood in patients with schizophrenia: a diagnostic algorithm based on a review. Acta Psychiatr. Scand. 106, 83–96.

HM Government, 2009. Work, recovery and inclusion: employment support for people in contact with secondary care mental health services. HM Government, London.

Kelson, M., 1996. Consumer involvement in the audit activities of the royal colleges and other professional bodies. College of Health, London.

Kutchins, H., Kirk, S.A., 1997. Making us crazy. Free Press, New York.

Laing, R.D., 1960. The divided self. Tavistock, London.

Levenson, J.L., Olbrisch, M.E., 1993. Psychosocial evaluation of organ transplant candidates. Psychosomatics 34, 314–323.

Link, B.G., Cullen, F.T., Struening, E.L., et al., 1989. A modified labeling theory approach to mental disorders: an empirical assessment. Am. Sociol. Rev. 54, 400–423.

Link, B.G., Phelan, J.C., 2001. Conceptualizing stigma. Br. J. Nurs. 27, 363–385.

Mental Health Foundation, 2000. Pull yourself together: a survey of the stigma and discrimination faced by people who experience mental distress. Mental Health Foundation, London.

Moncrieff, J., 2003. The politics of a new Mental Health Act. Br. J. Psychiatry 183, 8–9.

Phipps, L., 1997. Psychiatric evaluation and outcomes in candidates for heart

Psychiatry of learning disability

13

Jean O'Hara

CHAPTER CONTENTS

Introduction

What is learning disability? The UK Government's policy document 'Valuing People' (DoH 2001a) defines it as:

- A significantly reduced ability to understand new or complex information, to learn new skills (impaired intelligence), with
- a reduced ability to cope independently (impaired social functioning)
- which started before adulthood, with a lasting effect on development.

While the psychiatry of learning disability is a specialist field, 'Valuing People' makes it explicit that the NHS should be able to accommodate the needs of people with learning disabilities in mainstream services, with specialist support as appropriate. This 'integration' and 'social inclusion' has meant that the needs of people with learning disabilities must feature in the undergraduate and postgraduate training of all healthcare professionals (Box 13.1).

This chapter provides a core text to the understanding of learning disabilities and the generic and specialist mental health needs of this population. Other developmental aspects are covered elsewhere in this volume.

Definitions and terminology

In the UK, the Department of Health has adopted the term 'learning disability', although people themselves prefer 'learning difficulty'. (The reader should also be aware that 'learning difficulty' is used in education to cover a wider group of specific learning problems, such as dyslexia.) In the USA, the official term is 'mental retardation'; in developing countries, it is 'mental handicap', while in international literature, the term 'intellectual disability' has emerged.

International classification systems such as ICD-10 (WHO 1992) and DSM-IV (APA 1994) refer to 'mental retardation'. Mental impairment and severe mental impairment, previously

Box 13.1

The MRCPsych curriculum

The MRCPsych curriculum (RCPsych 2009) expects the following core subjects to be examined or assessed as part of a range of competency 'workplace-based assessments' with regard to the psychiatry of learning disability:

1. Stages of normal human development – including how cognitive and emotional development may influence the aetiology, presentation and management of mental health problems; gene-environment interactions with specific reference to intelligence; developmental issues in relation to cultural and economic backgrounds
2. Family relationships and parenting practices
3. Genetics and conditions associated with chromosome abnormalities
4. Mental health problems and mental illness (including good clinical practice, service provision, treatment options and issues of consent)
5. All aspects of risk assessment, risk management and contributory factors
6. Being a good communicator; working within multidisciplinary teams.

Box 13.2

WHO definitions of impairment, disability and handicap

- Impairment – a loss or abnormality of structure or function, including psychological functioning
- Disability – a restriction or lack of ability to perform an activity within the range considered normal for a human being
- Handicap – a disadvantage resulting from an impairment or disability that limits or prevents the fulfilment of a normal role.

defined in the Mental Health Act (1983), are not synonymous with learning disability.

The World Health Organization (WHO 1980) makes a distinction between impairment, disability and handicap (Box 13.2).

Historical overview

'... even if the nature went wrong, yet nothing has been wrong with the soul and the spirit'

(Paracelsus, sixteenth century Swiss physician)

Societies and historical periods have dealt with disability and handicap in different ways. In European history, the Spartans allowed weak infants to perish, while the Romans killed malformed children, and used 'defectives' for amusement. In the Middle Ages, witchcraft and belief in changelings often resulted in cruel treatment. It was during the reign of Edward I (1272–1307) that a distinction was made between the 'born fool' (learning disability) and the 'lunatic' (mental illness). Eighteenth century education theories led to attempts to educate the deaf and the 'wild boy of Aveyron'. In 1846, Seguin declared that 'while waiting for medicine to cure idiots, I have undertaken to see that they participate in the benefit of education'.

By the mid-nineteenth century, there was a greater scientific interest in the nature and the inheritance of abilities, clinical and behavioural symptoms and syndromes. The development of the IQ (intelligence quotient) test was hailed as a great scientific advance, and led to the 'discovery' of many 'mentally deficient people' who would not fit into the education system of the time.

In an attempt to provide more humane and protective care for those afflicted, and to prevent a 'national degeneracy', Victorian England created the first workhouses and asylums. An Idiots Act was passed in 1886 to care for 'idiots and imbeciles'. The 1910 General Election included a vigorous campaign 'discouraging parenthood in feeble-minded and other degenerate types' and for the building of separate institutions. The Mental Deficiency Act (1913) introduced compulsory certification for people admitted to institutions as 'mentally defective' (Ryan 1980).

Ideas of degeneration persisted, with the Nazi extermination of thousands of 'mentally handicapped' people, and the 'voluntary' sterilization of 'mentally defective' women in the UK, while such sterilizations became compulsory in many US states.

UK government policies and philosophy of care

In post-war Britain, asylums were incorporated in the newly formed National Health Service (1948). It resulted in the 'medicalization' of learning disability: residents became patients, 'treated from cradle to grave' by nurses and doctors, often in institutions far away from the local community. Over the years, it led to appalling physical and material conditions, as well as chronic understaffing. Scandals reached public awareness in 1967/8 through two newspaper articles, one in the *News of the World* about Ely Hospital, and the other in *The Guardian* about Harperbury Hospital. The government responded with the publication of its policy document, 'Better Services for the Mentally Handicapped', in 1971. Its core premise was that people with learning disability should not 'necessarily' be segregated from others. 'Normalization' of the physical environment and a normal living routine were essential components to care. Treating the person as an individual, and valuing his/her role within society (social role valorization) underpinned this social philosophy. However, the blanket adoption of normalization and ordinary life principles led, in some cases, to a denial of difference. Health needs were ignored or neglected in an 'anti-medical' stance, while community teams (community team for people with learning disabilities otherwise known as CTLD, or community learning disability team otherwise known as CLDT) adopted a social model of care where specialist skills were often denied and medical or psychiatric involvement marginalized.

Some 30 years later, the Government published 'Valuing People' (DoH 2001a), with its emphasis on valuing the person with a learning disability, including their human and civil rights, their right to live as ordinary citizens, to live in the community and access ordinary services, and to have a family life. It recognized the barriers to accessing the same healthcare as others and acknowledged that people with learning disabilities may have complex health needs requiring specialist knowledge and intervention. It also acknowledged their increased vulnerability to mental illness. More recent scandals have led to higher prioritization of physical healthcare for vulnerable groups (Michael Report, DH 2008b) and specific quality measures from health and social care organizations (Care Quality Commission, CQC 2009).

Aetiology and prevention

While much has been published on the causes of learning disability and interventions to prevent the birth of such an afflicted child, it is important to consider how society's 'pursuit of perfection' may impact on the life of an individual with learning disability and his/her family.

Globally, learning disability is associated with poverty, malnutrition and environmental factors. In the UK, 90% of the learning disabled population are only mildly disabled, and up to 60% will not have an identifiable cause for their disability. They are, however, more likely to have parents belonging to lower socioeconomic groups and to have experienced a socially disadvantaged environment.

It is customary for textbooks to list examples of the many prenatal, perinatal and postnatal causes of learning disability, including:

- Infective and inflammatory agents, e.g. the ToRCH infections (toxoplasmosis, rubella, cytomegalovirus and herpes)
- Toxic/metabolic factors, e.g. lead, maternal smoking in pregnancy, maternal alcohol consumption in pregnancy, drugs – prescribed and illicit
- Traumatic events pre- and perinatally, e.g. assisted deliveries, hypoxic events, prematurity, very low birthweight
- Chromosomal and genetic causes (Table 13.1)
- Endocrine disorders

- Maternal factors, e.g. anaemia, hypertension, bleeding during pregnancy
- Postnatal factors, e.g. encephalitis, meningitis, severe dehydration and electrolyte imbalance, head injuries, non-accidental injuries (violent shaking), hypoxia.

Psychological or 'reversible' causes include maternal and sensory deprivation, neglect and sexual abuse, leading to a failure to thrive in an infant or developmental delay in a child. Such experiences can lead to a 'secondary handicap' – a psychological defence that protects the self from unbearable memories. It may be the primary cause of the disability, or may exacerbate the experience of 'handicap' (Sinason 1992).

Epidemiological aspects and the IQ test

The total learning disabled population in England is about 1.2 million; 210 000 have severe or profound disabilities.

Intelligence is believed to follow a normal distribution, with the average at 100, although this is increasing. There is a smaller peak towards the lower end of the bell-shaped curve, to take account of those with severe learning disability caused by clear organic factors. Two standard deviations above and below the mean would encompass 95% of the population: i.e. 95% of the population would score between 70 and 130 on an IQ test. A score below 70 is defined as 'intellectual impairment', and below 50 is defined as severe intellectual impairment. Clearly, these are arbitrary cut-offs, but they give a prevalence rate of mild (2–3%) and severe (0.2–0.3%) intellectual impairment.

However, impaired intellectual functioning is only one factor in the definition of learning disability. It is important to assess social/adaptive skills, particularly in those with mild intellectual impairment and to be clear about the person's educational opportunities and personal history. In practice, this consideration is not of diagnostic importance in those presenting with severe disabilities.

IQ scores must therefore be interpreted with care, particularly as there are many different profiles of ability that give the same total IQ score. Non-verbal tests are used where English is not the primary language, but cultural sensitivity cannot be assumed. Performance is also affected by medication/drugs, mental state, concentration, motivation and the ability to complete tasks within a time frame.

Communication

The GMC's publication *Tomorrow's Doctors* (2002) highlights the importance of being able to communicate effectively with individuals, regardless of their disability (Box 13.3). People with learning disabilities may have cognitive difficulties such as slow reaction times, difficulty sustaining attention, and long- and short-term memory problems. Their language development may be:

Delayed: smaller vocabulary, limited grammar resulting in difficulty understanding and using the full range of tenses,

Table 13.1 Some chromosomal and genetic causes of learning disability

Chromosomal disorders

Autosomal	Down syndrome (trisomy 21)
Deletion/microdeletion	Prader–Willi syndrome (long arm – chromosome 15) Cri du chat syndrome (short arm – chromosome 5)
Sex-linked	Klinefelter syndrome (47XXXY) Turner syndrome (45XO)
Genomic imprinting	Prader–Willi syndrome (ch 15 – paternal origin) Angelman syndrome (ch 15 – maternal origin)

Single gene disorders

Dominant	Neurofibromatosis Tuberous sclerosis
Recessive	Inborn errors of metabolism, e.g. phenylketonuria
X-linked	Lesch–Nyhan (hyperuricaemia) Fragile X syndrome (Xq27) – CGG repeats

areas, which not only influence presentation but management options.

A hierarchical approach to diagnosis is adopted within learning disability psychiatry, in accordance with ICD-10 (Mental Retardation).

Axis I: Severity of learning disabilities

Axis II: Cause of learning disabilities; other associated medical conditions

Axis III: Psychiatric disorders

DC-LD Level A: Developmental disorders

DC-LD Level B: Psychiatric illness

DC-LD Level C: Personality disorders

DC-LD Level D: Problem behaviours

DC-LD Level E: Other disorders

Axis IV: Global assessment of psychosocial disability

Axis V: Associated abnormal psychosocial situations.

Work is underway to consider how best to include learning disabilities in ICD-II.

Treatment issues

The range of investigations and treatments available to the general population should also be made available to people with learning disabilities. It is important to acknowledge that access to healthcare is often dependent on others, and referrals may be made to services without the person's knowledge or agreement. Particular issues to consider include:

* Person-centred approach
* Consent and incapacitated adults
* Physical treatments
* Psychological treatments.

The decision to prescribe medication should follow a comprehensive assessment of the person's emotional and behavioural disturbance. The psychiatrist should try to resist 'knee-jerk' responses despite the pressure of crises presentations (Einfeld 2001). It is unusual for medication alone to be sufficient; drug treatment should be part of an integrated multidisciplinary care plan. Proper consideration needs to be given to informed consent (see below).

Antipsychotics

* Atypical antipsychotics are now the first drug of choice in the treatment of schizophrenia
* There is no good evidence that antipsychotic medication helps in managing challenging behaviour (systematic review of randomized controlled trials/RCTs)
* Lower level evidence suggests antipsychotic medication can reduce challenging behaviours but with significant side-effects. Approximately 25% can be treated effectively, 50% fairly effectively and the remaining 25% with intermittent success or not at all
* Akathisia is an important side-effect to consider, particularly as the person may be unable to describe the sense of restlessness and irritability. The resultant increase in

agitation may lead the psychiatrist to increase the dose of antipsychotic medication inappropriately
* The fatality rate of neuroleptic malignant syndrome in people with learning disabilities is twice that of the general population.

Antidepressants

* SSRIs have largely supplanted tricyclic antidepressants in the treatment of depression in people with learning disability
* SSRIs are widely used to treat repetitive behaviours, including ritualistic/stereotypic behaviours associated with autism and self-injurious behaviours (SIB)
* In practice, the availability of a liquid preparation often makes it easier to accept and administer, and may be the deciding factor in the choice of one SSRI over another.

Anxiolytics

* No specific studies available on the treatment of anxiety in people with learning disabilities
* Use of medication is similar to the general population, with the assumption that it acts in the same way and with the same results
* Benzodiazepines are commonly used in the treatment of epilepsy, but are not used for behavioural or emotional disturbance, as it frequently causes disinhibition and irritability in people with organic brain impairment.

Mood stabilizers

* Lithium, carbamazepine and valproate are used as mood stabilizers in the treatment of bipolar affective disorder
* The difficulties of monitoring side-effects of lithium, as well as serum lithium levels, in this population make carbamazepine and valproate the drugs of choice
* Lithium and carbamazepine have also been used in the treatment of impulsive, aggressive behaviours.

Other drugs

* People with learning disabilities are frequently on anti-epileptic drugs. These may have psychiatric side-effects
* Stimulants are used in the treatment of attention deficit hyperactivity disorder (ADHD)
* Anti-libidinal drugs are sometimes used as a last resort in the treatment of inappropriate sexual behaviours in men with learning disabilities who have sexually offended
* As in the general population, hypnotics may help with sleep problems in the short term, but it is more important to assess the reasons why sleep is disturbed, to establish good sleep hygiene and to treat any underlying physical, emotional, psychiatric or environmental cause.

Parents with learning disability

The reproductive rights of women with learning disabilities have been at risk for much of the twentieth century. They are now enshrined in human rights legislation, and reflected in

'Valuing People'. Parents with learning disabilities have special needs, while acknowledging that the needs of their children are paramount. Until the last decade, the literature has tended to concentrate on risk factors, the inadequacies of parenting skills, parenting assessments and the provision of parenting skills programmes to those at the mild or borderline range of intellectual functioning.

Children of learning-disabled parents are particularly vulnerable to removal from their natural parents. Care proceedings are often inaccessible to parents with learning disabilities. Research suggests that an IQ score below 65 means that children are invariably placed into care, while above this score, the outcome depends on the network of support available. All too often, services are patchy and constrained by resources. There is a will to act proactively with such families, and there has been recent recognition of the mental health needs of parents with learning disabilities, whether or not their child is removed into care (O'Keeffe & O'Hara 2008).

Growing older with learning disability

People with learning disabilities are an ageing population. The increased lifespan is in part due to advances in medical treatments, better nutrition and healthier lifestyles. It is reasonable to speculate that many older people with learning disabilities will experience significant psychiatric health needs, but there is little research data available (Cooper 1997). However, the prevalence of dementia is much higher than in the age-matched general population. This has been a relatively neglected area as much clinical and research attention has been given to the dementia of Down syndrome.

The barriers to accessing appropriate healthcare for people with learning disabilities are compounded when one is older in part due to forced 'retirement' from day centres and loss of contact with care managers as they 'transfer' into mainstream elderly services.

Learning disability and the law

People with learning disabilities and the criminal justice system

Intellectual impairment (i.e. low IQ, but not necessarily learning disabilities) is a risk factor for offending in both adults and juveniles. There is little evidence to suggest that the presence of learning disability predisposes to criminal behaviour. There are particular difficulties looking at the numbers convicted; it is generally considered that the prevalence rates for offenders with learning disabilities may be higher than the general population, especially among those convicted of arson or sexual offences. There is also a predominance of males among offenders with learning disability.

People receiving specialist learning disability services are unlikely to offend, partly because the offending behaviour is re-labelled as 'challenging behaviour' and therefore decriminalized. However, in the UK, people with learning disabilities are over-represented among those arrested and taken to police stations, especially those with mild disability. The Police and Criminal Evidence Act 1984 (PACE) seeks to protect vulnerable people during the interview process, and requires the presence of an appropriate adult.

People with learning disabilities are also victims of crime. The fact that they have learning disabilities may prejudice their chances of being judged to be a reliable witness. Prosecutions are therefore not very common. The Bradley Report (DH 2009b) emphasizes that all parts of the process must be more aware and sensitive to the special needs of this vulnerable population.

The Mental Health Act (1983): England and Wales – 2007 Amendments

* Admission to hospital for assessment and treatment under the amended Mental Health Act (1983) applies if the person with learning disabilities fulfils the criteria for compulsory admission.
* The categories of 'mental impairment' and 'severe mental impairment' have been removed from the amended MHA 1983. Mental disorder is now defined more broadly as 'any disorder or disability of mind' (with the exception of drug dependence). However, to detain a person with learning disability in the absence of another mental disorder, the learning disability must be associated with 'seriously irresponsible or abnormally aggressive behaviour'. Therefore, this will only apply to a minority of people with learning disability needing hospital treatment because of a severe behavioural problem. Before being subject to compulsory detention, there must be appropriate medical treatment available at the hospital in which the person is detained.
* Guardianship allows an individual to receive community care where it cannot be provided without the use of compulsory powers. It requires the person to reside in a specified place, attend for education, training and daycare and gives access to any medical practitioner, social worker or other person specified by the guardian. It cannot be used for compulsory medication. The 2007 amendments contain the additional power to convey the person to the place where they are required to live; unauthorized removal is a criminal offence carrying a prison sentence of up to 5 years.
* The new Supervised Community Treatment Orders (CTOs) were introduced to facilitate early discharge of patients and to treat people in the community in less restrictive settings. The Code of Practice gives some guidance on choosing between guardianship (social care-led), section 17 leave (short-term leave for up to 7 days) and CTOs (DH 2008a).

The Care Programme Approach (CPA)

The use of CPA in learning disability services is variable across the country, yet all those with mental health needs must be assessed for CPA. The situation is partly due to the current fragmentation and organization of learning disability services, some within a partnership trust, others within a primary care or mental health trust.

References

ADSS, 2005. Safeguarding adults: a national framework of standards for good practice and outcomes in adult protection work. Association of Directors of Social Services, London.

Ambalu, S., 1997. Communication. In: O'Hara, J., Sperlinger, A. (Eds.), Adults with learning disabilities: a practical approach for health professionals. John Wiley, Chichester.

AMRC, 2009. No health without mental health: the ALERT summary report. Academy of Medical Royal Colleges, London.

APA, 1994. Diagnostic and Statistical Manual of Mental Disorders, fourth ed. American Psychiatric Association, Washington DC.

Brown, H., 1997. Vulnerability issues. In: O'Hara, J., Sperlinger, A. (Eds.), Adults with learning disabilities: a practical approach for health professionals. John Wiley, Chichester.

Butt, J., Mirza, K., 1996. Social care and black communities. HMSO, London.

Carvill, S., 2001. Sensory impairments, intellectual disability and psychiatry. J. Intellect. Disabil. Res. 45, 467–483.

Cooper, S.A., 1997. Learning disabilities and old age. Advances in Psychiatric Treatment 3, 312–320.

CQC, 2009. Performance assessment 2009/10 – indicators for acute and specialist trusts. Care Quality Commission, London.

Deb, S., 1997. Behavioural phenotypes. In: Read, S.G. (Ed.), Psychiatry in learning disability. WB Saunders, London (Chapter 4).

DoH, 2000. No secrets: the protection of vulnerable adults. Guidance on the development and implementation of multi-agency policies and procedures. HMSO, London.

DoH, 2001a. Valuing people: a strategy for learning disabilities for the 21st century. HMSO, London.

DoH, 2001b. Families matter: counting families. HMSO, London.

DoH, 2001c. Nothing about us without us. HMSO, London.

DH, 2007. Services for people with learning disabilities and challenging behaviour or mental health needs, revised ed. (Mansell Report II). Department of Health, London.

DH, 2008a. Code of Practice, Mental Health Act 1983. The Stationery Office, London.

DH, 2008b. Healthcare for all. Report of the independent inquiry into access to healthcare for people with learning disabilities (Michael Report). Department of Health, London.

DH, 2009a. Services for adults with autistic spectrum conditions (ASC): good practice advice for primary care trusts and local authority commissioners. Department of Health, Social Care Policy and Innovation, London.

DH, 2009b. The Bradley Report: Lord Bradley's review of people with mental health problems or learning disabilities in the criminal justice system. Department of Health, London.

DH, 2009c. Valuing people now: a new three year strategy for people with learning disabilities – making it happen for everyone. Social Care Policy and Innovation, Department of Health, London.

DH, 2009d. New horizons: towards a shared vision for mental health. A consultation. Department of Health: Mental Health Division, London.

Einfeld, S.L., 2001. Systematic management approach to pharmacotherapy for people with learning disabilities. Advances in Psychiatric Treatment 7, 43–49.

Emerson, E., Barrett, S., Bell, C., et al., 1987. Developing services for people with severe learning difficulties and challenging behaviours. Institute of Social and Applied Psychology, Canterbury.

General Medical Council, 2002. Tomorrow's doctors: recommendations on undergraduate medical education. GMC, London.

HM Government, 2007. Putting people first: a shared vision and commitment to the transformation of adult social care. HM Government, London.

Hubert, J., Hollins, S., 2000. Working with elderly carers of people with learning disabilities and planning for the future. Advances in Psychiatric Treatment 6, 41–48.

Lecomte, J., Mercier, C., 2008. The WHO atlas on global resources for persons with intellectual disabilities: a right to health perspective. Salud Publica Mex. 50, S160–S166.

O'Hara, J., 2003. Learning disability and ethnicity: achieving cultural competence. Advances in Psychiatric Treatment 9, 166–174.

O'Hara, J., 2007. Interdisciplinary multi-modal assessment for mental health problems in people with intellectual disabilities. In: Bouras, N., Holt, G. (Eds.), Psychiatric and behavioural disorders in intellectual and developmental disabilities, second ed. Cambridge University Press, Cambridge, UK, pp. 42–61.

O'Hara, J., 2010. Healthcare and intellectual disability. In: O'Hara, J., McCarthy, J., Bouras, N. (Eds.), Intellectual disability and ill-health: a review of the evidence. Cambridge University Press, Cambridge, UK, pp. 3–16.

O'Keeffe, N., O'Hara, J., 2008. Mental health needs of parents with intellectual disability. Curr. Opin. Psychiatry 21, 463–468.

OPG, 2005. Office of the Public Guardian 2005, the Mental Capacity Act. The Stationery Office, London.

Reiss, S., 1994. Psychopathology in mental retardation. In: Bouras, N. (Ed.), Mental health and mental retardation: recent advances and practices. Cambridge University Press, Cambridge, UK.

Roy, A., 2000. The Care Programme Approach in learning disability psychiatry. Advances in Psychiatric Treatment 6, 380–387.

RCPsych: Royal College of Psychiatrists, 2001. Diagnostic criteria for psychiatric disorders for use with adults with learning disabilities/mental retardation. DC-LD Occasional Paper OP 48, Gaskell, London.

RCPsych, 2009. A competency based curriculum for specialist training in psychiatry: core module. Royal College of Psychiatrists, London.

Ruedrich, S., 2010. Mental illness. In: O'Hara, J., McCarthy, J., Bouras, N. (Eds.), Intellectual disability and ill-health: a review of the evidence. Cambridge University Press, Cambridge, UK, pp. 165–177.

Ryan, J., 1980. The politics of mental handicap. Penguin Books, Harmondsworth.

Sinason, V., 1992. Mental handicap and the human condition: new approaches from the Tavistock. Free Association, London.

Sovner, R., 1986. Limiting factors in the use of DSM-III criteria with mentally ill/mentally retarded persons. Psychopharmacol. Bull. 24, 1055–1059.

WHO, 1980. International Classification of Impairment, Disabilities and Handicaps. World Health Organization, Geneva.

WHO, 1992. The ICD-10 Classification of Mental and Behavioural Disorders. World Health Organization, Geneva.

Child and adolescent psychiatry

14

Nick Goddard

CHAPTER CONTENTS

Introduction

An understanding and knowledge of child and adolescent psychiatry is important not just for prospective child psychiatrists, but for all psychiatrists. Adults with mental health problems were once children and it is therefore necessary to know the relevance of problems in childhood. Additionally, many adults will also be parents and parental illness can adversely affect children.

Epidemiology

Several studies have looked at the epidemiology of child and adolescent mental health. As the child and adolescent population contains subjects at different stages of development, studies have focused on age groups of children. Broadly, the young population can be divided into: pre-school children, middle childhood and adolescence.

Pre-school children

One of the most informative studies in this age group is the pre-school to school study by Richman et al (1982). One in four 3-year-olds from a north-east London borough were selected randomly. The study involved an initial screening interview with assessments at 3, 4 and 8 years for those found to be 'positive' (i.e. above the cut-off point for a mental health problem) and a sample of screen 'negative' children.

- **Findings at 3 years old:** 7% had moderate–severe problems with a further 15% having mild problems. There was a slight excess of boys. Factors associated with psychiatric problems were learning delay, marital discord, low warmth and high criticism in the family, living in a large tower block, large family size and maternal depression.
- **Findings at 8 years old:** of the 3-year-olds with problems, 75% of the boys still had problems and about 50% of the girls. Hyperactivity and low intelligence predicted persistence in boys, though not in girls.

With age, the nature of the problems changed. At 3 years fears, sleep problems, soiling and overactivity were more common. These decreased with age and worries became more common in older children.

The study has implications for early intervention, as early childhood problems can persist, therefore intervention at an early stage seems indicated. It can be difficult, however, to detect problems at this age and predict which ones will persist.

Middle childhood

One of the main sources of information on problems in this age group comes from an elegant study carried out on the Isle of Wight by Rutter et al (1976). All 10–11 year-olds living on the (Iow) of Wight and attending a state school were included. Screening interviews were carried out with teachers and parents. Further assessments were then done on all children who scored above the cut-off point or who were known to have attended child and adolescent mental health services (CAMHS).

Findings of the Isle of Wight study were as follows:

- The prevalence of psychiatric problems was 6.8%.
- Emotional disorders accounted for 2.5% of the prevalence with a similar rate among boys and girls (boy:girl = 0.7:1). There were more only children and children from small families in the group.
- Mixed emotional and conduct disorders were more similar in characteristics to pure conduct disorder.
- Conduct disorder (CD) was present in 4% with an excess of boys (boy:girl = 4:1). Children from large families (>4 children) were over-represented.
- Specific reading difficulties (SRD) overlapped with CD, though mixed SRD/CD was more similar to pure SRD in its presentation.
- Physical disorders were a risk factor for psychiatric problems. In children with a physical disorder not affecting the brain, the proportion with psychiatric problems was 12%; in children with epilepsy the figure was 29% and 44% in those with cerebral palsy.
- Only 10% of children with psychiatric problems were attending child psychiatric services, with a further 10% receiving help from other services.

A similar study was later carried out in an inner London borough, in a deprived area of London. Compared with the IoW study, rates of psychiatric problems were double in the inner London borough study. This is believed to be due to increased rates of marital discord, parental illness, social disadvantage and a high pupil/teacher turnover in schools (Rutter et al 1975).

Adolescence

Epidemiological studies in adolescence are hard to compare because of differences in defining the age range, e.g. 11–19, 13–18. Therefore studies often examine adolescents of a particular age.

The Isle of Wight study was extended to follow up children at the age of 14–15 years and still living in or around the area. The findings were:

- Prevalence of problems was around 9% (2% more than at age 10), with a further 10% of adolescents self-reporting feelings of misery.
- Depressive disorders rose to 2% (an increase from 0.2% at age 10). School refusal also increased.
- Of adolescents who had a problem, about 50% had a problem at the age of 10. New problems were not associated with educational difficulties, were slightly more common in males and had fewer adverse family factors.

Similar studies have been carried in Dunedin (New Zealand), Christchurch (New Zealand) and Ontario (Canada). Some studies have found rates of psychiatric problems from 10% to 40%, although these high rates may be a product of diagnosis based on symptoms without a measure of the impact of the problem.

Classification

Both ICD-10 and DSM-IV have a multiaxial framework for child and adolescent psychiatric diagnoses. ICD-10 has six axes and DSM-IV five axes. Axis 1 in DSM-IV allows multiple diagnoses and encompasses both specific developmental disorders and psychiatric diagnoses (Box 14.1).

Where conditions occur in both childhood and adult life, then the main ICD-10 diagnostic category is used, e.g. depression, obsessive compulsive disorder (OCD). ICD-10 contains a section relating to conditions specific in their onset to childhood, e.g. hyperkinetic disorder, enuresis.

Hyperactivity

Hyperactivity, like depression, is a term with a variety of uses and meanings. To parents, it may mean that their child is always in trouble or has excess energy. Child psychiatrists view it as implying a difficulty with restlessness, poor concentration and impulsive behaviour. These conceptual difficulties have also been mirrored in ICD-9 and DSM-III, leading to Americans diagnosing *attention deficit disorder with hyperactivity* (ADDH) more frequently than the narrower *hyperkinetic disorder* previously used in Britain. ICD-10 (hyperkinetic disorder) and DSM-IV (attention deficit hyperactivity disorder ADHD) are now closer in their diagnostic guidelines. ADHD has perhaps become the most commonly used term.

Box 14.1

ICD-10 axis

1. Psychiatric diagnosis, e.g. conduct disorder
2. Specific developmental disorder, e.g. autism
3. Intellectual level, e.g. moderate learning disability
4. Medical diagnosis, e.g. diabetes
5. Psychosocial adversity, e.g. sexual abuse
6. Level of functioning, e.g. moderate social disability.

ICD-10 lists:
- Hyperkinetic disorder with a disturbance in attention and activity
- Hyperkinetic disorder with conduct disorder.

Epidemiology

Hyperkinetic disorder has a prevalence of 1–2%, occurring more frequently in boys (male:female = 3:1) (Taylor et al 1991). The slightly broader diagnosis of ADHD was found to occur in a UK-wide study in 3.62% of boys and 0.85% of girls (Ford et al 2003). Prevalence declines with age. At age 25, 15% of adults diagnosed with ADHD in childhood still fulfilled criteria, though 65% fulfilled criteria for ADHD in partial remission.

Features

Symptoms need to be present for at least 6 months with an onset before the age of 7 (though symptoms are usually present before 5 years old and frequently before 2 years old). Although there may be a long history of symptoms, the problem may not be recognized until the start of schooling, when the difficulties in attention and disruptive behaviour become more apparent.

Behaviour is characterized by restlessness (unable to sit still, fidgeting), poor attention (frequent changes of activity) and impulsive behaviour.

The behaviour should be evident in different settings, i.e. both at home and school.

Associated features

Pure ADHD is rare and the condition is often accompanied by other problems. Behaviour is often defiant, aggressive or antisocial. Social relationships can be impaired and at times, this includes perceived rudeness to adults. There is often co-morbid specific learning problems and a below average IQ. Development can also be affected, e.g. speech delay or clumsiness. Sleep problems frequently occur.

Aetiology

ADHD is a heterogenous disorder involving an interplay of genetic and environmental factors.

Genetic factors

Twin studies suggest that genetic factors account for 75% of ADHD symptoms. No single gene has been identified.

Environmental factors

Biological factors: various factors can affect brain development in perinatal life and early childhood and some have been linked with an increase risk of ADHD: maternal smoking, alcohol consumption, maternal use of heroin during pregnancy, very low birthweight, fetal hypoxia, brain injury and exposure to toxins

Seizures: 10–30% develop seizures, usually in adolescence.

Hyperactivity: hyperactive behaviour is common, with temper tantrums and aggressive behaviour. Food fads are also common and deliberate self-injurious behaviour (biting self) also occurs.

Differential diagnosis

- **Hearing impairment:** the unresponsiveness and language difficulties can be confused with deafness. Hearing tests should be carried out.
- **Asperger syndrome:** sometimes regarded as 'mild autism'. Asperger differs in that there is little language delay, an absence of the early aloofness and no stereotypies. There may be narrow or pedantic interests and often marked clumsiness.
- **Rett syndrome:** occurs in girls only. Typically, development regresses at 12 months with decreased head growth and characteristic hand-washing movements. The illness is progressive and affected individuals die by the age of 30 years.
- **Disintegrative psychosis (Heller syndrome):** onset is usually between 3–8 years with regression, autistic features and mental retardation.
- **Learning difficulty ± autistic features:** can be very similar, though lacks all the essential features.
- **Severe deprivation:** studies on deprived orphanage children, later adopted, suggest some continue to demonstrate autistic features.
- **Fragile X:** can present with similar features of gaze avoidance and social anxiety.
- **Developmental language disorder:** even with profound language problems, communication exists with gestures and reasonable social interaction, though there are overlapping cases.

Aetiology

Genetic: twin studies suggest a concordance of up to 90%. There is a recurrence rate of 3% in families with one affected child. While several genes are of interest, current research suggests that a broader phenotype of social, communication and/or behavioural difficulties is transmitted in a familial manner.

Neurobiology: most structures of the brain have been implicated, though there is as yet no clear pathology, interest has focused on the medial temporal lobe structures and the cerebellum. Affected individuals do have larger brains and head circumference (Bailey 1993).

Psychology: several competing theories exist:

- 'Theory of mind' – this describes the ability to think of other people's points of view and understand and predict their actions. Various stories are related or acted out, characteristically autistic individuals are unable to predict the actions of others (Baron-Cohen 1989).
- Inborn error in the ability to communicate and relate to others – this suggests that autistic children are less able to respond to social or affect-related information (e.g. tones of voice) than non-social input (e.g. train whistles).
- Deficit in executive function – an inability to plan and organize.

Immunization: recent controversy has centred on the role of immunization (in particular the MMR vaccine) as a causative agent for autism. The area remains highly controversial.

Treatment

Parental support: parents require support and education. Voluntary support groups can be helpful as can planned respite care.

Education: autistic children do well in a well-structured environment that has experience with autistic children.

Behaviour modification: a functional analysis of problem behaviour can then lead to modification using behavioural techniques, e.g. reducing temper tantrums.

Medication: anticonvulsants are required for seizure control. Stimulants may decrease the hyperactivity but can increase stereotypies. Low-dose atypical neuroleptics may decrease problem behaviours but can be harmful if used long term. There was a flurry of interest in the gut hormone secretin, but a series of randomized control trials has failed to demonstrate a significant benefit over placebo.

Prognosis

About half of sufferers acquire speech, although if there is no language development by the age of 5 years, then it is unlikely to develop. Some 10% of autistic adults are working and living independently. A poor prognosis is associated with lack of language development and an IQ <60.

School refusal

School refusal is very common, accounting for around 5% of referrals to child psychiatry. In itself, school refusal is not a diagnosis (i.e. not in ICD-10), but a reflection of underlying problems (Hersov & Berg 1980).

Epidemiology

School refusal has three age peaks:

- **5–7 years:** school-starting age (may be associated with separation anxiety)
- **11 years:** transfer to secondary school
- **14–16 years:** the Isle of Wight study found no cases at age 10, but by age 15, there were 15 cases (0.7% prevalence). The sex incidence is equal.

Features

Children refuse to go to school or return home after leaving. Not going to school can be upsetting for them (ego-dystonic) and there may be overt anxiety or somatic complaints. Such complaints are usually absent in holidays and at weekends (although they may return on Sunday evenings). Parents are aware of the non-attendance. The onset can be abrupt or gradual with a range of precipitants – bullying, reading difficulties, etc.

Associated features

Intelligence: usually of average intelligence and ability.

Family organization: families can be ineffective in ensuring a return to school. This may be related to over-involvement with the children (e.g. over-enmeshed mother), lack of consensus on behaviour management (e.g. ineffectual father) or the child may be considered 'special' (e.g. because of difficulties at birth).

Family size: there is no family size effect, although the youngest child may be at increased risk.

Underlying psychiatric problems

* Separation anxiety – in younger children, often unable to go anywhere without one or both parents
* Phobia – may be specific phobia (e.g. of buses, or fear of being bullied)
* Depression
* Substance misuse – characterized by a change of behaviour, apathy
* Schizophrenia – a rare cause in adolescence.

Differential diagnosis

* **Truancy:** differs from school refusal in that it is ego-syntonic (i.e. the child is not upset about not attending school) and willful; the parents are often unaware; and it is associated with other antisocial behaviour (and therefore linked with associated features of CD – male sex, social disadvantage, marital discord, etc.).
* **Physical illness:** a genuine physical illness may exist.

Treatment

Behavioural: if acute onset, then should aim for a rapid reintroduction to school. If chronic, then a graded programme of exposure to school life may be needed. Close liaison with education services is essential, and tuition units may help.

Family therapy: may change the family dynamics and empower the parents to aid the return to school. If a two-parent family, both parents working together are required.

Medication: generally of little value, unless there is an underlying psychiatric condition.

Prognosis

Two-thirds of school refusers return to school, with return being more likely if the child is younger, if less severe and there is early intervention. One-third may have persisting neurotic problems, and a very small proportion may develop agoraphobia in adulthood, although the link with school refusal is less than conclusive.

Elimination disorders

Difficulties in toileting are not uncommon and may be due to underlying developmental problems.

Encopresis

Strictly speaking, encopresis is the passage of normally formed stools in abnormal places, while soiling is the passage of semi-solid faeces. Practically speaking, they are synonymous.

Epidemiology

Bowel control is usually achieved by the age of 4 years. At age 7–8, the prevalence is 1.5% (2.3% boys, 0.7% girls) and at age 10, 1.0% (1.3% boys, 0.3% girls). By the age of 16, soiling is extremely rare. At all ages, soiling is more common in boys.

Aetiology

Various classifications of soiling have been devised (primary/secondary, retentive/non-retentive), although rarely does soiling occur in such a clear pattern. Failure to go to the toilet may result in constipation with overflow of semi-soiled faeces. More important is to determine what may be causing the problem:

* **Physical cause:** where bowel control has never been achieved, an underlying physical cause should be considered, e.g. Hirschsprung disease.
* **Phobia:** a fear of sitting on the toilet or of monsters in the toilet is not uncommon among young children; careful questioning may be required to elicit the problem.
* **Family difficulties:** chronic discord and chaotic family organization may lead to soiling in strange places. Also lack of appropriate toilet training can contribute.
* **Stress:** stressful life-events, e.g. bereavement, parental separation, can precipitate regression to soiling behaviour.

Treatment

Assessment: joint assessment involving a paediatrician may be required.

Medication: laxatives can be used to soften the stool and promote bowel opening.

Behaviour management: the use of star-charts and behavioural regimes promotes a normal toilet routine. Appropriate steps and goals should be decided upon.

Family therapy: therapy involving the whole family may help decrease anxiety and ensure consistency of approach.

Prognosis

Soiling usually resolves by adolescence. It can take up to 6 months to retrain the bowel wall.

Enuresis

Enuresis is the involuntary passage of urine in the absence of physical abnormalities after the age of 5 years. In *primary enuresis* children have never acquired bladder control. In *secondary enuresis*, bladder control was achieved for at least 6 months and then lost. The prognosis is worse for secondary enuresis but otherwise, the two have similar characteristics.

- *Nocturnal enuresis* (bed-wetting) is more common and associated with boys; 10–30% also have diurnal enuresis.
- *Diurnal enuresis* (day-time wetting) is associated with girls; 60–80% also have nocturnal enuresis.

Epidemiology

Nocturnal

At age 5, the prevalence is 10% (male:female = 1:1); at age 10, 2.5% (male:female = 1.6:1) and at age 15, 1% (male:female = 1.8:1).

Diurnal

2% of all 5-year-olds, with an excess of females.

Associated features

Urinary tract infections (UTI) in girls: 1% of all 5-year-olds have asymptomatic UTI, but in children with enuresis, 5% have UTIs.

Family history: 70% have a positive family history.

Stress: life events at the age of 3–4 years double the likelihood of enuresis.

Late toilet training: training after the age of 20 months is associated with enuresis.

Enuresis is not associated with deep sleep, and is not an epileptiform equivalent.

Treatment

Bedtime routine: general advice on a night-time routine (going to the toilet before sleep, restricting fluids) may help.

Behavioural: a star chart reward system is effective in 20–30% of cases. Most effective is the 'bell & pad' or enuresis alarm. Success rates of 50–100% within 2 months are reported, although 35% then relapse, which can be offset by 'overlearning' – repeating the procedure with a pre-bedtime fluid load.

Medication: desmopressin (DDAVP) – usually as a nasal spray – is effective, but relapse rates are high when discontinued. Tricyclic antidepressants also achieve dryness, but tolerance can develop and relapse rates are high. There is also the potential for toxicity.

Prognosis

Most children fully recover. Approximately 3% of enuretics are still wetting at age 20. Poor prognosis is associated with boys, low social status and nightly wetting.

Tics and Tourette syndrome

Tics are rapid, involuntary, repetitive, stereotyped, motor movements or phonic productions. ICD-10 classifies tics as a:

- Transient tic disorder
- Chronic motor or vocal tic disorder
- Combined vocal and multiple motor tic disorder (Gilles de la Tourette syndrome).

Simple tics

Simple tics such as blinks, grunts or sniffs are usually transitory, occurring in 10% of children, with an excess of boys. They resolve spontaneously.

Tourette syndrome

Tourette syndrome (TS) combines both motor and phonic tics. Motor tics usually start first, with a mean age of 7 years (range 2–15 years) and vocal tics from 8–15 years. A small proportion may exhibit coprolalia (swearing), echolalia, echopraxia and copropraxia.

Associated features

Co-morbid features are common with obsessive–compulsive disorder (OCD) found in 30–60% of cases and hyperactivity present in 25–50%.

Aetiology

TS runs in families along with OCD, possibly due to a dominant gene with incomplete penetrance.

Treatment

Support: families may require support and education to understand the condition.

Behavioural: relaxation may help, particularly with the stress associated with chronic tics.

Medication:
- ○ Low-dose haloperidol or pimozide decreases tic frequency
- ○ More recent interest has fixed on atypical neuroleptics
- ○ Clonidine
- ○ Clomipramine or SSRI.

Prognosis

Tics usually decrease in frequency in adolescence/adulthood, although they can persist (Bruun 1988).

Elective mutism

Electively mute children demonstrate a marked, emotionally determined selectivity in speaking. Speech occurs in some situations and not in others, e.g. at school. The disorder occurs in early childhood with an equal sex frequency.

Epidemiology

Around 1% in children of school-starting age, and 2–5/10 000 at age 7–8 years.

Associated features

Language difficulties: the diagnosis presupposes a near-normal level of comprehension and expression. A history of some speech delay is not uncommon, but the diagnosis requires fluent speech in some situations.
Socioemotional problems: often present, particularly social anxiety. Tics, depression, enuresis, encopresis and oppositional behaviour may also be present.

Aetiology

The cause of the mutism is not clear. Inherent personality factors such as shyness may interact with psychosocial factors. However, there is often a family history of social anxiety. The role of trauma, e.g. sexual abuse, may also contribute.

Treatment

Speech therapy assessment and intervention may help, particularly where articulation problems are present.
Behavioural work, usually in the school setting, aims to decrease social anxiety.
Medication: SSRIs may help, though further studies are required.

Prognosis

Mutism usually resolves, but the prognosis is worse if no improvement occurs in 6–12 months.

Suicide and deliberate self-harm

Suicide

Suicide is rare under the age of 12 and increases thereafter with age. Although suicide rates in adolescents are well beneath rates in adults, it is the second most common cause of death in adolescents. It occurs more commonly in males (male: female = 4:1) and there may be differences between ethnic groups. Between the ages of 5 and 14 years, the rate is 0.8/100 000, rising to 13/100 000 between 15 and 19 years old. Official figures are likely to under-report the true rate of deaths by suicide.

Associated features

Method: males tend to use more violent means: hanging, vehicle exhaust fumes, shooting (particularly in the USA). Females are more likely to use methods of overdose (particularly paracetamol).
Psychiatric disorder: high rates of depression are found along with anxiety and eating disorders.
Family history: increased rates of deliberate self-harm, depression and alcohol or substance misuse are found in the family.
Substance misuse: alcohol and drug misuse was found in one study to be a predictive factor for eventual suicide following deliberate self-harm.
Precipitant: often a recent crisis, e.g. school or police trouble, or arguments with parents or boy/girlfriends.
Imitation: there is some inconsistent evidence that recent exposure to suicide, either directly or in the media, may lead to similar acts. In residential settings, e.g. boarding schools, one suicide may lead to several other attempts by fellow pupils (so-called 'contagion').

Prevention

Discussion: up to 50% may discuss suicidal thoughts with someone, or be in contact with health professionals in the 24 h before death. All such contacts should be viewed as potential pre-suicide consultations.
Education: several 'suicide curricula' have been tried in schools, aiming to increase awareness, indirectly find cases and provide information. Results have been mixed.
Crisis services: telephone help lines, e.g. the Samaritans, provide point of contact at time of crisis.
Limiting access to methods: e.g. decreasing availability of paracetamol, fitting catalytic converters to vehicles.
Post-vention: this refers to an intervention after a suicide with the family and peers. By acting as a 'de-briefing', post-vention helps increase understanding and prevent imitation.

Deliberate self-harm

There is no current consensus on best terminology. Deliberate self-harm (DSH) refers to parasuicide and attempted suicide, and includes self-poisoning (overdose) and self-injury (cutting). DSH is much more common than suicide (up to 100 times more frequent), with self-poisoning being the most common method.

Epidemiology

Rates vary between studies. The incidence increases with puberty (before then it is more common in boys). Community studies suggest 8% of adolescents have made a DSH attempt, although only 2% receive medical attention. Up to 20% of adolescents may have had serious suicidal ideation. After puberty, it is more common in females (female:male = 7:1).

Associated features

Method: overdose is the most common form of DSH. Tablets used by children and adolescent may vary enormously from psychotropics to antibiotics. The most common medication used is paracetamol. DSH is often impulsive and therefore any medication easily available may be used.

Precipitant: often interpersonal conflicts – boy/girlfriend rows, family arguments and school problems. One-third of young people cannot identify any precipitant.

Past history: around 20% have made previous attempts.

Psychiatric problems: some studies suggest that over 50% of young people attempting DSH have depression. Usually, this is transient and the majority are not severely depressed.

Abuse: previous abuse may be more common among young people who deliberately self-harm.

Intent: can be difficult to assess in young people. Attempt is often impulsive, but can be a way of coping with a difficult situation. Should not be seen as a 'cry for help' from professionals. Intent should be assessed in terms of the amount of planning, precautions taken about being found, knowledge about the lethality of the method and leaving a suicide note.

Treatment

Assessment: of reasons, precipitants, intent, current suicidality, etc. The assessment of adolescents after DSH differs from adult assessments in that parents/carers should also be seen. Engaging the young person in the assessment process may also take some time.

Outpatient treatment: family therapy is often offered, though it is often hard to engage families. Individually, cognitive therapy or solution-based brief therapies may help. Longer-term psychotherapy may occasionally be required.
Compliance with follow-up is notoriously low (Brent 1997).

Outcome

Follow-up studies are very difficult. Up to 10% may repeat, usually within 1 year, and 1% may eventually commit suicide. Some studies suggest that this group are more prone to depression in adult life (e.g. Pfeffer et al 1994).

NICE guidelines (NICE 2004) make comprehensive recommendations regarding the assessment and treatment of DSH in young people, including the recommendation that all young people are admitted to a paediatric ward overnight and assessed by the child and adolescent mental health team the following day.

Schizophrenia

Schizophrenia in childhood and adolescence is uncommon, and when it does occur, the symptomatology is similar to that in adults. Incidence increases in puberty, although cases in younger

children are recorded. Diagnosis may be difficult initially, not least because the onset is often insidious.

Differential diagnosis of schizophrenia in children/adolescents

- **Alcohol and substance misuse:** may present with a similar picture of change of behaviour
- **Depression**
- **Schizoaffective disorder, other psychoses:** can be difficult to differentiate
- **Autism:** not very similar, with onset before 3 years, social impairment, language delay and ritualized behaviour. Neuroleptics are rarely useful in the treatment of autism.

Depression

Feeling miserable is not uncommon among children and even more so with adolescents. Depression, when present, is diagnosed using the same criteria as for adults. There have been protracted arguments over whether children can be depressed. Generally, from around the age of 8–9 years, children exhibit depressive symptomatology and the rate increases with adolescence. Somatic complaints may be more common, along with irritability. Appetite and sleep problems are less common, with less evidence of hopelessness.

NICE guidelines (NICE 2005) set out clear recommendations for the detection and treatment of depression in children and young people.

Epidemiology

The prevalence for pre-pubertal children is 1–2% and 2–5% for adolescents. In prepubertal children, the sex ratio is equal, but a similar pattern to adults occurs after puberty, with an excess proportion of females.

Treatment

Family therapy: e.g. 15 fortnightly sessions.

Individual therapy: cognitive behaviour therapy (CBT) and interpersonal therapy (IPT) have shown some benefits.

Medication: the evidence for the role of antidepressants is equivocal. Tricyclic antidepressants in one study were found to be as effective as placebo. Additionally, they have potential toxic side-effects. SSRIs may have a role, though further studies are required; only fluoxetine is currently indicated for use in young people under the age of 18 years. NICE (2005) recommend that fluoxetine is the first choice medication, being the only medication where the benefits have been found to outweigh side-effects. An increase in suicidal ideation has been linked with SSRI use and monitoring for suicidal ideas during treatment is recommended. Sertraline or citalopram are recommended as second line treatment. Medication should be given in combination with psychological therapy.

Prognosis

True depressive episodes can last up to 9 months and may recur. There is a subsequent increased risk for depression in adulthood (Harrington et al 1990).

Bipolar affective disorder

There has been a series of publications, mainly from the USA, on early-onset bipolar disorder. The literature in this area is confusing, mainly arising from the application of diagnostic criteria designed for adults to children and adolescents. The blurring of diagnostic boundaries has led to the suggestion that bipolar disorder in children may present as disruptive behaviour, irritability and temper tantrums (Biederman 1998).

Adult studies suggest that between 20% and 54% of people with bipolar disorder report symptoms in childhood. The lifetime prevalence of bipolar disorder for adolescents is about 1%.

NICE (2006) recommends that the same criteria as in adults are used in diagnosing bipolar 1 disorder in children and adolescents. In prepubertal children, mania must be present and irritability is not a core criterion. In adolescents, mania is also required, although irritability can be helpful if it is episodic and impairs function but it should not be a core diagnostic criterion.

Treatment can involve lithium, sodium valproate or carbamazepine, with some evidence for atypical neuroleptics (e.g. risperidone, olanzapine). Lithium is the only medication with a licence for the treatment of bipolar 1 disorder in the 12–18-year-old group; however, off-licence medications can be used where the use is justified. Mood stabilizers are being used in the USA on younger children who in the UK may receive alternative diagnoses and non-medication treatments.

Compared with adults, adolescents with bipolar disorder have a longer early course and can be more resistant to treatment. In a 5-year follow-up, 4% of young people remained ill, 44% had a relapse and 21% had a further two or more episodes (Strober et al 1995).

Child maltreatment

Child maltreatment or abuse is not a new phenomenon but has only relatively recently been seen as a child-health or welfare problem. Previously, 'abuse' was restricted to physical abuse ('the battered baby syndrome'), but now includes physical, sexual and emotional abuse, plus neglect.

The epidemiology of abuse is difficult due to definitional issues and sources of information. Around 4% of children under the age of 12 are brought to the attention of social services each year because of suspected abuse. In 1988, 3.5/1000 children under 18 years were on Child Protection Registers in England, with one in four registered for physical abuse and one in eight for emotional abuse.

Rates of child sex abuse vary according to the definition used, with studies finding incidence rates of 6–62% in females and 3–31% in males. Most studies find higher rates of abuse in girls (female:male = 2.5–5:1). Studies into ethnic differences are few; the available evidence suggests no differences in rates of sexual abuse between white and black women.

NICE (2009b) have published guidance summarizing the responsibilities of all who work with children and adolescents in considering possible child maltreatment and the responsibility to report suspected cases of maltreatment.

Physical abuse

Physical abuse usually presents with some form of injury, which is inferred to be non-accidental (NAI) in nature. Injuries consist of fractures, head injuries, burns, bruising, deliberate poisoning and sometimes deliberate suffocation.

Signs of NAI are not exact, but may include:

• A vague account of the accident
• The account is not compatible with the observed injury
• A delay in seeking help
• Parental affect does not reflect the level of anxiety expected
• The child's affect may be sad, withdrawn and frightened and the child may say something to arouse suspicion.

Characteristics of abused children and their families include:

• Unwanted pregnancy
• Low birthweight/separation from mother in the neonatal period
• Mental or physical handicap
• Restless baby, sleepless or crying non-stop
• Physically unattractive.

Parental risk factors include:

• Young, single parent
• Abused themselves as children
• Inconsistent or punishment-orientated discipline
• Adverse social circumstances: low income, social isolation, social stressors
• Large family.

Munchausen syndrome by proxy (factitious disorder by proxy – DSM IV)

First described by Meadow (1977), this syndrome describes a parent, usually mother, who fabricates illness in her child/children and presents for medical attention. Presentations are usually persistent and symptoms end when separated from the parent. Other children in the family are often, or have often been, presented with similar problems. Forms of presentation include seizures, smotherings, poisoning, apparent bleeding, temperatures and rashes.

Sexual abuse

The definition of child sexual abuse ranges from acts of exhibitionism to fondling to forced penetration. Cases that come to clinical attention are more likely to be severe. Children of all ages are abused and studies suggest a peak onset between the ages of 8 and 12. Alerting features can include: persistent or recurring dysuria, hepatitis B infection (with no clear vertical transmission), anogenital warts in a child or other sexually transmitted diseases, and unusual sexualized behaviours in a prepubertal child.

Most sexual abuse is committed by men, with 5–15% perpetrated by females. Often the perpetrator is known to the child. In intrafamilial abuse, fathers are the most common perpetrator. Stepfathers are over-represented in the figures and a girl living with a stepfather is reported as being six times more likely to be abused compared with one living with her biological father. Many of the studies into stepfathers are old and the findings may not apply to today's families.

Abuse outside the family often occurs with individuals known to the child. Stranger abuse also occurs (though is under-represented in studies) and is more likely to be directed at boys (Finkelhor 1979).

Neglect

Neglect includes a lack of providing for a child's physical needs and also not fulfilling his or her developmental and cognitive needs. Children may be inadequately fed, dressed and bathed or may be deprived of satisfactory contact with the parent or other children/adults.

Neglect may be evident on direct observation, although usually it is noticed by other family members or a teacher, or is inferred from the child's behaviour. Alerting features can include: severe and persistent infections (e.g. scabies), parents/carers who do not administer essential treatments for their child and faltering growth. Other forms of abuse often accompany neglect.

Emotional abuse

Physical abuse can result in visible injury, whereas emotional abuse is much harder to quantify. Emotional abuse is diagnosed if there is observable impairment in a child's mental or emotional functioning, evidenced by emotional or behavioural disorders and there is evidence that this is a result of rejection, deprivation of affection, exposure to domestic violence, inappropriate criticism or threats to the child. Alerting features can include: a fearful emotional state, habitual body rocking, indiscriminate contact, failure to seek comfort when distressed and a child who has age-inappropriate responsibilities that interfere with normal activities, e.g. not going to school because of having to care for a sibling.

Emotional abuse is not usually the only reason for seeking child protection. In extreme cases, it has been proposed that emotional abuse can effect growth and weight gain – non-organic failure to thrive (NOFT).

Management of abuse

Broadly speaking, the management of abuse occurs in three stages:
- **Stage 1:** Detection and disclosure
- **Stage 2:** Child protection and legal proceedings
- **Stage 3:** Support and therapeutic intervention.

Detection and disclosure

This is usually the responsibility of social services and involves interviewing the child, family and possibly the perpetrator. Interviewing the child has to occur with some skill, although there is good evidence that even young children's recall of past events is well developed. In cases of sexual abuse, anatomical dolls may be used but this can be controversial.

Child protection and legal proceedings

A decision to undertake legal proceedings may then be made. Children may be removed from their families either pending further investigations or with a view to long-term fostering or adoption. Psychiatric reports may be requested about the child, the parent's ability to parent or about the parents.

Support and therapeutic intervention

Work may be required to rehabilitate children with their families, or in cases where rehabilitation is not possible, to work to a new family placement. Therapeutic input may also be required to deal with the consequences of the abuse. Various models of abuse work have been tried, including individual, family and group therapy. In sexual abuse, working with the whole family including the perpetrator has had some success.

Outcome

In the short term, abuse can result in a change in a child's behaviour and emotional state. Children may be prone to mood swings, temper tantrums, wariness of strangers, etc. They can feel isolated, anxious and depressed. With sexual abuse, sexualized behaviour may develop. The specific consequences of physical abuse depend on the nature of the injury.

In the longer-term, abuse can have profound consequences on self-esteem, the ability to form satisfactory adult relationships and may also impact on parenting abilities. Sexual abuse in childhood, in particular, has been linked with the development of eating disorders, self-injury and depression in adults (see Ch. 25).

Child and adolescent mental health services

The Department of Health recommends that child and adolescent mental health services (CAHMS) are delivered according to the following 'tiered' model:
- **Tier 1:** Services delivered at the primary care level by GPs, health visitors, school nurses, teachers, etc.
- **Tier 2:** Unidisciplinary mental health services, i.e. a professional working alone without backup of a team, e.g. psychologists, nurses.
- **Tier 3:** Multidisciplinary team, usually located in the community or attached to a hospital; can consist of a child psychiatrist, child psychotherapist, social worker, psychologist, etc.

- **Tier 4:** Specialist services, includes adolescent inpatient units and highly specialized regional services.

CAMHS are therefore not just the province of the child psychiatrist, but delivered in a wide variety of settings, including voluntary agencies. Ideally, referrals should pass between the tiers as required and the main agencies – health, education and social services – should work together in the best interest of the child or adolescent.

The Royal College of Psychiatrists recommends that there should be 1.3 whole time equivalent (wte) consultants in child and adolescent psychiatry per 100 000 total population. In a population of 250 000, the British Psychological Society recommends 3.5 wte psychology posts. One psychotherapist is recommended per 100 000 and recommendations exist for other members of the multidisciplinary team.

Further reading

Goodman, R., Scott, S., 1997. Child psychiatry. Blackwell, London.

Rutter, M., Taylor, E. (Eds.), 2002. Child and adolescent psychiatry, fourth ed. Blackwell, Oxford.

References

Bailey, A.J., 1993. The biology of autism. Psychological Autism 23, 7–11.

Baron-Cohen, S., 1989. The autistic child's theory of mind: a case of specific developmental delay. J. Child. Psychol. Psychiatry 15, 315–321.

Biederman, J., 1998. Resolved: mania is mistaken for ADHD in prepubertal children: affirmative. J. Am. Acad. Child. Adolesc. Psychiatry 37, 1091–1093.

Brent, D.A., 1997. Practitioner review: the aftercare of adolescents with deliberate self-harm. J. Child. Psychol. Psychiatry 38, 277–286.

Bruun, R., 1988. The natural history of Tourette's syndrome. In: Cohen, D., Bruun, R., Leckman, J. (Eds.), Tourette's syndrome and tic disorders. Wiley, New York.

Connors, C.K., Epstein, J.K., March, J.S., et al., 2001. Multi-modal treatment of ADHD in the MTA: an alternative outcome analysis. J. Am. Acad. Child. Adolesc. Psychiatry 40, 159–167.

Finkelhor, D., 1979. What's wrong with sex between adults and children? Ethics and the problem of sexual abuse. Am. J. Orthopsychiatry 49, 692–697.

Ford, T., Goodman, R., Meltzer, H., 2003. The British Child and Adolescent Mental Health Survey 1999: the prevalence of DSM-IV disorders. J. Am. Acad. Child. Adolesc. Psychiatry 42, 1203–1211.

Harrington, R., Fudge, H., Rutter, M., et al., 1990. Adult outcome of childhood and adolescent depression. I. Psychiatric status. Arch. Gen. Psychiatry 47, 465–473.

Hersov, L., Berg, I. (Eds.), 1980. Out of school. Wiley, Chichester.

Meadow, R., 1977. Munchausen syndrome by proxy. The hinterland of child abuse. Lancet ii, 343–345.

MTA cooperative group, 1999a. A 14-month randomized clinical trial of treatment strategies for attention-deficit/hyperactivity disorder. The MTA cooperative group multimodal treatment study of children with ADHD. Arch. Gen. Psychiatry 56, 1073–1086.

MTA Cooperative Group, 1999b. Moderators and mediators of treatment response for children with attention-deficit/hyperactivity disorder; the multi-modal treatment study of children with attention-deficit/hyperactivity disorder. Arch. Gen. Psychiatry 56, 1088–1096.

NICE and National Collaborating Centre for Mental Health, 2004. Self-harm. The short-term physical and psychological management and secondary prevention of self-harm in primary and secondary care. NICE, London.

NICE, 2005. Depression in children and young people. Identification and management in primary, community and secondary care. NICE, London.

NICE, 2006. Bipolar disorder. The management of bipolar disorder in adults, children and adolescents in primary and secondary care. NICE, London.

NICE, 2009a. Attention deficit hyperactivity disorder. Diagnosis and management of ADHD in children, young people and adults. NICE, London.

NICE, 2009b. When to suspect child maltreatment. NICE, London.

Pfeffer, C.R., Hurt, S.W., Kakuma, T., et al., 1994. Suicidal children grow up: suicidal episodes and effects of treatment during

follow-up. J. Am. Acad. Child. Adolesc. Psychiatry 33, 225–230.

Richman, N., Stevenson, J.E., Graham, P., 1982. Pre-school to school: a behavioural study. Academic Press, London.

Robins, L.N., 1978. Sturdy childhood predictors of adult antisocial behaviour: replications from longitudinal studies. Psychol. Med. 8, 611–622.

Rutter, M., Cox, A., Tupling, C., et al., 1975. Attainment and adjustment in two geographical areas – I. The prevalence of psychiatric disorder. Br. J. Psychiatry 126, 493–509.

Rutter, M., Tizard, J., Yule, W., et al., 1976. Isle of Wight studies 1964–1974. Psychol. Med. 6, 313–332.

Strober, M., Schmidt-Lackner, S., Freeman, R., et al., 1995. Recovery and relapse in adolescent with bipolar affective illness: a naturalistic study. Am. J. Psychiatry 147, 457–471.

Swanson, J., Kraemer, H.C., Hinshaw, S.P., et al., 2001. Clinical relevance of the primary findings of the MTA; success rates based on the severity of ADHD and ODD at the end of treatment. J. Am. Acad. Child. Adolesc. Psychiatry 40, 168–179.

Taylor, E., Sandberg, S., Thorley, G., et al., 1991. The epidemiology of childhood hyperactivity. Maudsley Monographs no. 33. Oxford University Press, Oxford.

Timimi, S., Taylor, E., 2004. ADHD is best understood as a cultural construct. Br. J. Psychiatry 184, 8–9.

Volkmar, F.R., Lord, C., Bailey, A., et al., 2004. Autism and pervasive developmental disorders. J. Child. Psychol. Psychiatry 45, 135–171.

Personality disorders

15

Gwen Adshead   Caroline Jacob

CHAPTER CONTENTS

Introduction

'Personality disorder' is a term which has undergone several changes in the last decade, and continues to change. It is often described as a 'contentious' diagnosis; but it perhaps would be fairer to say that it is the *use* to which the term has been put which is contentious. In this chapter, we will set out a modern functional evidence-based account of normal personality, and then describe how personalities can become disordered. Different types of personality disorder are seen in different settings, and we will focus on those disorders which are most often seen in secondary and tertiary psychiatric care. We will conclude by describing the range of treatments currently available (and their evidence base); and set out some of the most interesting questions that are still areas of empirical uncertainty.

We have two main take-home messages for readers. First, 'personality disorder' is not a homogenous entity, any more than any other complex disorder. We do not speak of patients having 'cancer', without further explicating what type of cancer it is, what systems are affected and how far it has spread. Equally, just making a diagnosis of 'personality disorder' because a patient has behaved in an unreasonable, frightening or annoying way is clinically useless; such a diagnosis needs to be accompanied by some sort of psychological account of what the personality problem is and a history to back this up.

The other take-home message is that the word 'untreatable' has no place in the lexicon of psychiatrists; especially not for personality disorder. This term used to be a proxy for 'discharge them from my service' and had some legal authority; but the legal basis for this term has now disappeared from mental health legislation. There is now no justification for any good clinician to make statements like, 'He has a personality disorder, so he is untreatable'. Again, the analogy with oncology is fruitful: some types of tumour are aggressive, treatment resistant and can only use palliative care; whereas other types of neoplastic disease (especially when caught early) are milder, not so invasive or pervasive and respond well to intervention.

Normal personality

The term 'personality' comes from the Greek, 'persona', meaning 'mask'; referring to the masks that denoted the characters that actors played in the great dramas of Greek theatre. The sociologist Erwin Goffman (1956) has described how people interact with each other by 'acting' out roles; and our personalities define how we play those roles, and what parts we play. On this responses (Sarkar & Adshead 2006). Repeated exposure to chronic stress, fear and hostility impacts on the development of the right orbito-frontal cortex, which (together with the limbic system, hypothalamus and hippocampus) regulates negative emotions. Children raised in such risky environments form insecure attachments to their carers, which influence their personal beliefs about the social world, and their capacity for self-reflection and empathy (Siegal 2001). Some children may not be exposed to highly risky environments, but have risky genetic profiles, especially for Cluster B and C disorders (Caspi et al 2002).

Personality disorders tend to present in late childhood and early adolescence as children begin to develop a social network of relationships at school with peers and teachers outside the family. There are different developmental trajectories, and many children with early behavioural difficulties may improve with intervention and support. However, a proportion of those children with interpersonal behavioural problems will continue to show such behaviours into adulthood (Kim et al 2009).

Such a persistent trajectory has been best described in antisocial children; a subgroup of whom show early antisocial behaviour which persists into adolescence (usually as substance abuse and school drop-out) and then adulthood, where it is manifest as criminal rule breaking. A worse prognosis is associated with early (under 10) antisociality and conduct disorder; these children are thought to have a genetic profile that puts them at risk of antisocial personality traits such as callousness and lack of emotional response to others (Viding et al 2007).

A common risk factor for adult personality disorder is early childhood maltreatment or neglect (including emotional neglect) by carers (Johnson et al 1999). Both physical abuse and neglect are particularly associated with the development of antisocial personality disorder in adulthood. Sexual abuse (of a chronic nature) has been reported as being associated with the development of self-harming behaviours and borderline personality disorder. Combined types of maltreatment result in combined forms of personality disorder, and there is a generally a linear relationship between the amount of maltreatment and the severity of the personality disorder. Having said that, some individuals are exceptionally resilient and exposure to positive experiences during childhood and adolescence can reduce the risk of poor social outcomes (Werner 1993).

Personality disorders can also be acquired in adulthood if there is damage to the neural and psychological systems that regulate negative feelings, especially fear, anger and threat. Acquired personality disorders can be observed after traumatic brain injury, after extensive psychological trauma and as a consequence of chronic mental illness. Some personality disorders may only manifest when the individual engages in particular adult social roles, such as becoming a parent or a spouse.

Prognosis

Personality disorders can take a remitting and relapsing course. Some cases of mild personality disorder can remit completely in time, and with interventions. Other, more severe, conditions will persist well into the 6/7th decade (Mordekar & Spence 2008). In follow-up studies of both antisocial and borderline personality disorder, a third were shown to have remitted completely, a third were the same and a third were worse (Paris 2003).

Assessment

As with other disorders, a thorough history and mental state examination is essential. History-taking needs to include the following:

- Were parents affectionate or frightening? Was there domestic violence or substance misuse in the home?
- Family dynamics and experiences of separations or loss of attachments
- Family history of disturbance in parents that might have led to a fearful or stressful environment (psychiatric illness, alcoholism, drug misuse or imprisonment)
- Early (under 5) hospitalizations and/or serious illness in the child or family
- A detailed account of childhood and adolescence, especially friendships and rule breaking at school
- History of persistent neglect, physical or sexual abuse
- Any positive relationships with peers or adults outside the home
- Truanting (alone or with friends) and age at first rule breaking behaviour, especially any record of physical harm to others before age 15
- Any risky or self-harming behaviours (including substance misuse or eating disorder symptoms)
- Attitudes to professional help (including the present interview)
- Continuing substance misuse
- Medication and what has helped in past
- If evidence of criminality, does this include physical harm to others? Is the criminal behaviour escalating in severity? Is deception a key feature of offending (this may suggest psychopathic traits)
- Any positive resilience factors (including adult relationships, such as work or sport)?
- Check for co-morbid psychotic, affective and or organic illness.

Mental state assessment rarely reveals clear psychotic phenomena, although the interviewer may find him/herself unsure about the exact nature of what the patient experiences. It is not unusual for patients to describe persecutory thoughts and beliefs about others, usually carers or those in close relationships with them. Attitudes towards others may oscillate between highly positive and very negative poles. Patients frequently experience themselves as being let down or abused by others, and they may easily become highly aroused, angry and distressed during interviews with healthcare professionals.

Collateral history is *essential* for a valid diagnosis of personality disorder, if only to see whether their presentation to you is typical or unusual. One should gather as much information as possible from friends, relatives, other professionals and hospital records, and any others involved. A number of questionnaires are available for the evaluation of personality. These are listed in Box 15.2.

Box 15.2

Assessment of PD

Observer-rated structured interview

- International Personality Disorder – Examination (Loranger et al 1994)
- Diagnostic Interview for DSM-IV – Personality Disorders (Zanarini et al 1996)
- Structured Interview for DSM-IV – Personality Disorders (Pfohl et al 1997)
- Structured Clinical Interview for DSM-IV – Axis I Disorders (First et al 1997)
- Personality Disorder Interview–IV (Widiger et al 1995)

Self-rated questionnaire

- Personality Diagnostic Questionnaire (Hyler 1994)

Structured interview – other sources

- Standardized Assessment of Personality (Mann et al 1981)
- Personality Assessment Schedule (Tyrer 1979)
- Structured Dimensional Assessments

Observer-rated structured interview

- Schedule for Normal and Abnormal – Personality (Clark 1993)

Self-rated questionnaire

- Personality Assessment Inventory (Morey 1991)
- Minnesota Multiphasic Personality – Inventory II (Butcher et al 1989)
- Millon Clinical Multiaxial Inventory III (Millon & Davis 1997)
- Eysenck Inventory Questionnaire (Eysenck & Eysenck 1975)
- NEO Five-Factor Inventory (McCrae & John 1992)
- Unstructured Assessments

Interview based

- Clinical interview
- Psychodynamic formulation

Other

- Rorschach Test (Rorschach 1964)
- Thematic Apperception Test (Morgan & Murray 1935)

From Bannerjee et al 2009.

Management of personality disorders

As with any medical condition (particularly one which involves regulatory systems), there are some general points to consider in planning and delivering treatment for personality disorders:

- What sort of disorder is it?
- How severe is it?
- How far has it spread?
- Is there co-morbid illness?

Specifically it is useful to consider:

- What affects are predominant, if any?
- What behaviours manifest when, and what do they mean to this person?
- How impulsive is this person?
- How many social systems (e.g. police, family services, civil law, social service, health) are involved in their lives?
- Can the patient describe or name any of their feelings or thoughts?
- Do they have any history of enduring (over 12 months) attachments?
- What is their attitude to help-seeking or eliciting?
- Are they hostile to the vulnerable, or exploit trust?
- Do they have strengths, and if so, what are they?
- Are they actively psychotic, addicted or depressed?

Treatment interventions

Treatment options have radically altered since the first edition of this book. There is ample evidence that some types of personality disorder respond well to treatment; but the therapeutic intervention has to be matched to the disorder. Just as there is no one single disorder, there is no one single treatment approach; and people who are offered the wrong treatment will not get better

and may get worse. The rate of progress is usually slow (months or years, not weeks), and follow-up is necessary. The quality and consistency of the therapeutic relationship is clinically important in terms of outcome. The overall aim is to help this person take their own minds, and the minds of others, seriously.

Within the UK, there are now national guidelines for the treatment of BPD and ASPD (NICE 2009a,b). In patients with a mixed picture, it is best to look at the overall symptom and behaviour pattern, and work out a systematic problem-based approach. In general, problems of impulsivity and mood dysregulation need to start with a cognitive approach, whereas withdrawal, hostility and exploitation need a more reflective pro-social approach. Depending on the symptoms, crisis management may include carefully planned short-term use of medication, such as anxiolytics.

Of great importance is the therapeutic attitude of staff and the treatment environment. If a mental health service is generally hostile to people with personality disorder, and operates a model of care that requires patients to take medication passively and be grateful, then people with personality disorder will indeed be 'untreatable'. However, in a service where there is an emphasis on recovery, where staff understand that interpersonal dysfunction is the symptom that they have to manage and have training to support this way of working, and where agency is negotiated with patients, then therapeutic progress can be made with even quite severe personality disorder (Genders & Player 1995; Allen et al 2008). People may not completely recover from their personality disorder, but they may discover a new way of living with it which does not hurt themselves or others.

Personality disorder and risk

The majority of people with a diagnosis of personality disorder pose no risk to anyone but themselves. People with BPD, for example, are at increased risk of self-harming behaviours and completed suicide. But a minority of people with personality disorders, especially antisocial personality disorder, do pose a significant risk of severe harm to others. Studies of violent offending consistently show that having a personality disorder diagnosis (particularly ASPD) increases the risk (Alden et al. 2007; Wallace et al 1998), and the risk is greatly increased if the subject also has a severe mental illness and a history of substance misuse. High levels of personality disorder have been found in populations of violent offenders, especially men who have committed sexual homicide and/or child abusers.

When assessing risk, the key issues are how antisocial this person has been generally in their lives to date, and what sort of criminality or rule breaking they have carried out. Generally, offending patterns run true (burglars tend to keep burgling), but it is important to take a longitudinal view of acting out, and consider whether the seriousness of the behaviour is escalating. Any history of violence should be taken seriously, including family violence to partners, parents and children.

The amendments to the UK Mental Health Act 1983 (MHA) in 2007 now make it easier to detain people with a personality disorder. It is no longer necessary to categorize a type of mental disorder, nor is there any 'treatability' clause. For detention to be legal, 'appropriate treatment must be available for the treatment or prevention of deterioration of the mental disorder'. Treatment is broadly defined and may include nursing interventions and psychological therapies. However, real ethical and legal questions remain about whether it is right to detain someone with ASPD or BPD, if no specific treatment programmes are available to them, *purely* on the basis of risk to others.

Specific personality disorders

Rather than list a long succession of diagnostic criteria for every personality disorder, over the next section we have chosen to focus more closely on those personality disorders which will be encountered most frequently within clinical practice (and therefore within examination situations), namely emotionally unstable or borderline, dissocial or antisocial, paranoid and schizoid personality types.

The ICD-10 criteria for personality disorder diagnosis include the following:

Marked disharmonious attitudes and behaviour involving usually several areas of functioning, e.g. affectivity, arousal, impulse control, ways of perceiving and thinking and style of relating to others:

- The pattern of behaving is enduring and longstanding.
- The pattern of behaviour is pervasive and clearly maladaptive to a broad range of personal and social situations.
- The disorder leads to considerable personal distress (although this may not always be apparent until later in its course).
- The disorder is often (but not always) associated with significant problems in occupational and social performance.

In addition to these general criteria, each personality subtype is diagnosed by the presence of three or more of the listed features. The criteria for other specific personality disorders are

clearly outlined within DSM-IV or ICD-10 and readers are directed to reference their chosen classification text for details. The diagnostic criteria given in this chapter are drawn mostly from the ICD-10. However, as an aide-memoire, the DSM-IV cluster system is practically helpful in highlighting the main characteristics of the personality disorders featured within each grouping, and we have set this text out accordingly.

Emotionally unstable or borderline personality disorder (BPD: Cluster B)

ICD-10 describes general features for emotionally unstable personality disorder, but further differentiates the disorder into *impulsive* and *borderline* types. In clinical practice, the distinction between the two is rarely evident and subsequently scarcely used. Emotionally unstable personality disorder is more frequently diagnosed in females. It is prevalent in just under 1% of the general population (NICE 2009a, b). Healthcare professionals will probably most frequently encounter individuals with borderline personality disorder presenting in crisis with self-harm, suicide attempts and aggressive or violent outbursts (often via the police).

The main features of the disorder are:

- Marked impulsivity with no consideration for the consequences of actions or ability to forward plan
- Outbursts of anger and affective instability.

The more 'borderline' features are:

- Unstable self-image, aims and preferences (including sexuality)
- Chronic feelings of emptiness
- Unstable, intense relationships
- Fear of abandonment
- Episode of self-harm or suicide threats often in response to emotional crises.

The predominant 'impulsive' features are:

- Emotional instability
- Lack of impulse control
- Violence or threatening behaviour.

In addition to these 'official' diagnostic criteria, individuals with borderline personality disorder may present with dissociative states, paranoid thinking (extreme hypersensitivity to others' reactions) and parapsychotic symptoms such as hearing voices. Such 'voices' tend to take the form of highly persecutory and threatening voices that tell the patient to hurt themselves or someone else, or advise them that they are at risk from others. They wax and wane in intensity and may become much worse with depressed mood. Transient psychotic episodes can occur (or co-morbid psychotic illnesses) and substance misuse and eating disorders, especially bulimia nervosa, are common co-morbid diagnoses.

The marked affective component of this disorder means that individuals are vulnerable to developing co-morbid mood disorders or to be incorrectly diagnosed with a mood disorder, e.g. bipolar disorder, without true recognition of the more global difficulties present, particularly interpersonal and self-esteem related.

Kernberg (1967) describes key features of what he has termed 'borderline personality organization' as impaired reality testing, primitive defence mechanisms (splitting, projection and projective identification), characteristic object relations (idealized and devalued) and fragile sense of identity or identity diffusion. These features are responsible for much of the interpersonal dysfunction. Patients with BPD typically form instant and intensely positive relationships with others (including mental health professionals), which then turn abruptly negative and then oscillate between the two emotional poles.

Aetiology

There appears to be a strong link between experience of adverse events as a child, particularly sexual abuse and later development of BPD. Those with a mother who has a diagnosis of BPD are more at risk of developing BPD themselves; possibly because the effect of stress on gene expression, but more likely because of aberrant parenting by mothers with BPD (Hobson et al 2009).

In Kleinian theory, the BPD presentation is a result of the patient still being stuck in a primitive form of relating (i.e. akin to "paranoid-schizoid" modes of functioning) (see Chapter 37). In attachment theory, emotionally unstable personality disorder is a manifestation of insecure attachment, particularly the 'preoccupied' or insecure-ambivalent subtype. Attachment theory is a particularly useful theoretical model to understand the relational dynamics which arise when working with those with borderline personality disorder (Bateman & Fonagy 2006).

Management

Short-term/crisis management

As mentioned above, individuals with borderline personality disorder often present to health services in crisis.

In the case of self-harm or a suicide attempt, triage assessment of the individual should include an assessment of their capacity to consent to medical treatment and appropriate first aid, and medical management of any self-harm or overdose will take priority. Mental health assessment will focus primarily on risk management, specifically identifying triggers to the incident (often interpersonal conflicts resulting in overwhelming emotional states), risk factors relating to the self-harm or suicide attempt (see Ch. 22 for further information) and identification of co-morbid mental illness. In those who are known to services, there may be information available or a care plan in place to guide the management of any crisis presentation.

Unplanned hospital admissions following crises are generally considered to be unhelpful in these cases. The process of admission to a hospital environment often leads to heightened levels of emotional arousal and attachment-seeking behaviour by the service user as he/she tries to find containment and security. A complicated dynamic develops between the service user and hospital. The fantasy of 'total care' provided by the hospital environment may initially feel very secure, and the service user forms a positive attachment to the ward/team, which relieves their anxiety.

However, as the service user becomes more dependent, their own coping strategies become undermined and their anxiety rises. As the admission progresses, the service user may also begin to feel overwhelmed or trapped which can lead to further self-harm or acting out in an unconscious bid to 'reject' care. Conversely, at the time of discharge planning, significant anxiety relating to feelings of abandonment and rejection by the 'system' may be experienced, which can also result in risk-taking behaviour in a bid to prevent discharge. Staff teams may become caught up in relationship dynamics with the individual which enacts his/her own psychological difficulties. For example, staff teams become split, some members being idealized by the service user, while others are seen as 'bad' or 'uncaring' (Main 1957).

Provided the risk can be managed safely, early discharge into the community with prompt follow-up, for example by crisis teams, should be planned. It may be that the act of self-harm has 'relieved' the individual of their immediate uncontainable emotional state, but often these individuals are at chronic risk of self-harm and consequently at high risk of completed suicide. Those who are not under a mental health team or specialist service follow-up should be considered for referral. Brief psychological interventions such as problem-solving may be helpful and co-morbid mental illness should be treated. Other strategies such as 'crisis cards' have been used. Short-term use of sedative medication may be considered; the duration of time should be negotiated with the patient but medication should ideally be discontinued within a week.

Long-term management

Therapeutic relationship

The main long-term management for borderline personality disorder is psychological therapy (NICE 2009a). However, in order for an individual to be in a place to engage in therapy, it is important to stabilize any 'chaos' surrounding them, such as housing, support for childcare and drug and alcohol problems.

As we have noted, those with borderline personality disorder are extremely sensitive to the dynamics of interpersonal relationships and, within mental health services, establishment of a consistent and 'good enough' therapeutic relationship is key. A large number of those with a diagnosis of personality disorder have experienced childhood abuse and maltreatment from caregivers. This sets up very complicated dynamics when these individuals come into contact with professionals offering care. Many of those with borderline personality disorder are help-seeking, but do not seek help in the most effective way, e.g. not attending an appointment and then presenting in crisis late at night (Henderson 1974).

For effective management of staff splitting and other relational dynamics, emphasis should be placed on engagement with named, consistent members of staff. However, this needs to be managed sensitively, as this may also lead to dependency and staff burnout. Supervision and reflective practice for any staff members who work with those with personality disorder is essential (NIMHE 2003). Particular attention should be given to changes in staff contact such as holidays, staff leaving, etc. as transitions are risk periods.

Psychological interventions

It is now widely acknowledged that individuals with borderline personality disorder require long-term psychological therapy (over 12 months) and that short-term therapy (<6 months)

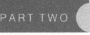

Interventions

There is a limited evidence base for the treatment of paranoid personality disorder.

Pharmacotherapy

Anecdotally, low dose antipsychotic medication may reduce levels of arousal and help prevent decompensation into acute psychotic episodes but the use of pharmacotherapy is not evidence-based.

Psychological interventions

It is likely that longer-term individual rather than group therapy will initially be required as the process of engagement and establishing trust within a therapeutic relationship will be challenging and will take time. The concept of group therapy may just be too overwhelming for an individual with paranoid personality disorder to consider. The long-term treatment goals should include increasing self-esteem, identifying and accepting feelings of vulnerability, establishing trust in others and verbalizing distress and feelings. In order to maximize engagement, clinicians should be transparent in their information-seeking and communication and attempt to avoid generating suspicion or feeling defensive themselves.

Cognitive therapy has been used in paranoid personality disorder (Beck et al 2004). The aim of therapy is to enhance self-esteem and social skills, followed by identification and challenge of the paranoid belief system and tendency to attribute blame, with development or more rational thinking styles.

Schizoid personality disorder (Cluster A)

ICD-10 diagnostic criteria include:

* Emotional coldness, detachment or flattened affect
* Little interest in sexual relationships
* Preoccupation with fantasy and introspection
* Limited capacity to express warmth, tenderness or anger and indifference to praise or criticism
* Lack of close friends and no desire to have confiding relationships
* Preference for solitary activities
* Insensitivity to prevailing social norms or convention.

Prevalence of schizoid personality disorder is reported to be about 0.8% of the general population in the UK (Coid et al 2006). Individuals may be at increased risk of developing schizoid personality disorder if there is a family history of schizoid personality disorder, schizotypal disorder or schizophrenia.

Differential diagnoses include the prodromal phase of schizophrenia, delusional disorder, schizotypal disorder, social phobia or a pervasive developmental disorder such as Asperger syndrome. There is an increased risk of developing co-morbid mental illness such as psychotic and anxiety disorders. Drug misuse or alcohol misuse may form part of the clinical presentation.

There are no well-established aetiological theories for schizoid personality disorder. Abuse or emotional neglect may predispose to developing the disorder. Individuals with schizoid personality disorder are essentially 'avoidant' of attachment. They build a rich and self-sufficient internal world which allows avoidance of external reality and any negotiation of interpersonal relationships, especially intimacy.

Management

Individuals with schizoid personality disorder do not tend to be help-seeking, and referrals may originate from family or healthcare professionals who are concerned about the person's 'eccentricity' or isolation, or from concern that psychosis may be present. Co-morbid diagnoses should be treated. Supportive therapy, problem-solving interventions or cognitive behavioural approaches to assist with social skills or to challenge cognitive belief systems patterns may be helpful (Beck et al 2004). There may be a case for monitoring the individual for a period of time, if there are concerns about social isolation or a prodrome of active psychotic breakdown.

'Things we wished we had known earlier'

Patients with personality disorders are often unpopular with mental health staff, largely because of the feelings they generate in us (Hinshelwood 1999). One of the professional competencies that every psychiatrist has to learn is how to deal compassionately and thoughtfully with patients who seek help but often rubbish it or reject it. There follows some practical thoughts we learned the hard way!

Challenging behaviour may be better understood as pathological 'care-eliciting' or attachment seeking behaviour.

Those with PD are sometimes called 'difficult' patients, but this usually describes how they make us feel, not who they are.

* Know your limits and maintain them with your patients.
* Do not give hugs to people with BPD, no matter how unkind or impolite it seems at the time.
* Attend regular supervision and use reflective practice or Balint groups.
* You cannot make everything better for these patients and you do not have to.
* Managing risk may mean managing other professionals' anxiety.
* People with personality disorders get physical and mental illnesses too, and get distressed.
* Do not patronize, challenge or compete with people with personality disorder.
* Make contracts but never go along with blackmail.
* If you refuse someone what they are asking, always offer something instead, e.g. 'I can't see you today but I will see you on X at Y o.clock'.
* Shame increases agitation and violence: do nothing that makes a person with personality disorder feel ashamed.
* Do not break off therapeutic attachments abruptly. Especially do not break off clinical relationships because you are angry or frightened; instead get help to manage the patient's continuing care.
* Practise sceptical compassion, and take nothing personally.
* Set appropriate therapeutic goals, and include damage limitation as one of them.

- Get help early from other colleagues: do not try and do it all by yourself.
- Be very, very cautious with anyone who says, 'You are the best psychiatrist I ever had; none of the others understand me'.

There is an increasing evidence base for the treatment of personality disorders, and there is no case for assuming that it is diagnosis with a hopeless prognosis. We hope to have conveyed in this chapter that working with personality disorder is sometimes difficult because the way that we see the world as healthcare professionals is not the way that people with personality disorders see the world. Each of us needs to develop a reflective stance so that we learn to ask questions and how to maintain dialogue and curiosity with people who may be ambivalent about seeking our help, but still hope that we will listen to them.

Further reading

Castillo, H., 2003. Personality disorder: temperament or trauma? Jessica Kingsley, London.

National Institute for Mental Health in England, 2002. Personality disorder: no longer a diagnosis of exclusion. Department of Health, Leeds.

Roth, A., Fonagy, P., 2002. What works for whom? A critical review of psychotherapy research, second ed. Guilford Press, New York.

References

Alden, A., Brennan, P., Hodgins, S., et al., 2007. Psychotic disorders and sex offending in a Danish birth cohort. Arch. Gen. Psychiatry 64, 1251–1258.

Allen, J.G., Fonagy, P., Bateman, A., 2008. Mentalizing in clinical practice. American Psychiatric Press, Washington.

APA: American Psychiatric Association, 1994. Diagnostic and statistical manual of mental disorders, fourth ed., text revision. American Psychiatric Association, Washington DC.

Bannerjee, P.J.M., Gibbon, S., Huband, N., 2009. Assessment of personality disorder. Advances in Psychiatric Treatment 15, 389–397.

Bateman, A., Fonagy, P., 2006. Mentalization-based treatment for borderline personality disorder. A practical guide. Oxford University Press, Oxford.

Bateman, A., Fonagy, P., 2008. 8-year follow-up of patients treated for borderline personality disorder: mentalization-based treatment versus treatment as usual. Am. J. Psychiatry 165, 631–638.

Bateman, A., Fonagy, P., 2009. Randomised controlled trial of outpatient mentalization based therapy vs structured clinical management for borderline personality disorder. Am. J. Psychiatry 166, 1355–1364.

Beck, A.T., Freeman, A., Davis, D. (Eds.), 2004. Cognitive therapy of personality disorders. second ed, Guilford Press, New York.

Bennett, A., Leschk, P., Heils, A., et al., 2002. Early experience and serotonin transporter gene variation interact to influence primate CNS function. Mol. Psychiatry 7, 118–122.

Bernstein, D., Useda, J., 2007. Paranoid personality disorder. In: O'Donohue, W., Fowler, K., Lilienfeld, S. (Eds.), Personality disorders: towards the DSM-V. Sage, New York.

Butcher, J.N., Dahlstrom, W.G., Graham, J.R., et al., 1989. Manual for the restandardized Minnesota Multiphasic Personality Inventory: MMPI–2. University of Minnesota Press, Minnesota.

Campbell, S., 2003. The feasibility of conducting an RCT at HMP Grendon. Online. Available: www.dspdprogramme.gov.uk/pdfs.

Carroll, A., 2009. Are you looking at me? Understanding and managing paranoid personality disorder. Advances in Psychiatric Treatment 15, 40–48.

Caspi, A., McClay, J., Moffitt, T., et al., 2002. The role of the genotype in the cycle of violence in maltreated children. Science 297, 851–854.

Clark, L.A., 1993. Manual for the schedule for nonadaptive and adaptive personality. University of Minnesota Press, Minneapolis.

Coid, J., Yang, M., Tyrer, P., et al., 2006. Prevalence and correlates of personality disorder in Great Britain. Br. J. Psychiatry 188, 423–431.

Dolan, B., Warren, F., Norton, K., 1997. Change in borderline symptoms one year after therapeutic community treatment for severe personality disorder. Br. J. Psychiatry 171, 274–279.

Dozier, M., Lomax, L., Tyrrell, C., et al., 2001. The challenge of treatment for clients with a dismissing state of mind. Attachment and Human Behaviour 3, 62–76.

Dunbar, R.I.M., 2003. The social brain: mind, language and society in evolutionary perspective. Annu. Rev. Anthropol. 32, 163–181.

Eysenck, H.J., Eysenck, S.B.G., 1975. Manual of the Eysenck Personality Questionnaire. Hodder & Stoughton, London.

Fazel, S., Danesh, J., 2002. Serious mental disorder in 23000 prisoners: a systematic review of 62 studies. Lancet 359, 545–550.

First, M.B., Spitzer, R.L., Williams, J.B., et al., 1997. Structured clinical interview for DSM-IV Axis I Disorders (SCID-I). American Psychiatric Association, Washington DC.

Genders, E., Player, E., 1995. Grendon: a study of a therapeutic prison. Oxford University Press, Oxford.

Goffman, E., 1956. The presentation of self in everyday life. University of Edinburgh Social Science Research Centre. Anchor Books, London.

Grant, B.F., Hasin, D.S., Stinson, F.S., et al., 2004. Prevalence, correlates, and disability of personality disorders in the United States: results from the national epidemiologic survey on alcohol and related conditions. J. Clin. Psychiatry 65, 948–958.

Hare, R.D., 1991. The Hare Psychopathy Checklist. Multi-health systems, New York.

Henderson, S., 1974. Abnormal care eliciting behaviour in man. J. Nerv. Ment. Dis. 15, 172–181.

Hobson, P., Patrick, M., Hobson, J., et al., 2009. How mothers with borderline personality disorder relate to their year old infants. Br. J. Psychiatry 195, 325–330.

Holmes, J., 1993. Attachment theory: a biological basis for psychotherapy. Br. J. Psychiatry 163, 430–438.

Hinshelwood, R.D., 1999. The difficult patient: the role of scientific psychiatry in understanding patients with chronic schizophrenia or severe personality disorder. Br. J. Psychiatry 174, 187–190.

Hyler, S.E., 1994. Personality Diagnostic Questionnaire–4 (PDQ–4). New York Psychiatric Institute, New York.

Johnson, J., Cohen, P., Brown, J., et al., 1999. Child maltreatment increases risk for personality disorder in early adulthood. Arch. Gen. Psychiatry 56, 600–606.

Kernberg, O., 1967. Borderline personality organization. Journal of the American Analytic Association 15, 641–685.

Kim, J., Cicchetti, D., Rogosch, F., et al., 2009. Child maltreatment and trajectories of personality and behaviour functioning: implications for development of personality disorder. Dev. Psychopathol. 21, 889–912.

Levy, K.N., Meehan, K.D., Kelly, K.M., et al., 2006. Change in attachment patterns and reflective function in an RCT of transference focussed therapy in borderline personality disorder. J. Consult. Clin. Psychol. 74, 1027–1040.

Lieb, K., Vollm, B., Rucker, G., et al., 2010. Pharmacotherapy for borderline personality disorder: Cochrane systematic review of randomised trials. Br. J. Psychiatry 196, 4–12.

Linehan, M.M., Armstrong, H., Suarez, A., et al., 1991. Cognitive-behavioral treatment of

Epidemiology

Anxiety disorders are the most common mental health disorders occurring in up to one-third of the population in their lifetime (Kessler et al 2005a,b, 2007).

Important surveys

As classification systems have improved (ICD-10 and DSM-IV), epidemiological studies have progressed. There have been many epidemiological studies over the past few decades, and a few are highlighted here for their contributions to epidemiology of anxiety disorders.

The National Psychiatric Morbidity Surveys of Great Britain estimated prevalence of psychiatric morbidity among adults aged 16–64 living in Great Britain. Experienced interviewers of the Office of Population and Censuses and Surveys (OPCS) interviewed 10 108 (79%) adults of 13 000 selected. Neurotic disorder was assessed using the Revised Clinical Interview Schedule (CIS-R) providing prevalence over a 1-week period. The overall prevalence of a neurotic disorder was 16%, with 12.3% in males and 19.5% in females. Individual neurotic disorders occurred more often in women; however the difference in panic disorder was small and non-significant (Jenkins et al 1997). Individual anxiety disorder prevalence rates are summarized in Table 16.1.

The National Morbidity Survey (NCS) and its replication (NCS-R) was a nationally representative household survey of people aged 15–54 in the USA. The NCS-R diagnoses are based on the World Mental Health Survey Initiative Version of the World Health Organization Composite International Diagnostic Interview (WMH-CIDI). It generates both ICD-10 and DSM-IV diagnoses. The lifetime estimate for anxiety disorders is 28.8% with a 12-month prevalence of 18.1% (Kessler et al 2005a,b). Individual anxiety disorder prevalence rates are summarized in Table 16.1. All individual anxiety disorders had an increased prevalence among women (Table 16.2) (NCS-R 2007).

The Epidemiologic Catchment Area Study (ECA) in the USA incorporated residents that were both institutionalized and living in the community. It was a large study, yielding 20 861 respondents overall. The diagnostic interview used in the ECA was the NIMH Diagnostic Interview Schedule (DIS) Version III yielding diagnoses categorized according to the DSM-III. Interviews took place between 1980 and 1985. The lifetime prevalence rate for any anxiety disorder was 14.6% and the 12-month prevalence rate was 12.6% (Regier et al 1998).

The variance in lifetime and 12-month prevalence rates among the ECA and NCS-R probably reflects the diagnostic instruments used and sampling differences. The chronic nature of anxiety disorders is indicated by the increased lifetime prevalence rate compared with the 12 months or 1 week prevalence rates.

Presentation

In general, all anxiety disorders develop relatively early in life. The median age of onset for anxiety disorders is 11 years, with 75% developing the conditions between 6 and 21 years. Separation anxiety disorder and specific phobia have an early age of onset (median age 7), whereas other anxiety disorders occur during later ages (median range 19–31) (Kessler et al 2005a). It is estimated that fewer than 40% of people with a lifetime psychiatric disorder receive professional treatment (Kessler et al 1994). For those who do seek treatment for anxiety disorders, there is a delay in presentation ranging from 9 to 23 years. Delay in presenting for treatment is particularly associated with those who develop the disorder at an early age, who are married, who have poor educational attainment, or who are members of racial or ethnic minorities (Wang et al 2005).

Co-morbidity

Epidemiological data suggests co-morbid psychiatric disorders are common and in fact more the rule rather than the exception. Kessler reported that three-quarters of those with a lifetime anxiety disorder have at least one other lifetime psychiatric disorder. Panic disorder had the highest co-morbidity of 92.3%. Table 16.3 summarizes rates of co-morbidity among people with lifetime anxiety disorders (Michael et al 2007).

Table 16.1 Prevalence (percentages) of anxiety disorders

Disorder	NPMS	ECA		NCS-R	
Prevalence	1 week	12 months	Lifetime	12 months	Lifetime
Any anxiety disorder	16	12.6	14.6	18.1	28.8
Generalized anxiety disorder	3.1	3.7	–	3.1	5.7
Simple (specific) phobia	1.1	9.1	10.1	8.7	12.5
Social phobia	–	4.2	2.8	6.8	12.1
Agoraphobia	–	5.8	5.2	0.8	1.4
Obsessive -compulsive disorder	1.2	2.1	2.5	1.0	1.6
Panic disorder	0.8	1.3	1.6	2.7	4.7
Post-traumatic stress disorder	–	1.9	–	3.5	6.8

Table 16.2 Male/female percentages of anxiety disorders

Disorder	NPMS		NCS-R			
Prevalence	1 week		12 months		Lifetime	
Sex	Male	Female	Male	Female	Male	Female
Any anxiety disorder	12.3	19.5	14.3	23.4	25.4	36.4
Generalized anxiety disorder	2.8	3.4	1.9	3.4	4.2	7.1
Simple (specific) phobia	0.7	1.4	5.8	12.2	8.9	15.8
Social phobia			6.1	8.0	11.1	13.0
Agoraphobia			0.8	0.9	1.1	1.6
Obsessive–compulsive disorder	0.9	1.5	0.5	1.8	1.6	3.1
Panic disorder	0.8	0.9	1.6	3.8	3.1	6.2
Post-traumatic stress disorder	–	–	1.8	5.2	3.6	9.7

Table 16.3 Lifetime psychiatric co-morbidity rates with an anxiety disorder

Any anxiety disorder	74.1%
Panic disorder	92.2%
Agoraphobia	87.3%
Social phobia	81.0%
Simple phobia	83.4%
Generalized anxiety disorder	91.3%
Post-traumatic stress disorder	81.0%

Kessler also reported an average odds ratio of 6.6 for an association between an anxiety and affective disorder, with particularly strong associations between affective disorders and generalized anxiety disorder or panic disorder (Kessler et al 2007). Around two-thirds of people with both affective and anxiety disorders reported the anxiety disorder developed first (Kessler et al 2007; Regier et al 1998).

Sociodemographic correlates

Women have a higher prevalence of anxiety disorders. They are also associated with being widowed, divorced or unmarried. Being unemployed, stay at home parents, having low levels of education and low income, are linked with anxiety (Michael et al 2007).

Classification of anxiety disorders

The DSM-IV and the ICD-10 contain the current classification of anxiety disorders (Box 16.1). They use a categorical approach that defines mental disorders based on specific features. The DSM-IV utilizes a five axes classification enabling the complexity of the mental illness to be captured. Both allow for dual

Box 16.1

DSM-IV-TR and ICD-10 classification of anxiety disorders

DSM-IV anxiety disorders
- Panic disorder without agoraphobia
- Panic disorder with agoraphobia
- Agoraphobia without a history of panic disorder
- Specific phobia
- Social phobia
- Obsessive–compulsive disorder
- Post-traumatic stress disorder
- Acute stress disorder
- Generalized anxiety disorder
- Anxiety disorder due to general medical condition
- Substance-induced anxiety disorder
- Anxiety disorder not otherwise specified

ICD-10 neurotic, stress-related and somatoform disorders
- Phobic anxiety disorders
- Other anxiety disorders
- Obsessive–compulsive disorder
- Reaction to severe stress, and adjustment disorders
- Dissociative (conversion) disorders
- Somatoform disorders
- Other neurotic disorders

diagnosis. There are 12 distinct categories of anxiety disorders in the DSM-IV. The ICD-10 has seven categories defined under the heading neurotic, stress-related and somatoform disorders (APA 2000; WHO 1992).

The American Psychiatric Association and the World Health Organization have begun revising the DSM-IV and ICD-10. Issues concerning revising include considerations regarding structure of the classifications, the relationship between categories and dimensions, sensitivity of thresholds for diagnosis and simplifying the diagnostic criteria to improve clinical utility (Andrews et al 2008).

Epidemiological studies have shown high co-morbidity of anxiety disorders with other anxiety and mood disorders (Kessler et al 1997). Therefore, they may be more appropriate as part of a broader category of internalizing disorders (Andrews et al 2008). Anxiety disorders share common elements such as fear and avoidance of situations, but differ on the specific content. Contamination may be the fear associated with OCD and spiders may be the fear associated with specific phobia. However, the stress and subsequent anxiety reducing actions are similar. In addition, anxiety and mood disorders often share categorical similarities such as hopelessness, easily fatigued, poor concentration, etc. And the social and psychological treatments for anxiety and mood disorders are often similar (Stein 2009).

The DSM-IV and ICD-10 classify mental disorders into categories; however, mental disorders exist on a continuum. The number of symptoms and the duration are necessary for diagnosing an anxiety disorder according the ICD-10 and DSM-IV criteria. These specific criteria can exclude those with debilitating illness. A dimensional approach might improve the reliability and validity of the classification. Present DSM-IV and ICD-10 is very comprehensive and clinically too cumbersome to be remembered by clinicians in diagnosis. Simplifying the diagnostic criteria may improve clinical usefulness of these classification systems (Andrews et al 2008).

Aetiology of anxiety disorders

The aetiology of anxiety disorders is multifaceted. Underlying risk factors and external stressors interplay in the development of anxiety disorders.

Psychological theories

Fear and anxiety are normal emotional states. Fear is a response to an impending identifiable danger. Anxiety is a state of chronic apprehension about future harm that may be unknown, internal or vague, characterized by tension, worry, negative affect and a feeling of insecurity (Grillon 2008). Psychological theories aim to explain causes and offer psychological treatment to anxiety disorders.

Learning theory

The case of Little Albert implicated classical conditioning as a mechanism to acquiring fears and phobias. Little Albert, an 11-month-old baby, was introduced to a loud sound (unconditioned stimulus) that resulted in fear (unconditioned response), a natural response. Then he was introduced to a rat (neutral stimulus) paired with the loud sound (unconditioned stimulus) resulting in fear (unconditioned response). Successive introductions of a rat (conditioned stimulus) resulted in fear (conditioned response) (Watson & Rayner 1920). Learning theory postulates that traumatic experiences are needed for developing phobic fears and anxiety disorders and that anxiety is a conditioned response to a specific environmental stimulus (Mineka & Oehlberg 2008).

Psychodynamic and psychoanalytic theory

Freud noted that a major drive for most people is the reduction in tension, and that a major cause of tension was anxiety. He identified three different types of anxiety. Reality anxiety is the most basic form of anxiety. It is based on fears of real and possible events. Moral anxiety is fear of violating values manifesting as feelings of guilt or shame. Neurotic anxiety, which has its place in modern-day anxiety disorders, is anxiety arising from unconscious fear that basic impulses of the Id (the primitive part of our personality) will take control of the person resulting in expressing the Id's desires and eventual punishment (Freud 1953–1974). Psychoanalytic treatment of anxiety disorders utilizes exploration of the unconscious and aims to increase personal awareness.

Cognitive psychology

The cognitive model of anxiety proposes a person's beliefs regarding danger predisposes individuals to focus their attention to threat, to make catastrophic interpretations of vague stimuli, and to engage in dysfunctional safety behaviours. The danger-orientated bias is present at all levels of processing (perception, interpretation and recall) and throughout all anxiety disorders (Beck 2005). Therefore cognitive behavioural therapy or CBT is a treatment that can be used in the treatment of all anxiety disorders.

Developmental precursors

There are some identifiable developmental precursors as risk factors for adult anxiety disorders. Childhood anxiety disorders, particularly separation anxiety disorder, overanxious disorder/GAD, social or specific phobia increases the risk for later developing anxiety disorders. Behavioural inhibition, a temperament trait of being sensitive and fearful, is a predictor of later social phobia and associated with other anxiety disorders. In anxiety sensitivity, normal physiological cues are interpreted as harmful, contributing to a 'fear of fear' cycle. Anxiety sensitivity is a predictor of later anxiety disorders. Negative affectivity is a predisposition to experience negative emotions or distress. It is a predictor of future psychopathology, including anxiety disorders (Hirshfelf-Becker et al 2008).

Neuropsychology

In animal studies, fear and anxiety are distinct responses to stimuli. Fear is a phasic response to imminent threat and it is mediated by the amygdala. Anxiety is a sustained state of apprehension to uncertain danger and it is mediated by the bed nucleus of the stria terminalis. The bed nucleus of the stria terminalis is a limbic forebrain structure that receives projections from the amygdala and in turn projects to hypothalamic and brainstem target areas that are associated with autonomic and behavioural responses to aversive stimuli (Walker et al 2003). These neural circuits are highly conserved across species, allowing inferences to be made from animal studies regarding anxiety and fear in humans (LeDoux 1995). Lesions to the amygdala have been shown to block measures of fear such as blood pressure elevation, heart rate changes, startle reflex and freezing (Hamm & Weike 2005).

Neuroanatomy

The amygdala is involved in processing fearful material and co-ordinating the autonomic threat response. It receives sensory information from the anterior thalamus and projects behavioural and autonomic nervous system responses to the motor area and brainstem. Increased amygdalar reactivity to threat cues has been documented in anxiety disorders (Mathew et al 2008). Recent data have focused on the altered anterior insular function as having a role in anxiety disorders. Patients experience an augmented signalling of the prospective human body state, thereby triggering an increase in anxiety (Paulus & Stein 2006). The prefrontal and parietal cortex along with the hippocampus and neocortex are also implicated in stress responses.

Genetics

Numerous genetic studies have highlighted the increased risk of anxiety disorders in first-degree relatives (Smoller et al 2009), who have an overall 4–6-fold increased risk of developing an anxiety disorder. Concordance rates for monozygotic twins range from 12% to 26% and from 4% to 15% for dizygotic twins. The heritability of anxiety disorders is in the modest range of 30–40%, which is significantly lower than schizophrenia and bipolar disorder. This indicates environmental factors play a considerable role (Hettema et al 2001). Research into the genetics of anxiety disorders over the period between 2002 and 2007 was considerably less than for other major psychiatric disorders. This may reflect the ever-evolving classification of anxiety disorders therefore making them difficult to categorize. Anxiety disorders are complex and share overlapping clinical dimensions with other psychiatric disorders (Smoller et al 2008).

Neurochemistry

Hormones

Exposure to stressful events during development has been shown to produce alterations in the hypothalamic-pituitary-adrenal axis (HPA) and in turn, act as a risk factor for developing anxiety and mood disorders (Gillespie et al 2009). The HPA axis is a hormonal system that is reactive to stress. The hypothalamus releases CRF, which stimulates the pituitary gland to disperse adrenocorticotropin-releasing hormone (ACTH) into the bloodstream. The adrenal cortex responds to ACTH by releasing glucocorticoids, in particular cortisol. Cortisol affects arousal, vigilance, attention and memory. A negative feedback system occurs when cortisol binds to glucocorticoid receptors in the hypothalamus and pituitary (Mathew et al 2008). Hypercortisolaemia and reduced negative feedback inhibition have been implicated in anxiety states (Holsboer 2003). Elevated CRF in anxiety states have also been reported (Mathew et al 2008).

Therapeutic techniques at the neurochemical level may act as primary prevention of anxiety disorders. CRF antagonists may reverse stress-related behaviours. Targeting aspects of memory associated with hyperarousal and trauma forms the rationale of treatments such as propranolol, a beta-blocker and mifepristone, a glucocorticoid receptor antagonist (Mathew et al 2008).

Neurotransmitters

Noradrenaline

People with anxiety disorders are thought to have poorly regulated adrenergic systems that cause an increase in noradrenaline release. Raised noradrenaline is associated with anxiety symptoms. Studies shows administering the α2-adrenergic antagonist yohimbine to rats increases noradrenaline release in several brain regions, especially the hypothalamus, amygdala and locus coeruleus (Tanaka et al 2000). In humans, yohimbine increased panic symptoms in healthy adults (Vasa et al 2009). This suggests that an increased release of noradrenaline in these specific brain regions provides a neurochemical mechanism for stress and anxiety. Conversely, clonidine (α2-receptor agonist) and prazosin (α1-receptor antagonist) cause a pharmacologic reduction of CNS noradrenergic activity. There is evidence they can play a useful role in treating sleep disturbance and hyperarousal in post-traumatic stress disorder (Boehnlein & Kinzie 2007).

Serotonin

Selective serotonin reuptake inhibitors have shown to have anti-obsessional qualities in the treatment of OCD. Other classes of psychotropic medication have little effect on OCD. Therefore, serotonin pathophysiology is implicated in OCD; however, clinical aetiological studies are inconclusive (Goddard et al 2008). In addition, SSRIs also have anti-anxiety affects and are used in the treatment of social phobia and generalized anxiety disorder.

GABA

GABA is the most widely implicated neurotransmitter in the pathophysiology of anxiety disorders. Evidence from the use of benzodiazepines supports the role of a relative deficiency in GABA neurotransmission (Numeroff 2003). Benzodiazepines enhance the activity of GABA and the GABA type A receptor. The hippocampus is rich in GABAergic neurons. The hippocampus is important in laying down memories and reduced hippocampal volume is associated with some anxiety disorders.

Neuropeptides

Neuropeptides are short-chain amino acids that act as neurotransmitters in the brain circuits associated with anxiety.

Cholecystokinin (CCK)

There is some evidence for increased sensitivity to exogenous cholecystokinin-tetrapeptide (CCK-4) in normal controls and general anxiety disorder, with the latter experiencing more distressing symptoms of anxiety (Koszychi et al 1993; Brawman-Mintzer et al 1997). However, patients with social phobia and OCD did not experience a worsening in their symptoms,

supported by the literature. MAOIs may be indicated in treatment refractory panic disorder (Roy-Byrne et al 2006). Benzodiazepines are used for their anti-anxiety affects; however, NICE guidelines contraindicate long-term use due to abuse potential (NICE 2004). Relapse rates when discontinuing medication are around 25–50% (Roy-Byrne et al 2006).

CBT is the most widely studied and validated psychotherapeutic treatment for panic disorder. However, it is often an underutilized treatment option. CBT educates patients about panic, helps correct misconceptions regarding panic symptoms and exposes patients to feared body sensations (palpations, dyspnoea), to lessen the fear response. Other less studied treatments include insight-oriented therapies, relaxation training without exposure, stress management, hypnosis, and eye-movement desensitization and reprocessing therapy (EMDR) (Roy-Byrne et al 2006).

Specific phobia

Specific phobia (SP) is a marked and persistent fear of clearly discernible, circumscribed objects or situations. When a person with specific phobia is exposed to the stimulus, it provokes an immediate anxiety response, usually in the form of a panic attack. The person recognizes the response is excessive or unreasonable and tries to avoid the stimulus. The DSM-IV-TR diagnostic criteria are summarized in Box 16.6 (APA 2000).

Interestingly, blood injury phobia initially presents with a rise in heart rate followed by a vasovagal bradycardia and frequently syncope. Other phobias cause persistent tachycardia (Marks 1988).

Epidemiology

Specific phobia is a common lifetime condition occurring in 9.4% to 12.5% in the general population (Regier et al 1998; Kessler et al 2005a; Stinson et al 2007). It is the most common psychiatric disorder (12.5%) (Kessler et al 2005a). Specific phobia is more common in females (NCS-R 2007, Stinson et al 2007). It is a highly co-morbid condition (83.4%) and strongly associated with alcohol and drug dependence (Michael et al 2007; Stinson et al 2007). Bipolar II is the most strongly related mood disorder to SP and panic disorder with agoraphobia was the anxiety disorder most highly associated. Being female, young and low income increases risk (Stinson et al 2007).

Course

The mean age of onset of specific phobia is 9.7 years and the mean duration of the episode is 20.1 years according to Stinson et al (2007). Magee et al (1996) reported 15 years as mean age of onset, and Kessler et al (2005a) reported 7 years as mean age of onset. Age 5 shows the highest onset of cases with another peak around 10 years. Animals and heights are the most prevalent phobic stimuli among respondents with lifetime specific phobia, with 50% reporting them. Only 8% report treatment specifically for specific phobia. The disability associated with specific phobia is less than mood disorders, but comparable with those with substance use disorders and other anxiety disorders. Most specific phobias involve multiple fears and an increasing number of fears are associated with greater disability, treatment seeking and co-morbidity with other psychiatric disorders (Stinson et al 2007).

Aetiology

Classical conditioning theory conceptualized the aetiology of phobias. The 'Little Albert' study (Watson & Rayner 1920) reported that pairing of a white rat (neutral stimulus) with a loud noise (aversive stimulus) produced a conditioned fear response when exposed to the rat in future occasions. To account for the simplicity of this model, Seligman (1971) further developed preparedness theory of fear acquisition. He postulated

---

Box 16.6

DSM-IV-TR diagnostic criteria for specific phobia

A. Marked and persistent fear that is excessive or unreasonable, cued by the presence or anticipation of a specific object or situation (e.g. flying, heights, animals, receiving an injection, seeing blood)

B. Exposure to the phobic stimulus almost invariably provokes an immediate response, which may take the form of a situationally bound or situationally predisposed panic attack. *Note*: In children, the anxiety may be expressed by crying, tantrums, freezing, or clinging

C. The persona recognizes that the fear is excessive or unreasonable. *Note*: In children this feature may be absent

D. The phobic situation(s) is avoided or else is endured with intense anxiety or distress

E. The avoidance, anxious anticipation, or distress in the feared situation(s) interferes significantly with the person's normal routine, occupational (or academic) functioning, or social activities or relationships, or there is a marked distress about having the phobia

F. In individuals under 18 years the duration is at least 6 months

G. The anxiety, panic attacks, or phobic avoidance associated with the specific object or situation are not better accounted for by another mental disorder, such as obsessive–compulsive disorder (e.g. fear of dirt in someone with an obsession about contamination); post-traumatic stress disorder (e.g. avoidance of stimuli associated with a severe stressor); separation anxiety disorder (e.g. avoidance of school); social phobia (e.g. avoidance of social situations because of fear of embarrassment); panic disorder with agoraphobia, or agoraphobia without a history of panic disorder.

Specify type

- Animal type
- Natural environment type (e.g. heights, storms, water)
- Blood-injection injury type
- Situational type (e.g. airplanes, elevators, enclosed places)
- Other type (e.g. fear of choking, vomiting, or contracting an illness; in children, fear of loud sounds or costumed characters).

humans are biologically prepared to develop fears of stimuli that threaten personal safety and phobias were a result of prepared learning.

Genetic factors appear to play a role and their contribution may vary according to symptom type. Bolton et al (2006) found in their twin study of 6-year olds a 60% heritability for SP. Adult heritability appears to be lower (25–59%) with environmental contribution playing a greater role (Kendler et al 1999, 2001). Blood injury phobias appear to have a more genetic contribution than other phobias (Kendler et al 1999; Fyer et al 1990).

Neuroimaging studies vary greatly in specific phobia with varying evidence for hyperactivation of the amygdala and subsequent reduction in activity after exposure therapy (Pull 2008).

Treatment

Psychological therapy is the mainstay of treatment in specific phobia. Most phobias respond to exposure, but it is associated with high dropout rates and low treatment acceptance. Systematic desensitization response is more moderate. Some studies suggest that virtual reality may be effective in flying and heights. Cognitive therapy is most helpful in claustrophobia. Applied tension is unique for blood-injection-injury phobia. This involves the patient rapidly and frequently tensing various muscle groups in his or her body, thereby creating a physiological state incompatible with fainting (Choy et al 2007).

Data on medication treatment are limited. Although benzodiazepines provide short-term relief from anxiety, there is no evidence for long-term reductions, and they may, in fact, precipitate a more profound rebound anxiety (Wilhelm & Roth 1997). There is some new evidence for the use of d-cycloserine as an augmentation treatment to exposure therapy in specific phobia (Hofmann et al 2006).

Social phobia

In social phobia, there is a marked and persistent fear of social or performance situations in which embarrassment may occur. Anxiety occurs when exposed to the social or performance situation. The person recognizes their fear is excessive or unreasonable and tries to avoid the situation. Individuals with social phobia experience concerns about embarrassment and are afraid that others will judge them to be anxious or weak. The DSM-IV-TR diagnostic criteria are summarized in Box 16.7 (APA 2000).

Epidemiology

Social phobia is a common disease, with varying lifetime prevalence rates in epidemiological studies. Lifetime prevalence rate in the ECA was 2.8% and in the NCS-R is 12.1% (Regier et al 1998; Kessler et al 2005a; Ruscio et al 2008a). Variations are associated with the measuring instruments (Ruscio et al 2008a). Co-morbidity is high ranging from 62.9% to 81%, depending on epidemiological study (Ruscio et al 2008a; Michael et al 2007). Co-morbidity, role impairment and treatment seeking are closely related to the number of social fears (Ruscio et al 2008a). In one epidemiologic study, over 50% of patients with social anxiety disorder did not complete secondary school, more than 70% were in the lowest two quartiles in terms of socioeconomic status, and approximately 22% were receiving welfare payments, suggesting they were unable to work (Schneier et al 1992). Lifetime social phobia is correlated with being younger than 60, previously married, and being unemployed or disabled (Ruscio et al 2008a).

Course

Social phobia begins in childhood or adolescence and has a chronic course. Patients report suffering from symptoms for many years before seeking treatment. Around two-thirds seek

---

Box 16.7

DSM-IV diagnostic criteria for social phobia

A. A marked and persistent fear of one or more social or performance situations in which the person is exposed to unfamiliar people or to possible scrutiny by others. The individual fears that he or she will act in a way (or show anxiety symptoms) that will be humiliating or embarrassing. *Note*: In children, there must be evidence of the capacity for age-appropriate social relationships with familiar people and the anxiety must occur in peer settings, not just in interactions with adults

B. Exposure to the feared social situation almost invariably provokes anxiety, which may take the form of a situationally bound or situationally predisposed panic attack. *Note*: In children, the anxiety may be expressed by crying, tantrums, freezing, or shrinking from social situations with unfamiliar people

C. The person recognizes that the fear is excessive or unreasonable. *Note*: In children, this feature may be absent

D. The feared social or performance situations are avoided or else are endured with intense anxiety or distress

E. The avoidance, anxious anticipation, or distress in the feared social or performance situations(s) interferes significantly with the person's normal routine, occupation (academic) functioning, or social activities or relationships, or there is marked distress about having the phobia

F. In individuals under age 18 years, the duration is at least 6 months

G. The fear or avoidance is not due to the direct physiological effects of a substance (e.g. a drug of abuse, a medication) or a general medical condition and is not better accounted for by another mental disorder (e.g. panic disorder with or without agoraphobia, separation anxiety disorder, body dimorphic disorder, a pervasive developmental disorder, or schizoid personality disorder)

H. If a general medical condition or another mental disorder is present, the fear in Criterion A is unrelated to it, e.g. the fear is not of stuttering, trembling in Parkinson disease, or exhibiting abnormal eating behaviour in anorexia nervosa or bulimia nervosa.

Specify if:

Generalized: if the fears include most social situations (also consider the additional diagnosis of avoidant personality disorder).

treatment; however, only about one-third ever receive treatment for social phobia. Unfortunately, there is an inverse relationship between number of fears and treatment offered. This suggests that those most debilitated by it are not receiving adequate input (Ruscio et al 2008a).

Aetiology

There is good evidence to suggest genetic factors play a role and the heritability ranges from 30% to 65%, depending on the study (Rapee & Spence 2004). It is suggested there is a dysfunction of postsynaptic serotonin receptors. People with social phobia are hypersensitive to challenges with caffeine, CO_2 and pentagastrin, all of which are anxiety inducing substances. Neuroimaging studies suggest a dysfunction of the striatal presynaptic dopamine transporter in social phobia (Den Boer 2000).

Temperamental factors associated with social phobia may be identified in infancy or early childhood. Behavioural inhibition to the unfamiliar has been implicated as a precursor to social phobia. It is an enduring tendency, occurring in 10–15% of white American children, to demonstrate fear, avoidance, or quiet restraint and reticence when exposed to unfamiliar situations, objects or people. In anxious adults and adolescents, parental overprotection, over affection, concern with the opinions of others, shame of their shyness and a tendency to use shaming as a discipline style, were reported. Conditioning events, such as experiencing a humiliating event or witnessing/hearing a fearful experience of others are associated with developing social phobia. Many adults with social phobia (44–58%) are able to identify a specific humiliating event at the onset or exacerbation of their disorder. Some (13–16%) reported observing a traumatic social event, while others reported (3%) acquiring their phobia through information transfer. The cognitive factors in social phobia portray a person who overestimates threats that are social-evaluative. The person predicts that he or she will experience criticism or disapproval, and will be socially incompetent and that catastrophic results will ensue (Ollendick & Hirschfeld-Becker 2002).

Treatment

Management of social phobia entails medication and psychological treatments. SSRIs have been shown to be efficacious along with clomipramine. There is some evidence for phenelzine; however, because of serious side-effects it is rarely used. Benzodiazepines have anxiolytic effects but are not recommended owing to their addictive properties and lack of long-term benefits and relapse when stopped. Beta-blockers have a role in those with performance anxiety, especially if physiological tremor suppression is an advantage. They have advantages over other medication because they do not sedate, impair concentration or induce dependence. However, they have not been shown to be beneficial in generalized social phobia. Other pharmacological approaches are demonstrating positive results, such as gabapentin, nefazodone and venlafaxine.

Psychological therapies include CBT to help people overcome anxiety reactions in social and performance situations

and to alter beliefs and responses that maintain this behaviour. CBT group therapy is also indicated (Den Boer 2000). Virtual reality therapy (VRT) is a new form of exposure-based therapy. The virtual environments used in the treatment reproduce four situations that people with social phobia feel the most threatening: performance, intimacy, scrutiny and assertiveness. The therapist helps the patient to learn adapted cognitions and behaviours that translate into real-life situations (Klinger et al 2004).

Obsessive–compulsive disorder

Obsessions are persistent ideas, thoughts, impulses, or images that are experienced as intrusive and inappropriate and that cause marked anxiety or distress. Obsessions are ego-dystonic; the content is alien, not within his or her own control, and not the kind he or she would expect to have. However, the person is able to recognize the obsessions are a product of his or her mind, not imposed from without. Compulsions are repetitive behaviours or mental acts with a goal to prevent or reduce anxiety or distress. An adult at some point will recognize that obsessions or compulsions are excessive or unreasonable. The diagnostic criteria for obsessive–compulsive disorder (OCD) are summarized in Box 16.8 (APA 2000). OCD is a symptomatically heterogeneous condition, in which various kinds of obsessions and compulsions exist (McKay et al 2004).

Classification controversies

Currently, OCD is classified in the DSM-IV-TR under anxiety disorders, whereas in the ICD-10 it is under neurotic, stress-related and somatoform disorders, as a separate disorder from other anxiety disorders. The DSM-V Work Group suggests removing OCD from anxiety disorders and placing it in obsessive–compulsive-related disorders (OCRDs). These disorders share obsessive and compulsive domains, which none of the other anxiety disorders possess. Other disorders possibly included would be obsessive compulsive personality disorder, Tourette syndrome, Sydenham/paediatric autoimmune neuropsychiatric disorders associated with streptococcal infection (PANDAS), trichotillomania, body dysmorphic disorder, autism, eating disorders, Huntington disease, Parkinson disease, schizo-obsessive disorder, impulse control disorders, and substance use disorders. There is evidence that these disorders share common features of phenomenology, co-morbidity, neurocircuitry, genetic factors and treatment response. Many of these disorders are under-studied and placing them in a category may help in screening and diagnosis and ultimately better treatment. Potential disadvantages for including OCD in OCRDs would be complicating treatment delivery and fragmenting existing anxiety clinics (Hollander et al 2008).

Epidemiology

Results from the initial NCS-R show OCD to have a lifetime prevalence rate of 1.6% and a 12-month prevalence rate of 1.0% (Kessler et al 2005a,b). Further assessment on a random 30% of the original NCS-R sample population was performed. This was

Box 16.8

DSM-IV-TR diagnostic criteria for obsessive–compulsive disorder

A. Either obsessions or compulsions:

Obsessions defined by (1), (2), (3) and (4):

(1) Recurrent and persistent thoughts, impulses, or images that are experienced, at some time during the disturbance, as intrusive and inappropriate and that cause marked anxiety or distress

(2) The thoughts, impulses, or images are not simply excessive worries about real-life problems

(3) The person attempts to ignore or suppress such thoughts, impulses, or images, or to neutralize them with some other thoughts or actions

(4) The person recognizes that the obsessional thoughts, impulses, or images are a product of his or her own mind (not imposed from without as in thought insertion).

Compulsions as defined by (1) and (2):

(1) Repetitive behaviours (e.g. hand-washing, ordering, checking) or mental acts (e.g. praying, counting, repeating words silently) that the person feels driven to perform in response to an obsession, or according to rules that must be applied rigidly

(2) The behaviours or mental acts are aimed at preventing or reducing distress or preventing some dreaded event or situation; however, these behaviours or mental acts either are not connected in a realistic way with what they are designed to neutralize or prevent or are clearly excessive.

B. At some point during the course of the disorder, the person has recognized that the obsessions or compulsions are excessive or unreasonable. *Note*: This does not apply to children.

---

done on a smaller sample due to the complexity of the OCD criteria and lengthy diagnostic interview. The lifetime and 12-month prevalence estimates for DSM-IV OCD were 2.3% and 1.2%, respectively. However, 28.2% of respondents reported experiencing obsessions or compulsions at some time in their lives. It was reported that 90% of those with lifetime OCD fulfill criteria for other psychiatric disorders. The most common co-morbid conditions are anxiety disorders (75.8%), mood disorders (63.3%), impulse-control disorders (55.9%) and substance use disorders (38.6%) (Ruscio et al 2008b). The female to male ratio for OCD is about 2:1 (NCS-R 2007).

Course

The mean age of onset of OCD is 19.5 years and the average length with the disorder is 8.9 years (Ruscio et al 2008b). It has a gradual onset and a continuous course (Pinto et al 2006). Males make up the majority who develop the OCD before the age of 10, while in adolescence, there is a female peak for acquiring the disorder. Very few people develop the disorder after age 30. In 65.3% of cases, those with OCD reported severe occupational, relationship and social impairment (Ruscio et al 2008b). OCD is considered to be among the 10 most disabling of all medical and psychiatric conditions in the world according to the World Health Organization, yet it takes on average 10 years from the appearance of symptoms to appropriate intervention (Pinto et al 2006).

Aetiology

Family and twin studies strongly support a genetic component in OCD. Van Grootheest et al (2005) in a review of the literature concluded that genetic influence on OC symptoms ranges from 27% to 47%. Suggestive genetic linkage peaks, regions that may contain a gene or genes for OCD have been generated. Exploring gene–gene interactions and gene–environment interactions along with alternative phenotypes, age at onset or co-morbid conditions may be key in locating genes in the pathogenesis of OCD (Grados & Wilcox 2007).

The serotonergic system has been implicated due to the anti-obsessional effects of SSRIs. OCD has been associated with hypersensitivity of postsynaptic serotonin receptors (Gross et al 1998). Neuroimaging studies have revealed dysfunctions of the dorsolateral, prefrontal, parietal regions, orbito-frontal cortex, anterior cingulate cortex, thalamus and caudate nucleus. It is suggested that the pathogenesis of OCD involves an imbalance between dorsal and ventral fronto-striatal circuits (Kwon et al 2009), and the dorsolateral prefrontal cortex is implicated in the inhibition of responses and in planning, organization and verification of previous actions (Abramowitz et al 2009).

The cognitive behavioural theory proposes that obsessions develop when patients attach particular meaning or significance to an intrusive thought. The person makes a catastrophic misinterpretation of the significance of the thought. CBT aims to change responsibility beliefs, thereby reducing distress and eliminate neutralizing responses (Salkovskis et al 1998).

Treatment

The mainstay of psychological treatment for OCD is cognitive-behavioural therapy involving exposure and response prevention. The exposure to anxiety provoking stimuli is systematic, repeated and prolonged. It urges the individual to perform compulsive rituals. Response prevention means to refrain from performing compulsive rituals. The aim is for the patient to recognize that his or her obsessional anxiety does not persist indefinitely and that avoidance behaviour and compulsive rituals are unnecessary for preventing harm (Abromowitz 2006).

If pharmacological treatment is warranted, SSRIs and pregabalin are first-line pharmacotherapy. Clomipramine is effective in OCD but has more side-effects than SSRIs. Higher doses of antidepressants are typically needed for anti-obsessional effects. Benzodiazepines can be used in treatment-resistant cases when there is no history of substance abuse disorders. Other treatments include irreversible and reversible MAO-Is and adjuvant atypical antipsychotics (Bandelow 2008).

(Rothbaum et al 2008). Mixed results for anticonvulsants have been demonstrated. Topiramate was not associated with improvement over placebo in one study; however, high drop-out rates were noted (Lindley et al 2007). Another study reported reductions in re-experiencing symptoms (Tucker et al 2007). The use of topiramate in adjunctive therapy was associated with reducing general symptoms of combat-related PTSD and reducing high-risk alcohol intake and nightmares (Alderman et al 2009). Divalproex was not shown to be effective as monotherapy and further studies are needed to determine the efficacy in combination with antidepressants (Davis et al 2008). Benzodiazepines were not shown to be effective in PTSD and should be avoided or used only for a short term because of potential addictive and depressive effects, and the possibility they may worsen symptoms of PTSD (Asnis et al 2004). Aerni and colleagues (2004) reported, in a pilot study using oral low dose cortisol, an improvement in re-experiencing symptoms and traumatic memories. Novel treatments, including pharmacoprevention are being studied. Propranolol, a beta-blocker, and gabapentin, an anxiolytic anticonvulsant, were administered within 48 h of injury to patients admitted to a surgical trauma centre. No significant benefit was shown over placebo in depressive or PTSD symptoms (Stein et al 2007).

Generalized anxiety disorder

Anxiety is a normal reaction that prepares one for fight or flight. It is an important biological response aimed to protect an individual. However, people with generalized anxiety disorder (GAD) tend to be anxious most of the time. The DSM-IV defines it as excessive anxiety and worry occurring for a period of at least 6 months, about a number of events. The individual finds it difficult to control the worry and it is accompanied by a feeling of restlessness, being easily fatigued, difficulty concentrating, irritability, muscle tension and disturbed sleep. The worries are not specifically related to anxiety caused by other anxiety disorders. The anxiety causes impairment in functioning. The intensity, duration or frequency of the anxiety is out of proportion to the actual impact of the feared event (APA 2000). The diagnostic criteria are featured in Box 16.10.

Epidemiology

The lifetime community prevalence rate of GAD approaches 6% in the NCS-R (Kessler et al 2005a). Twelve-month prevalence rates are between 3% and 4% (Regier et al 1998; Kessler et al 2005b). Females are nearly twice as likely to develop GAD over their lifetime (NCS-R 2007). GAD carries a high lifetime co-morbidity rate with other psychiatric disorders (92.3%) (Michael et al 2007). GAD co-morbidity rates have been reported in major depression (62.4%), dysthymia (39.5%), social phobia (34.4%) and drug abuse (27.6%). GAD is associated with being separated/widowed/divorced, age over 24 years, unemployment, or being in a low paying job (Wittchen et al 1994).

Aetiology

Hettema et al (2001) reviewed the genetics of GAD and found the heritability is in the range of 30–40%, with a significant proportion explained by individual environmental factors. Alterations in neurochemistry are implicated in the aetiology of GAD. Noradrenaline overactivity has been associated with GAD. Higher levels of catecholamines may lead to a downregulation of presynaptic $\alpha1$-adrenoreceptors (Sevy et al 1989). Serotonin is also thought to play a role in the pathogenesis of GAD. Although the aetiological role remains unknown, SSRIs are efficacious in the treatment of GAD suggesting serotonin neurotransmission reduces anxiety (Inoue et al 2004). Chiu et al (2001) provided evidence for dysregulation of peripheral benzodiazepine receptors in GAD. Decreased benzodiazepine function is implicated. The HPA axis appears over-stimulated

---

Box 16.10

DSM-IV-TR diagnostic criteria for generalized anxiety disorder

A. Excessive anxiety and worry (apprehensive expectation), occurring on more days than not for at least 6 months, about a number of events or activities

B. The person finds it difficult to control the worry

C. The anxiety and worry are associated with three (or more) of the following six symptoms (with at least some symptoms present for more days than not for the past 6 months).
   Note: one item only is required in children:
   a. Restlessness or feeling keyed up or on edge
   b. Being easily fatigued
   c. Difficulty concentrating or mind going blank
   d. Irritability
   e. Muscle tension
   f. Sleep disturbance (difficulty falling or staying asleep, or restless unsatisfying sleep)

D. The focus of the anxiety is not confined to features of an Axis I disorder, e.g. the anxiety or worry is not about having a panic attack (as in panic disorder); being embarrassed in public (as in social phobia); being contaminated (as in obsessive–compulsive disorder); being away from home or close relatives (as in separation anxiety disorder); gaining weight (as in anorexia nervosa); having multiple physical complains (as in somatization disorder) or having a serious illness (as in hypochondriasis), and the anxiety and worry do not occur exclusively during post-traumatic stress disorder.

E. The anxiety, worry, or physical symptoms cause clinically significant distress or impairment in social, occupational, or other important areas of functioning.

F. The disturbance is not due to the direct physiological effects of a substance (e.g. a drug of abuse, a medication) or a general medical condition (e.g. hyperthyroidism) and does not occur exclusively during a mood disorder, a psychotic disorder, or a pervasive developmental disorder.

in GAD and possible plays a role in perpetuating the disorder (Stein & Hollander 2010). Psychological factors also play a role in the aetiology. Negative life events appearing in an unexpected way, familial conflicts and abuses, separation during childhood, lack of social interactions, poor life satisfaction, and modelling a relative with an anxiety disorder are associated with GAD. The cognitive-behavioural approach has been widely studied and postulates several theories. Worry may function to help suppress images associated with negative thoughts. It is also suggested that deficit of attention might be responsible for excessive worry. Cognitive variables, such as intolerance of uncertainty, false beliefs about worry and cognitive avoidance, have been suggestive of maintaining GAD (Gosselin & Laberge 2003).

Course

Typically, GAD begins in early adulthood and has a chronic and persistent course and is associated with extensive psychiatric and medical co-morbidity. GAD often presents in a primary care setting, commonly with somatic symptoms, therefore it is important for primary care physicians to be aware of its existence. After treatment with CBT, relapse rates appear to be low

(Hidalgo & Davidson 2001). Patients with GAD use more services for a primary care provider or specialist than patients with other psychiatric disorders (Bereza et al 2009). GAD is a highly co-morbid disease (around 90%), and those with co-morbidities have increased psychological and social impairment, request additional treatment and have an extended course and poorer outcome (Nutt et al 2006).

Treatment

Combination psychological and pharmacological treatment is most effective for long-term benefit for patients with GAD. Psychological therapy, particularly relaxation, cognitive and cognitive-behavioural therapy has shown long-term benefits. Antidepressants, such as paroxetine and venlafaxine are effective as anxiolytics and also have benefits in targeting the often co-morbid depression. Buspirone and benzodiazepines have anxiolytic properties and are effective in the short term; however, both lack antidepressant effects (Gorman 2002). Benzodiazepines prescribed for more than 4 weeks can cause rebound anxiety and may lead to withdrawal symptoms (Rynn & Brawman-Mintzer 2004).

References

Abromowitz, J., 2006. The psychological treatment of obsessive-compulsive disorder. Can. J. Psychiatry 51, 407–416.

Abramowitz, J.S., Taylor, S., McKay, D., 2009. Obsessive-compulsive disorder. Lancet 374, 491–499.

Aerni, A., Traber, R., Hock, C., et al., 2004. Low-dose cortisol for symptoms of posttraumatic stress disorder. Am. J. Psychiatry 161, 1488–1490.

Alderman, C.P., McCarthy, L.C., Condon, J.T., et al., 2009. Topiramate in combat-related posttraumatic stress disorder. Ann. Pharmacother. 43, 635–641.

Andrews, G., Anderson, T.M., Slade, T., et al., 2008. Classification of anxiety and depressive disorders: problems and solutions. Depress. Anxiety 4, 274–281.

APA, 2000. Diagnostic and statistical manual of mental disorders, fourth ed., text revision (DSM-IV-TR). American Psychiatric Association, Washington DC.

Asnis, G.M., Kohn, S.R., Henderson, M., et al., 2004. SSRIs versus non-SSRIs in post-traumatic stress disorder; an update with recommendations. Drugs 64, 383–404.

Bandelow, B., 2008. The medical treatment of obsessive-compulsive disorder and anxiety. CNS Spectr. 13, 37S–46S.

Beck, A.T., 2005. The current state of cognitive therapy. Arch. Gen. Psychiatry 63, 953–959.

Bereza, B.G., Machado, M., Einarson, T.R., 2009. Systematic review and quality assessment of economic evaluations and quality-of-life studies related to generalized anxiety disorder. Clin. Ther. 31, 1279–1308.

Bisson, J., Andrew, M., 2007. Psychological treatment of post-traumatic stress disorder (PTSD). Cochrane Database Syst. Rev. (3): CD003388.

Bisson, J.I., Ehlers, A., Matthews, et al., 2007. Psychological treatments for chronic post-traumatic stress disorder. Br. J. Psychiatry 190, 97–104.

Boehnlein, J.K., Kinzie, J.D., 2007. Pharmacologic reduction of CNS noradrenergic activity in PTSD: the case for clonidine and prazosin. J. Psychiatr. Pract. 13, 72–78.

Bolton, D., Eley, T.C., O'Connor, T.G., et al., 2006. Prevalence and genetic and environmental influences on anxiety disorders in 6-year-old twins. Psychol. Med. 36, 335–344.

Brawman-Mintzer, O., Lydiard, R.B., Bradwejn, J., et al., 1997. Effects of the cholecystokinin agonist pentagastrin in patients with generalized anxiety disorder. Am. J. Psychiatry 154, 700–702.

Breslau, N., Kessler, R.C., 2001. The stressor criterion in DSM-IV posttraumatic stress disorder: an empirical investigation. Biol. Psychiatry 50, 699–704.

Breslau, N., Davis, G.C., Andreski, P., et al., 1997. Sex differences in posttraumatic stress disorder. Arch. Gen. Psychiatry 54, 1044–1048.

Bruce, S.E., Yonkers, K.A., Otto, M.W., et al., 2005. Influence of psychiatric co-morbidity on recovery and recurrence of generalized anxiety disorder, social phobia, and panic disorder: a 12 year prospective study. Am. J. Psychiatry 162, 1179–1187.

Chiu, S., Singh, A.N., Chiu, P., et al., 2001. Inverse agonist binding of peripheral benzodiazepine receptors in anxiety disorder. Eur. Arch. Psychiatry Clin. Neurosci. 251, 136–140.

Choy, Y., Fyer, A.J., Lipsitz, J.D., 2007. Treatment of specific phobia in adults. Clin. Psychol. Rev. 27, 266–286.

Davidson, J., Baldwin, D., Stein, D.J., et al., 2006. Treatment of posttraumatic stress disorder with venlafaxine extended release: a 6-month randomized controlled trial. Arch. Gen. Psychiatry 63, 1158–1165.

Davidson, J.R., Hughes, D., Blazer, D.G., et al., 1991. Post-traumatic stress disorder in the community: an epidemiological study. Psychol. Med. 21, 713–721.

Davis, L.L., Davidson, J.R., Ward, L.C., et al., 2008. Divalproex in the treatment of posttraumatic stress disorder: a randomized, double-blind, placebo-controlled trial in a veteran population. J. Clin. Psychopharmacol. 28, 84–88.

Den Boer, J.A., 2000. Social anxiety disorder/social phobia: epidemiology, diagnosis, neurobiology, and treatment. Compr. Psychiatry 41, 405–415.

Foa, E.B., 1997. Psychological processes related to recovery from a trauma and an effective treatment for PTSD. Ann. N.Y. Acad. Sci. 821, 410–424.

Foa, E.B., Zinbarg, R., Rothbaum, 1992. Uncontrollability and unpredictability in post-traumatic stress disorder: an animal model. Psychol. Bull. 112, 218–238.

Freud, S., 1953–1974. The standard edition of the complete psychological works of Sigmund

Freud (J. Strachey, Trans.), 24 vols. Hogarth, London.

Fyer, A.J., Mannuzza, S., Gallops, M.S., et al., 1990. Familial transmission of simple phobias and fears. A preliminary report. Arch. Gen. Psychiatry 47, 252–256.

Gillespie, C.F., Phifer, J., Bradley, B., et al., 2009. Risk and resilience: genetic and environmental influences of development of the stress response. Depress. Anxiety 26, 984–992.

Goddard, A.W., Shekhar, A., Whiteman, A.F., et al., 2008. Serotoninergic mechanisms in the treatment of obsessive-compulsive disorder. Drug Discov. Today 13 (7–8), 325–332.

Gorman, J.M., 2002. Treatment of generalized anxiety disorder. J. Clin. Psychiatry 63 (Suppl. 8), 17–23.

Gosselin, P., Laberge, B., 2003. Etiological factors of generalized anxiety disorder. L'Encephale 29, 351–361.

Grados, M., Wilcox, H.C., 2007. Genetics of obsessive-compulsive disorder: a research update. Expert Rev. Neurother. 7, 967–980.

Grillon, C., 2008. Models and mechanisms of anxiety: evidence from startle studies. Psychopharmacology 199, 421–437.

Gross, R., Sasson, Y., Chopra, M., et al., 1998. Biological models of obsessive-compulsive disorder; the serotonin hypothesis. In: Swinson, R.P., Antony, M.M., Rachman, S., et al. (Eds.), Obsessive-compulsive disorder: theory, research, and treatment. Guilford, New York, pp. 141–153.

Hamm, A.O., Weike, A.I., 2005. The neuropsychology of fear learning and fear regulation. Int. J. Psychophysiol. 57, 5–14.

Heim, C., Numeroff, C.B., 2001. The role of childhood trauma in the neurobiology of mood and anxiety disorders: preclinical and clinical studies. Biol. Psychiatry 49, 1023–1039.

Hettema, J.M., Neale, M.C., Kendler, K.S., 2001. A review and meta-analysis of the genetic epidemiology of anxiety disorders. Am. J. Psychiatry 158, 1568–1578.

Hidalgo, R.B., Davidson, J.R., 2001. Generalized anxiety disorder. An important clinical concern. Med. Clin. North Am. 85, 691–710.

Hirshfelf-Becker, D.R., Micco, J., Simoes, N.A., et al., 2008. High risk studies and developmental antecedents of anxiety disorders. Am. J. Med. Genet. 148C, 99–117.

Hofmann, S.G., Pollack, M.H., Otto, M.W., 2006. Augmentation treatment of psychotherapy for anxiety disorders with D-cycloserine. CNS Drug Rev. 12, 208–217.

Hollander, E., Braun, A., Simeon, D., 2008. Should OCD leave the anxiety disorders in DSM-V? The case for obsessive compulsive-related disorders. Depress. Anxiety 25, 317–329.

Holsboer, F., 2003. High-quality antidepressant discovery by understanding stress hormone physiology. Ann. N.Y. Acad. Sci. (Dec), 394–404.

Inoue, T., Li, X.B., Abekawa, T., et al., 2004. Selective serotonin reuptake inhibitor reduces conditioned fear through its effect in the amygdala. Eur. J. Pharmacol. 497, 311–316.

Jenkins, R., Lewis, P., Bebbington, T., et al., 1997. The National Psychiatric Morbidity Surveys of Great Britain – initial findings from the Household Survey. Psychol. Med. 27, 775–789.

Katschnig, H., Amering, M., 1998. The long-term course of panic disorder and its predictors. J. Clin. Psychopharmacol. 18, 6S–11S.

Katzman, M.A., Koszycki, D., Bradwejn, J., 2004. Effects of CCK-tetrapeptide in patients with social phobia and obsessive-compulsive disorder. Depress. Anxiety 20, 51–54.

Kendler, K.S., Karkowski, L.M., Prescott, C.A., 1999. Fears and phobias: reliability and heritability. Psychol. Med. 29, 539–553.

Kendler, K.S., Meyers, J., Prescott, C.A., et al., 2001. The genetic epidemiology of irrational fears and phobias in men. Arch. Gen. Psychiatry 58, 257–265.

Kessler, R.C., McGonagle, K.A., Zhao, S., et al., 1994. Lifetime and 12-month prevalence of DSM-III-R psychiatric disorders in the United States. Results from the National Comorbidity Survey. Arch. Gen. Psychiatry 51, 8–19.

Kessler, R.C., Sonnega, A., Bromet, E., et al., 1995. Posttraumatic stress disorder in the National Comorbidity Survey. Arch. Gen. Psychiatry 52, 1048–1060.

Kessler, R.C., Anthony, J.C., Blazer, D.G., et al., 1997. The US National Comorbidity Survey: overview and future directions. Epidemiol. Psichiatr. Soc. 6, 4–16.

Kessler, R.C., Berglund, P., Demler, O., et al., 2005a. Lifetime prevalence and age-of-onset distributions of DSM-IV disorders in the National Comorbidity Survey Replication. Arch. Gen. Psychiatry 62, 593–603.

Kessler, R.C., Chiu, W.T., Demler, O., et al., 2005b. Prevalence, severity, and co-morbidity of 12-month DSM-IV disorders in the National Co-morbidity Survey Replication. Arch. Gen. Psychiatry 62, 617–627.

Kessler, R.C., Chiu, W.T., Jin, R., et al., 2006. The epidemiology of panic attacks, panic disorder, and agoraphobia in the National Co-morbidity Survey Replication. Arch. Gen. Psychiatry 63, 415–424.

Kessler, R.C., Angermeyer, M., Anthony, J.C., et al., 2007. Lifetime prevalence and age-of-onset distributions of mental disorders in the World Health Organization's World Mental Health Survey Initiative. World Psychiatry 6, 168–176.

Klinger, E., Légeron, P., Roy, S., et al., 2004. Virtual reality exposure in the treatment of social phobia. Stud. Health Technol. Inform. 99, 91–119.

Koenen, K.C., Widom, C.S., 2009. A prospective study of sex differences in the lifetime risk of posttraumatic stress disorder among abused and neglected children grown up. J. Trauma Stress 22, 566–574.

Koszychi, D., Cox, B.J., Bradwejn, J., 1993. Anxiety sensitivity and response to cholecystokinin tetrapeptide in healthy volunteers. Am. J. Psychiatry 150, 1881–1883.

Kozlovsky, N., Matar, M.A., Kaplan, Z., et al., 2009. The role of the galaninergic system in modulating stress-related responses in an animal model of posttraumatic stress disorder. Biol. Psychiatry 65, 383–391.

Krystal, J.H., Deutsch, D.N., Charney, D.S., 1996. The biological basis of panic disorder. J. Clin. Psychiatry 57, 23S–31S.

Kwon, J.S., Jang, J.H., Choi, J.S., et al., 2009. Neuroimaging in obsessive-compulsive disorder. Expert Rev. Neurother. 9, 255–269.

LeDoux, 1995. Emotion: clues from the brain. Annu. Rev. Psychol. 46, 209–235.

Leon, A.C., Portera, L., Weissman, M.M., 1995. The social costs of anxiety disorders. Br. J. Psychiatry 27, 19S–22S.

Lepine, J.P., 2002. The epidemiology of anxiety disorders: prevalence and societal costs. J. Clin. Psychiatry 63, 4S–8S.

Lindley, S.E., Carlson, E.B., Hill, K., 2007. A randomized, double-blind, placebo-controlled trial of augmentation topiramate for chronic combat-related posttraumatic stress disorder. J. Clin. Psychopharmacol. 27, 677–681.

Magee, W.J., Eaton, W.W., Wittchen, H.U., et al., 1996. Agoraphobia, simple phobia, and social phobia in the National Comorbidity Survey. Arch. Gen. Psychiatry 53, 159–168.

Marks, I., 1988. Blood-injury phobia: a review. Am. J. Psychiatry 145, 1207–1213.

Marshall, R.D., Beebe, K.L., Oldham, M., et al., 2001. Efficacy and safety of paroxetine treatment for chronic PTSD: a fixed-dose, placebo-controlled study. Am. J. Psychiatry 158, 1982–1988.

Martin, E.I., Ressler, K.J., Binder, E., et al., 2009. The neurobiology of anxiety disorders: brain imaging, genetics, and psychoneuroendocrinology. Psychiatr. Clin. North Am. 32, 549–575.

Mason, J., Southwick, S., Yehuda, R., et al., 1994. Elevation of serum free triiodothyronine, total triiodothyronine, thyroxine-binding globulin, and total thyroxine levels in combat-related posttraumatic stress disorder. Arch. Gen. Psychiatry 51, 629–641.

Mathew, S.J., Price, R.B., Charney, D.S., 2008. Recent advances in the neurobiology of anxiety disorders: implications for novel therapeutics. Am. J. Med. Genet. 148C, 89–98.

McKay, D., Abramowitz, J.S., Calamari, J.E., et al., 2004. A critical evaluation of obsessive-compulsive disorder subtypes: symptoms versus mechanisms. Clin. Psychol. Rev. 24, 283–313.

Michael, T., Zetsche, U., Margraf, J., 2007. Epidemiology of anxiety disorders. Psychiatry 6, 136–142.

Mineka, S., Oehlberg, K., 2008. The relevance of recent developments in classical condition to understanding the etiology and maintenance of anxiety disorders. Acta Psychol. (Amst.) 127, 567–580.

NCS-R National Comorbidity Survey Replication, 2007. Update Jun 17: Lifetime prevalence of DSM-IV/WMH-CIDI disorders by sex and cohort. Online. Available: http://www.hcp.med.harvard.edu/ncs/ftpdir/table_ncsr_LTprevgenderxage.pdf.

Neylan, T.C., Lenoci, M., Samuelson, K.W., et al., 2006. No improvement of posttraumatic stress disorder symptoms with guanfacine treatment. Am. J. Psychiatry 163, 2186–2188.

NICE National Institute for Clinical Excellence, 2004. Anxiety: management of anxiety (panic disorder, with or without agoraphobia, and generalized anxiety disorder) in adults in primary, secondary and community care. National Collaborating Centre for Primary Care, London.

NICE National Institute for Clinical Excellence, 2005. Post-traumatic stress disorder (PTSD): the management of PTSD in adults and children in primary and secondary care. National Collaborating Centre for Primary Care, London.

Numeroff, C.B., 2003. Anxiolytics; past, present, and future agents. J. Clin. Psychiatry 64, 3S–6S.

Nutt, D., Argyropoulos, S., Hood, S., et al., 2006. Generalized anxiety disorder: a comorbid disease. Eur. Neuropsychopharmacol. 16 (Suppl. 2), S109–S118.

Ollendick, T.H., Hirshfeld-Becker, D.R., 2002. The developmental psychopathology of social anxiety disorder. Biol. Psychiatry 51, 44–58.

Paulus, M.P., Stein, M.B., 2006. An insular view of anxiety. Biol. Psychiatry 60, 383–387.

Pinto, A., Mancebo, E., et al., 2006. The Brown longitudinal obsessive compulsive study; clinical features and symptoms of the sample at intake. J. Clin. Psychiatry 67, 703–711.

Pull, C.B., 2008. Recent trends in the study of specific phobias. Curr. Opin. Psychiatry 21, 43–50.

Rapee, R.M., Spence, S.H., 2004. The etiology of social phobia: empirical evidence and an initial model. Clin. Psychol. Rev. 24, 737–767.

Raskind, M.A., Peskind, E.R., Hoff, D.J., et al., 2007. A parallel group placebo controlled study of prazosin for trauma nightmares and sleep disturbance in combat veterans with post-traumatic stress disorder. Biol. Psychiatry 61, 928–934.

Regier, D.A., Rae, D.S., Narrow, W.E., et al., 1998. Prevalence of anxiety disorders and their co-morbidity with mood and addictive disorders. Br. J. Psychiatry 193, 24S–28S.

Roberts, N.P., Kitchiner, N.J., Kenardy, J., et al., 2009. Multiple session early psychological interventions for the prevention of post-traumatic stress disorder. Cochrane Database Syst. Rev. (8):CD006869.

Rothbaum, B.O., Killeen, T.K., Davidson, J.R., et al., 2008. Placebo-controlled trial of risperidone augmentation for selective serotonin reuptake inhibitor-resistant civilian posttraumatic stress disorder. J. Clin. Psychiatry 69, 520–525.

Roy-Byrne, P.P., Stein, M.B., Russo, J., et al., 1999. Panic disorder in the primary care setting: co-morbidity, disability, service utilization and treatment. J. Clin. Psychiatry 60, 492–499.

Roy-Byrne, P.P., Stang, P., Wittchen, H.U., et al., 2000. Lifetime panic-depression co-morbidity in the National Comorbidity Survey, association with symptoms, impairment, course and help-seeking. Br. J. Psychiatry 176, 229–235.

Roy-Byrne, P.P., Craske, M.G., Stein, M.B., 2006. Panic disorder. Lancet 269, 1022–1032.

Ruscio, A.M., Brown, T.A., Chiu, W.T., et al., 2008a. Social fears and social phobia in the USA: results from the National Comorbidity Survey Replication. Psychol. Med. 38, 15–28.

Ruscio, A.M., Stein, D.J., Chiu, W.T., et al., 2008b. The epidemiology of obsessive-compulsive disorder in the National Comorbidity Survey Replication. Mol. Psychiatry 15, 53–63.

Rynn, M.A., Brawman-Mintzer, O., 2004. Generalized anxiety disorder: acute and chronic treatment. CNS Spectr. 9, 716–723.

Sadock, B.J., Sadock, V.A., 2008. Concise textbook of clinical psychiatry. Lippincott Williams & Wilkins, Philadelphia.

Salkovskis, P.M., Forrester, E., Richards, C., 1998. Cognitive-behavioural approach to understanding obsessional thinking. Br. J. Psychiatry Suppl. 35, 53–63.

Schneier, F.R., Johnson, J., Hornig, C.D., et al., 1992. Social phobia: co-morbidity and morbidity in an epidemiologic sample. Arch. Gen. Psychiatry 49, 282–288.

Seligman, M., 1971. Phobias and preparedness. Behav. Ther. 2, 307–320.

Sevy, S., Papadimitriou, G.N., Surmont, D.W., et al., 1989. Noradrenergic function in generalized anxiety disorder, major depressive disorder, and healthy subjects. Biol. Psychiatry 25, 141–152.

Shapiro, F., Maxfield, L., 2002. Eye movement desensitization and reprocessing (EMDR): information processing in the treatment of trauma. J. Clin. Psychol. 8, 933–946.

Smoller, J.W., Gardner-Shuster, E., Covino, J., 2008. The genetic basis of panic and phobic anxiety disorders. Am. J. Med. Genet. 148C, 118–126.

Smoller, J.W., Block, S.R., Young, M.M., 2009. Genetics of anxiety disorders: the complex road from DSM to DNA. Depress. Anxiety 26, 965–975.

Southwick, S.M., Krystal, J.H., Morgan, C.A., et al., 1993. Abnormal noradrenergic function in posttraumatic stress disorder. Arch. Gen. Psychiatry 50, 266–274.

Stein, D.J., Ipser, J.C., Seedat, S., 2006. Pharmacotherapy for post traumatic stress disorder (PTSD). Cochrane Database Syst. Rev. (25):CD002795.

Stein, M.B., 2009. Neurobiology of generalized anxiety disorder. J. Clin. Psychiatry 70 (Suppl. 2), 15–19.

Stein, M.B., Hollander, E., 2010. Textbook of anxiety disorders, second ed. American Psychiatric, Arlington.

Stein, M.B., Walker, J.R., Anderson, G., et al., 1996. Childhood physical and sexual abuse in a patient with anxiety disorders and in a community sample. Am. J. Psychiatry 153, 275–277.

Stein, M.B., Kline, N.Y., Matloff, J.L., 2002. Adjunctive olanzapine for SSRI-resistant combat-related PTSD: a double-blind, placebo-controlled study. Am. J. Psychiatry 159, 1777–1779.

Stein, M.B., Kerridge, C., Dimsdale, J.E., et al., 2007. Pharmacotherapy to prevent PTSD: results from a randomized controlled proof-of-concept trial in physically injured patients. J. Trauma Stress 20, 923–932.

Stinson, F.S., Dawson, D.A., Chou, S., et al., 2007. The epidemiology of DSM-IV specific phobia in the USA: results from the National Epidemiologic Survey on Alcohol and Related Conditions. Psychol. Med. 37, 1047–1059.

Tanaka, M., Yoshida, M., Emoto, H., et al., 2000. Noradrenaline systems in the hypothalamus, amygdala and locus coeruleus are involved in the provocation of anxiety: basic studies. Eur. J. Pharmacol. 405, 397–406.

Tucker, P., Trautman, R.P., Wyatt, D.B., et al., 2007. Efficacy and safety of topiramate monotherapy in civilian posttraumatic stress disorder: a randomized, double-blind, placebo-controlled study. J. Clin. Psychiatry 68, 201–206.

Van Grootheest, D.S., Cath, D.C., Beekman, A.T., et al., 2005. Twin studies on obsessive-compulsive disorder; a review. Twin Res. Hum. Genet. 8, 450–458.

Vasa, R.A., Pine, D.S., Masteen, C.L., et al., 2009. Effects of yohimbine and hydrocortisone on panic symptoms, autonomic responses, and attention to threat in healthy adults. Psychopharmacology (Berl.) 204, 445–455.

Vermetten, E., Vythilingam, M., Southwick, S.M., et al., 2003. Long-term treatment with paroxetine increases verbal declarative memory and hippocampal volume in posttraumatic stress disorder. Biol. Psychiatry 54, 693–702.

Walker, D.L., Toufexis, D.J., Davis, M., 2003. Role of the bed nucleus of the stria terminalis versus the amygdala in fear, stress, and anxiety. Eur. J. Pharmacol. 463, 1999–11216.

Wang, P.S., Berglund, P., Olfon, M., et al., 2005. Failure and delay in initial treatment contact after first onset of mental disorders in the National Co-morbidity Survey Replication. Arch. Gen. Psychiatry 62, 603–613.

Watson, J.B., Rayner, R., 1920. Conditioned emotional reactions. J. Exp. Psychol. 3, 1–14.

Weissman, M.M., Bland, R.C., Canino, G.J., et al., 1997. The cross-national epidemiology of panic disorder. Arch. Gen. Psychiatry 54, 305–309.

WHO, 1992. The ICD-10 Classification of mental and behavioural disorders. Clinical descriptions and diagnostic guidelines (ICD-10). World Health Organization, Geneva.

Wilhelm, F.H., Roth, W.T., 1997. Acute and delayed effects of alprazolam on flight phobics during exposure. Behav. Res. Ther. 35, 831–841.

Wittchen, H.U., Jacobi, F., 2005. Size and burden of mental disorders in Europe – a critical

Recommended structure of an ideal liaison service

A fuller description of the ideal structure and remit of a liaison psychiatry service can be found in the following documents published by the Royal College of Psychiatrists: 'No Health Without Mental Health' (Academy of Medical Royal Colleges & Royal College of Psychiatrists 2009) and 'Liaison Psychiatry and Psychological Medicine in the General Hospital' (Royal College of Psychiatrists 2007). According to these reports, a liaison service should include:

1. A service developed in consultation with non-psychiatrists (from the general hospital) and other psychiatrists (from the community providing catchment area and specialist psychiatric services)
2. An accessible system for collecting referrals, ideally a single point of referral
3. Simple protocols for the detection and management of psychiatric problems by general hospital staff
4. A well-organized medical record system, with standardized records of consultations for audit
5. Confidential facilities in the emergency department, wards and outpatients for interviews
6. Adequate staff, e.g. for a district general hospital with 600 beds, operating Monday–Friday 9am–5pm:
   ○ 1 consultant liaison psychiatrist – whole time
   ○ 1 senior nurse as team leader – whole time
   ○ 3 further senior nurses working as autonomous practitioners – whole time
   ○ 1 clinical (or health) psychologist – whole time
   ○ 1.5 × team administrator – whole time
   ○ Plus 1 non-career grade doctor and 2–3 senior nurses if older adults and people with learning disability are to be covered by the service
   ○ Plus doctors in training grades (ST4–6) and foundation trainees.

Clinical issues in liaison psychiatry

Psychiatric assessment of patients:

1. Conducting the consultation:
   ○ Discuss the case with referrer before seeing the patient to clarify the reason for referral and establish whether patient has been told of the referral
   ○ Review the medical notes
   ○ Ensure privacy for the interview
   ○ Consider gaining informant history from family or GP
   ○ Discuss assessment with referrer and establish ongoing medical responsibility
   ○ Liaise with nursing staff, GP and any relevant psychiatric teams.
2. Interviewing skills:
   ○ Address patient's feelings about psychiatric referral
   ○ Ask about physical symptoms and general medical history
   ○ Ask about psychological symptoms, using terms used by the patient if possible
   ○ Be aware of verbal and non-verbal cues of emotional distress and be empathic
   ○ Take a comprehensive but focused history and mental state examination
   ○ Remember to assess risk
   ○ Make a bio-psychosocial formulation of the patient's problems and use this to inform the management plan
   ○ Record your findings in medical notes.

Assessment of depression in the physically ill can be a particular problem, as somatic symptoms (e.g. fatigue, weight loss, insomnia, pain) may result from physical illness or depression. Assessment should therefore focus more on affective and cognitive symptoms (diminished interest or pleasure, psychomotor retardation/agitation, irritability, non-reactive mood, suicidal thoughts); depressed mood, morning depression and hopelessness provide good discrimination between depressed and non-depressed medically ill patients. Assessment tools such as the Hospital Anxiety and Depression Scale (HADS) (Zigmond & Snaith 1983) can be useful to monitor symptom severity and change – the HADS was specifically developed for use within the medically ill population.

Medically unexplained symptoms

Definitions

Many of the terms used in this area are interchangeable. Medically unexplained symptoms refer to symptoms that are disproportionate to identifiable physical disease. Somatization is the process by which people with psychological disorders present in non-mental health settings with somatic symptoms, which are not due to physical disease. Functional symptoms imply that there is an abnormality of functioning but no detectable physical pathology. Other terms include hysteria, somatoform and psychosomatic. Patients find the term functional most acceptable. The somatoform disorders, which are psychiatric conditions that usually involve the presentation of multiple medically unexplained symptoms, are covered in more detail below.

Somatic (or physical) symptoms are common and are the main reason why people seek medical care. Around a third of somatic symptoms that are seen in primary care can be classified as medically unexplained (Kroenke 2003), while the proportion is at least as high in secondary care clinics (Reid et al 2001).

Engagement issues

Patients with medically unexplained symptoms may be particularly reluctant to see a psychiatrist and may feel the referral means their doctor thinks there is nothing wrong with them. Referrers should always be encouraged to discuss with the patient that the referral is to a psychiatrist (rather than to another medical colleague as is sometimes done). Engaging the patient may be easier if the first consultation is in the medical clinic, possibly as a joint appointment with the physician, or in a specialized liaison psychiatry clinic. The psychiatrist should:

- Allow sufficient time
- Acknowledge the reality of their symptoms, recognize that their symptoms are not imaginary
- Take an exhaustive history of all symptoms to allow the patient to feel understood and to investigate precipitating and maintaining factors, while establishing a positive collaborative relationship
- Ask the patient about their past experience of contact with the medical system
- Acknowledge any fear of labelling and stigma
- Ensure good communication throughout the consultation, as previous experiences of medical consultations may have been negative.

Rule out anxiety and depression

Patients with anxiety or depression commonly present with physical rather than emotional symptoms, as these disorders can predispose, precipitate or perpetuate somatic symptoms. Both anxiety and depression are often experienced physically (e.g. anxiety can present with difficulty swallowing, stomach unease, sweaty palms; depression can present with weight loss, poor appetite, low energy). However, most patients will talk about the emotional symptoms of anxiety and depression if the topic is approached sensitively. Anxiety and depression should be treated in the usual way, for example by referring to NICE guidance (NICE 2007a, 2009).

Aetiology of medically unexplained symptoms

1. Predisposing factors:
   - Early childhood experience, e.g. lack of parental care, experience of parental illness as a child, childhood sexual abuse
   - Female gender
   - Personality traits, e.g. neuroticism, excessive health consciousness, somatic amplification (tendency to increased awareness of normal bodily sensations)
   - Genetic predisposition, e.g. in chronic fatigue syndrome, pain syndromes.
2. Precipitating factors:
   - Physical injury, e.g. in fibromyalgia
   - Infection, e.g. in chronic fatigue syndrome
   - Stressful events or life events, e.g. following disaster or trauma.
3. Perpetuating factors:
   - Neuroendocrine changes, e.g. in chronic fatigue syndrome, fibromyalgia
   - Deconditioning, e.g. in fibromyalgia
   - Central dysfunction, e.g. in conversion disorder
   - Illness beliefs, e.g. physical illness attributions, maladaptive coping strategies
   - Iatrogenic factors, e.g. doctors' fear of missing pathology may lead to inappropriate tests and treatments
   - Social factors, e.g. living environment, family views, financial reward and other secondary gain
   - Media influences, e.g. inaccurate internet information.

Consequences

- Inappropriate and expensive investigations and admissions
- Prescribed drug misuse
- Poor doctor–patient relationship
- Impact on family
- Disability and loss of employment
- Potentially harmful and inappropriate treatments
- 'Addiction' to healthcare system for social support.

Somatoform disorders

The somatoform disorders are considered to be psychiatric disorders and have in common the 'repeated presentation of physical symptoms, together with persistent requests for medical investigations, in spite of repeated negative findings and reassurances by doctors that the symptoms have no physical basis' (World Health Organization 1992). See Table 17.2 for a comparison of somatoform disorders as covered by current ICD-10 and DSM-IV diagnostic manuals.

Somatoform disorders have a confusing terminology with overlapping criteria; in clinical practice, it can be difficult to differentiate between different disorders but all encompass 'abnormal illness behaviour'. It is possible for one patient to fulfil diagnostic criteria for several somatoform disorders at one time (e.g. somatoform pain disorder and dissociative disorder), which has led to criticism of current diagnostic systems, and it is likely that future versions of the ICD/DSM will change how such disorders are defined (Kroenke et al 2007).

Epidemiology

The prevalence (frequency) of the specific somatoform disorders varies depending on the setting and the diagnostic criteria used. For example the population prevalence of strictly defined somatization disorder is around 0.5%, but rises to as much as

Table 17.2 Comparison of somatoform disorders: ICD-10 vs DSM-IV

ICD-10 Somatoform disorders (F45)	DSM-IV Somatoform disorders (300)
Somatization disorder	Somatization disorder
	Conversion disorder
Undifferentiated somatoform disorder	Undifferentiated somatoform disorder
Hypochondriacal disorders (includes body dysmorphic disorder)	Hypochondriasis
	Body dysmorphic disorder
Somatoform autonomic dysfunction	
Persistent somatoform pain disorder	Pain disorder
Other somatoform disorders	
Somatoform disorder, unspecified	Somatoform disorder, not otherwise specified

On the other hand, it is important to counter specific illness fears that the patient may hold (e.g. 'My symptoms mean I've got cancer') if that is not the case. This is why it is important to have asked the patient what they believe is wrong. Patients with high health anxiety will often attempt to elicit repeated reassurance, which fails to reassure for any length of time.

If there is evidence of anxiety or depression at first assessment, then this should be treated in the usual way. Doing so will often, although not always, lead to a significant improvement in the patient's somatic symptoms. A doctor that sees a patient with medically unexplained symptoms for follow-up has an important role in managing that patient's interaction with medical services. Even if doctors do not perceive themselves to be providing active therapy, they can be aware of potentially iatrogenic interventions, i.e. harm caused by doctors (Page & Wessely 2003). They can also provide regular follow-up that is not contingent on the patient being symptomatic, thereby discouraging the need for the patient to complain of symptoms in order to elicit care. It is sometimes possible to agree beforehand that only a certain proportion of the session will be devoted to discussing symptoms, and leave it to the patient to decide the content of the second half of the interview.

Psychotherapy

Overall CBT is known to be an efficacious treatment for the range of conditions loosely grouped under the somatoform disorders (Sumathipala 2007). CBT and similar therapies have shown specific usefulness in the treatment of hypochondriacal disorder, somatization disorder, CFS/ME, irritable bowel syndrome, fibromyalgia and burning mouth syndrome. CBT can be adapted for use in any of these disorders, but like most medical treatments relies on the patient being sufficiently motivated to participate. Evidence is lacking for useful psychotherapeutic treatments for conversion disorder, although preliminary studies have shown that CBT may be useful. Hypnotherapy or psychotherapy, in addition to CBT, are recommended for treatment of refractory irritable bowel syndrome (NICE 2008).

Pharmacotherapy

Overall there is evidence that antidepressant medication is useful in the treatment of somatoform disorders (Sumathipala 2007), although it is not possible to generally recommend the use of one type of antidepressant over another. For the functional somatic syndromes there are some specific recommendations, for example tricyclic antidepressants are effective in treating fibromyalgia and abdominal pain in irritable bowel syndrome. On the other hand, antidepressants have not been found to be useful in CFS/ME without co-morbid depression. In general, the effectiveness of antidepressants in these disorders increases if the patient has evidence of co-morbid depression or anxiety; however, medication is probably less effective than psychological approaches.

It is common to combine a psychotherapeutic and pharmacological approach to management of patients with medically unexplained symptoms. The patient may have strong feelings about treatment and these should be taken into consideration. It can be necessary to rationalize inappropriate medication, as some patients with somatoform disorders are prescribed medication that is unnecessary or even harmful. This needs to be done by (or in conjunction with) primary care and the rationale discussed with the patient in advance.

Special medical services

Specialist units in the general hospital often require specialized psychiatric services. Special links may be made between medical/surgical teams and liaison psychiatrists which help these units provide treatment more effectively. This is illustrated here by describing the role of liaison psychiatry in cancer care. The principles involved can be extended to other services such as neurology, diabetes, intensive care, plastic surgery and transplantation, although each specialty will have particular needs.

Psycho-oncology

Epidemiology

Cancer patients have a 3–4 times increased risk of psychiatric problems:

* 25–33% develop a generalized anxiety disorder, major depressive disorder or adjustment disorder within the first 2 years of diagnosis
* Up to 25% have body image problems after losing a body part or its function
* 25–33% have sexual problems
* 10–40% have an acute confusional state usually due to hypercalcaemia, brain metastases, drugs or infections.

Detection of these disorders is low by all hospital and primary care staff, partly due to patients not disclosing their problems and partly due to medical staff focusing on physical problems and using distancing strategies if patients try to discuss psychological issues.

Management

Psycho-oncology services can intervene by:

* Seeing referrals causing particular concern (the consultation approach discussed earlier) – but relying on referrals will miss most morbidity
* Training and supervising specialist nurses in recognition and treatment of psychological disorders using anxiety management and CBT, which can improve quality of life even in advanced cancers
* Supervising staff who run patient support groups
* Training doctors and nurses in cancer care to upgrade their psychological assessment skills, including breaking bad news effectively (see below)
* Arranging screening for psychological morbidity using instruments validated in cancer patients such as the Hospital Anxiety and Depression Scale or the Rotterdam Symptom Checklist (this should only be done where resources are available for further assessment and treatment).

Breaking bad news

Staff need to be aware of the following steps for breaking bad news:

1. Ensure a private consultation in a comfortable area with a relative or friend present
2. Check what the patient knows about their disease
3. Find out what the patient wants to know, e.g. by using a hierarchy of terms ('serious', 'tumour', etc.) and judging the patient's response ('you tell me what to do; I'll leave the details to you', indicating that the patient prefers to leave it to the expert). Patients may want a limited amount of information on the first consultation but staff should state that more information is available to them if and when they want it: 'if you want to know more in the future we can discuss it again then'.
4. Share the appropriate amount of information with the patient, clarifying and educating without jargon, giving information in small chunks and in writing; allow pauses for assimilation and acknowledge distress, asking for key concerns and discussing them in turn
5. Plan future consultations with the patient and summarize the present consultation.

Care of the dying and bereaved

There are several competing theories of bereavement (including psychoanalytic, stage, stress and social support theories). The stage theory is characterized as having five stages (Kübler-Ross 1970), although not all patients will pass through each stage. The stages are denial and isolation, anger, bargaining, depression and acceptance.

Patients who are close to dying may fear death, although this should not be assumed, and fear of becoming a burden or of pain may be more prominent. Regular talks to express fear and grief with a trusted health professional or diazepam to break a cycle of fear can be helpful. Adequate pain relief is also important. Psychiatric disorders such as depression or anxiety should be treated, however 'understandable' they may seem; patients with a terminal illness are at increased risk of suicide. Sedative antidepressants may be particularly helpful in patients with insomnia, and CBT can also improve quality of life. Paranoid states can be treated with antipsychotics and acute confusional states need assessment and management.

The psychiatrist's role is to advise the multidisciplinary team on assessment and management of the patient's and relatives' psychological needs and psychiatric complications, and support the multidisciplinary team who have to cope with their feelings of sadness and anger, which may lead to difficulties in staff interactions. Support should be available for close relatives when it is wanted, although the family may not be open to offers of help until after the patient has died.

The 'classic' stages of bereavement are:

- Numbness (lack of emotional reactivity)
- Acute 'pangs of grief' (anxiety and severe distress)
- Chronic background of depressive type symptoms (restlessness, poor concentration, poor memory, loss of appetite, weight and sleep, guilt, pseudohallucinations)
- Acceptance.

These stages are normal and the bereaved tend to complain more of physical symptoms than patients with depressive disorders and are less likely to feel suicidal. The professionals involved with the patient who has died should ensure transfer of care for relatives to others outside the hospital/hospice (e.g. GP or local psychiatrist when necessary), so that adjustment can be made to a life without the patient.

Bereavement and physical health

Mortality is increased in bereaved relatives, with heart disease as the most frequent cause of death. It is not clear whether this is due to increased smoking or changes in diet, or it may be the result of emotional factors more directly affecting the cardiovascular system. Increased mortality after bereavement is also due to liver cirrhosis, accidents and suicides. Newly bereaved people, particularly those under 65, consult their doctor more frequently than they did previously, for physical and psychological symptoms, possibly due to aggravation of pre-existing conditions (see Parkes 1996 for a full review).

Bereavement and psychiatric disorders

Bereavement is associated with an increased risk of depression, anxiety disorders, post-traumatic stress disorder after horrific types of bereavement, and a worsening of pre-existing alcohol misuse. Risk factors for these disorders include:

- The nature of the relationship
  - Spouse, child, loss of parent before age 20
  - Strength and security of relationship
  - Intensity of ambivalence
- Type of death, e.g. sudden and unexpected, or violent and horrific death
- Previous mental illness
- Other life events around the time of the bereavement
- Lack of social support
- Female
- Lack of religion or cultural factors influencing expression of grief.

The role of the liaison psychiatrist

- Training of A&E staff in breaking bad news
- Support for staff in frequent contact with the bereaved
- Provision of relevant information to those in contact with bereaved, e.g. information on CRUSE UK bereavement counselling service, at: http://www.crusebereavementcare.org.uk
- Appropriate treatment of patients referred with psychiatric disorder; patients avoiding grieving may benefit from 'guided mourning' (using exposure therapy); patients with chronic prolonged grief may benefit more from problem-focused therapy to promote re-integration into the world.

Eating disorders

18

Frances Connan   Rahul Bhattacharya

Introduction

Eating disorders (EDs) constitute a range of illnesses characterized by abnormal eating behaviour associated with emotional difficulties. Gull (1874) and Lasegue (1873) were the first clinicians to describe a disorder characterized by severe emaciation associated with amenorrhoea, which was inexplicable in terms of physical cause. The psychopathology of 'weight phobia' was incorporated much later. The first widely accepted criteria for anorexia nervosa (AN) were proposed by Russell in 1970 and emphasized the core features: (1) behaviour that produces weight loss; (2) fear of becoming fat; (3) associated endocrine/physiological disturbances. This view is reflected in the current ICD-10 and DSM-IV criteria. The syndrome of bulimia nervosa (BN) was first described by Russell in 1979 as an ominous variant of AN.

Diagnosis

It is now recognized that the majority of those presenting for help with EDs do not fit neatly into either category of AN or BN. Moreover, there is symptomatic and lifetime crossover between diagnostic categories (Table 18.1). For example, one-third of women with BN have a history of AN and an atypical eating disorder is a common outcome of AN. There are also common maintaining factors for AN, BN and atypical eating

disorders. These findings have led to the proposal of a transdiagnostic approach to EDs, in which it is suggested that they be classified as one disorder, with underweight and normal/overweight subtypes (Fairburn et al 2003). While there is some validity to this argument, it is not entirely satisfactory, as there is considerable evidence for restricting AN as a distinct and separate phenotype (Schmidt & Treasure 2006).

Overvaluation of weight and shape is present in many of those with AN, but some people do not report concerns

Table 18.1 Diagnosis of eating disorders

	ICD-10	DSM-IV
Anorexia nervosa (AN)	Code: 50.0 Significant weight loss, or in children a lack of weight gain, leading to a body weight of at least 15% below the normal or expected weight for age and height (BMI <17.5) Weight loss self-induced by avoidance of fattening food Dread of fatness as an intrusive overvalued idea, and a self-imposed low weight threshold Endocrine disorder with amenorrhoea/loss of sexual interest or potency (males), raised growth hormone and cortisol; reduced thyroid hormone level No subtypes classified	Refusal to maintain body weight over a minimal norm leading to body weight 15% below expected or failure to gain weight during growth Intense fear of gaining weight or becoming fat Disturbance in the way in which one's body weight, size or shape is experienced and undue influence of this on self-evaluation, or denial of the seriousness of the current low body weight Absence of three consecutive menstrual cycles (or if periods only occur following hormones) Subtypes: A. *Restricting type* B. *Binge/purging type*: binge eating or vomiting, misuse of laxatives, diuretics, enemas engaged in regularly during this episode
Bulimia nervosa (BN)	Code: F.50.2 Recurrent episodes of overeating with large amounts of food consumed in a short period of time Persistent preoccupation with eating and a strong desire, or sense of compulsion to eat Methods to counteract weight gain (at least one of): (1) vomiting, (2) purging (e.g. laxatives, enemas), (3) alternating periods of starvation, (4) use of drugs such as appetite suppressants, metabolic stimulants, diuretics Self-perception of being fat and a morbid fear of fatness No subtypes classified	Recurrent episodes of binge eating characterized by both: eating, in a discrete period of time (e.g. within any 2-h period), an amount of food that is definitely larger than most people would eat during a similar period of time and under similar circumstances; a sense of lack of control over eating during the episode, defined by a feeling that one cannot stop eating or control what or how much one is eating Recurrent inappropriate compensatory behaviour to prevent weight gain Self-induced vomiting Misuse of laxatives, diuretics, enemas, or other medications Fasting Excessive exercise The binge eating and inappropriate compensatory behaviour both occur, on average, at least twice a week for 3 months Self-evaluation is unduly influenced by body shape and weight The disturbance does not occur exclusively during episodes of anorexia nervosa Subclassification: *Purging* In purging type, the person has regularly engaged in self-induced vomiting or the misuse of laxatives, diuretics, or enemas *Non-purging* In non-purging type the person uses only fasting and excessive exercise to control weight
Other eating disorders	ICD-10 classifies eating disorders that do not fit in neatly in the above categories in two ways: *Atypical* variants: subthreshold AN or BN *Eating Disorder Unspecified*	DSM-IV classifies eating disorders who do not neatly fit into the above descriptions as: *Eating Disorder Not Otherwise Classified* (*EDNOS*) There is no 'atypical' variant category in DSM-IV
Binge eating disorder (BED)	BED is not recognized in ICD-10	Listed in the DSM IV-TR appendix: The disorder is characterized by episodes of binge eating without efforts to compensate by, e.g. food restriction, vomiting or laxative misuse

regarding weight or shape or the classical 'fear of fatness'. Instead, this group of people with AN describe being unable to eat due to feelings of fullness or bloating, a need for self-control and denial of hunger, or justify not eating by religious or aesthetic values. This is sometimes referred to as a 'non-fat phobic' variant of AN. This presentation is often (but not exclusively) seen among patients of non-Western cultural background and suggests that culture may have a pathoplastic effect on the presentation of AN. Indeed, AN is not a Western culture-bound syndrome: there are descriptions of AN in many non-Western cultures and earliest descriptions date back to the Middle Ages. Characteristic of AN is that the self-starvation is *motivated*, the desire to be thin being just one possible motivation of many (Schmidt & Treasure 2006).

Binge eating disorder

Since the introduction of binge eating disorder (BED) to DSM-IV as a provisional diagnosis, a body of research has been developed demonstrating its validity as a psychiatric nosology. A degree of clinical utility and validity has also been established and it is likely to be included as a distinct diagnostic category in DSM-V. In the USA, BED is more common in black and Latino populations, in which it is the commonest form of ED (Hudson et al 2007). Up to one-third of patients seeking treatment for obesity have BED. Most patients with BED report intense body disparagement and self-consciousness and want to lose weight, although they seem comfortable with aiming for average weight and do not have overvalued ideas about thinness. There is a strong association with clinical depression, with over 50% having a lifetime history.

Psychogenic vomiting

Psychogenic vomiting is described as episodes of vomiting after food without nausea. It is associated with psychological disturbance, often anxiety, but also dissociative and hypochondriacal disorders. The disorder occurs in childhood, and in women in early or middle adult life. In ICD-10, this is classified under vomiting associated with psychological disturbances.

Eating and feeding disorders in childhood

While typical AN and BN may present in childhood, atypical presentations and feeding disorders are more common. Food avoidance emotional disorder (FAED) has been described in which food is avoided for psychological reasons. The presentation is similar to that of AN, although the child acknowledges their low weight, and other medically unexplained symptoms are more common than in AN. The disorder is perhaps equivalent to non-fat phobic AN in adults. Some cases of food avoidance in childhood may be better understood as simple phobias.

Faddy eating is common in childhood, but when particularly severe and/or persisting beyond middle childhood, has been termed 'selective eating'. This has been described as a disorder in which the child limits the range of foods, often to less than 10 different types, and is extremely unwilling to try new foods (Nicholls et al 2001). When selective eating occurs in the context of a broader range of refusals, such as for walking and talking, pervasive refusal syndrome is a more appropriate diagnosis.

Substantial evidence exists for the concept of paediatric autoimmune neuropsychiatric disorders associated with streptococcal infection (PANDAS) underlying some cases of obsessive–compulsive disorder, tics and Tourette syndrome. Some evidence also exists for PANDAS-AN (Puxley et al 2008).

Differential diagnoses and psychiatric co-morbidity

Organic conditions

It is important to exclude medical conditions before diagnosing an ED. These include endocrine conditions, malignancies, inflammatory bowel conditions or malabsorption syndromes. Kallmann syndrome or pituitary hypogonadism is a rare but important differential diagnosis for pre-pubertal restrictive AN. In the absence of clinical signs or symptoms to indicate the need for other investigations, thyroid functions tests and an erythrocyte sedimentation rate (ESR) are usually sufficient to exclude organic causes.

Depression

Most studies have shown an increased prevalence of depression in patients with AN during acute illness and following recovery, with reported rates ranging from 36% to 68% (Berkman et al 2007). The diagnosis of depression at low weight is complicated because low mood, lack of energy, poor motivation, reduced enjoyment and poor concentration are also symptoms of starvation. Depressive symptoms prior to weight loss, persistence after weight gain and associated depressive cognitions are all suggestive of true co-morbidity, requiring treatment.

Half to two-thirds of those who suffer from BN will also develop major depression at some point in their life, with lifetime rates reported at 36–70% (Bulik et al 1996). Onset of depression may precede, succeed or may be simultaneous with BN, suggesting that neither is purely a secondary phenomenon of the other.

Anxiety disorders

A number of studies suggest a high lifetime prevalence of anxiety disorders, which often pre-date the onset of ED (Swinbourne & Touyz 2007). Social phobia (34%) and obsessive–compulsive disorder (OCD) (26%) are particularly prevalent in those with a history of AN. Obsessionality and compulsive routines are commonly associated with starvation, but tend to be related exclusively to food, eating, weight, shape and exercise. Cleaning and checking routines unrelated to ED concerns are suggestive of true OCD co-morbidity and tend to worsen with weight gain. PTSD may be a risk factor for BN (Brewerton 2007). Each of these co-morbidities requires specific treatment to achieve lasting recovery from ED.

Alcohol and drug misuse

A recent meta-analysis found significant associations between alcohol misuse and BN, BED and EDNOS, although there was no association with AN (Gadalla & Piran 2007). A small but significant association between drug misuse and BN, and to a lesser extent BED, has also been observed, with no such association with AN (Calero-Elvira et al 2009).

Personality disorder

In a clinic sample, 69% of ED patients met criteria for at least one personality disorder (mostly Cluster A (anxious, avoidant, dependent, OCPD) and cluster B (borderline, narcissistic, histrionic)), of whom 93% had another axis 1 diagnosis, including affective and substance misuse disorders (Braun et al 1994). In some patients, BN is only one of a variety of impulsive behaviours associated with borderline personality traits or disorder. 'Multi-impulsive bulimia nervosa' has been described as a subgroup of patients with high rates of excess alcohol consumption (22%), drug misuse (28%), stealing (21%), overdose (18%), self-cutting (15%) and sexual disinhibition (37%) (Lacey 1993). These women are more likely to have poor social adjustment and a history of sexual abuse.

Suicidality

Suicide attempts are observed in approximately 3–20% of patients with AN and in 25–35% of patients with BN. Clinical correlates of suicidality include purging behaviours, depression, substance misuse, and a history of childhood physical or sexual abuse. Assessment of suicidality should be routine, regardless of the severity of eating disorder or depressive symptoms (Franko & Keel 2006).

Psychoses

Food refusal and weight loss occasionally present as part of a psychotic disorder (affective or schizophrenia) with underlying delusions about food or eating, such as persecutory delusions about poisoning, or nihilistic delusions about bowel function.

Epidemiology

Epidemiological studies are limited by a number of methodological issues. For example, dieting, binge eating and weight and shape concern are prevalent among the general population, and may result in false positives on ED screening questions and thus overestimation of prevalence. Criteria and definitions of ED have also varied between studies.

AN has an estimated incidence of 8 per 100 000 population per year and prevalence is estimated at 0.3%. The majority of those affected are female (>90%) and prevalence among women in their late teens is estimated to be around 1%. Among high risk groups, such as ballet and modelling students, prevalence rates increase to 6.5–7%. Peak age of onset for AN is 16 years (Hoek & van Hoeken 2003).

For BN, incidence rates of 10–13 per 100 000 per year have been reported in primary care settings. Among young women, estimates of incidence rise to 52 per 100 000 per year. The prevalence of BN in Western women is approximately 1%, rising to over 5% if partial syndromes are included. Some 90% of sufferers are female. High risk groups include dieters, dancers and models. Prevalence is highest in cities, intermediate in urbanized areas and lowest in rural settings. Peak age of onset is 18 years (later than for AN), although there is some evidence that the peak is getting younger.

An upward trend was observed in the incidence of AN through the twentieth century up until the 1970s. Incidence in primary care in the UK remained relatively stable between 1988 and 2000, a finding replicated in Dutch data. In contrast to AN, the incidence of BN in primary care increased three-fold between 1988 and 1993, and then declined somewhat in the late 1990s (Currin et al 2005). It has long been recognized that the majority of people with bulimic type EDs never present for treatment and it therefore remains unclear to what extent these changes reflect increased help-seeking (possibly related to Princess Diana's disclosure of experience of BN) or true increased incidence.

Though AN and BN are the most commonly studied eating disorders, EDNOS is the commonest form of ED.

Aetiology

Interaction between genetic and environmental factors contributes to the aetiology of most psychiatric conditions. EDs are no exception and a multifactorial threshold model of causation has been proposed. Given the relatively low incidence of these disorders, prospective studies of causation are prohibitively expensive and difficult to conduct. The vast majority of studies have therefore been retrospective (with the associated problem of retrospective bias) and demonstrate associations, from which causality cannot be inferred. Persistence of putative risk factors after recovery from an ED increases the probability of a causal role, but the possibility that they are consequences, or scars, of the illness often cannot be excluded.

Anorexia nervosa

Genetic factors

There is now a substantial body of evidence supporting a role for genetic factors in the development of AN. Family studies show an increased rate of eating disorder (5–7%) among 1st-degree relatives of probands with either AN or BN, and there is evidence of shared liability for the disorders. The genotype can be passed through both maternal or paternal lines, although in most cases, the phenotype is not expressed. Phenotypic expression occurs most commonly in women of the same generation, with sisters being most commonly affected. Twin studies have consistently shown a higher level of concordance in identical compared to non-identical twins. Estimates of the genetic contribution to heritability range from 48% to 76%, but lack of power due to the low prevalence of AN is reflected in wide confidence intervals for these studies, spanning 0–95% (Slof-Op 't Landt et al 2005).

Multiple genes likely contribute to liability through a range of phenotypic features including regulation of appetite and weight and temperamental traits such as perfectionism, need for order and sensitivity to praise and reward (Wade et al 2008). There has been much interest in the search for candidate genes, with the serotonin system particularly relevant given the role of serotonin (5HT) in regulation of appetite and temperamental traits. The 5-HT2A receptor and brain derived neurotrophic factor (BDNF) genes are promising candidates, although to date, studies lack power and consistent replication (Monteleone & Maj 2008).

Systematic genome-wide scans based on families with two or more individuals with an ED (AN or BN) revealed initial linkage regions on chromosomes 1, 3 (for both AN and BN) and 4 (AN) (Hinney et al 2004).

Personality and psychological factors

Obsessive–compulsive personality disorder (OCPD) is a common co-morbidity with AN and there is some evidence of shared familial liability (Lilenfeld et al 1998). Furthermore, co-morbid OCPD predicts poor outcome. Among those without OCPD co-morbidity, prevalence of perfectionism, concern with exactness and symmetry, anxiety, rigidity and persistence is high. Starvation exacerbates these traits and dampens emotional experience, which may be highly reinforcing of self-starvation. Schmidt and Treasure (2006) have proposed a model for AN in which these traits are conceptualized as playing a central role in maintenance of the disorder, particularly of the restrictive subtype. Perfectionistic control of eating is thought to be driven by the need to avoid the expression and experience of intense negative emotions and to avoid closeness to others that might trigger such emotions. AN is associated with low novelty seeking, high harm avoidance, experiential avoidance (that is, avoidance of emotions, emotional memories and intimacy) and avoidant coping style. Such avoidance may contribute to shyness, feelings of shame, poor social comparison and sibling jealousy associated with AN. Indeed, avoidance may also be linked to overachievement associated with AN: striving for achievement may be motivated by anxiety to avoid undesirable outcomes, rather than to achieve desirable outcomes (Schmidt & Treasure 2006).

Family factors

Minuchin et al (1975) proposed the 'psychosomatic family' model, in which family characteristics of enmeshment, overprotectiveness, rigidity and lack of conflict resolution were thought to be specifically associated with AN. However, subsequent research has shown that in fact, there is no specific family style associated with AN, with the majority of families observed to be functioning normally (Eisler 2005). Levels of expressed emotion (EE) are elevated, although whether cause or the effect of feelings of helplessness and self-blame associated with the illness, remains to be demonstrated.

Families of those with AN report higher than expected levels of obstetric complications and loss prior to the birth of the child who goes on to develop AN. There is also an increased incidence of prematurity and birth complications in the birth histories of those with AN. These findings, alongside high parental trait anxiety, may contribute to heightened anxiety reported by parents during the perinatal period. It is perhaps not surprising in this context that AN is associated with insecure attachment, predominantly of an avoidant type, and some evidence of parental overprotection and over-control throughout the child's development. A lack of parental closeness and affection, lack of close friends in childhood, poor reflective function and impaired theory of mind may reflect a turning away from attachment needs in the face of heightened attachment anxiety (Connan et al 2003).

Adverse life events

A severe life event or difficulty has been reported directly preceding the onset of illness in 76% of cases (Schmidt et al 1997). Such events include lifecycle changes which revive separation anxieties (such as starting secondary school, puberty, leaving home, marriage, divorce, birth and death of close relative) and pudicity events (sexual disgust). Abuse in childhood is more common in the histories of those with AN than the general population, but less so than general psychiatric patients. It is therefore a nonspecific risk factor for AN (Fairburn et al 1999) and is associated with higher levels of general psychiatric co-morbidity.

Sociocultural factors

AN was once thought only to affect young women in Western affluent societies. However, the association between AN and high socioeconomic class is now known to have been due to referral bias in clinic samples, and community-based studies demonstrate no class association. In addition, AN has been reported in many non-Western cultural groups. Interestingly, a large case control study found that risk factors for dieting (parental obesity, premorbid obesity, teasing about weight and shape) did not increase the risk for AN (Fairburn et al 1999). While there is no evidence that a Western cultural overvaluation of thinness plays a causative role in AN, this may be an important cultural maintaining factor. For example, 'fat phobia' among a cohort of women with AN in Hong Kong was associated with worse prognosis (Lee et al 1993).

Biological factors

Neuroimaging studies have demonstrated atrophy of the brain in AN with associated widening of sulci and enlargement of ventricles. These changes are largely reversible, although some loss of grey matter may persist after recovery. Functional brain imaging has demonstrated increased activation in response to food cues in the orbitofrontal cortex and anterior cingulate region. These abnormalities are present in both AN and BN, and may contribute to the compulsive quality of eating disorders (Uher et al 2004). Unilateral temporal hypoperfusion has been observed in early onset AN (Lask et al 2005). Compared with

4. Biopsychosocial consequences of ED symptoms and behaviour, including low weight or obesity.

   ○ *Biological*:

     a. Starvation: feeling cold and tired, proximal muscle weakness (e.g. difficulty climbing stairs or getting up from chairs), dry skin, thinning of scalp hair, increased body hair, oedema, constipation, dizziness, headache, amenorrhoea in women or sexual dysfunction and reduced libido in men

     b. Compensatory behaviours: sore mouth and teeth, dental erosion, haematemesis, irritable bowel, fainting, dehydration, palpitations

     c. Obesity: shortness of breath, high blood pressure, high cholesterol, diabetes, osteoarthritis, sleep apnoea.

   ○ *Psychological*: low self-esteem, shame and guilt, low mood, anxiety, irritability, feeling 'numb' or unable to experience emotions (alexithymia), increased emotions, emotional lability, poor concentration, reduced enjoyment, obsessional thoughts or rituals, compulsions and disturbed sleep.

   ○ *Social*: isolation, social withdrawal or avoidance, parental/ spousal concern or conflict, eliciting closer care from others, time off job or school / university, specific advantages of low weight (e.g. for dancer/model/jockey/athlete).

Past psychiatric history

Explore the onset and evolution of ED:

- Premorbid eating behaviour and attitudes, premorbid weight
- Context and precipitating factors at onset
- Maximum and minimum weight (and BMI), pattern of fluctuations
- Evolution and course of ED behaviours
- Physical complications
- Psychiatric co-morbidity
- Treatment history.

Family and personal history

Elicit developmental history in the context of eating disorder, with particular reference to risk factors and maintaining factors for disorder:

- Family history: weight, psychiatric disorders, personality traits
- Birth history, e.g. obstetric difficulties
- Early relationships with carers (attachment), family interpersonal style (emotionally inexpressive, invalidating, critical, isolated) and family dynamics (enmeshment, poor parental relations, expressed emotion)
- Early development: separation anxiety and other childhood anxiety disorders, developmental adversity (separations, loss, abuse), childhood illness, feeding difficulties and special diets, sibling rivalry, over protectiveness (e.g. >11 years before sleeping away from home), peer relationships, teasing about weight and shape

- Psychosexual history: menarche, attitudes to menstruation and sex
- Premorbid personality traits: obsessional, perfectionist, rigid, compliant, avoidant; emotional instability, impulsivity; fear of abandonment, etc.
- Occupational history: schooling and achievement; impact of occupation on ED and vice versa.

Information gathering

Meeting with families, partners or friends may helpfully provide further information about the patient's behaviour, weight history, development, premorbid personality, psychosocial triggers for the illness and maintaining factors. In addition, this provides an important opportunity to engage the family or partner and assess family dynamics and interpersonal style. Some patients do not wish for significant others to be involved in their care and decline consent to share information. However, it should always be possible to negotiate contact with significant others to allow them to share their concerns with professionals and to obtain general information about eating disorders and treatment. When risk is high and significant others could contribute to risk management, it may be appropriate to breach confidentiality, but this should always be discussed with the patient and they should be informed of any information sharing.

The general practitioner (GP) is another valuable source of information and ongoing support for longer-term care. It may also be useful to make links with school or employer, with consent from the patient and/or family.

Physical review and examination

See Table 18.3.

Investigations

Full blood count, urea and electrolytes, bicarbonate, liver function tests, calcium, phosphate, ESR and thyroid function tests should be completed at assessment, with ECG and bone scan if indicated by severe or enduring weight loss respectively. Further monitoring should be provided regularly if there are indicators of high medical risk and in the early stages of refeeding (Table 18.4).

Psychological assessment instruments

- EDI (Eating Disorders Investigation): a well validated self-report questionnaire assessing eating attitudes and associated personality dimensions (Garner et al 1983).
- BITE (Bulimic Investigatory Test, Edinburgh): a self-report questionnaire widely used for bulimic features.
- EDE (Eating Disorders Examination): a structured interview to assess the psychopathology of eating disorders. Modified into EDE-Q self-report questionnaire (Fairburn & Beglin 1994).
- Morgan–Russell scales: measures outcome of anorexia nervosa in terms of physical status (weight, menstruation) and psychological status.

Table 18.3 Physical review and examination

Musculoskeletal	Measure height and weight (single layered clothing, ideally at a consistent time of day and on the same scale) and calculate BMI. BMI <15 is severe and <13.5 is critical weight loss. Risks are higher with rapid, acute weight loss. Short stature may arise from pathological fractures associated with osteoporosis or stunted growth if onset is pre-pubertal. Test for proximal myopathy (how much use of arms is needed to stand up from a squat)
Dermatological	Dry skin, dorsal finger calluses caused by injuries sustained while inducing vomiting (Russell's sign)
Dental	Loss of enamel, caries, abscesses (mainly due to vomiting, exacerbated by acidic or sugary foods and excessive brushing)
Cardiovascular system	Bradycardia, hypotension and postural hypotension are associated with low weight. Hypertension is associated with obesity. It is essential to use an appropriate sized cuff for accurate readings. A proportion of mortality results from acute arrhythmias secondary to prolonged QTc interval (starvation related) and/or electrolyte abnormalities. Clinically, collapse is more commonly due to hypovolaemic circulatory failure (as a result of dehydration) and/or reduced sympathetic response (postural hypotension). Idiopathic oedema and tachycardia are associated with refeeding syndrome. AN may be associated with mitral valve prolapse
Gastrointestinal system	Parotid enlargement and inflammation, oesophagitis, gastric tears (bleeding) are associated with purging behaviour. Delayed gastric emptying, peptic ulcers, gastric dilatation, constipation, paralytic ileus are associated with starvation. Irritable bowel syndrome may be associated with EDs and rectal prolapse with laxative misuse
Central nervous system	Confusion/fits/coma may result from low glucose or electrolyte imbalance (e.g. low sodium levels associated with water loading or low phosphate levels due to refeeding syndrome). Cognitive deficits in attention, concentration, memory, visuospatial analysis, new learning, judgement and problem-solving are associated with starvation

Table 18.4 Investigations and monitoring

Haematology	Normochromic, normocytic anaemia, reduced white cell count and reduced platelets associated with starvation
Erythrocyte sedimentation rate (ESR)	Is usually normal (an important test to exclude organic causes)
Urea and creatinine	Usually low in starvation. Elevated urea indicates dehydration. Elevated creatinine (or high normal in starvation) indicates renal impairment. Pre-renal failure and renal stones can arise from dehydration. Impaired renal filtration with reduced ability to concentrate urine and hypokalaemic nephropathy are also associated with ED
Hypokalaemia	Associated with purging behaviour, particularly at low weight
Hyponatraemia	Associated with rehydration after chronic dehydration, water loading (to falsify weight) or excessive water intake to reduce hunger
Low magnesium	Associated with potassium depletion (making the latter difficult to correct), or refeeding syndrome
Phosphate	Low levels are associated with refeeding syndrome during active weight gain, or bingeing at low weight. High phosphate may be associated with vomiting
Bicarbonate	Metabolic alkalosis associated with purging and hypokalaemia
Liver enzymes	May be raised in starvation
Protein	Usually normal. Low albumin is unusual and associated with poor prognosis
Amylase	Elevated levels usually indicate vomiting
Creatinine kinase (CK)	Elevated levels associated with excessive exercise/physical activity in starvation
Thyroid function tests	Important for differential diagnosis. Sick euthyroid associated with AN, and sometimes BN
ECG (electrocardiogram)	Monitor if severe low weight or purging with electrolyte abnormalities. Pre and post test if considering drugs which impact on QT interval
Bone density scan	Screen for osteoporosis if duration >1 year, monitor every 2 years
Pelvic ultrasound scan (PUS)	PUS can be useful for determination of healthy weight during recovery from AN. Multifollicular ovaries common and normal during weight restoration. Polycystic ovaries associated with BN

Treatment

General principles

The evidence base for treatment of the EDs is limited, particularly for AN and atypical eating disorders. Much of the NICE guidance (NICE 2004) is therefore reliant on expert clinical guidance, rather than robust randomized controlled trials (RCTs). General principles of care include the need to integrate medical, nutritional and psychological components of care, and to involve families, particularly for younger patients with AN. Principles of stepped care may also be useful, with guided self-help in primary care for those with mild disorders, specialist outpatient treatment for those with more severe disorders, and more intensive specialist treatment, such as inpatient and day-patient care, reserved for those with the most severe disorders.

Treatment adherence and effectiveness are likely to be improved by addressing social problems and treating co-morbid depression early. It is thought that starvation impairs efficacy of antidepressants via effects of low oestrogen on serotonin system function. Higher doses may therefore be needed, although this must be balanced against increased risk of side-effects such as QTc prolongation in underweight patients.

In the absence of evidence to guide the management of atypical eating disorders (EDNOS in DSM-IV) other than BED, it is recommended that the clinician considers following the guidance on the treatment of the eating problem that most closely resembles the individual patient's eating disorder (NICE 2004). Fairburn and colleagues have developed a transdiagnostic approach to cognitive behavioural therapy (CBT-E), in which all eating disorder diagnoses are treated with the same model of therapy. RCT data are now becoming available and in a large sample of ED patients with BMI >17.5, treatment outcome did not depend on ED diagnosis (Fairburn et al 2009). Other individual psychotherapy approaches included in the NICE guidance, such as cognitive analytic therapy (CAT) and interpersonal psychotherapy (IPT), are also transdiagnostic, with therapy formulation and delivery tailored to specific, individual presentations. As yet, there are no treatment trials specifically evaluating these therapies in atypical disorders.

Engagement and motivation

Many of those presenting for treatment are ambivalent about change. In one study, less than half those with AN presenting to a specialist service were in action phase, ready and willing to change. The remainder were in precontemplation or contemplation stages of motivation (Blake et al 1997). Many patients are sent by concerned families, partners or professionals. Others come with mixed feelings because they are concerned about negative consequences of bingeing and purging, but do not see the need to change valued aspects of their disorder, such as food restriction and weight control. An eating disorder may be experienced as the solution to unhappiness. Bingeing and vomiting may be experienced as allowing the sufferer to 'have her cake and eat it' in the pursuit of a thin ideal. AN may confer a sense of control, of feeling special and unique, or of being protected from the demands of an adult role in life (Serpell et al 1999). Fasting, bingeing and vomiting may be valued for emotion regulation. Each may provide temporary relief from unmanageable feelings, in much the same way as self-harm. An ED may also serve as a distance regulator in relationships, eliciting care, while preventing real closeness by dampening emotional experience and maintaining instead a focus on food and weight. Attempts to help may therefore be experienced as attacks on valued aspects of the self, and so resisted.

Ambivalence about change presents significant challenges to engagement and development of a therapeutic alliance. Motivational interviewing (MI), developed in the addictions field, provides a useful therapeutic approach for working with ambivalence. The evidence base for MI-based interventions remains poor in the EDs, with only a few preliminary, underpowered and often poorly designed studies. Nonetheless, MI is widely supported as an appropriate therapeutic stance and intervention.

MI aims to help professionals avoid confrontation and argument which build resistance, and to facilitate instead an empathic relationship in which commitment to change and self-efficacy can be developed. The key tenets are: (1) a collaborative rather than authoritarian approach; (2) honouring the patient's autonomy; (3) facilitating and strengthening the person's own motivation to change, rather than trying to instil motivation. Accurate empathy and increased patient commitment talk over the course of a session predict behaviour change. Intervention is matched to the patient's readiness, willingness and confidence in her ability to change. When these are low, the patient is offered an opportunity to explore the pros and cons of her ED. Open questions, empathic, reflective listening and affirmations are used to build rapport and to differentially evoke and strengthen the patient's own change talk. Arguments against change (sustain talk) are responded to with empathy, and concerns about physical and psychosocial wellbeing are affirmed and amplified. Psychoeducation is offered when the patient is receptive. Information about negative consequences of the ED can be personalized by including feedback about the results of physical health assessment and monitoring. As change talk increases, readiness to change can be increased by enhancing self-efficacy and developing discrepancy between current circumstances and future life goals. What might life be like in 5 years if things don't change? And what if they do change? As expressions of determination and commitment to change increase, the focus shifts away from exploration of ambivalence (which may detract from commitment talk) toward exploration of obstacles to change and the development of strategies, skills and action plans to support change. Enhancing self-efficacy and emphasizing choice remain important throughout (Miller & Rose 2009).

Theory and evidence suggest that MI is most important and effective when anger and resistance to change are high. Thus, instead of arguments and confrontation, the clinician can use the stance and skills of MI to find common ground with the patient in her own concerns about the impact of the illness on her physical health, career aspirations or social life. Even when options are limited, it is important and possible to collaborate in the process of generating choices and encouraging autonomy. The context can be set by drawing on higher authorities.

For example, the framework of the Mental Health Act does not permit us to allow people with AN to die from starvation. Nutrition is therefore not negotiable in severe starvation. In the in-patient setting, patient and clinician can then collaborate over the choice about how nutrition is taken, for example, as food, oral nutritional supplements, or by nasogastric (NG) feeding.

Psychoeducation

Sharing of information with patients, and their families where appropriate, is an important component of the early stages of treatment. Psychoeducation can be delivered as part of assessment and treatment sessions, and supported by self-help books, and resources provided by Beat (the leading UK ED charity), which include Web resources and support groups. Such resources help to lessen stigma, isolation and anxiety and increase knowledge and skills of patients and their families with which to support recovery. Evidence-based self-help books include: *Bulimia Nervosa: A Guide to Recovery* (Cooper 1993); *Getting Better Bit(e) by Bit(e)* (Schmidt & Treasure 1993); *Overcoming Binge Eating* (Fairburn 1995); and *Anorexia Nervosa: A survival guide for families, friends and sufferers* (Treasure 1997).

Components of psychoeducation include:

1. Cultural and psychological factors influencing weight and food habits
2. Physical/medical effects of starvation and weight control behaviours
3. Harm minimization (see below)
4. Biology of weight and food intake regulation and determination of healthy weight for the individual. There are significant genetic components to appetite and weight regulation which contribute to a 'set point' for an individual's healthy weight. Attempts to maintain weight below a set point maintain starvation syndrome (see below). Premorbid weight and family weight history help to guide negotiation of a healthy target weight, within the BMI range 20–25. When early onset has prevented attainment of a healthy weight, a BMI of 20–22 is recommended
5. Maintaining effects of starvation syndrome: food restriction and starvation cause anxiety, low mood, preoccupation with food and weight, body image disturbance, increased obsessionality and compulsivity, cognitive rigidity, excessive attention to detail (inability 'to see the wood for the trees') and hunger. All are important maintaining factors for EDs. Eating regularly reduces these symptoms and lessens the urge to binge
6. To gain 0.5 kg per week (recommended rate for outpatients), around 500 extra calories per day (3500/week) are needed
7. Negative reinforcement of refeeding: starvation causes delayed gastric emptying and elevated cortisol, such that increasing food intake is associated with feeling bloated, constipation and laying down of abdominal fat. Eating little and often improves bowel function and restoration of healthy weight restores normal distribution of fat stores
8. Carbohydrate restriction contributes to depressed mood (via tryptophan depletion) and possibly reduced satiety signalling, which may increase the urge to binge
9. Maintaining effects of the binge purge cycle. Bingeing causes guilt and low self-esteem. Vomiting gives temporary relief from those feelings, but lessens the motivation to stop bingeing. Insulin release in response to a binge causes hypoglycaemia after vomiting, which increases hunger and the urge to binge again
10. Laxatives and diuretics reduce weight temporarily through loss of water, but do not reduce calorie absorption. Stopping laxative or diuretic misuse is associated with oedema and electrolyte imbalance. Laxative cessation also causes feelings of bloating and constipation. Symptoms improve over time as normal water balance and bowel function are restored, although chronic use may cause permanent damage to bowels and kidneys. Advise to stop by reducing slowly.

Medical monitoring and management

Physical health monitoring and management

A care plan should be developed collaboratively with the patient, and their family when appropriate, in which the frequency and setting (often primary care) of physical health monitoring and management is agreed. When risk is high, boundaries for risk management should be discussed in advance, including sharing information about the circumstances in which it might be appropriate to break confidentiality or to consider use of the Mental Health Act (1983).

Weight should be monitored at every session and plotted on a graph in order to identify change trends over time. BMI markers on the chart help to maintain focus on the context of relative risk. As well as contributing to assessment of risk and progress, weight monitoring demonstrates that weight is taken seriously, which is just as important to normal and overweight patients as to those who are underweight.

The nature and frequency of physical health monitoring is determined by the symptom profile, stability of disorder and severity of medical compromise at assessment. Purging behaviour indicates a need for regular U&E monitoring, with greater frequency for those with abnormal results, escalating purging or falling weight. Blood pressure, pulse, temperature, FBC, U&E, glucose, LFT, calcium and phosphate and ECG monitoring is necessary for underweight patients. Phosphate monitoring is particularly important during the first few weeks of intensive refeeding and weight gain for underweight patients. Creatinine kinase monitoring may provide an objective, proxy measure for excessive activity levels. Again, charting all test results serially allows early detection of trends, which is particularly important when there is evidence of deterioration. Completion of medical risk assessment forms is also important when there are indicators of risk (see: eatingresearch.com for Maudsley medical monitoring and risk assessment forms). Bone density scans are recommended for those with a history of underweight, with monitoring every 2 years if low weight persists or there is evidence of osteoporosis. NICE guidance recommends an annual comprehensive physical health check in primary care for those with chronic AN. Pelvic ultrasound can be a useful investigation to enhance motivation for further weight gain

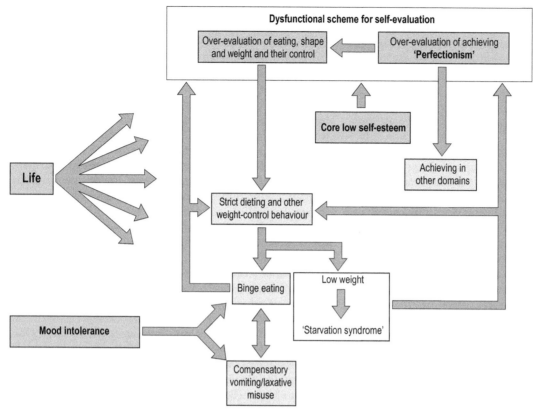

Figure 18.1 ● A schematic representation of the 'transdiagnostic' theory of the maintenance of eating disorders. 'Life' is shorthand for interpersonal life. (From Fairburn et al 2003.)

recently developed CBT-E for BN and EDNOS reports improved efficacy, with 51% of patients achieving symptom levels less than 1 standard deviation above the community mean at 60 week follow-up (Fairburn et al 2009).

CBT for eating disorders can be modified for use with children and adolescents, but there has been little systematic evaluation of the approach. In the only RCT of adolescent BN and EDNOS to date, CBT guided self-help produced more rapid reduction in bingeing, at lower cost and with greater acceptability than family therapy. Abstinence rates for bingeing and purging at 12 months were 36% and 41%, respectively (Schmidt et al 2007). This finding supports the NICE recommendation that children and adolescents with BN should be offered CBT-BN, adapted for age, with involvement of the family as appropriate. Internet-based CBT may be a useful first step for adolescents, with a level of symptom improvement similar to that achieved through guided self-help (Pretorius et al 2009).

For adult AN, there is some evidence that specialist therapies are more effective than non-specialist treatment or dietary advice alone, but little evidence of specific efficacy for CBT. CBT may reduce the risk of relapse after weight restoration, but in only two studies involving underweight patients had no clear benefit over a control group and was less effective than specialist supportive clinical management (Bulik et al 2007; McIntosh et al 2005).

Treatment studies of BED are limited in number and quality. There is moderate evidence for effectiveness of CBT tailored for BED, delivered in either individual or group format

(Brownley et al 2007). This intervention reduces the frequency and time spent binge eating, and may also reduce depressive symptoms. CBT does not significantly reduce weight, although weight stabilization is a good outcome, given the natural history of increasing weight trajectory. Self-help appears also to be effective, although there are no direct comparisons with CBT.

Interpersonal psychotherapy

Interpersonal psychotherapy (IPT) was first evaluated in the treatment of BN as a control condition for CBT. ED symptoms are not specifically addressed. The interpersonal context of the ED is investigated to identify interpersonal problems in one of 4 areas: interpersonal disputes, role transitions, grief or interpersonal deficits. Therapy then aims to facilitate change in the identified problem area and to develop skills with which to manage future interpersonal problems. It is now a well replicated finding that IPT is as effective as CBT, although much slower to take effect (Agras et al 2000). IPT is therefore the leading alternative to CBT for BN. It remains to be seen whether developments in CBT, such as CBT-E, improve efficacy against IPT. IPT was less effective than the specialist supportive clinical management in an RCT of psychological treatment for AN (McIntosh et al 2005).

One treatment trial has compared group IPT for BED with group CBT. As for BN, there was no difference in effectiveness at follow-up, but the effect of IPT was slower (Brownley et al 2007).

Cognitive analytic therapy (CAT)

CAT was developed by Anthony Ryle at Guy's Hospital in the 1980s as a means to convey a psychoanalytic model in a brief, time-limited, focused therapy that had broad applicability, including patients with severe borderline and narcissistic personality disorders (Ryle 1990). Kelly's construct theory and object relations theory have been integrated to develop interpersonal understanding that lies at the core of CAT (see also Ch. 37).

Relationship patterns are described as two poles of a dynamic in which self and other take reciprocal roles, such as controlling/rebellious, or abusive/abused. The reciprocity is important, reflecting the tendency to move dynamically between two reciprocal roles and to recruit others, or aspects of oneself, to the reciprocal pole of an active role. For example, abused children will often abuse themselves and others. Unhelpful patterns of relating to self and others arise from early experiences of care, and may be real (e.g. depriving/deprived) or compensatory phantasy (e.g. special, perfectly caring/special perfectly cared for). Maladaptive relationship patterns give rise to unmanageable affect and unmet needs, which may be managed by dysfunctional coping and symptoms. Problematic relationship patterns and dysfunctional coping are conceptualized as vicious cycles (called procedures in CAT) in which the same outcome or consequence persistently reinforces those problematic relationship patterns (and associated dysfunctional coping strategies, false assumptions and unmanageable feelings and needs). Procedures take the form of traps (e.g. striving to be perfect), snags (e.g. sabotaging good things because I do not deserve them) or dilemmas (e.g. either I am safe but alone, or close to another but risk being abused).

The process of CAT has three components: reformulation, recognition and revision. The aim of reformulation is to collaboratively develop an understanding of the maladaptive relationship patterns and procedures that maintain symptoms through maintenance of unhelpful beliefs and avoidance of painful emotions. Developing self-reflection, self efficacy and agency are important goals of CAT. Collaboration in the process of work toward shared goals is therefore essential. Shared 'target problems' are negotiated at the start of therapy, and help to maintain the focus on important symptoms (such as weight loss), as well as underlying intra and interpersonal problems (such as low self-esteem, perfectionism and placation). The reformulation is shared with the patient as an empathic *hypothesis*, in the form of a letter to the patient and a visual diagram (or 'map'). These use the patient's own words and metaphors in order to maintain emphasis on collaboration and empathic understanding. The map is then used as a tool to facilitate recognition of maladaptive relationship patterns and procedures explicitly in the here and now of the therapy relationship. It is only through here and now recognition that the patient and therapist create an opportunity for revision: the development of alternative, healthier ways of relating and of coping with overwhelming affect and needs there and then. The ending sessions, in which goodbye letters reviewing the progress of therapy and change are shared by patient and therapist, provide further opportunity for revision and change. A well managed ending may be particularly important and helpful for people with eating disorders, for whom separation and individuation can be difficult. The letters, map and follow-up sessions encourage the patient to continue to make use of the skills she has developed in her life outside therapy (Treasure & Ward 1997).

There has been one trial of CAT in AN, in which it was more effective than outpatient treatment as usual, with remission rate of around one-third with 20 sessions (Dare et al 2001). There have been no trials in BN or other eating disorders. Audit data suggests CAT may be effective for BN. It may therefore be a reasonable approach if assessment or trial of treatment suggests that CBT is unsuitable, particularly where there is significant personality disorder.

Psychodynamic models

Freud conceptualized anorexia nervosa as a means to avoid adult sexuality. Hilde Bruch (1973) developed this idea by conceptualizing a broader deficit in sense of self, identity and autonomy underlying AN. She hypothesized that core feelings of ineffectiveness in childhood are managed by perfectionism and excessive compliance, which through the approval of others confer a pseudo-sense of effectiveness. This orientation to please others impairs the child's capacity to develop a sense of herself and her own drives and feelings from within. The need to develop a more adult role and to manage sexual urges associated with adolescence are experienced as overwhelming, and self-starvation may be seen as a concrete solution to the need for self-control, identity, self-expression and self-efficacy. Thus core feelings of ineffectiveness come to be managed through control of the body. Bruch therefore hypothesized that change in AN can be achieved through development of an understanding of the meaning of self-starvation for the individual, leading to the development of alternative ways of experiencing the self and of self-expression than through AN. Therapy offers the opportunity to learn to put feelings and needs into words, to develop identity and autonomy, and to make use of relationships to manage feelings and needs, and thus no longer rely on a maladaptive relationship with food.

In object relations theory, AN is postulated to arise from the paranoid-schizoid position in which good (loving and gratifying) and bad (frustrating, persecutory and hated) aspects of the self and others cannot be integrated. Primitive defences of splitting and projection are employed to defend the good object against attack from the bad object. Understanding of the transference and counter-transference arising from these defences is helpful in managing the therapeutic relationship and avoiding collusion with AN patients, whatever the treatment modality.

Gianna Williams (1997) has described the term 'No Entry', by which she refers to the signs and behaviours that many patients with AN may manifest. Her proposal is that as infants, young people who develop an ED have been the recipients of the powerful projections of their parents, particularly their mothers. Such patients have not only lacked containment, but also perceived themselves as receptacles of unmetabolized phantasies and experiences projected into them by their parents. She refers to those patients who succeed in protecting themselves from this predicament by developing a 'no entry system of defences'. This line of thinking derives from Bion's notion of containment, according to which one of the functions of the mother is to receive and modify the projections of the infant. Such maternal containment may fail under certain circumstances and the child is then left to reintroject its own anxieties, unmodified and not understood. In addition, the mother may well project her own disturbed feelings into the child. The refusal to take in food is viewed as a misguided defence against taking in the unbearable feelings projected by the parent. In her vivid descriptions of patients suffering from AN, Marilyn Lawrence (2001, 2002) has written about the presence of the 'intrusive couple' and further developed ideas from Williams. Lawrence suggests that many women who suffer from AN have an intrusive object instated in their minds (which may not necessarily be the result of actual intrusions in external reality). She describes the intrusiveness of patients with AN in the transference and suggests that such patients very often harbour profound phantasies of intruding between the parents, with a wish to regain their special place with mother, untroubled by the presence of father. She also hypothesizes that the psychopathology underlying certain cases of AN leads to a failure in symbolization, and this failure in turn 'complicates the clinical picture, making such patients particularly difficult to think with about their difficulties'.

While classical psychoanalytic psychotherapy is not considered appropriate treatment for EDs, there is some evidence base for modified forms. In an RCT, focal psychodynamic psychotherapy (FAP), in which the therapist takes a non-directive stance and focuses upon the conscious and unconscious meaning of food in relationships, was more effective than treatment as usual. Like CAT and family therapy, FAP achieved a remission rate of around one-third. The duration of treatment for FAP and family therapy was 40 sessions, while CAT was 20 sessions (Dare et al 2001).

Family approaches

Family therapy

While there is no evidence to support a specific model of family dysfunction associated with AN, the structural family therapy model has endured and the Maudsley model has demonstrated efficacy for adolescent AN. As for other therapies, there has been a shift toward a maintenance model as more useful for guiding treatment. Families of all types become organized around AN, as they do around other chronic illnesses of adolescence, such as cystic fibrosis. AN comes to be accommodated and adaptive family behaviour is narrowed, such that families are unable to helpfully tackle the illness or manage normal family lifecycle changes. Thus, a family living with AN may understandably become less functional because of AN, and families should not be seen as the cause. The aim of family therapy is to make use of the adaptive mechanisms of individuals and the family to help the person with AN get better (Eisler 2005).

Maudsley model family therapy has four stages: engagement, challenging the symptoms, exploration of issues of individual and family development and ending sessions. Blame and guilt are addressed in engagement sessions, while exploring the role of AN in current family functioning. The focus is not on the cause of the problem, but on how to support recovery. Risk is

assessed and managed and psychoeducation offered. Family and individual strengths are explored and developed. AN is conceptualized as an external force that the child cannot resist, and that has invaded the family. For the family living with AN, time focus becomes narrowed to the here and now. In the second stage, the therapist therefore holds a broader timeframe and an expectation of change. The therapist does not have the answers, but facilitates the family finding their own solutions to the problem of feeding their child or sibling. Roles are clarified, parental alliance strengthened, age appropriate boundaries established and effective, open communication fostered. Once the family have established feeding and weight gain, the therapeutic work can move on to individual and family lifecycle issues: not as if dysfunction caused the problem, but as a normal need of the family that has been interrupted and affected by the presence of the illness. Ending sessions focus on consolidation and future plans (Eisler 2005).

There is moderate evidence of efficacy for this model in the treatment for adolescents' AN from a series of studies conducted at the Maudsley. At 5-year follow-up, 75% recovery rates are reported, with only 8% relapse rate after weight restoration (Eisler et al 2007). Conjoint family therapy was less effective than separated (family counselling and individual sessions with the patient) when maternal criticism was high. The model has also been adapted for delivery in multiple family day therapy and the outcome of an evaluation study is awaited. NICE guidance recommends family therapy as first-line treatment for adolescent AN and the markedly better treatment outcomes for adolescents than adults supports the NICE recommendation that early intervention is important. In adults, family therapy was more effective than individual supportive therapy as relapse prevention post-inpatient weight restoration for those with onset before the age of 19 and duration of illness less than 3 years (Russell et al 1987). As a standalone outpatient treatment, 40 sessions of family therapy had similar efficacy to CAT and focal psychodynamic, with remission rates of around one-third (Dare et al 2001).

The role of family therapy for people with BN is less established than for AN. The only RCT found family therapy to be less cost-effective and acceptable to adolescents than CBT guided self-help (Schmidt et al 2007).

Carer skills training

AN is associated with high carer distress and burden, and anxiety related emotional over-involvement and criticism (i.e. high expressed emotion (EE), of a level similar to that found in depression). It is therefore considered good practice to involve family and/or partners in treatment, both to support families and to reduce maintaining factors, and thus support recovery. The 'Maudsley eating disorder collaborative care skills workshops' is a novel approach in which staff and expert carers share with families the skills used by specialists nurses (including motivational interviewing skills). It is effective in reducing carer distress and EE (Sepulveda et al 2008). It remains to be seen whether this intervention improves outcome of AN. The model can also be delivered by the self-help book: *Skills-based Learning for Caring for a Loved One with an Eating Disorder: The New Maudsley Method* (Treasure et al 2007).

Inpatient and day-patient care (see Box 18.1)

A small RCT of inpatient vs outpatient treatment for young people with AN showed no advantage for inpatient treatment (Crisp et al 1991) and some advantages for outpatient treatment in terms of social adjustment. In another study, while severity of illness was an important predictor of poor outcome, receipt of inpatient care was of greater significance in multiple regression analyses (Gowers et al 2000). The possibility that inpatient care can be harmful must be taken seriously. Inpatient treatment should be a treatment of last resort, and outpatient treatment, of at least 6 months' duration, is therefore recommended for all patients, unless high medical or psychiatric risk or intolerable social circumstances necessitate admission. These data also call into question the assumption that restoration of healthy weight through external control improves the prospect of recovery. Weight gained through a patient's own volition and effort is probably more likely to be maintained. However, if a specialist outpatient treatment of reasonable duration does not restore weight, more intensive treatment should be considered, particularly if a patient expresses readiness and willingness to make use of more intensive support to gain weight. Options include adding family therapy to an established individual therapy, day-patient or inpatient care. Day-patient care may have the advantage of maintaining greater patient autonomy and connection with social context, although the intensity of care is unlikely to be sufficient for weight restoration for all patients. Except in emergencies, admission should be planned and prepared for in the outpatient setting, and psychological formulation and progress in therapy shared with the inpatient team. Continuity of therapy relationship through transitions in service levels may help patients to tolerate and make best use of more intensive treatment.

'People with anorexia nervosa requiring inpatient treatment should be admitted to a setting that can provide the skilled implementation of refeeding with careful physical monitoring (particularly in the first few days of refeeding) in combination with psychosocial interventions' (NICE 2004). The aim of admission for adults is to achieve weight restoration, reduce psychosocial maintaining factors and increase resilience. Individual and family therapies, as described above, should be offered as part of the package of care, preferably with continuity from outpatient care and through to further care post-discharge. Effective day-patient and inpatient care can only be delivered by a skilled multidisciplinary team. Specialist teams achieve better outcomes than non-specialist.

For adolescents, the aim of admission is to support the family in taking charge of their daughter's eating and weight gain. It is therefore essential to involve and collaborate with families as much as possible and to return to ongoing family therapy in the outpatient setting as soon as possible. This approach also helps to minimize the disruption to psychosocial development associated with admission.

Refeeding starts slowly with a low fibre, energy dense, phosphate rich diet (milk is an excellent source of phosphate) to reduce the risk of refeeding syndrome, including hypophosphataemia, hypokalaemia, hypomagnesaemia, oedema and heart failure (Mehanna et al 2008) and gastric dilatation, which can result in gastric perforation and death. Physical health monitoring is particularly important in the first 2 weeks of admission. A broad range of foods is then introduced and the quantity of food is slowly increased to 3000 calories per day with the aim of gaining 1–1.5 kg weight gain per week. There is some evidence that faster (around 1 kg per week), more consistent gain is associated with better outcome, perhaps because this reflects greater readiness and willingness of the patient to tolerate weight gain. It is helpful for patients to be aware of a healthy target weight band above which their weight will not be allowed to go, in order to lessen anxiety. For some patients with severe and enduring AN and a history of repeated admission, a lower plateau weight target may be agreed, but it is important not to negotiate compromise too early in admission. Assisted feeding against the will of the patient, usually by nasogastric (NG) but occasionally percutaneous endoscopic gastrostomy (PEG) feeding should only be considered as a last resort, and only in the context of informed consent, or appropriate legal powers (see below). Specialist advice should always be sought before considering compulsory admission and treatment. Meal support by skilled nurses significantly reduces the need for assisted feeding.

Specialist nursing care aims to achieve a balance between maintaining appropriate boundaries for behaviour and developing patient autonomy. A key nurse, or primary nurse, aims to establish a collaborative therapeutic alliance. This is particularly challenging in the presence of resistance to weight gain (driven by fear, anxiety and distress), and persistent, skilled efforts to avoid food and weight gain. The spirit and skills of motivational interviewing are particularly useful in this context. The nursing team support structured meals and develop a milieu in which peer support is encouraged and completing meals within agreed time limits and boundaries is considered a group task. Facilitating exploration and management of feelings provoked by eating is a core part of the process.

Psychological and occupational therapy is focused on eating behaviours, attitudes to weight and shape, healthy exercise and psychosocial maintaining factors. Individual therapy, family interventions and groups all play a part. Alongside nursing keywork, these interventions help to individualize care to match

Box 18.1

Indications for admission

- Physical compromise:
  - Syncope
  - Proximal myopathy
  - Hypoglycaemia
  - Severe electrolyte disturbance
  - Renal impairment
  - Severe low white cell count
  - Low platelet count
- Risk of suicide
- Co-morbid psychiatric condition requiring inpatient care
- Failed trial of evidence-based outpatient treatment
- Social or family situation unsuitable or unsafe to continue outpatient treatment.

as a funnel on the weight chart in order to monitor progress and lessen anxiety about excessive weight gain.

BN tends to improve during pregnancy, although a proportion of patients experience exacerbation or relapse, particularly if active during pregnancy. BN is associated with increased rate of miscarriage, fetal death and gestational diabetes. Past or present AN has been consistently associated with small for dates babies, an effect in part attributable to maternal smoking, and in part to low maternal weight pre pregnancy. A lifetime history of ED is also associated with high levels of anxiety and depression during pregnancy. Poor fetal nutrition and increased fetal exposure to glucocorticoids (associated with maternal anxiety and depression) have significant impact on prenatal metabolic programming and neuropsychiatric development, giving rise to increased risk for anxiety and stress related disorders, obesity and cardiovascular disease in later life (Micali & Treasure 2009).

In the postnatal period, problems with maternal adjustment are common and postnatal depression occurs in 40–60% of those with ED history. Increased risk is associated with active ED during pregnancy and past history of AN. The adverse effects of postnatal depression on child development are well established. Finally, a history of AN is associated with feeding difficulties, mothers having difficulty tolerating early infant expressions of autonomy through control of feeding (Micali & Treasure 2009).

Eating disorders in men

Males account for only 4–10% of those with eating disorders and presentation is similar to that in women. Men tend to have longer delay before seeking treatment and are more likely to be referred for medical investigations before diagnosis. One study found higher rates of homosexuality/bisexuality compared with female patients. This may reflect an increased contribution of physical appearance to self-esteem in male gay culture, giving rise to increased risk for ED (Carlat et al 1997).

Muscle dysmorphia has been described as a variant of body dysmorphic disorder in which men become preoccupied with muscularity. In contrast to healthy body builders, these men have significantly disturbed eating behaviour, greater risk of using anabolic steroids, high levels of body dissatisfaction, a tendency to see themselves as smaller than they are, high levels of anxiety and depression, low self-esteem and poor social and occupational functioning (Olivardia et al 2000). In many respects, this is a variant of BN, in which extreme muscle building behaviour is equivalent to extreme weight loss behaviour. While young women experience sociocultural pressure to be thin, the idealized body image for young men is lean, but muscular.

Night-time eating disorders

Night eating syndrome (NES) was identified for the first time in the 1950s and is characterized by 25% or more of daily food intake taken after the evening meal, with insomnia and conscious eating during the night. Sleep related eating disorder (SRED) is characterized by recurrent episodes of eating after an arousal from night-time sleep, with or without amnesia. SRED is frequently associated with other sleep disorders, in particular parasomnias. Topiramate may be an effective treatment for SRED. Both conditions are often chronic (Howell et al 2009).

References

Agras, W.S., Walsh, T., Fairburn, C.G., et al., 2000. A multicenter comparison of cognitive-behavioral therapy and interpersonal psychotherapy for bulimia nervosa. Arch. Gen. Psychiatry 57, 459–466.

Audenaert, K., Van, L.K., Dumont, F., et al., 2003. Decreased 5-HT2a receptor binding in patients with anorexia nervosa. J. Nucl. Med. 44, 163–169.

Becker, A.E., Burwell, R.A., Gilman, S.E., et al., 2002. Eating behaviours and attitudes following prolonged exposure to television among ethnic Fijian adolescent girls. Br. J. Psychiatry 180, 509–514.

Berkman, N.D., Lohr, K.N., Bulik, C.M., 2007. Outcomes of eating disorders: a systematic review of the literature. Int. J. Eat. Disord. 40, 293–309.

Blake, W., Turnbull, S., Treasure, J.L., 1997. Stages and processes of change in eating disorders. Implications for therapy. Clin. Psychol. Psychother. 4, 186–191.

Braun, D.L., Sunday, S.R., Halmi, K.A., 1994. Psychiatric co-morbidity in patients with eating disorders. Psychol. Med. 24, 859–867.

Brewerton, T.D., 2007. Eating disorders, trauma, and co-morbidity: focus on PTSD. Eat. Disord. 15, 285–304.

Brownley, K.A., Berkman, N.D., Sedway, J.A., et al., 2007. Binge eating disorder treatment: a systematic review of randomized controlled trials. Int. J. Eat. Disord. 40, 337–348.

Bruch, H., 1973. Eating disorders. Basic Books, New York.

Bulik, C.M., Sullivan, P.F., Carter, F.A., et al., 1996. Lifetime anxiety disorders in women with bulimia nervosa. Compr. Psychiatry 37, 368–374.

Bulik, C.M., Devlin, B., Bacanu, S.A., et al., 2003. Significant linkage on chromosome 10p in families with bulimia nervosa. Am. J. Hum. Genet. 72, 200–207.

Bulik, C.M., Berkman, N.D., Brownley, K.A., et al., 2007. Anorexia nervosa treatment: a systematic review of randomized controlled trials. Int. J. Eat. Disord. 40, 310–320.

Calero-Elvira, A., Krug, I., Davis, K., et al., 2009. Meta-analysis on drugs in people with eating disorders. Eur. Eat. Disord. Rev. 17, 243–259.

Capasso, A., Petrella, C., Milano, W., 2009. Pharmacological profile of SSRIs and SNRIs in the treatment of eating disorders. Curr. Clin. Pharmacol. 4, 78–83.

Carlat, D.J., Camargo Jr., C.A., Herzog, D.B., 1997. Eating disorders in males: a report on 135 patients. Am. J. Psychiatry 154, 1127–1132.

Claudino, A.M., Hay, P., Lima, M.S., et al., 2006. Antidepressants for anorexia nervosa. Cochrane Database Syst. Rev. (1), CD004365.

Connan, F., Campbell, I.C., Katzman, M., et al., 2003. A neurodevelopmental model for anorexia nervosa. Physiol. Behav. 79, 13–24.

Cooper, P.J., 1993. Bulimia nervosa: a guide to recovery. Robinson, London.

Crisp, A.H., Norton, K., Gowers, S., et al., 1991. A controlled study of the effect of therapies aimed at adolescent and family psychopathology in anorexia nervosa. Br. J. Psychiatry 159, 325–333.

Crow, S.J., Mitchell, J.E., Roerig, J.D., et al., 2009. What potential role is there for medication treatment in anorexia nervosa? Int. J. Eat. Disord. 42, 1–8.

Currin, L., Schmidt, U., Treasure, J., et al., 2005. Time trends in eating disorder incidence. Br. J. Psychiatry 186, 132–135.

Dare, C., Eisler, I., Russell, G., et al., 2001. Psychological therapies for adults with anorexia nervosa: randomised controlled trial of out-patient treatments. Br. J. Psychiatry 178, 216–221.

Dunican, K.C., DelDotto, D., 2007. The role of olanzapine in the treatment of anorexia nervosa. Ann. Pharmacother. 41, 111–115.

Eisler, I., 2005. The empirical and theoretical base of family therapy and multiple family day therapy for adolescent anorexia nervosa. J. Fam. Ther. 27, 104–131.

Eisler, I., Simic, M., Russell, G.F., et al., 2007. A randomised controlled treatment trial of two forms of family therapy in adolescent anorexia nervosa: a five-year follow-up. J. Child Psychol. Psychiatry 48, 552–560.

Fairburn, C.G., 1995. Overcoming binge eating. Guilford Press, Lynton.

Fairburn, C.G., Beglin, S.J., 1994. Assessment of eating disorders: interview or self-report questionnaire? Int. J. Eat. Disord. 16, 363–370.

Fairburn, C.G., Welch, S.L., Doll, H.A., et al., 1997. Risk factors for bulimia nervosa. A community-based case-control study. Arch. Gen. Psychiatry 54, 509–517.

Fairburn, C.G., Cooper, Z., Doll, H.A., et al., 1999. Risk factors for anorexia nervosa: three integrated case-control comparisons. Arch. Gen. Psychiatry 56, 468–476.

Fairburn, C.G., Cooper, Z., Shafran, R., 2003. Cognitive behaviour therapy for eating disorders: a 'transdiagnostic' theory and treatment. Behav. Res. Ther. 41, 509–528.

Fairburn, C.G., Cooper, Z., Doll, H.A., et al., 2009. Transdiagnostic cognitive-behavioral therapy for patients with eating disorders: a two-site trial with 60-week follow-up. Am. J. Psychiatry 166, 311–319.

Fittig, E., Jacobi, C., Backmund, H., et al., 2008. Effectiveness of day hospital treatment for anorexia nervosa and bulimia nervosa. Eur. Eat. Disord. Rev. 16, 341–351.

Franko, D.L., Keel, P.K., 2006. Suicidality in eating disorders: occurrence, correlates, and clinical implications. Clin. Psychol. Rev. 26, 769–782.

Gadalla, T., Piran, N., 2007. Co-occurrence of eating disorders and alcohol use disorders in women: a meta analysis. Arch. Womens Ment. Health 10, 133–140.

Garner, D.M., Olmsted, M.P., Garfinkel, P.E., 1983. Development and validation of multidimensional eating disorder inventory for anorexia nervosa and bulimia. Int. J. Eat. Disord. 48, 173–178.

Goebel-Fabbri, A.E., 2009. Disturbed eating behaviors and eating disorders in type 1 diabetes: clinical significance and treatment recommendations. Curr. Diab. Rep. 9, 133–139.

Goldbloom, D.S., Olmsted, M., Davis, R., et al., 1997. A randomized controlled trial of fluoxetine and cognitive behavioral therapy for bulimia nervosa: short-term outcome. Behav. Res. Ther. 35, 803–811.

Goldner, E.M., Srikameswaran, S., Schroeder, M.L., et al., 1999. Dimensional assessment of personality pathology in patients with eating disorders. Psychiatry Res. 85, 151–159.

Gowers, S.G., Weetman, J., Shore, A., et al., 2000. Impact of hospitalization on the outcome of adolescent anorexia nervosa. Br. J. Psychiatry 176, 138–141.

Gull, W.W., 1874. Anorexia nervosa (apepsia hysterica, anorexia hysterica). Transact. Clin. Soc. Lond. 7, 22–28.

Hay, P.P., Bacaltchuk, J., Stefano, S., et al., 2009. Psychological treatments for bulimia nervosa and binging. Cochrane Database Syst. Rev. (4), CD000562.

Hinney, A., Friedel, S., Remschmidt, H., et al., 2004. Genetic risk factors in eating disorders. Am. J. Pharmacoenomics 4, 209–223.

Hoek, H.W., van Hoeken, D., 2003. Review of the prevalence and incidence of eating disorders. Int. J. Eat. Disord. 34, 383–396.

Howell, M.J., Schenck, C.H., Crow, S.J., 2009. A review of nighttime eating disorders. Sleep Med. Rev. 13, 23–34.

Hudson, J.I., Hiripi, E., Pope Jr., H.G., et al., 2007. The prevalence and correlates of eating disorders in the National Comorbidity Survey Replication. Biol. Psychiatry 61, 348–358.

Jimerson, D.C., Mantzoros, C., Wolfe, B.E., et al., 2000. Decreased serum leptin in bulimia nervosa. J. Clin. Endocrinol. Metab. 85, 4511–4514.

Kaye, W., 2008. Neurobiology of anorexia and bulimia nervosa. Physiol. Behav. 94, 121–135.

Klump, K.L., Burt, S.A., McGue, M., et al., 2007. Changes in genetic and environmental influences on disordered eating across adolescence: a longitudinal twin study. Arch. Gen. Psychiatry 64, 1409–1415.

Lacey, J.H., 1993. Self-damaging and addictive behaviour in bulimia nervosa. A catchment area study. Br. J. Psychiatry 163, 190–194.

Lasegue, E.C., 1873. De l'anorexie hysterique. Archives General de Medecine 21, 385–483.

Lask, B., Gordon, I., Christie, D., et al., 2005. Functional neuroimaging in early-onset anorexia nervosa. Int. J. Eat. Disord. 37, S49–S51.

Lawrence, M., 2001. Anorexia, femininity and the intrusive object. Wiley, London.

Lawrence, M., 2002. Body, mother, mind: anorexia, femininity and the intrusive object. Int. J. Psychoanal. 83, 837–850.

Lee, S., Ho, T.P., Hsu, L.K., 1993. Fat phobic and non-fat phobic anorexia nervosa: a comparative study of 70 Chinese patients in Hong Kong. Psychol. Med. 23, 999–1017.

Lilenfeld, L.R., Kaye, W.H., Greeno, C.G., et al., 1998. A controlled family study of anorexia nervosa and bulimia nervosa: psychiatric disorders in first-degree relatives and effects of proband co-morbidity. Arch. Gen. Psychiatry 55, 603–610.

Mason, H.D., Key, A., Allan, R., et al., 2007. Pelvic ultrasonography in anorexia nervosa: what the clinician should ask the radiologist

and how to use the information provided. Eur. Eat. Disord. Rev. 15, 35–41.

McIntosh, V.V., Jordan, J., Carter, F.A., et al., 2005. Three psychotherapies for anorexia nervosa: a randomized, controlled trial. Am. J. Psychiatry 162, 741–747.

Mehanna, H.M., Moledina, J., Travis, J., 2008. Refeeding syndrome: what it is, and how to prevent and treat it. Br. Med. J. 336, 1495–1498.

Mehler, P.S., MacKenzie, T.D., 2009. Treatment of osteopenia and osteoporosis in anorexia nervosa: a systematic review of the literature. Int. J. Eat. Disord. 42, 195–201.

Micali, N., Treasure, J., 2009. Biological effects of a maternal ED on pregnancy and fetal development: a review. Eur. Eat. Disord. Rev. 17, 448–454.

Miller, W.R., Rose, G.S., 2009. Toward a theory of motivational interviewing. Am. Psychol. 64, 527–537.

Minuchin, S., Baker, L., Rosman, B.L., et al., 1975. A conceptual model of psychosomatic illness in children. Arch. Gen. Psychiatry 32, 1031–1038.

Monteleone, P., Maj, M., 2008. Genetic susceptibility to eating disorders: associated polymorphisms and pharmacogenetic suggestions. Pharmacogenomics 9, 1487–1520.

Mumford, D.B., Whitehouse, A.M., Platts, M., 1991. Sociocultural correlates of eating disorders among Asian schoolgirls in Bradford. Br. J. Psychiatry 158, 222–228.

NICE, 2002. The clinical effectiveness and cost effectiveness of surgery for people with morbid obesity. NICE, London.

NICE, 2004. Eating disorders: core interventions in the treatment and management of anorexia nervosa, bulimia nervosa and related eating disorders. NICE, London.

NICE, 2006. Obesity: the prevention, identification, assessment and management of overweight and obesity in adults and children. NICE, London.

Nicholls, D., Christie, D., Randall, L., et al., 2001. Selective eating: symptom, disorder or normal variant? Clin. Child Psychol. Psychiatry 6, 257–270.

Olivardia, R., Pope Jr., H.G., Hudson, J.I., 2000. Muscle dysmorphia in male weightlifters: a case-control study. Am. J. Psychiatry 157, 1291–1296.

Patton, G.C., Selzer, R., Coffey, C., et al., 1999. Onset of adolescent eating disorders: population based cohort study over 3 years. Br. Med. J. 318, 765–768.

Pretorius, N., Arcelus, J., Beecham, J., et al., 2009. Cognitive-behavioural therapy for adolescents with bulimic symptomatology: the acceptability and effectiveness of internet-based delivery. Behav. Res. Ther. 47, 729–736.

Puxley, F., Midtsund, M., Iosif, A., et al., 2008. PANDAS anorexia nervosa—endangered, extinct or nonexistent? Int. J. Eat. Disord. 41, 15–21.

Reas, D.L., Grilo, C.M., 2008. Review and meta-analysis of pharmacotherapy for binge-eating

disorder. Obesity (Silver Spring)
16, 2024–2038.

Riverside Health NHS Trust v Fox, 1994. 1 FLR
614–622.

Russell, G.F., Szmukler, G.I., Dare, C., et al.,
1987. An evaluation of family therapy in
anorexia nervosa and bulimia nervosa. Arch.
Gen. Psychiatry 44, 1047–1056.

Ryle, A., 1990. Cognitive analytical therapy:
active participation in change. A new
integration in brief psychotherapy. Wiley,
Chichester.

Schmidt, U., Treasure, J., 2006. Anorexia
nervosa: valued and visible. A cognitive-
interpersonal maintenance model and its
implications for research and practice. Br. J.
Clin. Psychol. 45, 343–366.

Schmidt, U., Treasure, J.L., 1993. Getting better
bit(e) by bit(e). A survival kit for sufferers of
bulimia nervosa and binge eating disorders.
Lawrence Erlbaum Associates, Mahwah NJ.

Schmidt, U., Tiller, J., Blanchard, M., et al.,
1997. Is there a specific trauma precipitating
anorexia nervosa? Psychol. Med.
27, 523–530.

Schmidt, U., Lee, S., Beecham, J., et al., 2007. A
randomized controlled trial of family therapy
and cognitive behavior therapy guided self-care
for adolescents with bulimia nervosa and
related disorders. Am. J. Psychiatry
164, 591–598.

Sepulveda, A.R., Lopez, C., Todd, G., et al., 2008.
An examination of the impact of 'the
Maudsley eating disorder collaborative care
skills workshops' on the well being of carers: a
pilot study. Soc. Psychiatry Psychiatr.
Epidemiol. 43, 584–591.

Serpell, L., Treasure, J., Teasdale, J., et al., 1999.
Anorexia nervosa: friend or foe? Int. J. Eat.
Disord. 25, 177–186.

Slade, P., 1982. Towards a functional analysis of
anorexia nervosa and bulimia nervosa. Br. J.
Clin. Psychol. 21, 167–179.

Slof-Op 't Landt, M.C., van Furth, E.F.,
Meulenbelt, I., et al., 2005. Eating disorders:
from twin studies to candidate genes and
beyond. Twin Res. Hum. Genet. 8, 467–482.

Strober, M., Freeman, R., Morrell, W., 1997. The
long-term course of severe anorexia nervosa in
adolescents: survival analysis of recovery,
relapse, and outcome predictors over 10–15
years in a prospective study. Int. J. Eat. Disord.
22, 339–360.

Sullivan, P.F., 1995. Mortality in anorexia
nervosa. Am. J. Psychiatry 152, 1073–1074.

Swinbourne, J.M., Touyz, S.W., 2007. The
co-morbidity of eating disorders and anxiety
disorders: a review. Eur. Eat. Disord. Rev.
15, 253–274.

Treasure, J., 1997. Anorexia nervosa: a survival
guide for families, friends and sufferers.
Psychology Press, Hove.

Treasure, J., Ramsay, R., 1997. Hard to swallow:
compulsory treatment in eating disorders.
Maudsley Discussion Paper. Institute of
Psychiatry, London.

Treasure, J., Smith, G., Crane, A., 2007. Skills
based learning for caring for a loved one with
an eating disorder: the new Maudsley model.
Routledge, London.

Treasure, J.L., Ward, A., 1997. Cognitive
analytic therapy in the treatment of
anorexia nervosa. Clin. Psychol. Psychother.
4, 62–71.

Uher, R., Murphy, T., Brammer, M.J., et al.,
2004. Medial prefrontal cortex activity
associated with symptom provocation in
eating disorders. Am. J. Psychiatry
161, 1238–1246.

Wade, T.D., Tiggemann, M., Bulik, C.M., et al.,
2008. Shared temperament risk factors for
anorexia nervosa: a twin study. Psychosom.
Med. 70, 239–244.

Wentz, E., Gillberg, I.C., Anckarsater, H., et al.,
2009. Adolescent-onset anorexia nervosa:
18-year outcome. Br. J. Psychiatry
194, 168–174.

Williams, G., 1997. Internal landscapes and
foreign bodies: eating disorders and other
pathologies. Tavistock Clinic Series,
Duckworth.

19

Schizophrenia and related disorders

Pádraig Wright   John E. Kraus

CHAPTER CONTENTS

Introduction

Schizophrenia is probably the single most important cause of chronic psychiatric disability. Fully half the beds in Europe's psychiatric hospitals are occupied by those afflicted with it.

Schizotypal, schizoaffective and persistent delusional disorders represent a heterogeneous group of illnesses that possess many of the features of schizophrenia, may be related to it aetiologically and are frequently difficult to distinguish from it clinically.

Schizophrenia

Definition of schizophrenia

In the absence of a biological marker, schizophrenia can only be defined by the nature and persistence of its clinical features (Box 19.1). Indeed, operational diagnostic systems such as the ICD-10 (WHO 1992) or DSM-IV (American Psychiatric Association 1994) require that a number of characteristic symptoms are present for at least 1 month (see Appendices 1 and 2 at the end of this chapter).

History of the concept of schizophrenia

Epilepsy, mania, dementia and depression are described in ancient writings but there are no unambiguous accounts of schizophrenia. Most physicians thought in terms of a unitary psychosis or *Einheitpsychose* until well into the nineteenth century. Thereafter, the concept of schizophrenia evolved through a number of steps. Partially accurate descriptions were provided by Haslam (1764–1844) and Pinel (1745–1826), while the description

However, when these patients were interviewed by psychiatrists associated with the US–UK Diagnostic Project using the Present State Examination, the frequency of schizophrenia was found to be the same in both cities. This result was confirmed by the World Health Organization (WHO) International Pilot Study of Schizophrenia (IPSS) (WHO 1973). However, the World Health Organization 10-country study found that the incidence of broadly defined schizophrenia varied up to four-fold between countries (Jablensky et al 1992).

There is some evidence that the incidence of schizophrenia has varied over time. Hare (1988) suggested that schizophrenia was uncommon before the nineteenth century, that its incidence peaked during the rapid industrialization of the nineteenth and early twentieth centuries, and that it is now again becoming uncommon. In keeping with this proposal, decreasing hospital admission rates for schizophrenia have been reported in the UK, Ireland and Australia. Der et al (1990), for example, examined the Mental Health Enquiry data for England and Wales and reported a 50% decline in first admissions to hospital for schizophrenia over three decades. This apparent reduction in incidence may result from changes in diagnostic practice or in the provision of health services, from improved treatments, or from alterations in background populations. Whether or not schizophrenia exhibits temporal variation remains unknown.

The 'season of birth effect' refers to the well-replicated epidemiological finding that schizophrenic patients are more likely by 7–15% to be born between February and May in the northern hemisphere and between June and October in the southern hemisphere (Mortensen et al 1999). It has been suggested that prenatal exposure to influenza epidemics may explain this finding (see Wright et al 1999 for review).

Sex and age

It is generally accepted that schizophrenia is equally common in males and females and Jablensky (1999) reported an equal cumulated risk for the sexes until the sixth decade of life from the IPSS. However, some investigators found an excess of narrowly defined schizophrenia in males (Hafner et al 1994) and male schizophrenic patients are more likely to experience obstetric complications and to exhibit impaired development during childhood (see below). Male schizophrenic patients are more likely to be hospitalized and are less likely to marry or have children than female patients, although the fertility of female patients is also substantially reduced compared to non-schizophrenic women. These differences may be accounted for by the greater severity of schizophrenia in men and the later onset of illness in women (see below).

Men with schizophrenia are diagnosed most frequently between the ages of 15 and 25 years, while the diagnosis is most likely to be made in women between the ages of 25 and 35 years (Hafner et al 1994). It is exceedingly rare for schizophrenia to be first diagnosed in men after the age of 45 years, while up to 10% of women are first diagnosed after this age (Goldstein et al 1989). Onset of illness between the ages of 40 and 60 has been called 'late-onset schizophrenia' (Howard & Reeves 2003), where the ratio of women to men is 2:1–4:1 (Lehmann 2003).

Social epidemiology

Schizophrenia is commoner in urban areas, in lower socioeconomic groups and in recent immigrants such as the Norwegian immigrants to the USA studied by Ødegaard (1932). These results may be explained by social deprivation and the stresses of immigration increasing the risk of developing schizophrenia. Alternatively, it may be that individuals in the prodromal or pre-psychotic phase of a schizophrenic illness are more likely to become socially or financially dependent, and either to migrate to cheap accommodation in urban centres, or to emigrate. This latter hypothesis, often referred to as 'downward drift', is supported by reports of schizophrenic patients being financially disadvantaged (McNaught et al 1997) and by Marshall's (1994) report that up to 40% of men and 65% of women living in hostels or homeless have schizophrenia. Further support for the hypothesis comes from reports of a higher incidence of schizophrenia in Afro-Caribbeans in the UK than in either the background UK population or in Afro-Caribbeans in Jamaica (Bhugra et al 1997), though this increased risk in black and minority ethnic groups is not entirely explained by socioeconomic status (Kirkbride et al 2008).

Clinical features of schizophrenia

The clinical features of schizophrenia are myriad (Tables 19.4–19.6). It is unusual for individual patients to exhibit more than a few of the vast array of schizophrenia symptoms at any point in time during their illness, and even in the course of a lifetime of schizophrenia it is an exceptional and unfortunate patient who experiences the majority of these symptoms. There is considerable phenomenological overlap in schizophrenia symptoms but they may be conveniently subdivided into delusions, hallucinations, formal thought disorders, passivity phenomena and affective abnormalities, and motor, cognitive and social abnormalities. The individual symptoms within these subdivisions are listed below, and are discussed in more detail in Chapter 6.

Less common features of schizophrenia include obsessive-compulsive symptoms (and indeed obsessive-compulsive disorder is an important differential diagnosis for schizophrenia), violence and aggression, and water intoxication (patients drink water excessively and develop polyuria and hyponatraemia). Seizures, coma and occasional deaths have been reported. The cause of water intoxication in schizophrenia is not known but may include response to delusions or hallucinations, or involvement of the hypothalamo–pituitary axis or other relevant brain structures in the underlying disease process (see Ch. 27).

The IPSS survey undertaken by the WHO determined the commonest symptoms exhibited by schizophrenic patients (WHO 1973; Table 19.4). These are discussed in Chapter 6 but some of them, along with several other schizophrenic symptoms, warrant detailed discussion, either because they are thought to be of specific importance in making a diagnosis of schizophrenia – Schneider's first rank symptoms – or because they are among the symptoms contributing to specific schizophrenic syndromes such as those described by Crow, Andreasen and Liddle.

Table 19.4 Symptoms of schizophrenia: delusions, hallucinations and formal thought disorders

Delusions	Hallucinations	Formal thought disorders[c]
Delusional mood/Wahnstimmung	Auditory	Over-inclusiveness/circumstantiality
Primary (autochthonous)	Somatic[a]	Concrete thinking
Paranoid	Visual[b]	Loosened associations/derailment
Somatic	Tactile[b]	Knight's move/vorbeireden
Religious	Olfactory[b]	Neologisms
Nihilistic	Gustatory[b]	Word salad/verbigeration
Grandiose		Tangentiality, illogicality
Complex/fantastic		Thought block
Pseudoscientific		Poverty of thought content
Mystical		

[a]Somatic hallucinations are not unusual in schizophrenia, are often sexual in nature, and are a component of somatic passivity, a Schneiderian first-rank symptom.
[b]Hallucinations other than auditory or somatic should always raise the suspicion of an organic disorder. Olfactory hallucinations in particular suggest a frontal lobe lesion or temporal lobe epilepsy.
[c]Formal thought disorder must, of necessity, be inferred from the patient's speech.

Table 19.5 Symptoms of schizophrenia: passivity phenomena and affective abnormalities

Passivity phenomena	Affective abnormalities
Thought insertion	Blunted/flattened affect
Thought broadcast	Incongruous affect
Thought withdrawal	Avolition
Made actions	Autism
Made impulses	Anxiety
Made feelings	Euphoria
Somatic passivity	Depression[a]

[a]Depression is common in schizophrenia either because of co-morbidity, side-effects of antipsychotic drugs, response to partial insight into the nature of the illness, or as an intrinsic component of the illness. Depressive symptoms can occur at any time during a schizophrenic illness but are thought to be most prominent in the early years of psychosis and are associated with a poor prognosis, with disease relapse and with suicide.

Schneider's symptoms of the first rank

Schneider considered the 11 symptoms described below to be of first-rank importance in differentiating schizophrenia from similar illnesses. However, while 58% of patients with a diagnosis of acute schizophrenia in the IPSS study did have one or more first-rank symptoms, these symptoms occur in almost 10% of non-schizophrenic patients (WHO 1973), while >20% of schizophrenic patients never exhibit even a single first-rank symptom (Mellor 1970). Schneider's symptoms of the first rank are as follows:

- **Thought insertion:** the patient believes that the thoughts he experiences are not the product of his own mind but have been inserted into it by an external agency, e.g. 'Thoughts are put into my mind by radio transmitters'.
- **Thought broadcast:** the patient believes that her private thoughts are readily available to others, e.g. 'My thoughts are also transmitted into other people's minds'.
- **Thought withdrawal:** the patient experiences an interruption in the flow of his thoughts and his mind is left completely blank, e.g. 'My thoughts were completely removed by something. My mind just stopped and was emptied'.
- **Thought echo:** two types of thought echo occur. In *écho de la pensée* the patient experiences his thoughts after thinking them as if hearing an echo, e.g. 'I think something, and then I hear my mind thinking it again and again'. In *Gedankenlautwerden* the patient experiences his thoughts as if he is hearing them simultaneously to thinking them, e.g. 'I hear myself thinking while I'm doing it'.
- **Delusional perception:** the patient develops a bizarre delusion in response to a real sensory perception, e.g. 'I saw the flower bulbs drop on the steps and immediately knew the manager of the factory was in love with me'.
- **Third-person auditory hallucinations – running commentary:** the patient experiences hallucinatory voices referring to him as 'he', e.g. 'Here he comes. There he goes. He's wearing that old grey coat again'.
- **Third-person auditory hallucinations – voices arguing:** the patient experiences two or more hallucinatory voices referring to her as 'he' in an argumentative manner, e.g. 'She's evil. She's excellent. Evil witch. She's a saint'.
- **Made feelings, impulses and actions:** these three first rank symptoms are experienced as arising without the patient's

volition and are outside his control, e.g. 'I don't hate him. They make me hate him'; 'The echo-rays make me want to move my arms upwards. They move me like a puppet' and 'Something speaks with my mouth and my lips. It's got my voice but it's not me'.

- **Somatic passivity:** the patient experiences bodily sensations in the absence of a stimulus (somatic hallucinations) and attributes these to an external force. Somatic passivity is also referred to as the experience of bodily influence, e.g. 'The radioactive emissions from Mars cause the muscles in my limbs to turn inside out. I can feel them turning all the time'.

Crow's Type 1 and 2 schizophrenia

Crow concluded in 1980 that the only consistently reported abnormality from postmortem investigations of brain tissue from schizophrenic patients was that of increased numbers of dopamine receptors. On the basis of this and other observations, he proposed a division of schizophrenia into a Type 1 and a Type 2 syndrome (Table 19.7). Subsequent research provides evidence that cognitive impairment and tardive dyskinesia occur most commonly in patients with the Type 2 syndrome and are infrequent in those with Type 1 schizophrenia.

Andreasen's positive and negative symptoms of schizophrenia

The division of schizophrenia into two syndromes based on whether symptoms are predominantly positive or negative was originally proposed by Hughlings-Jackson in 1931. Andreasen and Olsen (1982) subsequently provided a set of validated diagnostic criteria that facilitated the subdivision of patients into those with positive, negative or mixed schizophrenia (Box 19.2). The positive and negative symptoms they

Table 19.6 Symptoms of schizophrenia: motor, cognitive and social abnormalities

Motor abnormalities	Cognitive abnormalities	Social abnormalities
Catatonic stupor	Impaired insight	Impaired social skills
Catatonic excitement	Cognitive impairment	Odd appearance
Posturing		Perplexed facies
Flexibilitas cerea (waxy flexibility)		Impaired self-care
Catalepsy		Hoarding
Negativism		
Echopraxia		
Stereotypy		
Mannerisms		
Schnauzkrampf		
Mitmachen		
Mitgehen		
Forced grasping		
Automatic obedience		

Table 19.7 Crow's Type 1 and 2 schizophrenias

	Type 1	Type 2
Characteristic symptoms	Hallucinations, delusions, thought disorder (positive symptoms)	Affective flattening, poverty of speech, loss of drive (negative symptoms)
Type of illness in which most commonly seen	Acute schizophrenia	Chronic schizophrenia, the 'defect' state
Response to neuroleptics	Good	Poor
Outcome	Reversible	?Irreversible
Intellectual impairment	Absent	Sometimes present
Postulated pathological process	Increased dopamine receptors	Cell loss and structural changes in the brain

Box 19.2

Andreasen's positive and negative symptoms of schizophrenia

Positive symptoms

- Hallucinations
  - Auditory
  - Olfactory
  - Visual
- Delusions
  - Persecutory
  - Delusions of jealousy
  - Delusions of sin or guilt
  - Grandiose
  - Religious
  - Somatic ideas/delusions of reference
  - Delusions of being controlled
  - Delusions of mind reading
  - Delusions of thought broadcasting
  - Delusions of thought insertion
  - Delusions of thought withdrawal
- Bizarre behaviour
  - Clothing/appearance
  - Social/sexual
  - Aggressive/agitated
  - Repetitive/stereotyped
- Positive formal thought disorder
  - Derailment (loosened associations)
  - Tangentiality
  - Incoherence (word salad, schizophasia)
  - Illogicality
  - Circumstantiality
  - Pressure of speech
  - Distractible speech
  - Clanging
  - Inappropriate affect

Negative symptoms

- Affective flattening/blunting
  - Unchanging facial expression
  - Decreased spontaneous movement
  - Paucity of expressive gesture
  - Poor eye contact
  - Affective non-responsivity
  - Lack of vocal inflection
- Alogia
  - Poverty of speech
  - Poverty of content of speech
  - Blocking
  - Slow response to questions
- Avolition-apathy
  - Poor grooming and hygiene
  - Impersistence at work or school
  - Physical anergia
- Anhedonia-asociality
  - Few recreational interests/activities
  - Reduced sexual interest/activity
  - Inability to experience intimacy or closeness
  - Impaired relationships with friends and peers
- Attention
  - Social inattentiveness
  - Inattentiveness during mental state examination

---

defined are listed above. Mixed schizophrenia is diagnosed when patients do not meet the criteria for either positive or negative schizophrenia, or meet the criteria for both. Patients with positive-symptom schizophrenia exhibit adequate premorbid adjustment and global functioning, normal cognition and no evidence of cerebral atrophy, while patients with negative-symptom schizophrenia typically demonstrate poor premorbid adjustment, poorer global functioning, impaired cognitive function and cerebral atrophy.

Presentation of schizophrenia

Premorbid schizophrenia

Schizophrenic patients frequently exhibit subtle cognitive, intellectual, linguistic, motor, behavioural and social abnormalities many years before the onset of frank psychosis, termed the schizophrenia prodrome. Such premorbid dysfunction is reported retrospectively in 80–90% of cases by parents, teachers and patients as depression and anxiety, social withdrawal and apathy, odd or eccentric behaviour, suspiciousness and perceptual abnormalities. Jones et al (1995) prospectively confirmed such subjective reports in their study of almost 5000 individuals born in 1946 and subsequently evaluated on 11 occasions before the age of 16 years, and on nine further occasions before the age of 43 years. This research revealed that the 30 children who ultimately developed schizophrenia were: (1) slower in learning to walk; (2) noted by their mothers to prefer solitary play; (3) rated by their teachers as anxious and asocial at the age of 15 years; (4) rated themselves as lacking social confidence at the age of 13 years.

The concept of schizophrenia prodrome has led to efforts to prospectively identify those at ultra high risk (UHR) for schizophrenia, such that early treatment interventions might either prevent onset of frank psychosis or otherwise favourably affect the natural history of the illness. Psychological and pharmacological treatment interventions have been shown to improve symptoms and reduce transition to psychosis (McGorry and Warner 2002; Woods et al 2003). However, only 35–54% of those identified at UHR transition to psychosis over a 12-month period (Nelson et al 2008) and these patients are more sensitive to the adverse effects of antipsychotic drugs. Thus, standard pharmacological treatment cannot yet be recommended. Recently, neuroimaging coupled with clinical findings has been shown to better predict which patients might transition to psychosis (Schobel et al 2009). DSM-V proposes a new category termed Psychosis Risk Syndrome (Carpenter 2009); however, this diagnosis is not without controversy.

Poor performance on cognitive tests, especially non-verbal, verbal and mathematical tests, predicted schizophrenia at all evaluation points throughout childhood. In one study, blinded viewers observing home movies reliably identified children who subsequently developed schizophrenia. This and other studies provide powerful evidence that schizophrenic patients exhibit a range of childhood developmental, cognitive and social impairments when compared with children who either remain healthy or develop non-schizophrenic psychiatric illness. Patients with schizophrenia may present with an acute florid psychosis which develops over a few days or weeks, or following a more insidious onset of disease over many months or even over years. It is therefore clinically useful to differentiate between acute and chronic schizophrenia.

Acute schizophrenia

This may develop rapidly and *de novo* but is not infrequently preceded by a period of days or weeks in duration during which delusional mood (see Ch. 6), increasingly bizarre behaviour and progressively more severe abnormalities of speech and affect occur. These may be accompanied by declining personal, domestic, social and occupational competence. These latter characteristics may be evidenced by poor personal hygiene, failure to clean or change clothing, isolation within the family initially followed by increasingly marked loss of contact with family members and peers, homelessness, unacceptable social behaviour, poor work performance and loss of earning capacity.

Acute schizophrenia is characterized by symptoms that may be described as Schneiderian, Type 1 or positive schizophrenia. Thus auditory hallucinations, persecutory delusions, passivity phenomena and thought disorder are common. Catatonic features may also occur although these appear to be becoming less common in industrialized countries. Abnormalities of affect such as anxiety, depression or euphoria are common, and there is an increased risk of both violence and suicide. Recent studies indicate that the neuropsychological/cognitive deficits associated with schizophrenia are present prior to the first acute episode (Hawkins et al 2008). Insight is almost always impaired and few patients realize that they are ill, attribute their experiences to illness or recognize the need for treatment. Patients with acute schizophrenia may require urgent hospitalization in order to prevent danger to themselves or others, to undertake investigations and to initiate treatment.

Chronic schizophrenia

This is characterized by Bleulerian, Type 2, or negative symptoms. Thus avolition, affective abnormality (including depression), autism and poverty of speech occur. Patients with chronic schizophrenia do not care adequately for themselves and need repeated encouragement to wash, dress and eat. They remain inactive for long periods of time, undertake activities slowly, do not socialize, converse infrequently or are effectively mute, and may be incontinent. Insight is almost always impaired and violence and suicide may occur. Patients with chronic schizophrenia may be unable to live independently and frequently need help in order to ensure basic personal care and to prevent self-neglect.

It is generally accepted that general intellectual function is not compromised in chronic schizophrenia despite the fact that patients perform poorly on almost all cognitive tests. Payne (1973), for example, demonstrated that the mean IQ of 1284 schizophrenic patients was 96 and also provided some evidence of a decline from a normal mean IQ, based on academic and military records. In contrast, Russell et al (1997) reported no change in mean IQ over 20 years in 34 children initially evaluated for childhood psychiatric disorder who subsequently developed schizophrenia (although these individuals did have below-average IQs when first evaluated as children). These results suggest that IQ is below normal at or before the onset of schizophrenia and does not decline thereafter. This view is supported by a report of similar neuropsychological function in newly diagnosed and previously diagnosed patients, but of impaired function in both groups when compared to healthy subjects (Censits et al 1997).

Classification and diagnosis

Classification

The number and variety of symptoms and the variable course of schizophrenia has led to repeated attempts to subtype patients. The classic subtypes of schizophrenia – paranoid, hebephrenic and catatonic – are retained in both ICD-10 and DSM-IV (in which hebephrenia is referred to as disorganized schizophrenia) along with undifferentiated schizophrenia and will now be described (see also Appendices 3 and 4).

Paranoid schizophrenia

This is the commonest subtype and is characterized by prominent delusions (which may or may not be persecutory in content) and hallucinations, usually auditory. Thought disorders, affective abnormality and negative symptoms occur but are not prominent, while the course may be episodic, with partial or complete remission, or chronic.

Hebephrenic (disorganized) schizophrenia

This is characterized by affective abnormality, thought disorder, irresponsible and unpredictable behaviour and mannerisms. Hallucinations and delusions are inconspicuous, avolition and anhedonia common, and the course often one of progressive deterioration.

Catatonic schizophrenia

Psychomotor disturbances ranging from violent excitement to stupor and including posturing, negativism, waxy flexibly, automatic obedience and perseveration characterize this subtype. Visual hallucinations may occur in a dreamlike or oneiroid state.

ICD-10 also includes simple schizophrenia and post-schizophrenic depression as subtypes while both ICD-10 and DSM-IV include residual schizophrenia.

Simple schizophrenia

Negative symptoms develop slowly and progressively and without evidence of delusions or hallucinations. This uncommon subtype is diagnosed very infrequently.

Post-schizophrenic depression

This is characterized by the development of depressive symptoms such that antidepressant treatment is warranted and there is an increased risk of suicide in the aftermath of a schizophrenic episode. Schizophrenic symptoms may persist or be absent and post-schizophrenic depression may be difficult to differentiate from negative symptoms or the adverse effects of treatment. Post-psychotic depression is most common within the first five years of schizophrenia onset.

Residual schizophrenia

Negative symptoms progressively replace delusions, hallucinations and other positive symptoms and there is no evidence that these are caused by depression, dementia or other disorders.

It should be noted that it is often difficult to subtype schizophrenic patients and indeed the IPSS (WHO 1973) found no evidence that subtypes exist. Because of this and for other reasons, research may be conducted on subgroups of patients defined pragmatically, for example on the basis of whether or not they have a schizophrenic relative, respond to treatment, or have normal cerebral ventricles on neuroimaging.

Disorders similar to schizophrenia

These disorders confound the diagnosis of schizophrenia. They include schizotypal, schizoaffective and persistent delusional disorders, which will be discussed later in this chapter, and several other psychotic disorders that are similar to, but do not meet the diagnostic criteria for schizophrenia (Box 19.3). Discussion of these disorders is complicated by the numerous diagnostic terms available. ICD-10 nosology will therefore be used when possible and equivalent or similar diagnostic terms will be provided as appropriate.

Acute and transient psychotic disorders

These disorders significantly disrupt global functioning and are characterized by:

- An associated acute psychological stress, the putative precipitant
- An abrupt (within 48 h of the stress) or acute (within 2 weeks of the stress) onset
- Variable and rapidly changing (or polymorphic) schizophrenia symptoms, usually including delusions and hallucinations that resolve rapidly.

Characteristically, the delusions and hallucinations change in content and sensory modality from day to day or even hour to hour, and are associated with a fluctuating affective state. These disorders are thought to be more common in females and immigrants. Schneiderian first-rank symptoms may occur and it is not infrequently difficult to identify a precipitant. Synonyms for acute and transient psychotic disorders include brief psychotic disorders (DSM-IV), psychogenic psychosis, reactive psychosis, acute paranoid psychosis, *bouffée délirante* and cycloid psychoses.

Box 19.3

Psychiatric and non-psychiatric disorders that may mimic schizophrenia

Psychiatric

- Psychotic disorders
  - Affective psychoses
  - Schizoaffective psychosis
  - Acute and transient psychoses
  - Persistent delusional disorders
  - Cycloid psychoses
  - Induced delusional disorders
- Non-psychotic disorders
  - Schizotypal disorder
  - Personality disorders
  - Obsessive–compulsive disorder
  - Autism/Asperger syndrome
- Drug-induced psychosis
  - Alcoholic hallucinosis
  - Lysergic acid diethylamide (LSD)
  - Amphetamine
  - Cocaine
  - Cannabis
  - Ecstasy
  - Phencyclidine (PCP)
  - Levodopa
  - Steroids

Non-psychiatric

- Neurological disorders
  - Temporal lobe epilepsy
  - Other epilepsies
  - Cerebral tumours
  - Cerebrovascular accidents
  - Huntington disease
  - Dementia
- Infectious disorders
  - Neurosyphilis
  - Herpes encephalitis
  - HIV
- Autoimmune disorders
  - Hyperthyroidism
  - Hypothyroidism
  - Diabetes mellitus
  - Cushing disease/syndrome
  - Systemic lupus erythematosus
- Systemic disorders
  - Metachromatic leucodystrophy
  - Fever
  - Postoperative
  - Postpartum
  - Wilson disease
- Traumatic disorder
  - Head injury.

Induced delusional disorder

These uncommon psychotic disorders consist of delusions, usually persecutory or grandiose, shared by two or more people (*folie à deux*). Delusions are induced in one individual who has as close relationship with and is dependent upon another individual who is psychotic, most often because of schizophrenia. Typically the two individuals are isolated by geography, culture or language, and these factors make for presentation only after prolonged illness. Despite this, induced psychoses usually resolve when the individuals involved are separated.

Diagnosis

There are no diagnostic tests for schizophrenia and the diagnosis must be made on the basis of the presence of typical schizophrenia symptoms for a minimum duration of time and the exclusion of another psychiatric or non-psychiatric cause for the symptoms. Thus both ICD-10 and DSM-IV require that a minimum number of specific symptoms are apparent for at least 1 month and that there is no evidence of either a psychiatric disorder such as affective psychosis, or the effects of alcohol or psychoactive substances, or a disorder such as Huntington disease or hypothyroidism (Appendices 1 and 2).

inherited risk of schizophrenia when they studied the offspring of twins discordant for schizophrenia. They demonstrated that while the risk of schizophrenia was much less in the offspring of unaffected when compared to the offspring of affected dizygotic twins, the risk was similar in the offspring of unaffected when compared to the offspring of affected monozygotic twins. The risk of schizophrenia is greatest when:

- Close relatives are affected
- Several relatives are affected
- Female relatives are affected
- Affected relatives have early-onset schizophrenia
- Affected relatives have severe schizophrenia
- A monozygotic sibling has schizophrenia.

The approximate lifetime risks of schizophrenia for various degrees of genetic relatedness to a schizophrenic individual are shown in Table 19.9 (Gottesman 1991). The risk is highest in the offspring of parents who both have schizophrenia, where up to two thirds of offspring develop a psychiatric illness (Gottesman et al 2010). These data underpin the importance of familial aetiological factors but do not differentiate between genetic and environmental familial effects – environment sharing increases with degree of relatedness and monozygotic twins share the same uterus for the same period of time.

Adoption studies were performed in order to exclude environmental factors in heritability. About 10% of the offspring of schizophrenic individuals who are adopted by non-schizophrenic parents develop schizophrenia (Kety 1983) while there is no increase in schizophrenia among the offspring of healthy individuals adopted by schizophrenic parents (Wender et al 1974). These results clearly favour genetic heritability of the disease.

Molecular genetics

It is extremely unlikely that a single gene is responsible for schizophrenia because it is impossible to assign a classic Mendelian model of inheritance to a disease with monozygotic twin concordance of <100% and in which >60% of patients do not have an affected relative. Single-gene (monogenic or single major locus) genetic models have therefore given way to polygenic (schizophrenia results from the combined effects of several predisposing genes) or polygenic/multifactorial (schizophrenia results from the combined effects of both several predisposing genes and a number of triggering environmental factors) models. An important implication of the polygenic/multifactorial model is that schizophrenia may result from genes alone, from the interaction of genes and environmental insults such as obstetric complications or head injury, or from environmental insults alone, and the clinical picture may differ in each case (Box 19.4). The

Box 19.4

Genetic, genetic/environmental and environmental models of schizophrenia

Genetic
- Patient has close relative(s) with schizophrenia
- Patient inherits sufficient predisposing genes to cause schizophrenia

Genetic/environmental
- Patient may or may not have close relative(s) with schizophrenia
- Patient inherits insufficient predisposing genes to cause schizophrenia
- Patients experience insufficient environmental insults to cause schizophrenia
- The combined effects of insufficient predisposing genes and insufficient environmental insults are sufficient to cause schizophrenia

Environmental
- Patient has no close relative(s) with schizophrenia
- Patient experiences sufficient environmental insults to cause schizophrenia.

Table 19.9 Lifetime schizophrenia risks for degrees of genetic relatedness to a schizophrenic

Relative	Lifetime risk of schizophrenia (%)	Degree of genetic relatedness
(General population)	(1)	(–)
Spouse of patient	2	Unrelated
First cousin of patient	2	3rd
Nephew/niece of patient	4	2nd
Grandchild of patient	5	2nd
Child of patient, other parent healthy	13	1st
Child of patient, other parent with schizophrenia	46	1st
Sibling of patient	9	1st
Sibling of patient, one of patient's parents has schizophrenia	17	1st
Dizygotic twin sibling of patient	17	1st
Monozygotic twin sibling of patient	48	1st
Parent of patient	6	1st

polygenic/multifactorial model is currently the subject of international collaborative efforts to identify the responsible genes and environmental factors (see elsewhere in this volume).

Chromosome 6p24–22 was the focus of much research when the first edition of this volume was published (Mowry et al 1995; see Wright et al 2000 for review). A number of plausible susceptibility genes were reported during the past decade and several of the reports were replicated. The reported associations are as follows:

- The neuregulin 1 (NRG1) gene at chromosome 8p12–21 in Icelandic (Stefansson et al 2002), Scottish (Stefansson et al 2003) and Han Chinese (Li et al 2004) populations
- The dysbindin (DTNBP1) gene at chromosome 6p22 in Irish (Straub et al 2002) and German (Schwab et al 2003) populations
- The novel G72 gene at chromosome 13q34 in French–Canadian and Russian populations (Chumakov et al 2002)
- The D-amino acid oxidase (DAAO) gene at chromosome 12q24 in a French–Canadian population (Chumakov et al 2002)
- The regulator of G protein signalling 4 (RGS4) gene at chromosome 1q21–22 in American and Indian populations (Chowdari et al 2002)
- The proline dehydrogenase (PRODH) gene at chromosome 22q11 (Ma et al 2007)
- The catechol-o-methyltransferase (COMT) gene at chromosome 22q11 (Shifman et al 2002)
- The disrupted in schizophrenia gene 1 (DISC1) at chromosome 1q32–42 in Scottish, Finnish, British, Icelandic and Taiwanese populations (Chubb et al 2008)
- The phosphodiesterase 4B gene (PDE4B) at chromosome 1p31 in Scottish (Pickard et al 2007), Japanese (Numata et al 2008) and Scandinavian (Kähler et al 2010) populations.

Implication of the COMT gene is highly plausible given the dopamine hypothesis of schizophrenia and the role of COMT in degrading dopamine. Implication of the other genes listed above is less obvious. However, schizophrenia is thought to be a neurodevelopmental disorder and NRG1, DTNBP1, DISC1 and RGS4 may play a role in neurodevelopment. Furthermore, the products of many of the genes listed modify glutamatergic neurotransmission and thus the findings may support the glutamate hypothesis of schizophrenia (see Harrison & Owen 2003, for review). Consistent with these concepts, a recent investigation of microdeletions and microduplications in schizophrenic patients revealed mutations that affected signalling networks important in neurodevelopment, including ERBB4, a neuregulin receptor and SLC1A3, a glutamate transporter (Walsh et al 2008).

Neurostructural, neurochemical and neurofunctional brain changes

Neurostructural brain changes

Neuropathological and neuroimaging studies of schizophrenia have a long history. Alzheimer (1913) described cortical atrophy in the brains of some of Kraepelin's patients after death; Jacobi and Winkler reported enlarged ventricles in schizophrenic patients using pneumoencephalography in 1927; Ingvar and Franzen demonstrated hypoperfusion of the frontal cortex using a gamma camera and Xenon-133 in 1974 (Jacobi & Winkler 1927; Ingvar & Franzen 1974). Contemporary research in these fields benefits from both technical innovation and operationalized diagnosis.

The brains of schizophrenic patients weigh slightly less than those of control subjects. Harrison et al (2003), for example, reported that the mean brain weight of 540 schizophrenia subjects was 2% lighter than that of 794 controls. Structural neuroimaging provides evidence that the brains of schizophrenic patients also have slightly larger third and lateral ventricles than brains from age- and sex-matched controls (Lawrie & Abukmeil 1998). Ventricular enlargement is present at disease onset in patients who have not been treated with antipsychotic drugs (Harrison 1999), does not progress, is commoner in patients without a schizophrenic relative, and only occurs in the affected twins of monozygotic twins discordant for disease (Suddath et al 1989).

About 15% of schizophrenic patients have widened sulci and narrowed gyri at postmortem examination, and reduced numbers of neurons and specific subpopulations of neurons have been reported (Akbarian et al 1993). Basal ganglia enlargement may be caused by treatment with older antipsychotic drugs because it is reversed by treatment with clozapine and does not appear to occur in patients treated with clozapine from onset of disease (Chakos et al 1995). Recent evidence suggests that basal ganglia enlargement may be largely confined to male patients (Heitmiller et al 2004).

Bogerts et al (1985) reported smaller hippocampi, parahippocampi and amygdalae in some schizophrenic patients at postmortem and these results have been confirmed with MRI (Suddath et al 1989). Reduced numbers, reduced size and disorientation of the hippocampal pyramidal neurons and heterotopy of parahippocampal pre-alpha cells have also been reported. Recent MRI studies found smaller thalami, hippocampi and superior temporal lobes bilaterally (Flaum et al 1995), and Pakkenberg (1990) has reported reduced numbers of thalamic neurons. Gliosis, a marker of brain insult, was reported in schizophrenic brains by Alzheimer but has largely not been confirmed by modern studies. The neuropathology of schizophrenia has been extensively reviewed by Harrison (1999, 2004) and Harrison et al (2003).

Neurochemical brain changes

Almost every brain chemical has been implicated in an aetiological theory of schizophrenia but only the dopamine, serotonin, excitatory amino acid (EAA) and phospholipid membrane hypotheses merit detailed description. The transmethylation hypothesis warrants brief mention as the first biochemical theory of schizophrenia. It derives from the fact that mescaline, an hallucinogen, is an orthomethylated metabolite of dopamine and proposes that abnormal methylation of brain monoamines produces an endogenous hallucinogen, dimethyl tryptamine. However, while methyl group donors, e.g. methionine, can exacerbate schizophrenia, methyl group acceptors, e.g. nicotinic acid, are not effective antipsychotics.

The dopamine hypothesis

The dopamine hypothesis derives from the data listed in Box 19.5 and states that schizophrenia is caused by excess dopaminergic activity in mesolimbic and cortical brain regions. The

Box 19.5

Research findings supporting the dopamine hypothesis of schizophrenia

- Amphetamine releases dopamine at the synapse and causes positive symptoms of schizophrenia in non-schizophrenic individuals
- Levodopa increases central dopamine concentrations and causes positive symptoms of schizophrenia in non-schizophrenic individuals
- Disulfiram inhibits dopamine metabolism and exacerbates schizophrenia
- All effective antipsychotic drugs are dopamine D_2 receptor antagonists
- Only the a isomer of flupentixol is a D_2 receptor antagonist and an effective antipsychotic; the b isomer is not a D_2 antagonist and is clinically inactive (Johnstone et al 1978)
- Antipsychotic efficacy correlates significantly with D_2 receptor occupancy (Sunahara et al 1993)
- Increased (Wong et al 1986) and asymmetrical (Farde et al 1990) brain D_2 receptor densities have been reported in living schizophrenic patients, using PET
- Increased concentrations of D_2 receptors (Lee & Seeman 1980) and of dopamine (Mackay et al 1982) have been found in postmortem brain tissue from schizophrenic patients.

Box 19.6

Research findings in conflict with the dopamine hypothesis of schizophrenia

- Amphetamine, levodopa and disulfiram do not produce negative schizophrenic symptoms
- Antipsychotic drugs are not exclusively 'anti-schizophrenic' and are effective in other disorders
- Antipsychotic drugs are ineffective in about 30% of patients with schizophrenia
- Antipsychotics block D_2 receptors within hours but antipsychotic efficacy is not apparent for days or weeks
- Normal concentrations of dopamine and D_2 receptors (Gur & Pearlson 1993) have been found in postmortem brain tissue from schizophrenic patients
- Normal brain D_2 receptor densities have been reported in living schizophrenic patients (Farde 1997).

research findings listed in Box 19.6 conflict with the dopamine hypothesis. Nonetheless, the fact that every effective antipsychotic drug blocks dopamine D_2 receptors is powerful evidence of the importance of dopamine in the pathogenesis of schizophrenia. Contemporary investigations of the dopamine hypothesis focus on:

- The influence of dopamine receptor subtypes and their genetic variants on response/non-response to treatment via their relative distributions in various brain structures (Sunahara et al 1993)
- Response/non-response to antipsychotic treatment and D_2 receptor occupancy (Pilowsky et al 1997)

- The role of the D_3 receptor in both the aetiology of schizophrenia and response to antipsychotic drugs (Kerwin & Owen 1999)
- The fast dissociation hypothesis of atypical antipsychotic efficacy and safety, which postulates that while D_2 receptor occupancy is responsible for antipsychotic effect, rapid dissociation from the D_2 receptor (rather than occupancy of $5HT_{2A}$ or other receptors) accounts for extrapyramidal safety (Kapur & Seeman 2001) (see Ch. 39).

The serotonin hypothesis

The serotonin hypothesis states that schizophrenia is caused by excess serotonergic activity in the brain and is based on the two key research findings:

- That lysergic acid diethylamine (LSD) and psilocybin, $5HT_{2A/2C}$ receptor agonists, cause positive symptoms of schizophrenia in non-schizophrenic individuals
- That newer antipsychotics such as clozapine, olanzapine and risperidone are potent $5HT_{2A}$ receptor antagonists.

However, LSD produces visual hallucinations which are uncommon in schizophrenia, older antipsychotics block serotonin receptors and newer antipsychotics are potent D_2 receptor antagonists. Recent investigations suggest that midbrain serotonergic neurons may modulate limbic and cortical dopaminergic systems and several newer antipsychotics have greater affinity at the $5HT_{2A/2C}$ receptor than at the D_2 receptor. Recent investigations of the serotonin hypothesis have concentrated on the influence of serotonin receptor subtypes and their genetic variants on response/non-response to treatment (Arranz et al 1995) and on functional neuroimaging of these receptors in patients treated with various antipsychotic drugs (Busatto & Kerwin 1997).

The excitatory amino acid hypothesis

The EAAs include glutamate and aspartate and the EAA hypothesis of schizophrenia states that insufficient EAAs or their kainate, quisqualate or N-methyl-D-aspartate (NMDA) receptors are implicated in schizophrenia (see Ch. 39). Low cerebrospinal fluid levels of glutamate were reported by Kim et al (1980), and Deakin et al (1989) found reduced numbers of glutamate receptors in temporal cortex from schizophrenic patients. The hypothesis is further supported by the finding that a single dose of phencyclidine (PCP) (a non-competitive NMDA receptor antagonist) can produce positive and negative schizophrenic symptoms in non-schizophrenic individuals and exacerbations of schizophrenia in stable patients, and that kainate and NMDA receptors are reduced in number in postmortem temporal cortex from schizophrenic patients (Royston & Simpson 1991).

The phospholipid membrane hypotheses

The function of neuronal membranes may be modified by alterations in their phospholipid and cholesterol composition. Horrobin (1999) has therefore proposed a phospholipid membrane hypothesis of schizophrenia based on abnormalities of phospholipid metabolism in both brain and red blood cells and clinical trials of omega 3 fatty acids have been undertaken (Emsley et al 2003).

Neurofunctional brain changes

The frontal hypoperfusion reported by Ingvar and Franzen (1974) was confirmed by contemporary PET studies. Over 10 years ago, Sedvall (1990) concluded that PET results in schizophrenia demonstrated decreased brain metabolism overall with particularly decreased frontal metabolism, and increased left-hemisphere metabolism with particularly increased left temporal lobe metabolism. These results appear to be independent of treatment. More recently, Erritzoe et al (2003) reviewed PET and single proton emission tomography (SPET) research and concluded that investigations consistently demonstrated increased presynaptic striatal dopaminergic activity and that this was associated with positive symptoms and a good response to antipsychotic drugs.

Magnetic resonance spectroscopy (MRS) has been used in addition to PET and SPET to study brain function in schizophrenia. Most ^{1}H MRS studies have found reduced N-acetyl-aspartate in frontal and temporal cortex (Cecil et al 1999) while ^{31}P studies have reported reduced phosphomonoesters and increased phosphodiesters (Frangou & Williams 1996). The exact meaning of these findings is unclear at present.

Attempts to correlate symptomatology and functional neuro-imaging data have been undertaken. Thus Liddle et al (1992) reported that each of his three syndromes of chronic schizophrenia was associated with a specific pattern of regional cerebral blood flow (rCBF), while McGuire et al (1993) demonstrated hyperperfusion of Broca's area in patients experiencing auditory hallucinations. This latter work has been extended by Shergill et al (2000) who reported that auditory hallucinations were associated with activation in a network of cortical and subcortical areas (inferior frontal/insular, anterior cingulate and temporal cortex bilaterally, right thalamus and inferior colliculus and left hippocampus and parahippocampal cortex) rather than in a single area.

Functional neuroimaging has also demonstrated that schizophrenic patients show impaired activation of the frontal lobes when undertaking tests of frontal lobe function (Velakoulis & Pantelis 1996) and Rodriguez et al (1996) demonstrated higher rCBF in the thalamus and left basal ganglia of clozapine-responsive schizophrenic patients compared to clozapine non-responders.

Abnormalities of event-related evoked potentials, skin conductance and smooth pursuit (and other) eye movements have been reported in schizophrenic patients and these abnormalities are being increasingly incorporated into models of the disease, of treatment response and of prognosis. For example:

- Jeon and Polich (2003) undertook a meta-analysis of P300 and schizophrenia and concluded that the P300 effect size was of reduced amplitude and greater latency in schizophrenia than in healthy controls, and that the latency effect increases with disease duration.
- Dawson and Schell (2002) reviewed studies of skin conductance and schizophrenia and concluded that abnormally high electrodermal arousal and reactivity is predictive of poor outcome in at least some patients.
- Lee and Williams (2000) reviewed available studies and concluded that dysfunction of smooth pursuit eye movements was a trait marker for schizophrenia and was evident in patients' 1st-degree relatives.

The neurodevelopmental hypothesis of schizophrenia

Neurodevelopmental hypotheses of schizophrenia proposed by Weinberger (1987), Murray and Lewis (1987), Murray (1994) and others state that a proportion of schizophrenia commences with impaired fetal or neonatal neurodevelopment and not with the onset of psychotic symptoms in early adulthood. Support for the neurodevelopmental hypothesis is provided by:

- The excess of structural brain abnormalities and underlying cytoarchitectural anomalies described in schizophrenia (see above)
- The excess of congenital brain abnormalities reported in schizophrenic patients (Lewis et al 1988)
- The increased frequency of craniofacial and dermatoglyphic minor physical anomalies reported in schizophrenia, which is significant because both brain and skin develop from primitive neuroectoderm (Griffiths et al 1998)
- The lower than average IQ and subtle psychomotor, behavioural, personality and social abnormalities described in schizophrenia (see above)
- The nonspecific neurological soft signs that occur in more than 50% of schizophrenic patients, the abnormal smooth pursuit eye movements that occur in patients and their relatives, and the reduced amplitude and greater latency of event-related evoked potentials described in schizophrenic patients.

Environmental factors are implicated in neurodevelopmental schizophrenia because only the schizophrenic members of disease-discordant monozygotic twin pairs exhibit dilated ventricles. Such environmental factors may include obstetric complications, prenatal viral infections and prenatal malnutrition. However, the vast majority of individuals who experience obstetric complications do not develop schizophrenia. The neurodevelopmental hypothesis therefore implicates predisposing genes and states that environmental factors such as obstetric complications and prenatal viral infections cause the neurostructural, neurochemical and neurofunctional brain changes of schizophrenia in genetically predisposed individuals.

The treatment of schizophrenia

The treatment of schizophrenia is largely psychopharmacological. Repeated double-blind trials have demonstrated that antipsychotic drugs both alleviate acute episodes and prevent recurrences of schizophrenia more effectively than either placebo or general tranquillizers (Gilbert et al 1995). More recently, it has been recognized that optimized psychopharmacological treatment also facilitates a range of educational, psychological and social interventions.

General treatment of schizophrenia

Treating acute episodes of schizophrenia

The advantages of hospitalization for many patients with first episodes or any significant relapse of schizophrenia are summarized below (Box 19.7). Antipsychotic (AP) treatment with a single AP drug should be initiated as soon as the diagnosis of schizophrenia

---

Box 19.7

Some advantages of hospitalization in the treatment of schizophrenia

- A period of safe, medication-free observation is possible
- Thorough investigation and definitive diagnosis are facilitated
- Data on personal development, premorbid personality, medical and psychiatric history, education and occupation may be collected and collated
- Social evaluation may be undertaken
- Security and safety may be provided
- Respite is provided to family/relatives
- Antipsychotic treatment may be initiated, dosage titrated and efficacy/safety evaluated, and education of the patient and family/relatives about schizophrenia and its treatment may be undertaken.

---

is established because there is evidence that the duration of untreated psychotic symptoms determines time to recovery, extent of recovery and risk of relapse (Loebel et al 1992). Agitated and/or anxious patients may also require oral or parenteral benzodiazepines. Severely ill patients who are agitated and/or unwilling to accept oral AP therapy may require a parenterally administered antipsychotic drug (see below and Chs 36 and 39).

Atypical AP drugs have been recommended as first-line treatment for almost all patients with schizophrenia by the National Institute for Health and Clinical Excellence (NICE 2002, 2010). Treatment should commence with an adequate dose of a single atypical AP drug. If this is ineffective after 2–3 weeks the dose should be increased and treatment continued for a further 2–3 weeks. If treatment remains ineffective this drug should be discontinued, a second atypical AP drug should be prescribed and the same two-stage process repeated. If the second atypical AP drug proves ineffective, treatment with clozapine should be commenced. If the first atypical AP drug is not tolerated the patient should be switched to a second atypical AP drug. If this is not tolerated the patient should be switched to clozapine. Partial or non-response to AP therapy may indicate:

- Misdiagnosis
- Co-morbidity
- Non-compliance
- Inadequate dosage
- Inadequate duration of treatment
- Concurrent use of psychotomimetic drugs
- Inefficacy.

These problems may be addressed by reassessment of diagnosis and exclusion of co-morbidity, by use of liquid or parenteral preparations to enhance compliance, by increasing dosage, by waiting and/or by careful monitoring to exclude abuse of psychotomimetic drugs. An alternative AP drug should be prescribed if these problems have been addressed and response remains inadequate.

Preventing recurrences of schizophrenia

The relapse rate in untreated schizophrenic patients may be as high as 100% over 1–2 years, so once an acute episode has resolved, virtually all patients should receive maintenance therapy

(Davis 1985). It is well established that risk of recurrence never disappears, even after many years of stability, and maintenance therapy will be lifelong for the great majority of patients (Davis et al 1994). Maintenance AP drugs may be administered orally or by long acting depot injections (see below).

Benzodiazepines may be a useful adjunct to AP drugs for some agitated or anxious patients and adjunctive lithium may be beneficial to patients with affective symptoms. Antidepressant treatment including ECT may be appropriate for patients with post-schizophrenic depression, which is associated with an increased risk of suicide and may be difficult to differentiate from extrapyramidal side-effects or from negative symptoms. Once effective AP maintenance therapy has been established, patients may be discharged from hospital and a range of educational, psychological and social interventions commenced (see below).

Treatment-resistant schizophrenia

The majority of schizophrenic patients respond adequately to AP treatment. However, it has been estimated that approximately 30% respond inadequately and 10% of patients show no response. Many of these patients fulfill the Kane et al (1988) criteria for treatment resistance and have functioned poorly for at least 5 years, have severe psychopathology and have not responded to at least three periods of treatment with AP drugs from at least two different classes of AP in doses equivalent to 1 g of chlorpromazine per day for at least 6 weeks' duration (assuming compliance).

Apparent treatment resistance may be caused by non-compliance, use of psychotomimetic agents, co-morbid illness or disease severity. These causes may be addressed by ensuring compliance (choose drug and dosage that minimizes adverse effects, consider depot formulations), preventing use of psychotomimetic drugs (when possible), treating co-morbid psychiatric or non-psychiatric disease, modifying dosage or changing to another AP from a different chemical class. However, a proportion of patients will remain severely ill, despite these efforts. There is clear evidence that such patients may respond to clozapine (Lieberman et al 1994). This should be commenced – with appropriate haematological monitoring – as soon as treatment resistance is established because outcome is determined by duration of psychosis before effective treatment is instituted (see above).

Primary treatment resistance in which symptoms have never been adequately controlled must be differentiated from secondary treatment resistance in which previously well controlled symptoms suddenly or gradually re-emerge. In patients with secondary treatment resistance consideration must always be given to co-morbid cerebral tumour, dementia or other pathology.

Atypical and typical antipsychotic drugs

Newer or atypical AP drugs such as olanzapine, quetiapine and risperidone have largely replaced older typical AP drugs such as haloperidol in the management of schizophrenia in developed countries. The main advantage atypical AP drugs have over typical AP drugs is their reduced propensity to cause adverse effects. Thus they:

- Are less likely to cause extrapyramidal adverse-effects because they have less affinity for nigrostriatal dopamine D_2 receptors (atypical antipsychotics reduce spontaneous firing in A10 neurons, typical antipsychotics reduce firing in both A9 and A10 neurons)
- Are less likely to cause hyperprolactinaemia and associated adverse effects because they have less affinity for tuberoinfundibular dopamine D_2 receptors
- Have relatively high serotonin $5HT_{2A}$ to dopamine D_2 receptor binding ratios.

Atypical and typical antipsychotic drugs are equally effective against positive symptoms. Atypical AP drugs may be somewhat more effective in treating negative, affective and cognitive symptoms (Bilder et al 2002). As noted above, NICE has recommended atypical AP drugs for almost all patients with schizophrenia. However, typical AP drugs have a place in the treatment of patients who have responded to them previously. Furthermore, a randomized controlled trial of 1500 patients with schizophrenia treated with either typical (perphenazine) or atypical (olanzapine, quetiapine, risperidone, ziprasidone) AP drugs, the CATIE study, found that differences between them were modest: 64% of olanzapine, 74% of risperidone, 75% of perphenazine, 79% of ziprasidone and 82% of quetiapine treated patients discontinued treatment before 18 months (Lieberman et al 2005).

Rapidly acting intramuscular injections

Patients who are agitated and/or unwilling to accept oral antipsychotic therapy may require a rapidly acting parenterally administered AP drug. Such a requirement no longer necessitates the use of typical AP drugs because rapidly acting intramuscular formulations of aripiprazole and olanzapine are now available in the UK (Wright et al 2001). An intramuscular formulation of ziprasidone is also available in a number of countries (Brook 2003). Intramuscular formulations of atypical AP drugs are much less likely to cause acute dystonia and other extrapyramidal adverse effects. This reduces the distress experienced by patients during what is an already highly distressing period and may facilitate the patient/doctor relationship and long-term adherence to prophylactic AP therapy. NICE have made the following important treatment recommendations about the care of schizophrenic patients who are agitated (2002; see also Ch. 39):

- Oral administration of medication is preferred to parenteral administration.
- Intramuscular administration of medication is preferred to intravenous administration.
- The intramuscular drugs recommended are haloperidol, lorazepam and olanzapine.
- A single drug is preferred to a combination of drugs whenever possible.
- If haloperidol (or another typical AP drug) is administered intramuscularly, an anticholinergic drug should also be administered in order to reduce the risk of acute dystonia and other extrapyramidal side-effects.

Long-acting intramuscular injections

Patients who adhere poorly to long-term prophylactic AP therapy may benefit from a long-acting or depot parenterally administered antipsychotic drug. Such a requirement no longer

necessitates the use of typical antipsychotic drugs because depot formulations of olanzapine and risperidone are now available in the UK (Hosalli & Davis 2003).

An algorithm for the psychopharmacological treatment of schizophrenia is presented in Figure 19.1. In using this treatment algorithm, the term efficacy refers not only to adequate control of positive symptoms but also to significant alleviation of negative and affective symptoms. Isolated control of positive symptoms may therefore warrant a change of treatment if negative or affective symptoms persist.

Extrapyramidal syndromes: side-effects of antipsychotic drugs or symptoms of schizophrenia?

The principal adverse effects of AP drugs are discussed in Chapter 39. Acute dystonia, parkinsonism, akathisia, tardive dyskinesia and neuroleptic malignant syndrome may be a component of the schizophrenia syndrome because they were described before the advent of AP drugs and have been reported in schizophrenic patients who have never been treated with AP drugs (Waddington 1989). However, typical AP drugs greatly increase risk for these disorders.

Acute dystonia (fixed contortions of the muscles of the head, neck and upper limbs) occurs immediately or within a few days of treatment with an AP drug, especially in young male patients. Parkinsonism (bradykinesia, mild rigidity and tremor) may only develop after many weeks of treatment and is commonest in older female patients. Both may be treated by anticholinergic/antimuscarinic drugs (which rapidly alleviate acute dystonia if administered parenterally) and/or reducing antipsychotic dosage. Prophylactic anticholinergic treatment should be avoided as it may lead to dependency and may be associated with increased risk of tardive dyskinesia. Akathisia (distressing psychological restlessness and undirected movement) usually develops during the first few days or weeks of treatment.

Tardive dyskinesia is a syndrome of abnormal involuntary movements, typically choreoathetoid and usually complex, rapid and stereotyped. Choreiform lip pursing, tongue protrusion and sucking and chewing movements occur in 80% of cases. Limbs are less often affected and trunk muscles and muscles of respiration only rarely. Patients are often unaware of the movements or are able to suppress them if requested to do so, and are free of them when sleeping. Risk factors for tardive dyskinesia include antipsychotic drugs, increasing age, female sex, organic brain damage and diabetes mellitus. The incidence of tardive dyskinesia is about 5% per year, and the prevalence between 20% and 25%, in patients receiving AP treatment. Aetiological theories, which do not explain the preferential involvement of orofacial muscles, include striatal dopamine receptor supersensitivity (long-term administration of AP causes partial blockade of dopamine receptors which then compensate physiologically by becoming supersensitive to available dopamine), dopaminergic excess/cholinergic deficiency and/or free radical cytotoxicity. There is no effective treatment for tardive dyskinesia and reducing dosage of or discontinuing AP drugs may exacerbate the disorder. However, the risk of tardive dyskinesia is significantly less with clozapine and transfer of patients from typical antipsychotics to clozapine or another atypical AP is a useful treatment strategy.

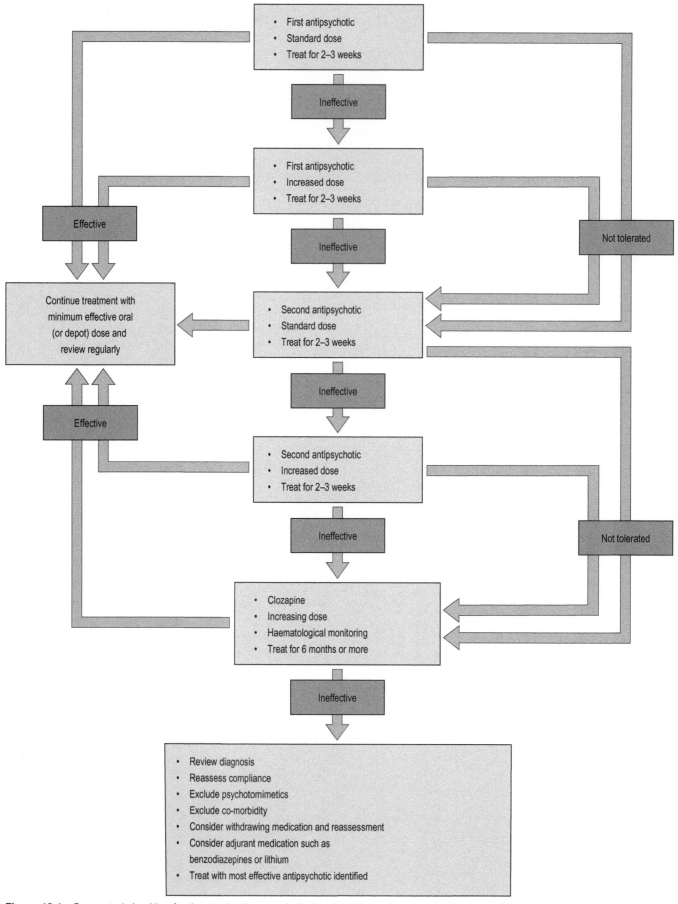

Figure 19.1 • Suggested algorithm for the psychopharmacological treatment of schizophrenia. The terms first and second antipsychotic ideally refer to two different atypical antipsychotics (e.g. olanzapine followed by risperidone). In less ideal circumstances, these terms may also refer to a typical and an atypical antipsychotic (e.g. haloperidol followed by olanzapine) or to two typical antipsychotics from two different classes (e.g. chlorpromazine followed by haloperidol). Clozapine should be reserved for treating patients who are treatment resistant or intolerant. The term (or depot) is used because some patients must currently be treated with depot typical antipsychotics and because depot atypical antipsychotics are not widely available.

The neuroleptic malignant syndrome consists of extrapyramidal symptoms (rigidity), fluctuating consciousness (delirium, stupor) and autonomic lability (hyperthermia, tachycardia, hypo- or hypertension, sweating, pallor, salivation and urinary incontinence). It is rare, most often develops within a few weeks of initiating or altering AP therapy, and has a mortality rate of 10–20%. Marked elevation of creatinine phosphokinase occurs and aldolase, liver enzymes and white cells may also be raised. Thromboembolism and renal failure caused by myoglobinuria secondary to muscle necrosis are common and if untreated, death may occur from cardiovascular collapse, respiratory failure or secondary pneumonia (see Ch. 39).

Educational, psychological and social interventions in schizophrenia

Education of patients and their relatives about schizophrenia and its treatment represents good clinical practice and should occur on an ongoing basis. Patients and their relatives should also be advised about and referred to appropriate support organizations.

Cognitive therapy (see Ch. 38) may focus on the alleviation of individual psychotic symptoms or on the global treatment of schizophrenia. The alleviation of auditory hallucinations by treating them as negative automatic thoughts, and of delusions by challenging their inherent illogicality by repeated questioning has been reported (see, e.g. Shergill et al 1998). Controlled trials of cognitive therapy in the global treatment of schizophrenia have been undertaken by Kemp et al (1996), who reported improved compliance and global functioning and by Garety et al (1994), who reported reduced general symptomatology and improved social functioning in drug-resistant psychosis. It seems likely that as these techniques develop they will be combined with psychopharmacology and that specific patients and/or psychotic symptoms will be targeted.

Brown et al (1962) found that schizophrenic patients were more likely to relapse if discharged to families exhibiting 'high expressed emotion' (hostility, critical comments and emotional over-involvement), especially if they were exposed to these families for more than 35 h per week. Relapse was much less likely in low-expressed emotion families or families that expressed warmth and positive remarks. Leff et al (1985) demonstrated the interaction between expressed emotion and antipsychotic medication in schizophrenic relapse (Table 19.10), and in a controlled trial, they also showed the effectiveness of family intervention therapy consisting of education about schizophrenia and its treatment, communication training and

Table 19.10 The interaction between relapse rates in schizophrenia, exposure to high-expressed emotion (EE) for <35 or >35 h per week, and treatment with antipsychotic medication

	Low EE	High EE	
		<35 h	>35 h
Antipsychotic	12%	15%	53%
No antipsychotic	15%	42%	92%

support for relatives, in alleviating the effects of high expressed emotion (see also Ch. 7).

Course and outcome in schizophrenia

Course

Perhaps 20% of patients who initially receive a diagnosis of schizophrenia experience a single acute episode, recover fully, and thereafter lead a reasonably fulfilling life. Other patients (particularly males) experiencing a similar acute episode may remain institutionalized and have a life of chronic psychosis punctuated by frequent exacerbations of illness or ended prematurely by suicide. This variability in course and outcome may occur because:

- Patients who experienced favourable outcomes were incorrectly diagnosed and did not have schizophrenia
- Patients receive different treatments or respond differentially to the treatments they receive
- Schizophrenia is a heterogeneous group of psychotic illnesses with variable prognoses, or
- The course and outcome of schizophrenia, in common with many other diseases, is extremely variable.

Irrespective of the cause of these variations, it is generally accepted that schizophrenia follows one of the four courses described by Shepherd et al (1989) in their report of a 5-year follow-up study of 49 schizophrenic patients (Table 19.11).

Outcome

Schizophrenia is traditionally thought of as a disease characterized by progressive deterioration – the dementia of dementia praecox. However, it may be that this deterioration is caused by institutionalization or medication. Schizophrenic patients scored at least 2 standard deviations below the mean for a chronically hospitalized physically ill comparison sample on a range of clinical cognitive tests (Owens & Johnstone 1980) and this

Table 19.11 The course of schizophrenia

Course	Symptoms	Interepisodic impairment	Patients (%)
Course 1	Single episode of acute schizophrenia	No residual impairment	22
Course 2	Recurrent episodes	No or slight impairment	35
Course 3	Recurrent episodes	Significant, non-progressive impairment	8
Course 4	Recurrent episodes	Significant, progressive impairment	35

Wallace et al (2004) recently compared criminal convictions in 2861 people with schizophrenia and an equal number of control subjects over a 25-year period in the Australian state of Victoria. Schizophrenic patients had more criminal convictions overall and were more likely to have been convicted of both any criminal offense (21.6% vs 7.8%) and a violent offence (8.2% vs 1.8%). Furthermore, criminal conviction was more likely in patients with substances abuse problems than in those without (68.1% vs 11.7%).

Apart from the crimes themselves, schizophrenia cost the English criminal justice system £1 million in 2004/2005 (Mangalore & Knapp 2007).

Schizotypal disorder

Schizotypal disorder is characterized by eccentric behaviour and unusual thinking and affect. It resembles schizophrenia but characteristic schizophrenic symptoms do not occur. Typical symptoms of schizotypal disorder include eccentricity and aloofness, social withdrawal, paranoid quasi-delusional ideas, magical thinking, obsessive ruminations, depersonalization and derealization, visual and somatic illusions, metaphorical and over-elaborate speech, and transient auditory hallucinations.

Schizotypal disorder is commoner in individuals with a schizophrenic relative and is usually thought of as a schizophrenia spectrum disorder. It behaves like a personality disorder (and indeed is classified as such in DSM-IV) with no clear time of onset, a chronic course with fluctuating intensity of symptoms, and no acute episodes or periods of remission. Schizotypal disorder may occasionally progress to schizophrenia in which case it should probably be retrospectively rediagnosed as prodromal schizophrenia.

Schizoaffective disorder

Differentiating between schizophrenia and affective disorder is often difficult because many symptoms, including Schneiderian first-rank symptoms, are common to both schizophrenia and affective disorder and because depression commonly occurs with schizophrenia. Schizoaffective disorder may be diagnosed when schizophrenic and affective symptoms are episodically, equally and simultaneously prominent. Patients with schizoaffective disorder have an excess of relatives with affective psychosis and the disorder may be thought of as either a schizophrenia spectrum or an affective spectrum disorder.

Schizophrenic symptoms may coexist with manic, depressive or both manic and depressive symptoms in schizoaffective disorder. Schizomanic disorders are associated with a family history of affective disorders, are usually florid with grossly disturbed behaviour; negative symptoms rarely evolve and patients respond to mood-stabilizing drugs and recover rapidly. Schizodepressive disorders are associated with a family history of schizophrenia, are markedly less florid, patients may develop chronic negative symptoms and response to treatment is variable. Mixed schizoaffective disorder is said to be present when schizophrenic, depressive and manic symptoms coexist.

Persistent delusional disorders

Persistent delusional disorders may occur in isolation or within the context of a schizophrenic or other psychosis and may be conveniently classified into eponymous and non-eponymous groups (Table 19.13). The eponymous disorders are described in Chapter 23, while the non-eponymous disorders will be discussed here. These disorders are characterized by a persistent, often lifelong, non-bizarre delusion or set of related delusions, most usually arising insidiously in midlife or later. Transient auditory hallucinations may occur but schizophrenic symptoms are incompatible with the pure diagnosis. Affect, thought and behaviour are globally normal but patients' attitudes and actions in response to their delusions are appropriate and may lead to dangerousness in disorders such as Othello syndrome.

Paranoia and paraphrenia are controversial entities that were separated from dementia praecox by Kraepelin, who described paranoia as a persistent systematized delusion arising in later life without evidence of either hallucinations or a deteriorating course, and paraphrenia as an identical syndrome to paranoia but with hallucinations. Kretschmer (1927) considered paranoia a reaction to stress in predisposed individuals (*Der sensitive Beziehungswahn*) while ICD-10 classifies paranoia, (late) paraphrenia and *Der sensitive Beziehungswahn* as persistent delusional disorders that require symptoms of at least 3 months' duration for their diagnosis.

Delusional dysmorphophobia and paranoia querulans are also included as persistent delusional disorders in ICD-10. Patients with delusional dysmorphophobia are convinced that some physical feature, usually of their head or of a secondary sexual characteristic, is abnormal in shape or size and may repeatedly seek cosmetic surgery to correct the imagined deformity (see Chapter 17). Paranoia querulans is characterized by repeated and prolonged litigation, most often against local or national government authorities, following an imagined or minor event. Some patients in this category undertake elaborate social, religious or political missions and may behave violently towards their imagined opponents.

The treatment of persistent delusional disorders is extremely difficult – patients lack insight and may interpret attempts to help as persecution. Assessment of dangerousness (Ch. 36) is extremely important and compulsory admission may be required. Antipsychotic, anxiolytic and mood-stabilizing drugs may be useful.

Table 19.13 Eponymous and non-eponymous persistent delusional disorders

Eponymous	Non-eponymous
de Clerambault syndrome (erotomania)	Paranoia
Othello syndrome (morbid jealousy)	(Late) paraphrenia
Capgras syndrome (*l'illusion des sosies*)[a]	*Der sensitive Beziehungswahn*
Ekbom syndrome (delusion of infestation)	Delusional dysmorphophobia
Fregoli syndrome	Paranoia querulans

[a]Literally 'illusion of doubles'; delusion of doubles is a more accurate phenomenological description.

References

Akbarian, S., Vinuela, A., Kim, J.J., 1993. Distorted distribution of nicotinamide adenine-dinucleotide phosphate diaphorase neurons in temporal lobe of schizophrenics implies anomalous cortical development. Arch. Gen. Psychiatry 50, 178–187.

Alzheimer, A., 1913. Beitrage zur pathologischen Anatomie der Dementia praecox. Allgemeine Zeitschift fur Psychiatrie und gerichtliche Medizin 70, 810–812.

American Psychiatric Association, 1994. Diagnostic and Statistical Manual of Mental Disorders, fourth ed. APA, Washington DC.

Andreasen, N.C., Olsen, S., 1982. Negative v positive schizophrenia. Am. J. Psychiatry 39, 789–794.

Arranz, M., Collier, D., Sodhi, M., 1995. Association between clozapine response and allelic variation in the 5HT2A receptor gene. Lancet 346, 281–282.

Bateson, G., Jackson, D., Haley, J., et al., 1956. Towards a theory of schizophrenia. Behav. Sci. 1, 251–264.

Bhugra, D., Leff, J., Mallett, R., et al., 1997. The first contact of patients with schizophrenia with psychiatric services: social factors and pathways to care in a multiethnic population. Psychol. Med. 29, 475–483.

Bilder, R.M., Goldman, R.S., Volavka, J., et al., 2002. Neurocognitive effects of clozapine, olanzapine, risperidone, and haloperidol in patients with chronic schizophrenia or schizoaffective disorder. Am. J. Psychiatry 159, 1018–1028.

Bleuler, E., 1911. Dementia praecox or the group of schizophrenias (translated edition 1950). International University Press, New York.

Bogerts, B., Meertz, E., Schonfeldt-Bausch, R., 1985. Basal ganglia and limbic system pathology in schizophrenia. A morphometric study of brain volume and shrinkage. Arch. Gen. Psychiatry 42, 784–791.

Brook, S., 2003. Intramuscular ziprasidone: moving beyond the conventional in the treatment of acute agitation in schizophrenia. J. Clin. Psychiatry 64 (Suppl. 19), 13–18.

Brown, A.S., Derkits, E.J., 2010. Prenatal infection and schizophrenia: a review of epidemiologic and translational studies. Am. J. Psychiatry 167, 261–280.

Brown, G.W., Birley, J.L., 1968. Crisis and life change at the onset of schizophrenia. J. Health Soc. Behav. 9, 203–224.

Brown, G.W., Monck, E.M., Carstairs, G.M., et al., 1962. Influence of family life on the cause of schizophrenia. Br. J. Prev. Soc. Med. 16, 55–68.

Busatto, G.F., Kerwin, R.W., 1997. Perspectives on the role of serotonergic mechanisms in the pharmacology of schizophrenia. J. Psychopharmacol. 11, 3–12.

Carpenter, W.T., 2009. Anticipating DSM-V: should psychosis risk become a diagnostic class? Schizophr. Bull. 35, 841–843.

Cecil, K.M., Lenkinski, R.E., Gur, R.E., et al., 1999. Proton magnetic resonance spectroscopy in the frontal and temporal lobes of neuroleptic naive patients with schizophrenia. Neuropsychopharmacology 20, 131–140.

Censits, D.M., Ragland, J.D., Gur, R.C., et al., 1997. Neuropsychological evidence supporting a neurodevelopmental model of schizophrenia: a longitudinal study. Schizophr. Res. 24, 289–298.

Chakos, M.H., Lieberman, J.A., Alvir, J., 1995. Caudate nuclei volumes in schizophrenic patients treated with typical antipsychotics and clozapine. Lancet 345, 456–457.

Chowdari, K.V., Mirnics, K., Semwal, P., et al., 2002. Association and linkage analyses of RGS4 polymorphisms in schizophrenia. Hum. Mol. Genet. 11, 1373–1380.

Chubb, J.E., Bradshaw, N.J., Soares, D.C., et al., 2008. The DISC locus in psychiatric illness. Mol. Psychiatry 13, 36–64.

Chumakov, I., Blumenfeld, M., Guerassimenko, O., et al., 2002. Genetic and physiological data implicating the new human gene G72 and the gene for D-amino acid oxidase in schizophrenia. Proc. Natl. Acad. Sci. U.S.A. 99, 13675–13680.

Cooper, J.E., Kendell, R.E., Gurland, B.J., et al., 1972. Psychiatric diagnosis in New York and London. Maudsley Monograph no. 20. Oxford University Press, London.

Crow, T.J., 1980. Molecular pathology of schizophrenia: more than one disease process. Br. Med. J. i, 66–69.

Davis, J.M., 1985. Maintenance therapy and the natural course of schizophrenia. J. Clin. Psychiatry 46, 18–21.

Davis, J.M., Metalon, L., Watanabe, M.D., 1994. Depot antipsychotic drugs: place in therapy. Drugs 47, 741–773.

Dawson, M.E., Schell, A.M., 2002. What does electrodermal activity tell us about prognosis in the schizophrenia spectrum? Schizophr. Res. 54, 87–93.

Deakin, J.F.W., Slater, P., Simpson, M.D.C., 1989. Frontal cortical and left temporal glutamatergic dysfunction in schizophrenia. J. Neurochem. 52, 1781–1786.

Der, G., Gupta, S., Murray, R.M., 1990. Is schizophrenia disappearing? Lancet 335, 513–516.

Emsley, R., Oosthuizen, P., van Rensburg, S.J., 2003. Clinical potential of omega-3 fatty acids in the treatment of schizophrenia. CNS Drugs 17, 1081–1091.

Erritzoe, D., Talbot, P., Frankle, W.G., et al., 2003. Positron emission tomography and single photon emission CT molecular imaging in schizophrenia. Neuroimaging Clin. N. Am. 13, 817–832.

Evans, J.J., Chua, S.E., McKenna, P.J., et al., 1997. Assessment of the dysexecutive syndrome in schizophrenia. Psychol. Med. 27, 635–646.

Farde, L., 1997. Brain imaging of schizophrenia – the dopamine hypothesis. Schizophr. Res. 28 (2–3), 157–162.

Farde, L., Wiesle, F.A., Stone-Elander, S., 1990. D2 dopamine receptors in neuroleptic naive schizophrenic patients. Arch. Gen. Psychiatry 47, 213–219.

Faris, R.E.L., Dunham, H.W., 1939. Mental disorders in urban areas. Chicago University Press, Chicago.

Flaum, M., Swayze, V.W., O'Leary, D.S., 1995. Effects of diagnosis, laterality and gender on brain morphology in schizophrenia. Am. J. Psychiatry 152, 704–111.

Frangou, S., Williams, S.C., 1996. Magnetic resonance spectroscopy in psychiatry: basic principles and applications. Br. Med. Bull. 52, 474–485.

Garety, P.A., Kuipers, L., Fowler, D., et al., 1994. Cognitive behaviour therapy for drug resistant psychosis. Br. J. Med. Psychol. 67, 259–271.

Gilbert, P., Harris, M.J., McAdams, L.A., 1995. Neuroleptic withdrawal in schizophrenic patients: a review of the literature. Arch. Gen. Psychiatry 52, 173–188.

Gilmore, J.H., Fredrik Jarskog, L., Vadlamudi, S., et al., 2004. Prenatal infection and risk for schizophrenia: IL-1beta, IL-6, and TNFalpha inhibit cortical neuron dendrite development. Neuropsychopharmacology 29, 1221–1229.

Goldberg, E.M., Morrison, S.L., 1963. Schizophrenia and social class. Br. J. Psychiatry 109, 785–802.

Goldstein, J.M., Tsuang, M.T., Farone, S.V., 1989. Gender and schizophrenia: implications for understanding the heterogeneity of the illness. Psychiatry Res. 28, 243–253.

Gottesman, I.I., 1991. Schizophrenia genesis: the origins of madness. Freeman, New York.

Gottesman, I.I., Bertelsen, A., 1989. Confirming unexpressed genotypes for schizophrenia. Risks in the offspring of Fischer's Danish identical and fraternal discordant twins. Arch. Gen. Psychiatry 46, 867–872.

Gottesman, I.I., Laursen, T.M., Bertelsen, A., et al., 2010. Severe mental disorders in offspring with 2 psychiatrically ill parents. Arch. Gen. Psychiatry 67, 252–257.

Griffiths, T.D., Sigmundsson, T., Takei, N., et al., 1998. Minor physical anomalies in familial and sporadic schizophrenia: the Maudsley family study. Journal of Neurology and Psychiatry 61, 56–60.

Gur, R.E., Pearlson, G., 1993. Neuroimaging in schizophrenia research. Schizophr. Bull. 19, 337–353.

Hafner, H., Boker, W., 1982. Crimes of violence by mentally abnormal offenders (H. Marshall, Trans.). Cambridge University Press, Cambridge.

Hafner, H., Reimann, H., 1970. Spatial distribution of mental disorders in Mannheim. In: Hare, E.H., Wing, J.K. (Eds.), Psychiatric epidemiology. Oxford University Press, London.

Hafner, H., Maurer, K., Loefler, 1994. The epidemiology of early schizophrenia: influence of age and gender on onset and early course. Br. J. Psychiatry 164 (Suppl. 23), 29–38.

Hall, W., Degenhardt, L., Teesson, M., 2004. Cannabis use and psychotic disorders: an update. Drug Alcohol Rev. 23, 433–443.

Hare, E., 1988. Schizophrenia as a recent disease. Br. J. Psychiatry 153, 521–531.

Harrison, P.J., 1999. The neuropathology of schizophrenia. A critical review of the data and their interpretation. Brain 122, 593–624.

Harrison, P.J., 2004. The hippocampus in schizophrenia: a review of the neuropathological evidence and its pathophysiological implications. Psychopharmacology (Berl.) 174, 151–162.

Harrison, P.J., Owen, M.J., 2003. Genes for schizophrenia? Recent findings and their pathophysiological implications. Lancet 361, 417–419.

Harrison, P.J., Freemantle, N., Geddes, J.R., 2003. Meta-analysis of brain weight in schizophrenia. Schizophr. Res. 64, 25–34.

Hawkins, K.A., Keefe, R.S., Christensen, B.K., et al., 2008. Neuropsychological course in the prodrome and first episode of psychosis: findings from the PRIME North America Double Blind Treatment Study. Schizophr. Res. 105, 1–9.

Hebephrenia, 1871. A contribution to clinical psychiatry by Dr. Ewald Hecker in Görlitz.

Heila, H., Isometsa, E.T., Henriksson, M.M., et al., 1997. Suicide and schizophrenia: a nationwide psychological autopsy study on age and sex specific clinical characteristics of 92 suicide victims with schizophrenia. Am. J. Psychiatry 154, 1235–1242.

Heitmiller, D.R., Nopoulos, P.C., Andreasen, N.C., 2004. Changes in caudate volume after exposure to atypical neuroleptics in patients with schizophrenia may be sex-dependent. Schizophr. Res. 66, 137–142.

Hollingshead, A.B., Redlich, F.C., 1958. Social class and mental illness: a community study. J. Psychosom. Res. 11, 213–218.

Horrobin, D.F., 1999. Lipids and schizophrenia. Br. J. Psychiatry 175, 88.

Hosalli, P., Davis, J.M., 2003. Depot risperidone for schizophrenia. Cochrane Database Syst. Rev. (4), CD004161.

Howard, R., Reeves, S., 2003. Psychosis and schizophrenia-like disorders in the elderly. J. Nutr. Health Aging 7, 410–411.

Ingvar, D.H., Franzen, G., 1974. Abnormalities of cerebral blood flow distribution in patients with chronic schizophrenia. Acta Psychiatr. Scand. 50, 425–462.

Jablensky, A., 1999. The concept of schizophrenia: pro et contra. Epidemiol. Psichiatr. Soc. 8, 242–247.

Jablensky, A., Sartorius, N., Ernberg, G., et al., 1992. Schizophrenia: manifestations, incidence and course in different cultures. A World Health Organization ten-country study. Psychol. Med. Monogr. Suppl. 20, 1–97.

Jacobi, W., Winkler, H., 1927. Encephalographische Studien auf chronisch schizophrenen. Arch. Psychiatr. Nervenkr. 81, 299–332.

Jacobs, S., Myers, J., 1976. Recent life events and acute schizophrenia psychosis: a controlled study. J. Nerv. Ment. Dis. 162, 75–87.

Jaspers, K., 1913. General Psychopathology - Volumes 1 & 2.

Jeon, Y.W., Polich, J., 2003. Meta-analysis of P300 and schizophrenia: patients, paradigms, and practical implications. Psychophysiology 40, 684–701.

Johnstone, E.C., Crow, T.J., Frith, C.D., et al., 1978. Mechanism of the antipsychotic effect in the treatment of acute schizophrenia. Lancet i, 848–851.

Jones, P.B., Murray, R.M., Rodgers, B., 1995. Childhood risk factors for adult schizophrenia in a general population birth cohort at age 43 years. In: Mednick, S.A., Hollister, J.M. (Eds.), Neural development and schizophrenia. Plenum Press, New York.

Kahlbaum, K.L., 1863. Die Gruppierung der psychischen Krankheiten und die Eintheilung der Seelenstörungen: Entwurf einer historisch-kritischen Darstellung der bisherigen Eintheilungen und Versuch zur Anbahnung einer empirisch-wissenschaftlichen Grundlage der Psychiatrie als klinischer Disciplin. Danzig: Kafemann.

Kähler, A.K., Otnaess, M.K., Wirgenes, K.V., et al., 2010. Association study of PDE4B gene variants in Scandinavian schizophrenia and bipolar disorder multicenter case-control samples. Am. J. Med. Genet. B Neuropsychiatr. Genet. 153B, 86–96.

Kane, J., Honigfeld, G., Singer, J., 1988. Clozapine for the treatment resistant schizophrenia: a double blind comparison with chlorpromazine. Arch. Gen. Psychiatry 45, 789–796.

Kapur, S., Seeman, P., 2001. Does fast dissociation from the dopamine D2 receptor explain the action of atypical antipsychotics? A new hypothesis. Am. J. Psychiatry 158, 360–369.

Kemp, R., Hayward, P., Applewhaite, G., et al., 1996. Compliance therapy in psychotic patients: randomised controlled trial. Br. Med. J. 312, 345–349.

Kerwin, R., Owen, M., 1999. Genetics of novel therapeutic targets in schizophrenia. Br. J. Psychiatry 38 (Suppl.), 1–4.

Kety, S., 1983. Mental illness in the biological and adoptive relatives of schizophrenic adoptees: findings relevant to genetic and environmental factors in etiology. Am. J. Psychiatry 140, 720–727.

Kim, J.S., Kornhuber, H.H., Schmidt-Burgk, W., et al., 1980. Low cerebrospinal fluid glutamate in schizophrenic patients and a new hypothesis of schizophrenia. Neurosci. Lett. 400, 330–344.

Kirkbride, J.B., Barker, D., Cowden, F., et al., 2008. Psychoses, ethnicity and socio-economic status. Br. J. Psychiatry 193, 18–24.

Kraepelin, E., 1893. Psychiatrie: Ein kurzes Lehrbuch fur Studirende und Aerzte. Vierte, vollstandig umgearbeitete Auflage. Leipzig: Abel Verlag.

Kraepelin, E., 1896. Psychiatrie. Ein Lehrbuch fur Studierende und Arzte. 5, Auflage. A. Abel, Leipzig.

Kraepelin, E., 1919. Dementia praecox and paraphrenia. Churchill Livingstone, Edinburgh.

Kretschmer, E., 1927. Der sensitive Beziehungswahn. In: Hirsch, S.R., Shepherd, M. (Eds.), Themes and variations in European psychiatry. Wright, Bristol.

Lawrie, S.M., Abukmeil, S.S., 1998. Brain abnormality in schizophrenia. A systematic and quantitative review of volumetric magnetic resonance imaging studies. Br. J. Psychiatry 172, 110–120.

Lee, K.H., Williams, L.M., 2000. Eye movement dysfunction as a biological marker of risk for schizophrenia. Aust. N.Z. J. Psychiatry 34 (Suppl.), S91–S100.

Lee, T., Seeman, P., 1980. Elevation of brain neuroleptic dopamine receptors in schizophrenia. Am. J. Psychiatry 137, 135–144.

Leff, J.P., Kuipers, L., Berkowitz, R., et al., 1985. A controlled trial of interventions in the families of schizophrenic patients: two-year follow up. Br. J. Psychiatry 146, 594–600.

Lehmann, S.W., 2003. Psychiatric disorders in older women. Int. Rev. Psychiatry 15, 269–279.

Leucht, S., Barnes, T.R., Kissling, W., et al., 2003. Relapse prevention in schizophrenia with new-generation antipsychotics: a systematic review and exploratory meta-analysis of randomized, controlled trials. Am. J. Psychiatry 160, 1209–1222.

Lewis, G., David, A., Andreasson, S., et al., 1992. Schizophrenia and city life. Lancet 340, 137–140.

Lewis, S.W., Reveley, M.A., David, A.S., 1988. Agenesis of the corpus callosum and schizophrenia. Psychol. Med. 18, 341–347.

Liddle, P.F., 1987. The symptoms of chronic schizophrenia. A re-examination of the positive-negative dichotomy. Br. J. Psychiatry 151, 145–151.

Liddle, P.F., Friston, K.J., Frith, C.D., 1992. Patterns of cerebral blood flow in schizophrenia. Br. J. Psychiatry 160, 179–186.

Lidz, R.W., Lidz, T., 1949. The family environment of schizophrenic patients. Am. J. Psychiatry 106, 332–345.

Lieberman, J.A., Safferman, A.Z., Pollack, S., 1994. Clinical effects of clozapine in chronic schizophrenia: response and predictors of outcome. Am. J. Psychiatry 151, 1744–1752.

Lieberman, J.A., Stroup, T.S., McEvoy, J.P., et al., 2005. Effectiveness of antipsychotic drugs in patients with chronic schizophrenia. N. Engl. J. Med. 353, 1209–1223.

Li, T., Stefansson, H., Gudfinnsson, E., et al., 2004. Identification of a novel neuregulin 1 at-risk haplotype in Han schizophrenia Chinese

patients, but no association with the Icelandic/
Scottish risk haplotype. Mol. Psychiatry
9, 698–704.

Loebel, A.D., Lieberman, J.A., Alvir, J.M., 1992.
Duration of psychosis and outcome in first
episode schizophrenia. Am. J. Psychiatry
149, 1183–1186.

Ma, X., Sun, J., Yao, J., et al., 2007. A quantitative
association study between schizotypal traits
and COMT, PRODH and BDNF genes in a
healthy Chinese population. Psychiatry Res.
153, 7–15.

Mackay, A.V.P., Iversen, L.L., Rosser, M., 1982.
Increased brain dopamine and dopamine
receptors in schizophrenia. Arch. Gen.
Psychiatry 39, 991–997.

Mangalore, R., Knapp, M., 2007. Cost of
schizophrenia in England. J. Ment. Health
Policy Econ. 10, 23–41.

Marshall, E.J., 1994. Homelessness and
schizophrenia. Schizophrenia Monitor 4, 1–4.

Mayer-Gross, W., 1932. Die Schizophrenie. In:
Bumke's handbuch der geisteskrankheiten,
vol. 9, Springer, Berlin.

McGorry, P.D., Warner, R., 2002. Consensus on
early intervention in schizophrenia. Schizophr.
Bull. 28, 543–544.

McGuire, P.K., Shah, G.M., Murray, R.M., 1993.
Increased blood flow in Broca's area during
auditory hallucinations in schizophrenia.
Lancet 342, 703–706.

McKenna, P.J., 1995. General intellectual
function in schizophrenia. Schizophrenia
Monitor 5, 1–5.

McNaught, A.S., Jeffreys, S.E., Harvey, C.A.,
et al., 1997. The Hampstead
schizophrenia survey 1991 2: Incidence
and migration in inner London. Br. J.
Psychiatry 170, 307–311.

McNeil, T.F., 1995. Perinatal risk factors and
schizophrenia: selective review and
methodological concerns. Epidemiology
Review 17, 107–112.

Mellor, C.S., 1970. First rank symptoms of
schizophrenia. Br. J. Psychiatry 117, 15–23.

Meltzer, H.Y., Baldessarini, R.J., 2003. Reducing
the risk for suicide in schizophrenia and
affective disorders. J. Clin. Psychiatry
64, 1122–1129.

Morel, B.A., 1852. Études cliniques: traité,
théorique et pratique des maladies mentales.
Vol. 1. Nancy.

Moore, T.H., Zammit, S., Lingford-Hughes, A.,
et al., 2007. Cannabis use and risk of
psychotic or affective mental health
outcomes: a systematic review. Lancet
370, 319–328.

Mortensen, P.B., Juel, K., 1993. Mortality and
causes of death in first admitted schizophrenic
patients. Br. J. Psychiatry 163, 183–189.

Mortensen, P.B., Pedersen, C.B., Westergaard, T.,
et al., 1999. Effects of family history and place
and season of birth on the risk of
schizophrenia. N. Engl. J. Med. 340, 603–608.

Mowry, B.J., Nancarrow, D.J., Lennon, D.P.,
et al., 1995. Schizophrenia susceptibility and
chromosome 6p24-22 (letter). Nat. Genet.
11, 233–234.

Murphy, H.B.M., Raman, A.C., 1971. The
chronicity of schizophrenia in indigenous
tropical people. Br. J. Psychiatry
118, 489–497.

Murray, R.M., 1994. Neurodevelopmental
schizophrenia: the rediscovery of dementia
praecox. Br. J. Psychiatry 165, 6–12.

Murray, R.M., Lewis, S.W., 1987. Is
schizophrenia a neurodevelopmental disorder?
Br. Med. J. 295, 681–682.

Nelson, B., Yung, A.R., Bechdolf, A., et al., 2008.
The phenomenological critique and self-
disturbance: implications for ultra-high risk
('prodrome') research. Schizophr. Bull.
34, 381–392.

NICE National Institute for Clinical Excellence,
2002. Schizophrenia: core interventions in the
treatment and management of schizophrenia
in primary and secondary care. Online.
Available: www.nice.org.uk (accessed
26.05.04).

NICE National Institute for Clinical Excellence,
2010. Guideline on core interventions in the
treatment and management of schizophrenia
in adults in primary and secondary care,
updated edition. NICE, London.

Nordentoft, M., Hjorthøj, C., 2007. Cannabis use
and risk of psychosis in later life. Lancet
370, 293–294.

Norman, R.M., Malla, A.K., 1993. Stressful life
events and schizophrenia: a review of the
research. Br. J. Psychiatry 162, 161–166.

Numata, S., Ueno, S., Iga, J., et al., 2008. Positive
association of the PDE4B (phosphodiesterase
4B) gene with schizophrenia in the Japanese
population. J. Psychiatr. Res. 43, 7–12.

Ødegaard, Ø., 1932. Emigration and insanity. Acta
Psychiatr. Scand. 4 (Suppl.), 1–206.

Owens, D.G.C., Johnstone, E.C., 1980. The
disabilities of chronic schizophrenia – their
nature and the factors contributing to their
development. Br. J. Psychiatry 136, 384–393.

Pakkenberg, B., 1990. Pronounced reduction of
total neuron number in mediodorsal thalamic
nucleus and nucleus accumbens in
schizophrenics. Arch. Gen. Psychiatry
47, 1023–1028.

Payne, R.W., 1973. Cognitive abnormalities. In:
Eysenck, H.J. (Ed.), Handbook of abnormal
psychology. Pitman, London.

Pickard, B.S., Thomson, P.A., Christoforou, A.,
et al., 2007. The PDE4B gene confers sex-
specific protection against schizophrenia.
Psychiatr. Genet. 17, 129–133.

Pilowsky, L.S., Mulligan, R.S., Acton, P.D., 1997.
Effects of clozapine and typical antipsychotics
on striatal and limbic D2/D2-like receptors
in vivo by 123I epidepride. Schizophr. Res.
24, 181.

Rodriguez, V.M., Andree, R.M., Castejon, M.J.P.,
et al., 1996. SPECT study of regional cerebral
perfusion in neuroleptic resistant
schizophrenic patients who responded or did
not respond to clozapine. Am. J. Psychiatry
153, 1343–1346.

Royston, M.C., Simpson, M.D.C., 1991. Postmortem neurochemistry of schizophrenia. In:
Kerwin, R.W., Dawbarn, D., McCulloch, J.

et al., (Eds.), Neurobiology and psychiatry.
Cambridge University Press, Cambridge.

Rudin, E., 1916. Studien uber Vererbung und
Entstehung geistiger Storungen. I. Zur
Vererung und Neuentstehung der Dementia
Praecox. Springer, Berlin.

Russell, A.J., Munro, J.C., Jones, P.B., et al., 1997.
Schizophrenia and the myth of intellectual
decline. Am. J. Psychiatry 154, 635–639.

Sartorius, N., Jablensky, A., Korten, A., 1986.
Early manifestations and first contact
incidence of schizophrenia in different
cultures. A preliminary report on the
initial evaluation phase of the WHO
collaborative study of determinants of
outcome of severe mental disorders. Psychol.
Med. 16, 909–928.

Schneider, K., 1959. Clinical psychopathology.
Grune and Stratton, New York.

Schobel, S.A., Lewandowski, N.M.,
Corcoran, C.M., et al., 2009. Differential
targeting of the CA1 subfield of the
hippocampal formation by schizophrenia and
related psychotic disorders. Arch. Gen.
Psychiatry 66, 938–946.

Schwab, S.G., Knapp, M., Mondabon, S., et al.,
2003. Support for association of schizophrenia
with genetic variation in the 6p22.3 gene,
dysbindin, in sib-pair families with linkage and
in an additional sample of triad families. Am. J.
Hum. Genet. 72, 185–190.

Sedvall, G., 1990. Current status of PET imaging
in schizophrenia. In: Stefanis, C.,
Sladtos, C.R., Rabivilas, A.D. (Eds.),
Psychiatry – a world perspective. Elsevier,
Amsterdam.

Shepherd, M., Watt, D., Falloon, I., 1989. The
natural history of schizophrenia: a five-year
follow up study of outcome and prediction in a
representative sample of schizophrenics.
Psychol. Med. Monogr. Suppl. 15, 1–46.

Shergill, S.S., Murray, R.M., McGuire, P.K.,
1998. Auditory hallucinations: a review of
psychological treatments. Schizophr. Res.
32, 137–150.

Shergill, S.S., Brammer, M.J., Williams, S.C.,
et al., 2000. Mapping auditory hallucinations
in schizophrenia using functional magnetic
resonance imaging. Arch. Gen. Psychiatry
57, 1033–1038.

Shifman, S., Bronstein, M., Sternfeld, M., et al.,
2002. A highly significant association between
a COMT haplotype and schizophrenia. Am. J.
Hum. Genet. 71, 1296–1302.

Stefansson, H., Sigurdsson, E.,
Steinthorsdottir, V., et al., 2002. Neuregulin 1
and susceptibility to schizophrenia. Am. J.
Hum. Genet. 71, 877–892.

Stefansson, H., Sarginson, J., Kong, A., et al.,
2003. Association of neuregulin 1 with
schizophrenia confirmed in a Scottish
population. Am. J. Hum. Genet. 72, 83–87.

Straub, R.E., Jiang, Y., MacLean, C.J., et al., 2002.
Genetic variation in the 6p22.3 gene
DTNBP1, the human ortholog of the mouse
dysbindin gene, is associated with
schizophrenia. Am. J. Hum. Genet.
71, 337–348.

Appendix 3
ICD-10 Diagnostic subtypes of schizophrenia

- Paranoid schizophrenia
- Hebephrenic schizophrenia (disorganized in DSM-IV)
- Catatonic schizophrenia
- Undifferentiated schizophrenia
- Post-schizophrenic depression
- Residual schizophrenia
- Simple schizophrenia
- Other schizophrenia
- Schizophrenia, unspecified.

Appendix 4
DSM-IV Diagnostic subtypes of schizophrenia

- Paranoid schizophrenia
- Disorganized schizophrenia (hebephrenic in ICD-10)
- Catatonic schizophrenia
- Undifferentiated schizophrenia
- Residual schizophrenia.

Unipolar depression

Anthony Cleare   Abebaw Fekadu   Lena Rane

CHAPTER CONTENTS

Introduction

Depression represents a considerable public health burden, with a lifetime incidence approaching 20%. There is evidence that the incidence and prevalence of depression have been increasing in recent decades. The WHO estimates that depression is the fourth most important cause of disability worldwide, and that by 2020, it will be the second most important.

Clinical features

Phenomenology of depression

The core feature of the clinical syndrome of depression is persistent and pervasive low mood and/or anhedonia. Many other characteristic features make up the full syndrome; they can be divided into behavioural, emotional, cognitive and biological features. Severe cases are associated with the development of psychotic features.

Behavioural features

* Psychomotor retardation or agitation
* Altered facial expression such as mouth turned down, exaggerated facial lines, lack of facial expressivity
* Self-neglect and social withdrawal.

Emotional features

* Low mood, distinct from ordinary unhappiness qualitatively (depth and pervasiveness) and quantitatively (DSM-IV TR requires >2 weeks)
* Tearfulness
* Loss of interest in activities that would normally have given pleasure
* Inability to feel pleasure (*anhedonia*)
* Loss of reactivity of mood to external events
* Irritability
* Anxiety: psychological and physical components.

Cognitive features

Form of thought
* Slow speed of thought
* Reduced speed and latency of speech
* Reduced volume of speech
* Reduced tonal modulation and expressivity in speech
* Subjective impairment in concentration, registration and recall, paralleled by objective impairment in psychometric testing. Memory disturbance may be severe and resemble dementia (*depressive pseudodementia*).

Content of thought
* Thought content reflects the abnormality in mood, with negative or depressive cognitions: negative views of self (*self-blame*), the world (*negativism*) and the future (*pessimism*)
* Milder forms include a vague pessimistic outlook and a tendency to worry unnecessarily
* Moderate cases may show hopelessness, worthlessness and excessive guilt. Patients may be unable to distract themselves from these repetitive thoughts (*depressive ruminations*)
* Distorted views of the future may lead to predictions of disaster and suicidal thoughts or behaviour.

Biological symptoms

* Diurnal variation of mood (usually, but not always, worse in the morning)
* Sleep disturbance: *early morning waking* (*or late insomnia*) is the classic disturbance, but initial (early) insomnia and restless/disturbed sleep (middle insomnia) are common
* Loss of appetite
* Weight loss (DSM-IV TR specifies 5% as significant)
* Loss of libido
* Fatigue and generalized lassitude (*anergia*)
* Constipation
* Amenorrhoea.

Reversed biological features may be present, i.e. hypersomnia (increased sleep), increased appetite and weight gain. *Atypical depression* is a syndrome with reversed biological features, preserved mood reactivity, extreme (leaden) anergia, and interpersonal rejection sensitivity.

Psychotic features

* Delusions: in severe depression, cognitive distortions give way to delusions that are in keeping with the depressed mood (*mood congruent*). Common content involves guilt, poverty and hypochondriasis. The patient may feel he/she is being persecuted, which sometimes, but not always, is viewed as deserved.
* Hallucinations: auditory hallucinations may occur, classically second person accusatory; hallucinations in other sensory modalities can also occur.
* *Cotard syndrome* characteristically occurs in elderly patients, where severe depression results in nihilistic delusions, often with hypochondriacal content, such as a belief that the bowel has rotted away.

Subtypes and variants of the depressive syndrome

Melancholic depression

While most agree that depression is a heterogeneous condition, there have been innumerable attempts to subdivide depression according to symptom patterns. Most studies of depression have identified a group of patients characterized by certain symptoms: early morning waking, weight loss, poor appetite, anhedonia and agitation. This symptom grouping has been variously labelled as *core, endogenous, nuclear* and *melancholic* depression, the latter now being ensconced within DSM-IV. Early conceptualizations of this category noted that patients were said to show a preferential response to antidepressants and ECT, and to show more dysfunction of biological correlates of depression such as the dexamethasone suppression test. Few good studies have made direct comparisons between melancholic depression and other types, preventing firm conclusions from being drawn.

Although initial descriptions of depression were based on inpatients with melancholic and psychotic features, in current practice, where the large majority of patients come from the community, this group actually represents the minority of cases of depression. Most patients have milder symptoms, day-to-day fluctuation of mood, initial insomnia and prominent features of anxiety. Results attempting to define these have been conflicting:

- **Newcastle classification:** Roth and colleagues separated out two groups of depressed patients using multiple regression analysis, and argued that the melancholic and neurotic groups were distinct.
- **Kendell's classification:** Kendell was unable to demonstrate that a point of rarity exists between the two forms and proposed that depression represented a continuum with varying degrees of melancholic and neurotic symptoms (Kendell 1976).
- **Paykel's classification:** Paykel (1971) separated four groups of patients using cluster analysis:
  - Psychotic depressives (i.e. melancholic)
  - Anxious depressives (middle-aged, moderate depressive symptoms plus anxiety)
  - Hostile depressives (young, hostile)
  - Younger depressives with personality disorders.

More recently, Kendler (1997) used twin pairs to demonstrate that DSM-IV-defined melancholia was associated with an increased genetic loading, as well as increased co-morbidity with anxiety disorders (but not alcohol dependence or bulimia), a more severe and recurrent illness course and lower levels of neuroticism. Thus, while it represented a valid subtype associated with a particularly high familial liability, the data best supported a quantitative, rather than qualitative, distinction, in keeping with Kendell's description.

DSM-IV depression

Kendler also used this sample to ask whether the DSM-IV criteria of requiring five symptoms to diagnose major depressive disorder was appropriate or represented an arbitrary cut-off (Kendler & Gardner 1998). Three DSM criteria were studied:

- Presence of five out of nine symptoms
- Duration of symptoms >2 weeks
- Severity of symptoms or associated functional impairment.

Both severity and number of symptoms in one twin were associated in a linear fashion with risk of depression in the co-twin. This relationship was not found with duration. Using criteria below the threshold for DSM major depression on each of the three measures were all good predictors of future depressive risk, both in individuals and their co-twin. The authors concluded that the DSM-IV criteria are of little use in predicting personal or genetic risk of depression, and that depressive illness is likely to lie on a continuum.

Psychotic depression

The clinical importance of separating out psychotic depression relates primarily to the implications for treatment and prognosis. Some authors have argued that psychotic depression represents a separate and distinct category, based on clinical, genetic, treatment response and biological features. Evidence for this is discussed later in this chapter.

Atypical depression

Atypical depression has been used in the past to mean a number of different conditions, including non-endogenous depression, depression secondary to another condition, depression associated with anxiety or panic, and depression with reversed biological features. However, as the concept has evolved, atypicality has been more tightly defined, and is now included within DSM-IV. It is defined as a subtype of depressive disorder characterized by reversed biological symptoms (e.g. hypersomnia, hyperphagia and variation of mood worse in the evening), preserved mood reactivity, extreme ('leaden') anergia and chronic interpersonal rejection sensitivity. Atypical depression does appear to be a valid concept. Sullivan and colleagues (Sullivan et al 1998) used data from the large US National Comorbidity Survey, and identified six depressive syndromes, two of which corresponded to mild atypical depression and severe atypical depression respectively. A study of female twin pairs also found an atypical depression syndrome; furthermore, individuals tended to have the same syndrome on each recurrence and the concordance of syndrome type was greater in monozygotic than in dizygotic pairs (Kendler et al 1996). Importantly, atypical depression probably responds more favourably to monoamine oxidase inhibitors than to tricyclic antidepressants.

Somatization

Epidemiological studies show that physical symptoms are strongly associated with depression; furthermore, patients frequently present with such symptoms rather than emotional symptoms. The physical symptoms may be medically explained, i.e. they represent a co-morbid physical illness (physical illness is associated with increased rates of depression). More frequently, they represent medically unexplained, or functional symptoms. Such symptoms may represent the biological disturbance in depression, such as loss of weight or sleep disturbance, or the process of *somatization*. Somatization is a complex phenomenon, dealt with in more detail in Chapter 17, but includes components of heightened symptom production (i.e. via the effects of autonomic arousal), heightened symptom perception (via symptom focusing), abnormal interpretation of symptoms (as representing physical illness), excessive response to symptoms leading to disability (e.g. avoidance behaviour) and seeking medical help. Frequent presentations include fatigue and weakness, headache, gastrointestinal disturbance, chest symptoms, dizziness or pain. Longitudinal studies show that these often precede the emergence of frank affective symptoms. As usual, this process represents a spectrum, and psychiatrists (and other doctors) may need to move gently in the shift of focus from physical to psychological symptoms in order to avoid alienating patients with more extreme tendencies to somatization.

prevalence of depression was 10% (8% in males, 13% in females) and the lifetime prevalence 17% (13% in males, 21% in females). Dysthymia was diagnosable in 6% of the population (5% in males, 8% in females). A recent study, the NCS-R, using DSM-IV criteria for depression, found 12-month rates of 6.6% and lifetime rates of 16.2% (Kessler et al 2003).

The peak age of onset is 20–40 years for unipolar depression and 50–70 years for psychotic depression. There are some suggestions of a bimodal peak in unipolar depression with the second peak occurring in the 50s (Eaton et al 1997). There is a female predominance of approximately 2:1 in unipolar depression, the reasons for which are not clear, and may in part be due to a greater willingness to admit to depressive symptoms, or social reasons such as greater subjection to sexual abuse and domestic violence, or biological factors such as the influence of sex hormones. The excess of unipolar depression in women decreases with age, particularly in those over 55 years (Bebbington 1998). Using the Present State Examination, 15% of Camberwell (inner city London) women are depressed compared with 8% in the Hebrides (rural Scotland). There is international variation in rates: lifetime rates range from 1.5% in Taiwan to 19% in Beirut, with annual rates ranging from 0.8% in Taiwan to 5.8% in New Zealand (Weissman et al 1996). Such cross-national variation has been repeatedly replicated (Andrade et al 2003; Simon et al 2002) and is unlikely to be due to 'category fallacy' (i.e. due to cross-cultural difference in the nature and validity of unipolar depression) (Simon et al 2002).

There appears to have been a real rise in both the incidence and prevalence of depression in industrialized countries during the last three decades, believed to be a cohort effect (Kessler et al 2003; Andrade et al 2003; Klerman & Weissman 1989). This is true for both men and women.

Aetiology

Neurobiological components

Genetics

It has long been clear that there is a significant genetic component to unipolar depression. Evidence for this comes from studies utilizing a variety of genetic research methodology. Family studies show increased familial risk and the earlier the age of onset, the higher the familial risk. Late onset affective disorder has a lower genetic loading. Twin studies in unipolar depression show concordance rates of approximately 40–50% in monozygotic and 25% in dizygotic twins (McGuffin et al 1991; Price 1968). The MZ concordance rates seem to be lower for community sampled depression or neurotic depression, suggesting a lesser biological component in these cases (McGuffin et al 1996). Adoption studies in unipolar depression have found increased rates of illness in biological relatives compared to adopted relatives of probands (Mendlewicz & Rainer 1977).

In terms of the mode of inheritance, there is no compelling evidence of true Mendelian transmission. Although a few studies have reported linkage, none have been adequately replicated. It is probable that there are many genes implicated in mediating differing aspects of the overall genetic predisposition.

How then do these genes confer risk? First of all, there is little support for the suggestion that a higher personal genetic loading leaves an individual needing less environmental stress to become depressed (Tennant 2002). Instead, it is the tendency to become depressed in response to life events that is inherited (Kendler et al 1995). The situation is further complicated by the recent findings that there is a significant genetic component to life events themselves (Kendler & Karkowski-Shuman 1997). Thus, both the tendency to suffer adversity and to respond to it by becoming depressed have genetic components. Moreover, a functional polymorphism in the promoter region of the 5-HTT transporter gene was found to moderate the influence of adverse life events on the development of depressive symptoms (Caspi et al 2003).

However, it has also been observed that there is a tendency for each recurrence of depression to be less dependent on precipitating stress, a phenomenon likened to 'kindling' (see later). Kendler and colleagues (2001) used a large twin pair sample to discover that genetic risk tended to place people in a 'pre-kindled' state rather than speeding up the process of kindling.

It is now clear that there is genetic variation in several biological systems that have important roles in brain homeostasis, linked to the occurrence of polymorphic variation in gene alleles. Various studies have shown that certain polymorphisms at the serotonin (5HT) receptor subtypes (e.g. $5HT_{2C}$ receptor), of tryptophan hydroxylase (the rate limiting enzyme for the synthesis of 5HT) or the 5HT transporter are associated with depression. There is a functional significance of the different alleles: certain polymorphisms are associated with different rates of production of the 5HT receptor or 5HT transporter m-RNA, or differential capacity of the transporter for the reuptake of 5HT into the neuron. Such genetic variation could therefore provide a link between the genetics of depression and the 5HT hypothesis of depression (see below).

Future genetic research may also integrate elements of post-transcriptional changes and modifications, so-called *proteomics* – much of the expression of genetic risk appears to be dependent on what happens during this post-transcriptional period.

Neurochemistry

Brain neurochemistry has long been studied in the search for the biological basis of depression, dating from the original finding that monoamine depletion by the drug reserpine caused depression. The observation that the newly developed antidepressants (monoamine oxidase inhibitors and tricyclic antidepressants) enhanced synaptic monoamine levels and that there were reduced monoamine breakdown products (5HIAA, HVA and MHPG) in the cerebrospinal fluid (CSF) of depressed subjects led to the monoamine hypothesis of depression. This theory stated that there is a deficiency of noradrenaline (NA) (norepinephrine), dopamine and/or 5HT at monoaminergic synapses. From this original hypothesis, several proposed biological models of depression have developed.

Serotonergic theories

Coppen (1967) originally proposed the 5HT hypothesis of depression, suggesting that 5HT was the specific monoamine involved in depression. Classically, several pieces of evidence are cited to support the theory that many aspects of 5HT physiology may be dysregulated in depression (Maes & Meltzer 1995). It should be noted that there are at present no ways to measure directly the amount of 5HT present in brain synapses.

First, there is evidence of a reduced availability to the brain of the 5HT precursor tryptophan: there are reduced plasma levels of tryptophan and evidence of an enhanced alternative route of tryptophan catabolism via the kynurenine pathway in the liver.

Second, there are changes in the normal uptake mechanisms for 5HT: evidence for this comes from the finding of a reduced uptake of 5HT into the platelets, which act as a model of the neuronal 5HT transporter system.

Third, there are changes in the status of 5HT receptors in depression. Early work relied on the use of brains obtained from patients who had died by suicide. Several studies found increased $5HT_2$ receptors, which was felt to result from low 5HT synaptic content, and reduced $5HT_{1A}$ hippocampal and amygdala binding. A further approach has been the use of neuropharmacological challenge paradigms to test the integrity of neurotransmitter systems, or receptor sensitivity. Standardized drug challenges are given, ideally centrally acting and selective, and a physiological response is measured, such as hormone release or temperature change. The magnitude of the response is taken as an index of the activity of the system challenged. Many, although by no means all, of these studies have reported impairments in depression. One example is of a blunted prolactin response to fenfluramine, a drug that leads to release of presynaptic 5HT. Other positive examples include a blunted prolactin response to the 5HT precursor L-tryptophan, and a blunted response to the serotonin reuptake inhibitor clomipramine.

Fourth, the technique of tryptophan depletion (TD) suggests that there may be a *causal* relationship between 5HT changes and depression. The TD paradigm involves oral administration of a mixture of amino acids without tryptophan; this leads to a rapid fall in plasma tryptophan since protein synthesis stimulated as a result of the drink utilizes the available tryptophan. This reduction in plasma levels, together with competition from the other ingested amino acids, leads to lowered brain tryptophan entry, and reduced 5HT synthesis. TD in unmedicated depressed subjects has not revealed consistent results, perhaps because the 5HT system is maximally dysregulated (Delgado et al 1994). On the other hand, TD depletion induces a temporary state of depressive symptomatology in those at increased vulnerability to depression, including patients with a personal (Smith et al 1997) or family (Benkelfat et al 1994; Klaassen et al 1999) history of depression and females (Ellenbogen et al 1996). This is powerful evidence of a causal link between reduced serotonergic function and depression, rather than merely a cross-sectional association. TD may also be of predictive utility, since the presence of a positive (i.e. mood-lowering) effect of TD in those in remission from depression is associated with a higher rate of relapse in the following 12 months (Moreno et al 2000). Thus, certain individuals may have a biological vulnerability to short-term depressogenic effects of reduced brain 5HT availability, which places them at increased risk of future major depression, possibly as a response to other biological or environmental causes of reduced 5HT availability.

One anomaly in the TD literature is the observation that the mood lowering effect of tryptophan depletion does not occur to a significant degree in remitted depressed patients receiving continuation treatment with desipramine, a noradrenergic specific tricyclic antidepressant (Delgado et al 1999). They do, however, experience a transient relapse if noradrenaline (norepinephrine) synthesis is inhibited, while, conversely, those who responded to SSRIs are not affected by noradrenaline (norepinephrine) depletion (Delgado et al 1993).

Fifth, and finally, recent neuroimaging techniques have been utilized to visualize directly brain 5HT changes in depression. PET and SPET imaging can use radiolabelled ligands to measure receptor binding (a product of receptor density and receptor sensitivity) for specific neurochemical targets in the different brain regions.

The status of brain $5HT_2$ receptors has not been clarified by these techniques; receptor binding has been found to be increased, normal or decreased in different studies. The largest study (Yatham et al 2000) used PET and the $5HT_2$ receptor ligand [18F]setoperone in 20 drug-free patients with major depression and 20 matched healthy controls. The main finding was that depressed patients showed a marked global reduction in receptor binding (between 22% and 27% in various regions). Differences from previous studies may have been due to the shorter duration of drug free period in this study (2 weeks). There remains difficulty reconciling the accumulating finding of reduced binding with the fact that effective antidepressant treatments lead to further downregulation of $5HT_2$ receptors (Sheline & Mintun 2002).

The assessment of the status of brain $5HT_{1A}$ receptors in depression was assessed using the PET radioligand [11C] WAY-100635 in a group of 25 depressed patients, 15 of whom were unmedicated, and 10 of whom were rescanned after treatment with a selective serotonin reuptake inhibitor antidepressant (Sargent et al 2000). There was a generalized reduction in $5HT_{1A}$ receptor binding throughout the cortex. This was also present in the medicated subjects, however, and not altered by prospective treatment with an SSRI. The authors hypothesize a trait reduction in $5HT_{1A}$ receptors that is unaffected by treatment. Results of another study support the reduction in $5HT_{1A}$ binding, particularly in the mesiotemporal cortex (hippocampus–amygdala) and the midbrain (raphe nuclei) (Drevets et al 1999).

It has been pointed out that measuring receptor numbers may not represent receptor function. A neuroimaging paradigm attempting to assess receptor function extends the neuropharmacological challenge paradigms already described above. Thus, it is possible to measure changes in neural activity in different brain regions using functional imaging with PET or f-MRI after the administration of neuropharmacological challenges. Such serotonergically mediated changes in neural activity after fenfluramine administration are markedly reduced in major depression, suggesting downregulated central 5HT receptors (Mann et al 1996). However, a study using the more specific d-isomer of fenfluramine could not replicate this finding (Meyer et al 1998).

One argument against the significance of serotonergic changes in depression comes from observations that either specific behaviours (e.g. suicide) and/or enduring character traits (e.g. impulsivity) may be more closely related to 5HT function. Thus, while initial studies found reduced concentrations of the

5HT breakdown product 5HIAA in CSF from depressed patients, there have been recent suggestions that this is linked more specifically to suicide, impulsivity or aggression (Maes & Meltzer 1995). A further issue is whether or not the serotonergic changes are state or trait related. While the impaired serotonergic responses to neuropharmacological challenge tests usually normalize after successful treatment of depression, the reduced $5HT_{1A}$ receptor binding seen with PET does not (Sargent et al 2000). This suggests that some of the observed changes in depression may indeed be trait markers, and more closely linked to vulnerability or personality than to depressive state.

Noradrenergic theories

Many effective antidepressants (e.g. desipramine, nortriptyline and reboxetine) are potent inhibitors of the reuptake of noradrenaline (norepinephrine), with little effect on 5HT reuptake. Indeed, several studies found that low urinary levels of the noradrenaline (norepinephrine) metabolite MHPG predict a favourable response to tricyclic antidepressants (Schatzberg & Schildkraut 1995). Neuroendocrine challenge studies have also found evidence of reduced noradrenergic function in depression. For example, reduced GH responses to clonidine (Checkley et al 1981) and desipramine (Siever 1987) suggest impaired α2-receptor function, and abnormality that may persist into recovery of depression and thus may represent a trait marker (Siever et al 1992). Postmortem and platelet studies also provide some support for changes in α- and β-adrenergic receptors (Schatzberg et al 2002). Finally, in a novel (though highly invasive) study, concentration gradients for the main catecholamines and their metabolites were calculated using simultaneous sampling of brachial artery and internal jugular vein blood. In patients with treatment-resistant depression, there was a reduced concentration gradient for norepinephrine and its metabolites and for the dopamine metabolite homovanillic acid, but no differences in 5HT or its metabolite 5HIAA. These results provide further evidence of reduced noradrenaline (norepinephrine) availability in the brain, particularly in severe, resistant forms of depression (Lambert et al 2000).

Further support for noradrenergic dysfunction in depression comes from the use of the challenge drug clonidine in combination with PET imaging; this suggests functionally impaired presynaptic α2-adrenoceptors as well as regionally supersensitive postsynaptic cortical α2-adrenoceptors (Fu et al 2001).

Dopaminergic theories

Interest in the dopaminergic system has been stimulated by the introduction of bupropion, an antidepressant that works primarily on dopamine reuptake. There is some evidence of a reduced GH response to the dopamine receptor agonist apomorphine, but results are inconsistent, and there is little other work to date on the dopamine system in unipolar depression (Willner 1995). Levels of the breakdown product of dopamine, homovanillic acid (HVA), are reduced in the CSF of depressed subjects.

Cholinergic theories

Studies have shown an enhanced GH response to the anticholinesterase drug pyridostigmine, a measure of acetyl choline receptor function. Further evidence comes from the observation of reduced rapid eye movement latency and increased REM sleep in depression, effects that may represent increased cholinergic activity. Furthermore, depressed patients show supersensitivity to REM sleep effects of cholinergics. Janowsky proposed the cholinergic-adrenergic balance theory of depression, hypothesizing that increased cholinergic function and reduced noradrenergic function were both important in generating symptoms in depression (Janowsky & Overstreet 1995).

GABAergic theories

There is a reduced GH response to baclofen, a GABA-B receptor agonist, suggesting reduced GABA receptor activity in depression (O'Flynn & Dinan 1993). Plasma GABA may also be low (Schatzberg et al 2002).

Interactions of monoamines

There is now increasing evidence that drugs that affect one neurotransmitter system can also affect another through downstream effects. If one looks simply at 5HT, there are innumerable examples. Thus, $5HT_{1D}$ receptors may act in an inhibitory manner on neurons releasing other neurotransmitters. Similarly, α1-receptors on serotonergic cell bodies act to increase cell firing and 5HT release, while α2-receptors are present on serotonergic nerve terminals and are inhibitory to 5HT release. Serotonergic neurons project to other areas of the brain where they can inhibit dopaminergic function (Moghaddan & Bunney 1990). The 5HT transporter protein is thought to interact with the ability of α2-receptors to inhibit 5HT cell firing (Blier et al 1990). Finally, noradrenaline (norepinephrine) reuptake inhibition is potentiated in the presence of simultaneous 5HT reuptake inhibition (Engleman et al 1995).

It is likely that a number of neurotransmitter alterations are present in depression. The clinical relevance of this may be reflected in the finding that drugs that act on both 5HT and noradrenaline (norepinephrine), such as amitriptyline (Barbui & Hotopf 2001) and venlafaxine (Smith et al 2002), may have slightly enhanced efficacy in the treatment of depression.

Neuroendocrinology

Hypothalamo-pituitary-adrenal axis

The hypothalamo-pituitary-adrenal or HPA axis (Fig. 20.1) mediates the response of the body to stress, and has been a focus of biological research into depression, given the close link to stress. Research using 24-hour collections of blood, urine or saliva has clarified that about 50% of depressed patients show a picture of hypercortisolaemia. However, there is considerable variability in these findings: rates are higher in those with features of DSM-IV melancholic depression, strong somatic symptoms or psychosis (Belanoff et al 2001), while those with predominant features of atypical depression are often found to have the opposite picture, a shift towards hypocortisolaemia (see below).

Assessing the HPA axis is made problematic by the fact that cortisol is a pulsatile hormone with a strong diurnal rhythm, and is released in stressful circumstances, such as blood sampling. This has necessitated more detailed methods of endocrinological assessment. The test most widely used in depression research has been the dexamethasone suppression test (DST).

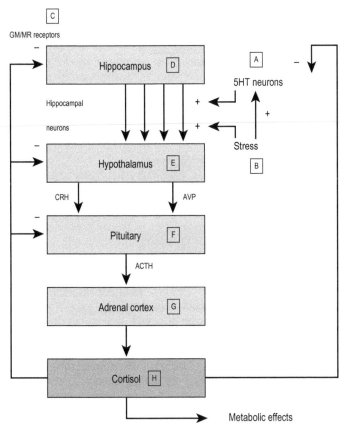

Figure 20.1 • Schematic representation of the control of the hypothalamo-pituitary-adrenal (HPA) axis. CRH, corticotrophin releasing hormone; ACTH, corticotrophin; AVP, arginine vasopressin; MR, mineralocorticoid receptors; GR, glucocorticoid receptors. Abnormalities in this axis in depression are shown in Box 20.3.

Box 20.3

HPA axis abnormalities in depression (Fig. 20.1)

A: Decreased 5HT neuronal function

B: Increased incidence of life events

C: Impaired hippocampal fast (rate-sensitive) feedback

D: Shrunken hippocampal structures

E: Raised CRH levels in the cerebrospinal fluid; impaired negative feedback by dexamethasone

F: Impaired pituitary ACTH response to CRH administration; this may represent downregulated CRH receptors or negative feedback from high cortisol levels. Pituitary hypertrophy

G: Hypertrophied adrenal cortices

H: Hypercortisolism.

Dexamethasone is a synthetic glucocorticoid that suppresses hypothalamic corticotrophin-releasing hormone (CRH) and pituitary corticotrophin (ACTH) release via its effects on glucocorticoid receptors (Fig. 20.1) and hence suppresses plasma cortisol release. In a proportion of depressed individuals such suppression fails to occur. This observation has led to the development of the dexamethasone suppression test (DST). There are variants of the test, but the most widely used in depression involves administering dexamethasone 1 mg at 11 p.m., and measuring plasma cortisol at 8 a.m., 4 p.m. or 11 p.m. Non-suppression of cortisol below a defined laboratory reference range represents a positive test. Rates of non-suppression vary, but average around 60–70% in melancholic depression and 30–40% in other forms of depression. The test is not specific, however, since non-suppression is also associated with schizophrenia (20%), old age, Alzheimer disease, weight loss (including anorexia nervosa) and a number of drugs (such as anticonvulsants). Proponents of the test note that it measures the responsiveness of the specific glucocorticoid receptors in the hypothalamus and pituitary glands, and gives an indication of glucocorticoid receptor resistance.

More recently, the combined dexamethasone-CRH test has been developed. The effect of CRH in stimulating ACTH and cortisol release is markedly attenuated after dexamethasone administration in healthy individuals. However, if glucocorticoid receptors are downregulated, the dexamethasone has less effect, and the CRH response is less attenuated. In depression, this test proved more able to distinguish depressed subjects from healthy individuals than the simple DST (Heuser et al 1994). Box 20.3 outlines the specific findings of various other endocrine tests applied to components of the HPA axis.

These studies show that, in a substantial proportion of depressed patients, there is oversecretion of cortisol and downregulation of glucocorticoid receptors. There are also several reasons for thinking that cortisol hypersecretion could be causally related to depression. Raised cortisol secretion in endogenous Cushing disease is associated with depression in between 50–85% of cases; this depression usually resolves when cortisol levels decrease after treatment of Cushing's. Even in non-Cushing depression, reducing the levels or effect of cortisol by administering cortisol synthesis inhibitor drugs such as metyrapone or ketoconazole, using CRH receptor antagonists or using glucocorticoid receptor antagonists can alleviate depression (Murphy 1997). Furthermore, cortisol has been shown to be associated with several other biological changes when present in abnormally high concentrations. For example, cortisol has strong, primarily inhibitory effects on neuronal 5HT neurotransmission; given the links between 5HT neurotransmission and mood changes already discussed, this is a mechanism by which 5HT neurotransmission could become dysregulated. There are also suggestions that prolonged periods of high cortisol can lead to hippocampal atrophy – indeed, in Cushing disease, the decreased hippocampus size can be correlated with plasma cortisol levels and cognitive impairment. Recent studies also suggest hippocampal atrophy in depression (Sheline & Mintun 2002).

Cortisol could also provide links between psychological risk factors for depression and the observed biological changes. For example, since cortisol is the main stress hormone, it is easy to see how it might mediate between life events and biological changes in depression. Similarly, adverse circumstances in childhood, such as losing parents or suffering abuse, are predisposing factors for depression. They are also linked to long-term alterations of the stress response both in childhood (De Bellis et al 1994) and in later adulthood (Heim et al 2000) irrespective of the actual presence of depression. Thus, it is also possible to use the HPA axis changes as a biological link between early life stresses and an increased vulnerability to stress and depression.

cortex (Elliott et al 1997) and left caudate (Elliott et al 1997), while the induction of sadness in healthy individuals leads to similar changes (Mayberg et al 1999). Depressed subjects also demonstrate an attenuated neural response to neutral or happy objects, but a relatively enhanced one to sad objects, in the same brain regions (Elliott et al 2002). This may represent a neural substrate underlying the negative cognitive bias in depression. It has recently been demonstrated that this abnormal emotional processing in which certain brain areas are over-responsive to negative stimuli such as sad faces is reversed by antidepressant therapy (Fu et al 2004).

However, certain neural changes are not specific to depression, and are present in other psychiatric conditions. It has been suggested these abnormalities are more closely related to specific psychological dysfunctions, such as psychomotor retardation (Bench et al 1993) or depressive pseudodementia (Dolan et al 1992), rather than diagnosis.

Of interest is the potential for clinical application of these findings. Some studies have also been able to show that some pre-treatment abnormalities reverse with treatment. The most consistent finding has been of increased activation of the subgenual prefrontal cortex during an acute depressive state which decreases following successful antidepressant treatment (Mayberg et al 1999, 2000). Other studies have taken a more complex look at dysfunction in the functional connections between brain regions, i.e. brain networks, rather than individual brain areas. Thus, one study revealed a complex picture of cortical and subcortical changes associated with treatment response to fluoxetine, with increases in the dorsal prefrontal cortex but decreases in the hippocampus (Mayberg et al 2000).

As described earlier, a proportion of subjects with remitted depression relapse after tryptophan depletion. The depressive relapse during tryptophan depletion produces a similar pattern of brain abnormalities as seen in a major depressive episode, both at rest and during a cognitive task (Bremner et al 1997; Smith et al 1999). These studies help link changes in 5HT function with changes in activity in specific brain areas during depressive relapse. Also of note is a study showing that blocking the synthesis of noradrenaline (norepinephrine) can also precipitate a temporary relapse in some recovered depressed patients and that this also results in similar brain changes as in the acute state (Bremner et al 2003). Thus, different neurochemical mechanisms may be related to common neural changes in depressive relapse.

Cellular factors

Kindling

Neurons show a process of *kindling*, whereby the seizure threshold is gradually lowered when they are repeatedly subjected to convulsions or electrical stimuli; eventually, the cells can become autonomously firing. Post (1992) has suggested that this phenomenon might underlie the tendency for episodes of affective disorder to require fewer provoking life events, or become more refractory, with passing time. He proposes that anticonvulsants prevent this progression by preventing kindling. There is some evidence that this phenomenon occurs in unipolar depression. A study from Virginia (Kendler et al 2000) followed

up over 2000 community-based female twin pairs over 9 years, and found that each episode of depression was followed by an increased subsequent risk of a further episode of depression. This was an essentially linear relationship up to nine episodes, after which the rate was constant. They also found that the risk that each life event a person experienced would be followed by depression decreased with each successive depressive episode, i.e. each successive episode of depression was less stress-related. These findings are based on a sound methodology and are supportive of the presence of a process similar to kindling. However, the specific mechanisms underlying this effect remain unclear, although investigation into links with the transcription or expression of peptides and neural growth factors is ongoing.

Intracellular signalling

There is evidence that antidepressants are able to modify intracellular signalling, for example by enhancing the cyclic AMP pathway activation occurring after serotonergic receptor stimulation (Duman et al 1997). It has been hypothesized that G proteins, important signal transducers in the phosphoinositol system, are overactive in depression; they are also potentially important in the mechanism of action of lithium. Several growth factors and neurotrophins are altered in depression, and may be important in neuronal changes seen in depression. Antidepressants also have effects on the expression of these factors. A new cellular model of depression is evolving in which there are felt to be impairments in signalling pathways that regulate neuroplasticity and cell survival (Manji et al 2001).

Immunology

Psychosocial stress can have an effect on the immune system. Thus, bereavement, marital disturbance and examinations are associated with findings such as reduced natural killer (NK) cell activity, reduced lymphocyte proliferation, and altered white cell counts. While the results in depression are often confusing, given the variety of measures used, in general there is a reduction in indices of immunocompetence as represented by NK cell activity and mitogen-induced lymphocyte proliferation. The degree to which these immunological observations result from other changes in depression, such as the HPA axis and behavioural factors like sleep, remains unclear.

Interferon treatment is strongly associated with the onset of depressive symptoms and illness, and can be a problematic complication in those treated for disorders such as melanoma and hepatitis. The mechanism is unclear, but may be linked to effects on the HPA axis or 5HT metabolism. Treatment with SSRIs can improve symptoms (Musselman et al 2001).

Sleep studies

Depression is associated with a number of abnormalities of sleep, including reduced REM latency, decreased deep sleep, and increased REM sleep (and therefore dreaming/nightmares), as shown by EEG changes. These effects may represent increased cholinergic activity. Depressed patients show supersensitivity to REM sleep effects of cholinergics and serotonergics. Sleep deprivation and selective REM sleep deprivation may result in temporary improvement in mood. Antidepressants reduce total REM sleep and reduce REM latency independent of their antidepressant effect.

Neurobiology of atypical depression

In view of the relatively recent addition of atypical depression to the psychiatric nosology, few data exist on the similarities and differences between typical and atypical depression. One of the most frequently observed differences relates to the hypothalamo-pituitary-adrenal axis. While hypercortisolaemia is characteristic of melancholic major depression (see below), several studies have now suggested that atypical depression is associated with hypocortisolaemia. Gold and colleagues have suggested that, while typical major depression can be characterized by an excessive activation of both the physiological stress systems, the locus coeruleus-noradrenergic system and the hypothalamo-pituitary-adrenal axis, the opposite changes are present in atypical depression (Gold et al 1995). Some support for this is provided by studies showing that the control of noradrenergic function is relatively preserved in atypical compared to typical depression (Asnis et al 1995). Gold and colleagues (1995) suggest that it is diminished central corticotrophin-releasing hormone (CRH) activity that is specifically related to the symptoms of hypoarousal of the syndrome. Support that it is low CRH rather than low cortisol that is related to the atypicality syndrome comes from one detailed study of Cushing syndrome, in which cortisol is high and CRH low, where atypical depression was the predominant depressive syndrome (Dorn et al 1995). Studies of serotonergic function are lacking, though one study suggested that platelet 5HT function is unaltered in atypical depression (Owens & Nemeroff 1994).

Neurobiology of psychotic depression

There is some evidence that there may be biological differences between psychotic depression and non-psychotic depression in terms of a more disturbed HPA axis (see above), increased dopamine turnover (i.e. higher homovanillic acid (HVA) levels in the CSF) and different patterns of disturbance of 5HT pathways (Wheeler Vega et al 2000). Overall, however, a separation on the basis of neurobiology remains premature.

Psychological components

Psychodynamic

The psychoanalytic view of depression was first developed from the similarities and differences between grief and depression, for example Freud's essay on 'mourning and melancholia'. Thus, the emphasis was on the importance of loss, which may be external (bereavement or separation) or an internally represented loss (an ideal or abstraction). Depression resulted when feelings of love and hostility were present at the same time (ambivalence), with hostility re-directed inwards. Loss of or threat to self-esteem was also emphasized by later writers. Klein suggested that depression was more likely if infants failed successfully to pass through 'the depressive position', when an infant learns to assimilate certain aspects of loss and restitution.

Cognitive

The cognitive theory of depression, as first described by Beck (1967), suggests that the cognitive distortions and errors that accompany depression are not just reflections of the lowered mood, but are instrumental in the origin and persistence of the disorder. For example, depressed people have substantial distortions of memory, with access to pleasant memories reduced and to unpleasant memories facilitated. Such distortions serve to amplify low mood. Cognitive theorists identify several specific errors in the thinking of depressed patients, described in Box 20.5.

In addition, Beck theorized that people develop *schema* – characteristic ways of interpreting and looking at the world, based upon development, learning, genetics, etc. These are then instrumental in bringing about cognitive distortions and hence depression. Although earlier studies indicated better efficacy in moderate depression, more recent studies have suggested that cognitive therapy may be as effective as medication for severely depressed outpatients (DeRubeis et al 1999).

Behavioural

Seligman (1975) developed a paradigm of chronic stress in animals, and found that some animals lose their capacity to act and avoid the stress. *Learned helplessness* was his term for the situation when reward or punishment is independent of any actions of the animal. This is also associated with similar behavioural, endocrine and neurochemical changes to those found in depressed people.

In a cognitive–behavioural formulation, Lewinsohn and colleagues (1970) proposed that a normal mood state depends upon positive behavioural rewards, which may result from job or marital satisfaction, while distressing experiences are associated with negative rewards, and hence depression.

Clinically, behavioural factors may be relevant to understanding the maintenance of some depressive illnesses. Patients may become stuck in a situation of reduced motivation to undertake activities, and hence experience less rewarding experiences. Similarly, there may be other important forces reinforcing unhelpful behaviours such as overprotective or under-supportive partners.

Box 20.5

The cognitive theory of depression

1. Automatic negative thoughts – regarding past, present and future (the cognitive triad: worthlessness, helplessness and hopelessness)
2. Negative expectations
3. Cognitive distortions:
   i. Arbitrary inference – assuming events to have negative implications
   ii. Selective abstraction – concentrating on only the negative aspects of events
   iii. Magnification – attaching undue importance to insignificant matters
   iv. Minimization – underestimating good performance or events
   v. Overgeneralization – extensive conclusions drawn from single incidents
   vi. Personalization.

up longer term difficulties such as low self-esteem as well as more acute changes related to depression. Other widely used scales are the General Health Questionnaire (GHQ) and the Hospital Anxiety and Depression Scale (HADS). The HADS has been designed to be used in those with physical illnesses, while the GHQ is well validated in primary care populations.

Thus, choice of scale depends upon the specific purpose required and the time available; however, it is probably true that some degree of objective rating of the effects of treatment is desirable in the management of depression, yet remains rarely implemented by psychiatrists outside of the domains of research.

Differential diagnosis

The main differentials for milder illness are anxiety, dysthymia, OCD or personality disorder. For more severe illnesses, dementing and psychotic illnesses become more important differentials. Organic illness should always be considered in the differential diagnosis.

Normal sadness/bereavement

Normal sadness lacks the other features of the syndrome. Bereavement may have many features of the syndrome, but is regarded as normal unless prolonged (>2 months in DSM-IV) or unusually severe, with features such as profound retardation, suicidal ideas or psychosis. Transient auditory and visual hallucinations of the dead person occur normally in about 10% of cases.

Anxiety disorders

It is clear that mild depression shows a large overlap with generalized anxiety disorder. Although in some cases it will be possible to distinguish the two by history (e.g. anxiety only occurring in the setting of a depressive illness) or examination (predominance of one set of symptoms over the other), in many mild cases it is neither practical nor necessary to differentiate between the two; most studies show a good response to antidepressants in both groups. ICD-10 recognized this by including the category of mixed anxiety and depression. Depression is a frequent occurrence in the natural history of agoraphobia, but less so in social and specific phobias.

Obsessive–compulsive disorder

Premorbid obsessional personality traits are a risk factor for depression. Furthermore, obsessional symptoms occur in 20–30% of patients with depression, most of whom do not have premorbid obsessional symptoms. Conversely, 35% of those with obsessive-compulsive disorder will also meet criteria for major depression.

Persistent affective disorders (dysthymia)

The Epidemiological Catchment Area (ECA) study showed that about half of subjects with dysthymia also suffered from recurrent major depression. Dysthymia does not therefore necessarily exclude a past or present diagnosis of depression if the severity criteria are met.

Personality disorder

Although this is a major differential, the presence of a premorbid personality disorder does not lessen the likelihood of depression; rather, the opposite is true. Patients with a personality disorder, or personality traits such as obsessionality or neuroticism, have an increased vulnerability to depression. Similarly, maladaptive personality traits may be more prominently expressed when patients are depressed, and there is some evidence that they are reversible on resolution of depressive symptoms.

Non-affective psychosis

Depressive symptoms are common in schizophrenia. The relative contribution of mood disorder must be determined in anyone presenting with predominantly paranoid features in order not to misdiagnose a psychotic depression. Psychotic features in depression are mood-congruent, i.e. related to themes of punishment, guilt, illness or nihilism. Post-schizophrenic depression is common after the acute psychosis; the best treatment is uncertain at present, but it may respond to antidepressants or antipsychotics.

Organic disorders

Dementia

Depressive pseudodementia may be mild, or severe and difficult to distinguish from organic dementia. Box 20.7 gives the main distinguishing features.

It is likely that there is an overlap in this separation. A large proportion of elderly patients with depression show evidence of cortical atrophy and enlarged ventricles. Thus, even in pseudodementia, there may be a significant organic component; indeed, there is some evidence that patients who develop pseudodementia while depressed have a higher incidence of organic dementia at follow-up. If in doubt, the patient should be treated as depressed. A PET study measuring cerebral blood flow

Box 20.7

Distinguishing true and pseudodementia

- Illness features that favour a diagnosis of depression or depressive pseudodementia:
  - Rapid onset
  - Distressed affect
  - Fluctuating cognitive deficit and patient's complaint of this
  - Islands of normality, with no dyspraxia or dysphasia
  - Past or family history of affective disorder
- Illness features that favour a diagnosis of dementia:
  - Normal sleep/wake cycle
  - No diurnal variation in symptoms
  - Gradual onset, with prominent memory disturbance, and focal features, such as apraxia, agnosia and dysphasia

showed that depressive pseudodementia showed features distinct from either depression or dementia, namely decreases in the left anterior medial prefrontal cortex and increases in the cerebellar vermis (Dolan et al 1992).

Others

A variety of medical conditions may be associated with depressive symptoms (Box 20.8). Similarly, many drugs may produce depressive symptoms (Boxes 20.9, 20.10). Organic factors must be considered in all cases of depression.

The Royal College of General Practitioners prospective contraception study suggests a small increase in the risk of depression with oestrogen doses >35 μg daily (Kay 1984). Kendler's twin study suggested that the tendency to develop depressive symptoms on the oral contraceptive was strongly genetic, but different from the genes controlling baseline susceptibility to depression (Kendler et al 1988).

Box 20.8

Organic causes of a depressive syndrome

Endocrine: disorders of cortisol, thyroxine or parathormone production; hypopituitarism; hypoglycaemia
Infections: glandular fever, syphilis, AIDS, encephalitis
Neurological: stroke, Parkinson disease, multiple sclerosis, brain tumours (classically meningioma), trauma, cerebral lupus
Carcinoma: common non-metastatic manifestation, especially pancreatic carcinoma, which may otherwise remain occult, and lung carcinoma
Nutritional: deficiencies of folate, nicotinamide (pellagra), vitamins B$_{12}$, B$_1$ (thiamine), B$_6$
Other: cerebral ischaemia, myocardial infarction.

Box 20.9

Drugs associated with depressive syndromes

Cardiovascular: methyldopa, reserpine, beta-blockers, clonidine, diuretics, digoxin
Endocrine: steroids, oral contraceptive (see text)
Neurological: L-Dopa, bromocriptine
Others: interferon alpha, pentazocine, indometacin, chloroquine, mefloquine
On withdrawal: psychostimulants (e.g. amphetamines, cocaine), benzodiazepines
Alcohol: cause and consequence.

Box 20.10

Prevalence of psychiatric side-effects of exogenous corticosteroid therapy

- Depression – 32%
- Mania – 22%
- Mixed affective symptoms – 6%
- Schizophreniform psychosis/delusional disorder – 11%
- Delirium – 8%.

Management

General management

The general management of depression must include consideration of the following:

- The need for inpatient or day-patient admission:
  a. In favour:
    - Allowing patient and family a breathing space
    - Danger of suicide
    - Inadequate nutrition and lack of self-care
  b. Against:
    - Stigma of hospitalization
    - Undermining of ability to cope
    - Institutionalization
- The use of the Mental Health Act
- Assessment using multidisciplinary team
- Risk.

Treatments

Pharmacological

Antidepressant medications are effective in moderate to severe depressive episode. The recent guideline from the National Institute for Clinical Excellence (NICE 2009) suggests that antidepressant medications should not be used to treat mild depression, but should be reserved for people with past history of moderate or severe depression, and in cases where the mild symptoms are chronic or unresponsive to initial non-medication treatment options such as low-intensity psychosocial interventions. A stepped care model is recommended in which duration and severity of the depressive disorder is considered in the treatment decision (Table 20.1).

More detail on indications, contraindications, side-effects, therapeutic effects and drug interactions of the various drugs that may be used in the treatment and prophylaxis of affective disorders are discussed in detail in Chapter 39. The general principles behind drug treatment strategies only are summarized here.

If antidepressant drugs are to be prescribed, the following principles should be observed:

- In view of the risk of overdose, outpatients should be assessed frequently and short supplies of drugs prescribed. Most tricyclic antidepressants are dangerous in overdose, and newer drugs may be preferred where there is concern.
- Prompt assessment following the initiation of antidepressants is also important given the possible increased risk of suicide in the early stages of treatment with an SSRI, particularly in those under 30.
- Patients (and their relatives) should be warned about the delay in treatment response, otherwise they may stop the treatment as ineffective.
- The nature and duration of likely side-effects should be described to aid adherence to treatment as well as to keep patients well-informed. Some patients may prefer some

Table 20.1 The stepped care model (adapted from the NICE guideline)

Symptom severity	Intervention	Level of care
Suspected depression	Assessment, monitoring and support and psychoeducation	Primary care
Persistent subthreshold depression, mild to moderate depression	Low-intensity psychosocial intervention, medication, referral	Primary care
As above with poor treatment response; moderate and severe depression	Medication, high-intensity psychosocial intervention, referral	Primary care and/or secondary care
Severe and complex depression; associated potential risk	Medication, high-intensity psychosocial intervention, combination therapy, ECT, inpatient care	Secondary care and/or tertiary care

potential side-effect profiles to others. Also, if sedative drugs are to be used, the effects on driving and the sedative interaction with alcohol should be explained. Some measures show amitriptyline to be as cognitively impairing as alcohol above the legal limit.

- The non-addictive nature of antidepressants should be stressed, as patients will frequently harbour a fear of addiction and subsequently not comply. However, patients should be warned of the possibility of discontinuation effects on abruptly stopping antidepressants, particularly those with a short half-life.
- Elderly patients may be more prone to develop problematic side-effects on older tricyclics, especially anticholinergic and hypotensive effects, and thus SSRIs or newer agents may be preferred.
- Medically ill: many antidepressants are contraindicated in heart disease, epilepsy, etc. Also, most SSRIs inhibit some of the cytochrome P450 liver enzymes and may interact with many liver metabolized drugs.
- Occupation: patients who operate machinery or drive should not be given sedative drugs.
- Agitated depression: anxiety or agitation within depression responds to antidepressant treatment. It is not necessary routinely to give sedative drugs in most cases as sedative and anxiolytic effects are pharmacologically distinct.
- Pregnancy: if drugs are necessary, older tricyclics are preferred as there is more experience of their use, although more data and experience is also now emerging with SSRIs.

Physical

Electroconvulsive therapy

ECT is discussed in detail in Chapter 40. Patients with severe depression in whom a rapid response is needed, such as life-threatening states (dehydration, physical complications, stupor or suicidal behaviour) or postpartum, should be considered early for ECT. Otherwise, ECT is reserved for patients resistant to other treatments. Unlike antidepressants, ECT causes upregulation of postsynaptic $5HT_2$ receptors. Other effects (e.g. normalization of the reduced prolactin response to fenfluramine) are the same. ECT is clearly efficacious for the short-term treatment of depression (Geddes 2003). However, the caveats to ECT use include a number of contraindications, side-effects, patient acceptability and the tendency to relapse.

Sleep deprivation

Deprivation of sleep, and particularly REM sleep, is associated with substantial improvement in mood, although it is not usually a sustained response. Nevertheless, a positive response to sleep deprivation is predictive of future response to other somatic treatments.

Transcranial magnetic stimulation

Transcranial magnetic stimulation uses a strong and rapidly changing magnetic field to stimulate electrical activity in neurons. Early results suggest that it is effective compared to a sham procedure, and induces neurochemical changes similar to ECT, but its role in resistant cases of depression remains unproven.

Vagus nerve stimulation

Vagus nerve stimulation involves surgically attaching an electrode to the vagus nerve in the neck in order to stimulate afferent pathways into the brain. Primarily used as a treatment for refractory epilepsy, it may have some antidepressant properties in resistant cases.

Light therapy

Bright light has been shown to be effective in several placebo-controlled studies of seasonal depression. Morning light is more effective than evening light, and leads to a phase advance of the sleep–wake cycle and dim-light melatonin onset. The exact treatment protocols differ, but those found to be effective include 1.5 h per day of 6000 lux bright light starting at 6.00 a.m. There is evidence that serotonergic mechanisms may be important in the effectiveness of light treatment (Lam et al 1996). What remains unclear is the selection of which patients will respond, the regimens which are consistently most effective and the effect size of the treatment in comparison with other potential treatments.

Exercise

Aerobic exercise has beneficial effects on mood, and has been shown in at least one RCT to be of benefit in treating depression.

Neurosurgery

Neurosurgery for mental disorders (NMD, formerly psychosurgery), is described in detail in Chapter 40. This is rarely used, but can be performed for cases of severe, intractable depression using strict controls under the Mental Health Act, including fully informed consent and a second opinion. There are several techniques, including the use of diathermy and radioactive iridium implants in operations such as subcaudate tractotomy. Approximately one-third of patients are reported to gain marked benefit, one-third mild benefit and one-third no benefit. Side-effects can include personality changes of a frontal lobe nature and epilepsy. *Deep brain stimulation* is a recently developed neurosurgical procedure in which functional (and reversible) lesions can be induced. Its use in depression remains experimental only.

Psychological

Behavioural therapy

Behavioural treatments such as problem-solving techniques are effective in mild depression, and supported by several RCTs. Techniques such as behavioural activation and occupational therapy can be very useful adjuncts to treatment. In recent meta-analyses (Ekers et al 2008; Mazzucchelli et al 2009), behavioural activation has been shown to be superior in efficacy to control conditions and supportive therapy and to be similar to that of cognitive therapy.

Cognitive therapy

Cognitive therapy aims to alter the disturbed cognitions discussed above. Trials in outpatients have shown it to be as effective for mild to moderate depression in the short term as antidepressants. Other studies have suggested it may reduce relapse (Blackburn & Moore 1997; Fava et al 1998). Brief versions of cognitive therapy may be effective in primary care (Scott et al 1997) and postnatally (Appleby et al 1997).

Psychotherapy

Supportive psychotherapy should be part of the treatment of all depressed patients, with the following aims:

- Empathic, supporting relationship
- Ventilation of distress
- Education about nature of disorder
- General semi-directive counselling.

Brief focused therapies such as described by Malan (1976) may be useful. Dynamic psychotherapy is not a treatment for acute depression, but may help selected patients subject to recurrent depression modify some predisposing factors and develop insight into preventing certain precipitating factors.

Interpersonal therapy

Depression is viewed as a disorder of interpersonal relationships, regardless of aetiology. Therapy aims at symptom relief and a more effective approach to relationships. Reduced frequency therapy is an effective prophylaxis to reduce relapse (Frank et al 2007). There is some evidence that IPT may be effective on a group basis.

Couple therapy

Couple therapy has been shown to be a useful and effective therapy for depression where there is a degree of discord within the relationship, or where aspects of the relationship are felt to be a maintaining factor in a depressive illness.

Mindfulness-based cognitive therapy (MBCT)

MBCT was developed with the aim of preventing depressive relapse. It includes breathing exercises and meditation to help participants become more aware of the present moment and reduce depressive ruminations.

Social

Effective treatment of depression requires close attention to social factors. Patients may benefit from advice on, or help with, changing adverse social situations such as financial, housing and employment difficulties. Family relationships may need attention and, if indicated, specific family therapy. The meaning of a social situation may be modified by cognitive therapy.

Relative efficacy of treatments

The relative efficacy of treatments is under-researched or suffers from the use of underpowered trials. There is no convincing evidence that any antidepressant or class of antidepressants is more effective than another. While some older meta-analytic reports suggested a slightly increased rate of response or remission for the dual 5HT and noradrenergic drugs amitriptyline (Barbui & Hotopf 2001) and venlafaxine (Smith et al 2002), a recent meta-analysis comparing 12 new generation antidepressants has suggested sertraline and escitalopram may be more efficacious and acceptable (Cipriani et al 2009). This study does not consider the potential impact of gender on differential response and acceptability, which was shown to be an important factor in treatment response. In a study comparing sertraline and imipramine among patients with chronic depression, sertraline was shown to be more acceptable and more efficacious among women whereas this was the case for imipramine among men (Kornstein et al 2000).

A systematic review of RCTs, mostly in secondary care, suggests that cognitive therapy is at least as effective as antidepressant therapy (and behavioural therapies) in mild to moderate depression (Gloaguen et al 1998). There was also evidence that cognitive therapy was superior to non-directive therapy. The NIMH trial found no clear difference in efficacy between interpersonal psychotherapy and cognitive therapy, although later analyses suggested that there was overlap in the therapies actually received in that study. Several RCTs in primary care suggest that problem solving therapy is as effective as drugs. Evidence regarding the efficacy of non-directive counselling remains poor (Churchill et al 1999). The combination of antidepressants and cognitive therapy or interpersonal therapy affords a slight benefit over either alone, particularly in more severely ill patients (Thase et al 1997). A large RCT of a combination of an antidepressant and a form of cognitive therapy in chronic depression (mean duration 8 years) showed clear benefits over either therapy alone, in terms both of symptoms and of function (Keller et al 2000).

Some studies have looked at ways of improving the effectiveness in practice of the various therapies, and have shown that it is possible to improve outcome through means of standardized care pathways (including factors such as improved patient education, telephone follow-up and support to the primary care physician).

Barbui, C., Hotopf, M., 2001. Amitriptyline v. the rest: still the leading antidepressant after 40 years of randomised controlled trials. Br. J. Psychiatry 178, 129–144.

Beardsley, G., Goldstein, M.G., 1993. Psychological factors affecting physical condition. Endocrine disease literature review. Psychosomatics 34, 12–19.

Bebbington, P.E., 1998. Sex and depression. Psychol. Med. 28, 1–8.

Beck, A., 1967. Depression: clinical, theoretical and experimental aspects. University of Pennsylvania Press, Philadelphia.

Belanoff, J.K., Kalehzan, M., Sund, B., et al., 2001. Cortisol activity and cognitive changes in psychotic major depression. Am. J. Psychiatry 158, 1612–1616.

Bench, C.J., Friston, K.J., Brown, R.G., et al., 1993. Regional cerebral blood flow in depression measured by positron emission tomography: the relationship with clinical dimensions. Psychol. Med. 23, 579–590.

Benkelfat, C., Ellenbogen, M.A., Dean, P., et al., 1994. Mood-lowering effect of tryptophan depletion. Enhanced susceptibility in young men at genetic risk for major affective disorders. Arch. Gen. Psychiatry 51, 687–697.

Blackburn, I.M., Moore, R.G., 1997. Controlled acute and follow-up trial of cognitive therapy and pharmacotherapy in out-patients with recurrent depression. Br. J. Psychiatry 171, 328–334.

Blazer, D., Kessler, R., Swartz, M., 1998. Epidemiology of recurrent major and minor depression with a seasonal pattern. The National Comorbidity Survey. Br. J. Psychiatry 172, 164–167.

Blier, P., Galsin, A.M., Langer, S.Z., 1990. Interaction between serotonin uptake inhibitors and alpha-2 adrenergic heteroceptors in the rat hypothalamus. J. Pharmacol. Exp. Ther. 254, 236–254.

Bloch, M., Schmidt, P.J., Danaceau, M.A., et al., 1999. Dehydroepiandrosterone treatment in mid-life dysthymia. Biol. Psychiatry 45, 1533–1541.

Bowlby, J., 1980. Attachment and loss, Vol. 3. Loss: sadness and depression. Basic Books, New York.

Bremner, J.D., Innis, R.B., Salomen, R.M., et al., 1997. Positron emission tomography measurement of cerebral metabolic correlates of tryptophan depletion-induced relapse. Arch. Gen. Psychiatry 54, 364–374.

Bremner, J.D., Vythilingam, M., Ng, C.K., et al., 2003. Regional brain metabolic correlates of a-methylparatyrosine-induced depressive symptoms: implications for the neural circuitry of depression. J. Am. Med. Assoc. 289, 3125–3134.

Brody, A.L., Saxena, S., Stoessel, P., et al., 2001. Regional brain metabolic changes in patients with major depression treated with either paroxetine or interpersonal therapy: preliminary findings. Arch. Gen. Psychiatry 58, 631–640.

Brown, E.S., Woolston, D.J., Frol, A., et al., 2004. Hippocampal volume, spectroscopy, cognition and mood in patients receiving corticosteroid therapy. Biol. Psychiatry 55, 538–545.

Brown, G., Harris, T., 1978. The social origins of depression. Tavistock, London.

Brown, G.W., Harris, T.O., Peto, J., 1973. Life events and psychiatric disorders: the nature of the causal link. Psychol. Med. 11, 159–176.

Burt, D.B., Zembar, M.J., Niederehe, G., 1995. Depression and memory impairment: a meta-analysis of the association, its pattern, and specificity. Psychol. Bull. 117, 285–305.

Campbell, S., Marriott, M., Nahmias, C., et al., 2004. Lower hippocampal volume in patients suffering from depression: a meta-analysis. Am. J. Psychiatry 161, 598–607.

Caspi, A., Sugden, K., Moffit, T.E., et al., 2003. Influence of life stress in depression: moderation by polymorphism in the 5-HTT gene. Science 301, 386–389.

Chan, C.H., Janicak, P.G., Davis, J.M., et al., 1987. Response of psychotic and nonpsychotic depressed patients to tricyclic antidepressants. J. Clin. Psychiatry 48, 197–200.

Checkley, S., 1996. The neuroendocrinology of depression and chronic stress. Br. Med. Bull. 52, 597–617.

Checkley, S.A., Slade, A.P., Shur, P., 1981. Growth hormone and other responses to clonidine in patients with endogenous depression. Br. J. Psychiatry 138, 51–55.

Churchill, R., Dewey, M., Gretton, V., et al., 1999. Should general practitioners refer patients with major depression to counsellors? A review of current published evidence. Nottingham Counselling and Antidepressants in Primary Care (CAPC) Study Group. Br. J. Gen. Pract. 49, 738–743.

Cipriani, A., Furukawa, T.A., Salanti, G., et al., 2009. Comparative efficacy and acceptability of 12 new-generation antidepressants: a multiple-treatments meta-analysis. Lancet 373, 746–758.

Coppen, A., 1967. The biochemistry of affective disorders. Br. J. Psychiatry 113, 1237–1264.

Coryell, W., Schlesser, M., 2001. The dexamethasone suppression test in suicide prediction. Am. J. Psychiatry 158, 748–753.

Crimlisk, H.L., Bhatia, K., Cope, H., et al., 1998. Slater revisited: 6 year follow up study of patients with medically unexplained motor symptoms. Br. Med. J. 316, 582–586.

De Bellis, M., Chrousos, G., Dorn, L., et al., 1994. Hypothalamic-pituitary-adrenal axis dysregulation in sexually abused girls. J. Clin. Endocrinol. Metab. 78, 249–255.

de Groot, J.C., de Leeuw, F.E., Oudkerk, M., et al., 2000. Cerebral white matter lesions and depressive symptoms in elderly adults. Arch. Gen. Psychiatry 57, 1071–1076.

Delgado, P.L., Miller, H.L., Salomon, R.M., et al., 1993. Monoamines and the mechanism of antidepressant action: effects of catecholamine depletion on mood of patients treated with antidepressants. Psychopharmacol. Bull. 29, 389–396.

Delgado, P.L., Price, L.H., Miller, H.L., et al., 1994. Serotonin and the neurobiology of depression. Effects of tryptophan depletion in drug-free depressed patients. Arch. Gen. Psychiatry 51, 865–874.

Delgado, P.L., Miller, H.L., Salomon, R.M., et al., 1999. Tryptophan-depletion challenge in depressed patients treated with desipramine or fluoxetine: implications for the role of serotonin in the mechanism of antidepressant action. Biol. Psychiatry 46, 212–220.

DeRubeis, R.J., Gelfand, L.A., Tang, T.Z., et al., 1999. Medication versus cognitive therapy for severely depressed outpatients: Mega-analysis of four randomized comparisons. Am. J. Psychiatry 156, 1007–1013.

Dolan, R.J., Bench, C.J., Brown, R.G., et al., 1992. Regional cerebral blood flow abnormalities in depressed patients with cognitive impairment. J. Neurol. Neurosurg. Psychiatry 55, 768–773.

Dorn, L.D., Burgess, E.S., Dubbert, B., et al., 1995. Psychopathology in patients with endogenous Cushing's syndrome: 'atypical' or melancholic features. Clin. Endocrinol. (Oxf.) 43, 433–442.

Drevets, W.C., 2001. Neuroimaging and neuropathological studies of depression: implications for the cognitive-emotional features of mood disorders. Curr. Opin. Neurobiol. 11, 240–249.

Drevets, W.C., Frank, E., Price, J.C., et al., 1999. PET imaging of serotonin 1A receptor binding in depression. Biol. Psychiatry 46, 1375–1387.

Duman, R.S., Heninger, G.R., Nestler, E.J., 1997. A molecular and cellular theory of depression. Arch. Gen. Psychiatry 54, 597–606.

Eaton, W.W., Anthony, J.C., Gallo, J., et al., 1997. Natural history of Diagnostic Interview Schedule/DSM-IV major depression. The Baltimore Epidemiologic Catchment Area follow-up. Arch. Gen. Psychiatry 54, 993–999.

Ebmeier, K.P., Donaghey, C., Steele, J.D., 2006. Recent developments and current controversies in depression. Lancet 367, 153–167.

Ekers, D., Richards, D., Gilbody, S., 2008. A meta-analysis of randomised trials of behavioural treatments of depression. Psychol. Med. 38, 611–623.

Ellenbogen, M.A., Young, S.N., Dean, P., et al., 1996. Mood response to acute tryptophan depletion in healthy volunteers: sex differences and temporal stability. Neuropsychopharmacology 15, 465–474.

Elliott, R., Baker, S.C., Rogers, R.D., et al., 1997. Prefrontal dysfunction in depressed patients performing a complex planning task: a study using positron emission tomography. Psychol. Med. 27, 931–942.

Elliott, R., Rubinsztein, J.S., Sahakian, B.J., et al., 2002. The neural basis of mood-congruent processing biases in depression. Arch. Gen. Psychiatry 59, 597–604.

Engleman, E.A., Perry, K.W., Mayle, D.A., et al., 1995. Simultaneous increases in extracellular monoamines in microdialysates from hypothalamus of conscious rates by duloxetine, a dual serotonin and norepinephrine uptake inhibitor. Neuropsychopharmacology 12, 287–296.

Fava, G.A., Raffnelli, C., Grandi, S., et al., 1998. Prevention of recurrent depression with cognitive behavioural therapy: preliminary findings. Arch. Gen. Psychiatry 55, 816–820.

Fekadu, A., Wooderson, S., Markopoulo, K., et al., 2009. What happens to patients with treatment-resistant depression? A systematic review of medium to long term outcome studies. J. Affect. Disord. 116, 4–11.

Frank, E., Kupfer, D.J., Buysse, D.J., et al., 2007. Randomized trial of weekly, twice-monthly and monthly interpersonal psychotherapy as maintenance treatment for women with recurrent depression. Am. J. Psychiatry 164, 761–767.

Frasure Smith, N., Lesperance, F., Talajic, M., 1995. Depression and 18-month prognosis after myocardial infarction. Circulation 91, 999–1005.

Fu, C.H., McGuire, P.K., 1999. Functional neuroimaging in psychiatry. Philos. Trans. R. Soc. Lond. B Biol. Sci. 354, 1359–1370.

Fu, C.H., Reed, L.J., Meyer, J.H., et al., 2001. Noradrenergic dysfunction in the prefrontal cortex in depression: an [15O] H$_2$O PET study of the neuromodulatory effects of clonidine. Biol. Psychiatry 49, 317–325.

Fu, C.H., Williams, S.C., Cleare, A.J., et al., 2004. Attenuation of the neural response to sad faces in major depression by antidepressant treatment: a prospective, event-related functional magnetic resonance imaging study. Arch. Gen. Psychiatry 61, 877–889.

Geddes, J., 2003. Efficacy and safety of electroconvulsive therapy in depressive disorders: a systematic review and meta-analysis. Lancet 361, 799–808.

Geddes, J.R., Carney, S.M., Davies, C., et al., 2003. Relapse prevention with antidepressant drug treatment in depressive disorders: a systematic review. Lancet 361, 653–661.

George, M.S., Ketter, T.A., Parekh, P.I., et al., 1997. Blunted left cingulate activation in mood disorder subjects during a response interference task (the Stroop). J. Neuropsychiatry Clin. Neurosci. 9, 55–63.

Gloaguen, V., Cottraux, J., Cucherat, M., et al., 1998. A meta-analysis of the effects of cognitive therapy in depressed patients. J. Affect. Disord. 49, 59–72.

Gold, P.W., Licinio, J., Wong, M.L., et al., 1995. Corticotropin releasing hormone in the pathophysiology of melancholic and atypical depression and in the mechanism of action of antidepressant drugs. Ann. N.Y. Acad. Sci. 771, 716–729.

Harris, B., Othman, S., Davies, J.A., et al., 1992. Association between postpartum thyroid dysfunction and thyroid antibodies and depression. Br. Med. J. 305, 152–156.

Heim, C., Newport, D.J., Heit, S., et al., 2000. Pituitary-adrenal and autonomic responses to stress in women after sexual and physical abuse in childhood. J. Am. Med. Assoc. 284, 592–597.

Henderson, S., Byrne, D.G., Duncan-Jones, P., 1982. Neurosis and the social environment. Academic Press, London.

Heuser, I., Yassouridis, A., Holsboer, F., 1994. The combined dexamethasone/CRH test: a refined laboratory test for psychiatric disorders. J. Psychiatr. Res. 28, 341–356.

Hotopf, M., Carr, S., Mayou, R., et al., 1998. Why do children have chronic abdominal pain, and what happens to them when they grow up? Br. Med. J. 316, 1196–1199.

Howland, R.H., 1993. Thyroid dysfunction in refractory depression: implications for pathophysiology and treatment. J. Clin. Psychiatry 54, 47–54.

Jacoby, R.J., Levy, R., 1980. Computerised tomography in the elderly 3: affective disorder. Br. J. Psychiatry 136, 270–275.

Janowsky, D.S., Overstreet, D.H., 1995. The role of acetylcholine mechanisms in mood disorders. In: Kupfer, D.J., Bloom, F.E. (Eds.), Psychopharmacology: the fourth generation of progress. Raven Press, New York, pp. 945–956.

Joffe, R., Marriott, M., 2000. Thyroid hormone levels in recurrence of major depression. Am. J. Psychiatry 157, 1689–1691.

Judd, L.L., Paulus, M.J., Schettler, P.J., et al., 2000. Does incomplete recovery from first lifetime major depressive episode herald a chronic course of illness? Am. J. Psychiatry 157, 1501–1504.

Kay, C.R., 1984. The Royal College of General Practitioners' Oral Contraception Study: some recent observations. Clin. Obstet. Gynaecol. 11, 759–786.

Keller, M.B., McCullough, J.P., Klein, D.N., et al., 2000. A comparison of nefazodone, the cognitive behavioral-analysis system of psychotherapy, and their combination for the treatment of chronic depression. N. Engl. J. Med. 342, 1462–1470.

Kendell, R.E., 1976. The classification of depressions: a review of contemporary confusion. Br. J. Psychiatry 129, 15–28.

Kendler, K.S., 1997. The diagnostic validity of melancholic major depression in a population-based sample of female twins. Arch. Gen. Psychiatry 54, 299–304.

Kendler, K.S., Gardner, C.O., 1998. Boundaries of major depression: an evaluation of DSM-IV criteria. Am. J. Psychiatry 155, 172–177.

Kendler, K.S., Karkowski-Shuman, L., 1997. Stressful life events and genetic liability to major depression: genetic control of exposure to the environment? Psychol. Med. 27, 539–547.

Kendler, K.S., Martin, N.G., Heath, A.C., et al., 1988. A twin study of the psychiatric side effects of oral contraceptives. J. Nerv. Ment. Dis. 176, 153–160.

Kendler, K.S., Kessler, R.C., Walters, E.E., et al., 1995. Stressful life events, genetic liability, and onset of an episode of major depression in women. Am. J. Psychiatry 152, 833–842.

Kendler, K.S., Eaves, L.J., Walters, E.E., et al., 1996. The identification and validation of distinct depressive syndromes in a population-based sample of female twins. Arch. Gen. Psychiatry 53, 391–399.

Kendler, K.S., Thornton, L.M., Gardner, C.O., 2000. Stressful life events and previous episodes in the etiology of major depression in women: an evaluation of the 'kindling' hypothesis. Am. J. Psychiatry 157, 1243–1251.

Kendler, K.S., Thornton, L.M., Gardner, C.O., 2001. Genetic risk, number of previous depressive episodes, and stressful life events in predicting onset of major depression. Am. J. Psychiatry 158, 582–586.

Kendler, K.S., Hettema, J.M., Butera, F., et al., 2003. Life event dimensions of loss, humiliation, entrapment, and danger in the prediction of onsets of major depression and generalized anxiety. Arch. Gen. Psychiatry 60, 789–796.

Kessler, R.C., McGonagle, K.A., Zhao, S., et al., 1994. Lifetime and 12-month prevalence of DSM-III-R psychiatric disorders in the United States. Results from the National Comorbidity Survey. Arch. Gen. Psychiatry 51, 8–19.

Kessler, R.C., Berglund, P., Demler, O., et al., 2003. The epidemiology of major depressive disorder: results from the National Co-morbidity Survey Replication (NCS-R). J. Am. Med. Assoc. 289, 3095–3105.

Klaassen, T., Riedel, W.J., van Someren, A., et al., 1999. Mood effects of 24-hour tryptophan depletion in healthy first-degree relatives of patients with affective disorders. Biol. Psychiatry 46, 489–497.

Klerman, G.L., Weissman, M.M., 1989. Increasing rates of depression. J. Am. Med. Assoc. 261, 2229–2235.

Kornstein, S.G., Schatzberg, A.F., Thase, M.E., et al., 2000. Gender differences in treatment response to sertraline versus imipramine in chronic depression. Am. J. Psychiatry 157, 1445–1452.

Kupfer, D.J., Frank, E., Perel, J.M., et al., 1992. Five-Year Outcome for Maintenance Therapies in Recurrent Depression. Arch. Gen. Psychiatry 49, 769–773.

Lambert, G., Johansson, M., Ågren, H., et al., 2000. Reduced brain norepinephrine and dopamine release in treatment-refractory depressive illness: evidence in support of the catecholamine hypothesis of mood disorders. Arch. Gen. Psychiatry 57, 787–793.

Lam, R.W., Zis, A.P., Grewal, A., et al., 1996. Effects of rapid tryptophan depletion in patients with seasonal affective disorder in remission after light therapy. Arch. Gen. Psychiatry 53, 41–44.

Lee, A.S., Murray, R.M., 1988. The long-term outcome of Maudsley depressives. Br. J. Psychiatry 153, 741–751.

Lewinsohn, P.M., Weinstein, M.S., Alpere, T.A., 1970. A behavioural approach to the group treatment of depressed persons: a methodological contribution. J. Clin. Psychol. 26, 525–532.

Maciejewski, P.K., Zhang, B., Block, S.D., et al., 2007. An empirical examination of the stage theory of grief. J. Am. Med. Assoc. 297, 716–723.

Maes, M., Meltzer, H., 1995. The serotonin hypothesis of major depression. In: Bloom, F.E., Kupfer, D.J. (Eds.), Psychopharmacology. Fourth generation of progress. Raven Press, New York, pp. 933–944.

Malan, D., 1976. The frontier of brief psychotherapy. Plenum Medical, New York.

Manji, H.K., Drevets, W.C., Charney, D.S., 2001. The cellular neurobiology of depression. Nat. Med. 7, 541–547.

Mann, J.J., Malone, K.M., Diehl, D.J., et al., 1996. Demonstration in vivo of reduced serotonin responsivity in the brain of untreated depressed patients. Am. J. Psychiatry 153, 174–182.

Mayberg, H.S., Liotti, M., Brannan, S.K., et al., 1999. Reciprocal limbic-cortical function and negative mood: converging PET findings in depression and normal sadness. Am. J. Psychiatry 156, 675–682.

Mayberg, H.S., Brannan, S.K., Tekell, J.L., et al., 2000. Regional metabolic effects of fluoxetine in major depression: serial changes and relationship to clinical response. Biol. Psychiatry 48, 830–843.

Mazzucchelli, T., Kane, R., Rees, C., 2009. Behavioural activation treatments for depression in adults: a meta-analysis and review. Clin. Psychol. Sci. Pract. 16, 383–411.

McGuffin, P., Katz, R., Rutherford, J., 1991. Nature, nurture and depression: a twin study. Psychol. Med. 21, 329–335.

McGuffin, P., Katz, R., Watkins, S., et al., 1996. A hospital-based twin register of the heritability of DSM-IV unipolar depression. Arch. Gen. Psychiatry 53, 129–136.

Mendlewicz, J., Rainer, J.D., 1977. Adoption study supporting genetic transmission in manic–depressive illness. Nature 268, 327–329.

Meyer, J.H., Kennedy, S., Brown, G.M., 1998. No effect of depression on [(15)O]H$_2$O PET response to intravenous d-fenfluramine. Am. J. Psychiatry 155, 1241–1246.

Michelson, D., Stratakis, C., Hill, L., et al., 1996. Bone mineral density in women with depression. N. Engl. J. Med. 335, 1176–1181.

Moghaddan, B., Bunney, B.S., 1990. Acute effects of typical and atypical antipsychotic drugs on the release of dopamine from prefrontal cortex, nucleus accumbens, and striatum of the rat: an in vivo microdialysis study. J. Neurochem. 54, 1755–1760.

Moreno, F.A., Heninger, G.R., McGahueya, C.A., et al., 2000. Tryptophan depletion and risk of depression relapse: a prospective study of tryptophan depletion as a potential predictor of depressive episodes. Biol. Psychiatry 48, 327–329.

Murphy, B.E., 1997. Antiglucocorticoid therapies in major depression: a review. Psychoneuroendocrinology 22, S125–S132.

Musselman, D.L., Lawson, D.H., Gumnick, J.F., et al., 2001. Paroxetine for the prevention of depression induced by high-dose interferon alfa. N. Engl. J. Med. 344, 961–966.

Nemeroff, C., 1996. The corticotropin-releasing factor (CRF) hypothesis of depression: new findings and new directions. Mol. Psychiatry 1, 336–342.

Nemeroff, C.B., Evans, D.L., 1989. Thyrotropin-releasing hormone (TRH), the thyroid axis, and affective disorder. Ann. N.Y. Acad. Sci. 553, 304–310.

Nemeroff, C.B., Simon, J.S., Haggerty, J.J., et al., 1985. Antithyroid antibodies in depressed patients. Am. J. Psychiatry 150, 1728–1730.

NICE, 2009. Depression: the treatment and management of depression in adults. National Institute for Health and Clinical Excellence, London. Online. Available: http://www.nice. org.uk/nicemedia/pdf/ Depression_update_FULL_GUIDELINE.pdf (accessed 12.12.09.).

O'Flynn, K., Dinan, T.G., 1993. Baclofen-induced growth hormone release in major depression: relationship to dexamethasone suppression test result. Am. J. Psychiatry 150, 1728–1730.

Owens, M.J., Nemeroff, C.B., 1994. Role of serotonin in the pathophysiology of depression: focus on the serotonin transporter. Clin. Chem. 40, 288–295.

Parker, G., Roy, K., Hadzi-Pavlovic, D., et al., 1992. Psychotic (delusional) depression: a meta-analysis of physical treatments. J. Affect. Disord. 24, 17–24.

Parkes, C.M., 1998. Editorial. Bereave. Care 17, 18.

Paykel, E.S., 1971. Classification of depressed patients: a cluster analysis derived grouping. Br. J. Psychiatry 118, 275–288.

Paykel, E.S., 1978. Contribution of life events to causation of psychiatric illness. Psychol. Med. 8, 245–253.

Paykel, E.S., Ramana, R., Cooper, Z., et al., 1995. Residual symptoms after partial remission: an important outcome in depression. Psychol. Med. 25, 1171–1180.

Paykel, E.S., Scott, J., Teasdale, J.D., et al., 1999. Prevention of relapse in residual depression by cognitive therapy: a controlled trial. Arch. Gen. Psychiatry 56, 829–835.

Petrides, G., Fink, M., Husain, M.M., et al., 2001. ECT remission rates in psychotic versus nonpsychotic depressed patients: a report from CORE. J. ECT 17, 244–253.

Piccinelli, M., Wilkinson, G., 1994. Outcome of depression in psychiatric settings. Br. J. Psychiatry 164, 297–304.

Post, R.M., 1992. Transduction of psychosocial stress into the neurobiology of recurrent affective disorder. Am. J. Psychiatry 149, 999–1010.

Price, J., 1968. The genetics of depressive behaviour. In: Coppen, A., Walk, S. (Eds.), Recent developments in affective disorders 2. British Journal of Psychiatry Special Publication, pp. 37–54.

Reimherr, F.W., Amsterdam, J.D., Quitkin, F.M., et al., 1998. Optimal length of continuation therapy in depression: a prospective assessment during long-term fluoxetine treatment. Am. J. Psychiatry 155, 1247–1253.

Rush, A.J., Trivedi, M.H., Wisniewski, S.R., et al., 2006. Acute and longer-term outcomes in depressed outpatients requiring one or several treatment steps: A STAR*D report. Am. J. Psychiatry 163, 1905–1917.

Sargent, P.A., Kjaer, K.H., Bench, C.J., et al., 2000. Brain serotonin1A receptor binding measured by positron emission tomography with [11C]WAY-100635: effects of depression and antidepressant treatment. Arch. Gen. Psychiatry 57, 174–180.

Schatzberg, A.F., Schildkraut, J.J., 1995. Recent studies on norepinephrine systems in mood disorders. In: Bloom, F.E., Kupfer, D.J. (Eds.), Psychopharmacology. The fourth generation of progress. Raven Press, New York, pp. 911–920.

Schatzberg, A.F., Garlow, S.J., Nemeroff, C.B., 2002. Molecular and cellular mechanisms in depression. In: Davis, K.L., Charney, D., Coyle, J.T. et al., (Eds.), Neuropsychopharmacology. The fifth generation of progress. Lippincott, Williams & Wilkins, Philadelphia, pp. 1039–1050.

Scott, C., Tacchi, M.J., Jones, R., et al., 1997. Acute and one-year outcome of a randomised controlled trial of brief cognitive therapy for major depressive disorder in primary care. Br. J. Psychiatry 171, 131–134.

Seligman, M.E.P., 1975. Helplessness: on depression, development and death. Freeman, San Francisco.

Sheline, Y.I., Mintun, M.A., 2002. Structural and functional imaging of affective disorders. In: Davis, K.L., Charney, D., Coyle, J.T. et al., (Eds.), Neuropsychopharmacology. The fifth generation of progress. Lippincott, Williams & Wilkins, Philadelphia, pp. 1065–1080.

Siever, L.J., 1987. Role of noradrenergic mechanisms in the etiology of the affective disorders. In: Meltzer, H.Y. (Ed.), Psychopharmacology. The third generation of progress. Raven Press, New York.

Siever, L.J., Trestman, R.L., Coccaro, E.F., 1992. The growth hormone response to clonidine in acute and remitted depressed male patients. Neuropsychpharmacology 6, 165–177.

Simon, G.E., Goldberg, D.P., von Korff, M., et al., 2002. Understanding cross-national differences in depression prevalence. Psychol. Med. 32, 585–594.

Smith, D., Dempster, C., Glanville, J., et al., 2002. Efficacy and tolerability of venlafaxine compared with selective serotonin reuptake inhibitors and other antidepressants: a meta-analysis. Br. J. Psychiatry 180, 396–404.

Smith, K.A., Fairburn, C.G., Cowen, P.J., 1997. Relapse of depression after rapid depletion of tryptophan. Lancet 349, 915–919.

Smith, K.A., Morris, J.S., Friston, K.J., et al., 1999. Brain mechanisms associated with depressive relapse and associated cognitive impairment following acute tryptophan depletion. Br. J. Psychiatry 174, 525–529.

Solomon, D.A., Keller, M.B., Leon, A.C., et al., 1997. Recovery from major depression. Arch. Gen. Psychiatry 54, 1001–1006.

Starkman, M.N., Gebarski, S.S., Berent, S., et al., 1992. Hippocampal formation volume, memory dysfunction, and cortisol levels in patients with Cushing's syndrome. Biol. Psychiatry 32, 756–765.

Sullivan, P.F., Kessler, R.C., Kendler, K.S., 1998. Latent class analysis of lifetime depressive symptoms in the national co-morbidity survey. Am. J. Psychiatry 155, 1398–1406.

Taylor, D., Paton, C., Kerwin, R.W., 2009. The South London and Maudsley NHS Trust; Oxleas NHS Foundation Trust: Prescribing guidelines, tenth ed. Informa Healthcare, London.

Taylor, W.D., Steffens, D.C., MacFall, J.R., et al., 2003. White matter hyperintensity progression and late-life depression outcomes. Arch. Gen. Psychiatry 60, 1090–1096.

Tennant, C., 2002. Life events, stress and depression: a review of recent findings. Aust. N.Z. J. Psychiatry 36, 173–182.

Thakore, J.H., Richards, P.J., Reznek, R.H., et al., 1997. Increased intra-abdominal fat deposition in patients with major depressive illness as measured by computed tomography. Biol. Psychiatry 41, 1140–1142.

Thase, M.E., Simons, A.D., Reynolds, C.F.D., 1993. Psychobiological correlates of poor response to cognitive behavior therapy: potential indications for antidepressant pharmacotherapy. Psychopharmacol. Bull. 29, 293–301.

Thase, M.E., Dube, S., Bowler, K., et al., 1996. Hypothalamic-pituitary-adrenocortical activity and response to cognitive behavior therapy in unmedicated, hospitalized depressed patients. Am. J. Psychiatry 153, 886–891.

Thase, M.E., Greenhouse, J.B., Frank, E., et al., 1997. Treatment of major depression with psychotherapy or psychotherapy-pharmacotherapy combinations. Arch. Gen. Psychiatry 54, 1009–1015.

Videbech, P., Ravnkilde, B., 2004. Hippocampal volume and depression: a meta-analysis of MRI studies. Am. J. Psychiatry 161, 1957–1966.

Weissman, M.M., Bland, R.C., Canino, G.J., et al., 1996. Cross-national epidemiology of major depression and bipolar disorder. J. Am. Med. Assoc. 276, 293–299.

Wheeler Vega, J., Mortimer, A., Tyson, P.J., 2000. Somatic treatment of psychotic depression: review and recommendations for practice. J. Clin. Psychopharmacol. 20, 504–519.

WHO, 1992. ICD-10 Classification of mental and behavioural disorders. WHO, Geneva.

Willner, P., 1995. Dopaminergic mechanisms in depression and mania. In: Bloom, F.E., Kupfer, D.J. (Eds.), Psychopharmacology. The fourth generation of progress. Raven Press, New York, pp. 921–931.

Wolkowitz, O.M., Reus, V.I., Keebler, A., et al., 1999. Double-blind treatment of major depression with dehydroepiandrosterone. Am. J. Psychiatry 156, 646–649.

Yatham, L.E., Liddle, P.F., Shiah, I.S., et al., 2000. Brain serotonin2 receptors in major depression: a positron emission tomography study. Arch. Gen. Psychiatry 57, 850–858.

Young, A.H., Gallagher, P., Porter, R.J., 2002. Elevation of the cortisol-dehydroepiandrosterone ratio in drug-free depressed patients. Am. J. Psychiatry 159, 1237–1239.

Zheng, D., Macera, C.A., Croft, J.B., et al., 1997. Major depression and all-cause mortality among white adults in the United States. Ann. Epidemiol. 7, 213–218.

Bipolar disorders

21

Paul Mackin   Allan Young

CHAPTER CONTENTS

Table 21.1 Clinical features of hypomania and mania

	Hypomania	Mania
Appearance	May be unremarkable Demeanour may be cheerful	Often striking Clothes may reflect mood state Demeanour may be cheerful Dishevelled and fatigued in severe states
Behaviour	Increased sociability and disinhibition	Overactivity and excitement Social disinhibition
Speech	May be talkative	Often pressured with flight of ideas
Mood	Mild elation or irritability	Elated or irritable Boundless optimism Typically no diurnal pattern May be labile
Vegetative signs	Increased appetite Reduced need for sleep Increased libido	Increased appetite Reduced need for sleep Increased libido
Psychotic symptoms	Not present Thoughts may have an expansive quality	Thoughts may have an expansive quality Delusions and second-person auditory hallucinations may be present, often grandiose in nature 10–20% have Schneiderian first rank symptoms
Cognition	Mild distractibility	Marked distractibility. More marked disturbance in severe states
Insight	Usually preserved	Insight often lost, especially in severe states

is a manifestation of the rapid influx of thoughts, and patients give accounts of thoughts flooding the mind. When the individual is difficult to interrupt as a result of an incessant desire to talk and express these thoughts, speech is referred to as *pressured*. A more severe disorder of thinking manifested in speech is *flight of ideas* in which there is a logical connection between two sequential ideas, but the goal of conversation is not maintained and is difficult to follow. Flight of ideas often arises out of an extreme degree of distractibility and inappropriate responses to environmental cues. *Puns* and *clang associations* may also punctuate conversation. Although the form of speech may be disordered, important differences exist, which differentiate the patterns of speech characteristic of mania and schizophrenia. In schizophrenia, there is often a breakdown in association between ideas such that there appears to be no understandable connection between the chain of thoughts and the listener is often left feeling confused and bewildered.

Mood

An altered mood state is the core feature of mania and hypomania. Classically, mood is thought to be elated but frequently, it is irritable. The importance of an awareness of the manifestations of hypomanic and manic mood states cannot be overstated as many individuals presenting with irritability, rather than euphoric mania, are incorrectly diagnosed as suffering from unipolar depression with potentially disastrous consequences if treated only with antidepressant drugs. When elated, the individual appears inappropriately cheerful and may experience boundless optimism. Elated mood has an infectious quality, and is often

accompanied by religious or metaphysical preoccupations. Irritability, however, may predominate, which is intensely distressing and may result in irascible verbal and/or behavioural outbursts and in extreme cases, violence may occur. Although during a manic or hypomanic episode mood may change throughout the day, it usually does not show the diurnal pattern characteristic of depression. The mood may, however, be labile and frequently shift between elation and tearful dysphoria or irritability.

Vegetative signs

Appetite is frequently increased during hypomania and mania but this is not invariably accompanied by increased food intake. Indeed, the converse may occur resulting in weight loss as a consequence of reduced oral intake and increased motor activity. Sleep disturbance is characteristic, and individuals describe a reduced need for sleep and as such, are often resistive to suggestions that they retire to bed. Initial insomnia occurs and sleep may last for only 2–3 hours, after which energetic activity is resumed. Libido is often increased and there may be increased sexual interest and activity. Individuals may engage in impulsive and reckless liaisons and disregard issues such as birth control. Counselling and, if appropriate, pregnancy testing or referral to a sexual health clinic, should be offered to individuals if necessary.

Psychotic and related symptoms

Thoughts frequently have an expansive quality, which is congruent with the prevailing mood state, and are often grandiose in nature. These thoughts may be overvalued inasmuch as they preoccupy the individual and are pursued beyond the bounds of reason, but are not held with delusional intensity. When delusional ideas exist they may be of a grandiose or persecutory nature. Common grandiose themes are religious conversion or salvation, personal wealth or influence, and royal descent. Persecutory delusions may arise out of a belief that others are trying to frustrate the individual's plans. The content of the delusional idea(s) is often not stable and changes over a period of days. Delusions of reference and passivity phenomena may also occur, and it is estimated that Schneiderian first rank symptoms occur in 10–20% of manic episodes.

Auditory hallucinations are the most common perceptual disturbance occurring during a manic episode. Generally, they are mood-congruent and in the second person, such as God addressing the individual and offering instructions for world salvation. Reports exist of visual hallucinations occurring during mania, again typically taking the form of a religious scene, but visual hallucinations should alert the clinician to the possibility of an organic brain syndrome.

Cognition

Marked distractibility is common during mania. The immediate environment may provide a rich source of stimulation, which may frustrate any attempts to interview the individual. Orientation is usually preserved except in the most severe cases, but attention and concentration are often impaired. More subtle cognitive impairments, particularly in the realm of executive functioning, have been identified in recent years, but sophisticated neuropsychological testing is required to identify these abnormalities (see below).

Insight

The degree of impaired insight depends on the severity of the episode. Hypomania is often characterized by relatively preserved insight, and it is not uncommon for individuals to recognize a shift into hypomania and to seek medical intervention. In severe mania, however, insight is lost completely and any intervention is met with disdain and resistance. The use of statutory powers, such as those conferred by the Mental Health Act, are often required in order to offer appropriate treatment in the safest environment.

Manic stupor

Following the advent of effective pharmacological treatment of mania, the occurrence of manic stupor is now rare. When it does occur, it may follow from a period of manic excitement, or more rarely in the transition between depressive stupor and mania. Characteristically, the individual is immobile and mute with a serene facial expression or one suggestive of elation. On recovery the events during the stuporose period are recalled, and descriptions are given of rapid thoughts typical of mania.

Mixed states

Periods of depression and (hypo)mania are the hallmark of bipolar disorders. The switch between depression and mania occurs within a variable time frame with or without an intervening period of euthymia. Symptoms of mania and depression, however, may occur concurrently, and the term 'mixed state' is best reserved for such situations. For example, an individual my appear overactive with pressured speech and flight of ideas, but at the same time be experiencing profoundly negative and morbid thoughts. Females are more frequently represented in the group of mixed states, and using broad definitions, more than two-thirds of individuals with bipolar disorder have a mixed state at least once during the course of the illness.

Cyclothymia

Cyclothymia is often referred to as a persistent disorder of mood and is associated with significant distress and/or impairment of functioning. It is characterized by numerous hypomanic episodes and periods of depression that do not meet criteria for a diagnosis of bipolar disorder or recurrent (major) depressive disorder (see below). Mood swings often are not related to life events, and diagnosis can be difficult in the absence of clear and detailed accounts of symptoms and their chronology. The picture is also frequently complicated by substance misuse.

Classification

Box 21.2 shows the classification of bipolar disorders in ICD-10 and DSM-IV. Although the two systems share common features, there are important differences, which are discussed in more detail below.

ICD-10

Full diagnostic criteria are given in Appendix 1 at the end of this chapter.

Hypomania

Hypomania is defined in ICD-10 as elevated or irritable mood that is abnormal for the individual and is sustained for at least 4 days. Features such as over-familiarity, increased activity or talkativeness, distractibility, or reduced sleep should also be present, but these symptoms are not present to the extent that they lead to severe social disruption of work or result in social rejection. Criteria for a manic episode should not be met, nor should hallucinations or delusions be present.

Mania

Mania is defined as elevated, expansive or irritable mood that must be sustained for at least 1 week. Accompanying symptoms may include increased activity or talkativeness, flight of ideas, disinhibition, reduced sleep, grandiosity or reckless behaviour, which lead to severe interference with personal functioning in daily living. Mania may occur without or with psychotic symptoms, which may be mood-congruent or mood-incongruent. Typical mood-congruent hallucinations would take the form of voices telling the individual that he/she had superhuman powers. Mood-incongruent psychotic symptoms may include voices speaking about affectively neutral topics, or delusions of persecution.

Box 21.2

The classification of bipolar disorders in ICD-10 and DSM-IV

ICD-10

Mood (affective) disorders

- Hypomania
- Mania
  - Without psychotic symptoms
  - With psychotic symptoms
- Bipolar affective disorder
  - Current episode hypomanic
  - Current episode manic
  - Current episode depression[a]
  - Current episode mixed
- Persistent mood (affective) disorders
- Cyclothymia.

DSM-IV

Mood disorders

Mood episodes

- Hypomanic episode
- Manic episode

Bipolar disorders

Bipolar I disorder[d]

- Single manic episode[b]
- Most recent episode hypomanic
- Most recent episode manic[b]
- Most recent episode mixed[b]
- Most recent episode depressed[b]

Bipolar II disorder[d]

- Current episode hypomania
- Current episode depressed[c]

Cyclothymic disorder.

[a]Specified as mild, moderate or severe, with or without psychotic features.
[b]Specified as mild, moderate, severe without psychotic features, severe with psychotic features, in partial remission, in full remission.
[c]Severity and presence of psychotic features are specified.
[d]Rapid cycling may be used as a course modifier.

Bipolar affective disorder

The minimum ICD-10 criteria for diagnosing bipolar affective disorder are two separate mood episodes, one of which must be hypomania, mania or a mixed affective state. The current episode must be specified, and may be one of the following: hypomania; mania without psychotic symptoms; mania with psychotic symptoms; mild or moderate depression; severe depression without psychotic symptoms; severe depression with psychotic symptoms; mixed episode; or in remission.

Cyclothymia

In ICD-10, cyclothymia is classified under persistent mood (affective) disorders, and is defined as a persistent instability of mood involving numerous periods of depression and mild elation, none of which is sufficiently severe or prolonged to justify a diagnosis of bipolar affective disorder or recurrent depressive disorder. The period of instability of mood must be of at least 2 years' duration.

DSM-IV

Full diagnostic criteria are given in Appendix 2 to this chapter.

Hypomania

A hypomanic episode is defined as a distinct period during which there is an abnormally and persistently elevated, expansive, or irritable mood that lasts at least 4 days. Additional symptoms, such as inflated self-esteem, decreased need for sleep, distractibility or increase in goal-directed activity, must be present. The episode should not be severe enough to cause marked impairment in social or occupational functioning, or necessitate hospitalization, nor should there be psychotic features.

Mania

In DSM-IV a manic episode is defined as a distinct period of abnormally and persistently elevated, expansive or irritable mood, lasting 1 week (or any duration if hospitalization is necessary). Accompanying symptoms may include inflated self-esteem, sleep disturbance, pressure of speech and excessive involvement in pleasurable activities. The mood disturbance is sufficiently severe to cause marked impairment in occupational functioning or in usual social activities or relationships with others, or to necessitate hospitalization to prevent harm to self or others. Psychotic features may be present.

Bipolar disorders

Within the DSM-IV classification, bipolar disorders are subdivided into bipolar I disorder, bipolar II disorder, cyclothymia and bipolar disorder not otherwise specified (NOS).

Bipolar I disorder

The essential feature of bipolar I disorder is a clinical course characterized by the occurrence of one or more manic episodes, or mixed episodes. Often individuals have also had one or more major depressive episodes. The current episode may be specified as: mild; moderate; severe without psychotic features; severe with psychotic features; in partial remission; in full remission; with catatonic features or with postpartum onset. The type of mood episode (hypomania, mania, depression or mixed) should also be specified.

Bipolar II disorder

The essential feature of bipolar II disorder is a clinical course that is characterized by the occurrence of one or more major depressive episodes accompanied by at least one hypomanic episode. The presence of a manic or a mixed episode precludes the diagnosis of bipolar II disorder. Specifiers for current episodes are similar to those for bipolar I disorder.

Cyclothymic disorder

DSM-IV defines cyclothymic disorder as a chronic, fluctuating mood disturbance involving numerous periods of hypomanic symptoms and numerous periods of depressive symptoms. These symptoms should not meet full criteria for a manic episode or a major depressive episode, and should be present for at least 2 years (1 year in children and adolescents).

Differential diagnoses

Both depressive and manic disorders include schizophrenic illnesses and organic brain syndromes as possible differential diagnoses. The differential diagnosis of depressive disorders is considered elsewhere in this volume, and the following account highlights the important conditions from which manic disorders must be distinguished.

The differential diagnosis of manic disorders (Box 21.3) includes:

- Cyclothymia
- Schizophrenia
- Organic brain syndromes
- Illicit substance misuse
- Iatrogenic causes.

Cyclothymia

As referred to above, cyclothymia shares many of the characteristics of manic-depressive illness, but the severity and duration of symptoms are not sufficient to make a diagnosis of mania or recurrent depressive disorder. In order to make a diagnosis of cyclothymia, careful attention must be given to the history of the mood instability, and a corroborative account from a family member or close friend can assist in distinguishing the two disorders. Notwithstanding, a proportion of individuals with cyclothymia will go on to develop frank bipolar disorder (see below).

Schizophrenia

Differentiating mania from schizophrenia can be a difficult diagnostic problem, particularly in an acute setting with an unfamiliar patient. Both conditions share similar clinical features

Box 21.3

The differential diagnoses of manic states

- Cyclothymia
- Schizophrenia
- Organic brain syndromes
  - Degenerative conditions
  - Cerebrovascular disease
  - Epilepsy
  - Multiple sclerosis
  - Brain injury
  - Space-occupying lesions
  - HIV/AIDS
  - Other cerebral infections
  - Cerebral inflammatory conditions
- Illicit substance and alcohol misuse
- Iatrogenic causes
  - Dopamine agonists
  - Corticosteroids
  - Thyroid hormones
  - Anticholinergics.

such as psychomotor disturbance, thought disorder and psychotic phenomena. Schneider's first rank symptoms occur in 10–20% of individuals with mania, and their presence should not necessarily point to a diagnosis of schizophrenia. However, delusional beliefs and auditory hallucinations are typically less stable in manic disorders. A previous history of depression or (hypo)mania, or a family history of bipolar disorder may assist in making the diagnosis.

Organic brain syndromes

The presence of symptoms suggestive of mania, particularly in an older patient without previous affective disturbance, should alert the clinician to the possibility of an organic brain syndrome. Careful examination of the mental state, including thorough cognitive assessment may indicate organic pathology. Frontal lobe pathology, such as fronto-temporal dementia or Pick's disease, may manifest as a coarsening of social skills or marked disinhibition that may mimic a manic syndrome. Cerebrovascular insults or head injury resulting in brain damage may produce an organic mood disorder characterized by a change in mood or affect, usually accompanied by a change in the overall level of activity. Space-occupying lesions may cause significant mood disturbance, as well as worsening the course of an already established bipolar illness. The rise in the incidence of HIV infection should prompt careful investigation, particularly in younger individuals who present with atypical features.

Illicit substance misuse

A number of recreational drugs can cause affective and behavioural disturbance, which may mimic mania. A careful history of illicit substance use together with urine drug-screening may be helpful in reaching a diagnosis. Typically, the symptoms associated with drug misuse subside when the substance is withdrawn, unlike manic symptoms which persist. Co-morbid substance misuse is a significant problem for many individuals with established bipolar disorder, and continued use often destabilizes the illness and either prolongs recovery or precipitates relapse.

Iatrogenic causes

Prescribed medication can cause states resembling mania. Corticosteroids, especially in high doses can produce elated mood states as well as depression. Dopamine agonists and L-dopa may also cause pathological mood changes which may be difficult to distinguish from mania.

Epidemiology

The lifetime risk of bipolar disorder depends upon the diagnostic criteria used. The rate is usually quoted as approximately 1%, similar to that of schizophrenia. Lifetime prevalence rates of bipolar I and bipolar II disorders have both been estimated at approximately 1%, giving a combined prevalence of 2%. The

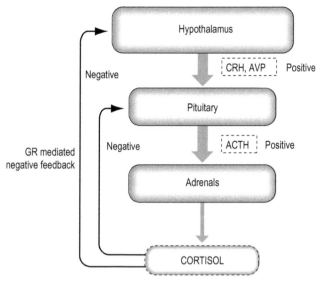

Figure 21.1 • The hypothalamic-pituitary-adrenal (HPA) axis. CRH, corticotropin-releasing hormone; AVP, arginine vasopressin; ACTH, adrenocorticotropin hormone; GR, glucocorticoid receptor.

Cortisol has a number of central and peripheral effects which are mediated via glucocorticoid receptors.

The activity of the HPA axis is highly regulated. Secretory cells within the paraventricular nucleus receive neuronal inputs from a number of brain regions including the amygdala, hippocampus and nuclei within the midbrain. The HPA axis also has an autoregulatory mechanism mediated by cortisol. Endogenous cortisol binds to glucocorticoid receptors in the HPA axis and acts as a potent negative regulator of HPA activity. These regulatory mechanisms are important in determining basal levels and circadian fluctuations in cortisol levels. Changes in glucocorticoid receptor number or function may be important in altering the homeostatic function of the HPA axis observed in healthy individuals.

Abnormalities of the HPA axis in depression have been well described. Plasma cortisol levels of patients with depression are higher than those of healthy controls. This observation has been consistently replicated, and studies have shown that HPA hyperactivity, as manifested by hypersecretion of CRH, increased cortisol levels in plasma, urine and cerebrospinal fluid, exaggerated cortisol responses to ACTH, and enlarged pituitary and adrenal glands, occurs in individuals suffering from severe mood disorders. Hypersecretion of CRH causing hypercortisolaemia may be a result of impaired feedback mechanisms resulting from glucocorticoid receptor abnormalities. Evidence of glucocorticoid receptor function abnormalities has been demonstrated in postmortem studies of patients with severe mood disorders. Reduced glucocorticoid receptor messenger RNA (mRNA) has been demonstrated in the hippocampi of individuals with unipolar and bipolar affective disorders, and there is accumulating evidence to suggest that antidepressant and mood-stabilizing drugs stimulate glucocorticoid receptor mRNA thus enhancing HPA autoregulation resulting in reduced CRH secretion and cortisol levels. The role of the HPA axis in bipolar disorders, and the place of antiglucocorticoid drugs as therapeutic agents in the management of these disorders are the focus of ongoing research activity (see below).

The hypothalamic-pituitary-thyroid axis

Abnormalities of thyroid function occur in mood disorders. Subclinical hypothyroidism is seen in a significant proportion of depressed patients, and an even higher proportion of those with treatment-resistant depression. T_3 (tri-iodothyronine) and T_4 (thyroxine) supplementation has been shown to enhance the effects of standard antidepressant treatment with regard to response rate and time to recovery, and may be particularly beneficial in those with treatment-resistance.

In mania, there are also abnormalities of thyroid function which include subclinical hypothyroidism and reduced pituitary responsiveness to thyrotropin-releasing hormone. Thyroid dysfunction has frequently been implicated in rapid cycling bipolar disorder, and is one of the most consistent findings within this subpopulation of those with bipolar illness. Thyroid supplementation may also be of some benefit in the treatment of rapid cycling.

Neuropathological studies

Studies of neuropathological changes in mood disorders, unlike studies in schizophrenia, are in their infancy. Findings are preliminary, and in many cases, inconsistent. Methodological difficulties with these studies, such as retrospective design, do not allow for straightforward interpretation of the available data, but these early studies have provided an impetus towards further investigation using suitable methodology. We await with interest further insights into the neuropathology of mood disorders, but a number of potentially important preliminary findings are briefly discussed below (Baumann & Bogerts 2001).

Increased brain weight, thicker parahippocampal cortex and smaller temporal horns have been described in a postmortem study of individuals with affective disorders compared with schizophrenic illnesses. Adding support to the suggestion that patients with mood disorders may have structural abnormalities in the parahippocampal cortex is another postmortem study, which showed a reduction in cortex size in suicide victims compared with non-psychiatric controls. Cytoarchitectural studies have also revealed malformations in the entorhinal lamination in patients with bipolar disorder and major depression. Additionally, further evidence of abnormalities of temporal lobe structure in bipolar disorder is provided by the reported reduction of non-pyramidal neurons in the CA2 region of the hippocampus of patients with bipolar disorder and schizophrenia. These studies add weight to the evidence provided by magnetic resonance imaging (MRI) studies, which have suggested temporal lobe pathology to exist not only in schizophrenia, but also in bipolar disorders.

The prefrontal lobe, the medial prefrontal cortex and the anterior cingulate cortex have also attracted attention in attempts to identify neuroanatomical abnormalities in mood disorders. Decreased cortical and laminar thickness have been demonstrated in the dorsolateral prefrontal cortex in patients with bipolar disorder and major depressive disorder, and volume reduction together with fewer glial cells have been observed in the subgenual prefrontal cortex (part of the anterior cingulate cortex) in familial mood disorders.

MRI studies have also identified a variety of other structural brain abnormalities in patients with bipolar disorder. Cerebral

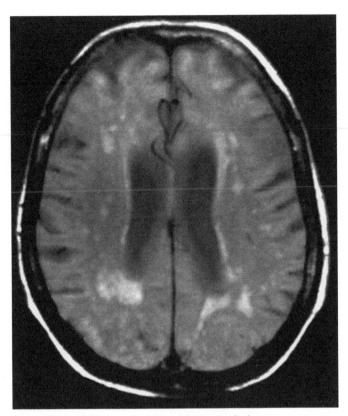

Figure 21.2 • MRI scan showing white matter lesions.

white matter lesions, as shown in Figure 21.2, have attracted particular attention, and a recent study has revealed that subcortical white matter lesions are associated with poor outcome in bipolar disorder (Moore et al 2001). The significance of these lesions in the aetiology of bipolar disorders, or as course modifiers, remains to be elucidated.

Taken together, these findings provide convincing evidence that mood disorders are associated with diverse neuroanatomical changes which may be indicative of circumscribed neurodevelopmental disturbances. An excellent review of the neuropathology of mood disorders can is given by Harrison (2002).

Psychological theories

A variety of psychological theories of the aetiology of depression and mania have been posited and, although there is evidence to support the use of some psychological treatments for depression, the aetiological significance of psychological theories of depression, and in particular mania, is controversial.

Loss is central to the psychodynamic view of the precipitant of depression and mania. Freud believed that the loss of an ambivalently loved object resulted in turning against the self. In depression this results in anxiety, guilt and possibly suicidality; in mania the ego is released from oppressive domination by the super-ego. Melanie Klein proposed the term *manic defence*, which she suggested to be a defence mechanism employed by the ego to protect against the psychic pain of depression and anxiety. Omnipotent control, triumph and contempt result and prevent the process of reparation. Few psychiatrists now

attach aetiological significance to these theories, but they may be useful in understanding the content of the ideas that often characterize the manic state.

Course and outcome

Illness course

Initial presentation

Bipolar illness often becomes clinically manifest in the late teenage years, although a substantial number of individuals are initially misdiagnosed with unipolar depression. Such misdiagnosis may have serious consequences if antidepressant drugs are used without mood-stabilizing agents. The proportion of 'false unipolars' in the diagnosis of unipolar depressive disorder has been estimated to be between 10.7% and 28.4% (Goodwin & Jamison 1990). Patients presenting for the first time with depressive symptoms should be carefully investigated for a history suggestive of (hypo)mania.

There is good agreement in the literature that the peak onset occurs in the 20s (between 25 and 30) (Goodwin & Jamison 1990), and the mean age of first hospitalization is at around the age of 26 years. Frequently, there have been previous episodes of affective disturbance that have not required admission to psychiatric inpatient facilities. With the increasing implementation of community-based psychiatric assessment and treatment services that are able to provide intensive home-based treatment and support, some of these admissions may be avoided. Those experiencing severe manic or depressive episodes, with their attendant risks of self-harm and social disruption are, however, likely to continue to require inpatient care.

In females, there is a secondary peak of mania occurring around the age of 45–50 years, which has caused some to speculate about the role of hormonal influences in this group of individuals. First onset of mania in late life is likely to be associated with organic brain disease and is often referred to as 'secondary mania'. Such individuals should be investigated for vascular, infective, inflammatory or degenerative disorders as well as space-occupying lesions and iatrogenic causes.

Number of episodes

Bipolar disorder is a chronic and recurrent condition, and the average number of mood episodes has been estimated to be 10. There is, however, huge variation with many individuals experiencing many more then 10 episodes in their lifetime. There are individuals who experience only one episode in a lifetime, but these are exceptions. The vast majority of patients have numerous mood episodes, but the patterns of mood disturbance in bipolar I and bipolar II disorders are different. Bipolar I disorder, the classic manic-depressive psychosis, is characterized by episodes of frank mania and depression, usually at well-spaced intervals. The defining characteristic of bipolar II disorder is the occurrence of hypomanic, but not manic, episodes. It is now clear that the major burden of illness in bipolar II disorder is depression, rather than hypomania, which has important treatment implications, particularly with regard to the use of antidepressant medication.

Frequency of episodes and length of cycles

The frequency of episodes can be estimated by evaluating the number and length of cycles. A cycle is defined as the time from one episode to the onset of the next. A variation in cycle length usually reflects variations in the length of intervals between episodes, as the length of episodes within an individual is often relatively stable. Survival analysis has shown that the first cycle is usually longer, and the second cycle shorter than all the others; later episodes usually arise at irregular intervals.

Length of episodes

The duration of depressive episodes in both unipolar and bipolar patients exceeds that of manic episodes. The duration of episodes of mania prior to the advent of effective pharmacological intervention was typically 3–12 months. It appears that duration of episodes is dependent on a number of factors, of which the most important is response to pharmacological treatment. The duration of a full depressive episode is typically 2–5 months, and that of manic episodes is on average 2 months (Goodwin & Jamison 1990). Within individuals, the length of mood episodes is often relatively stable, although as the illness progresses, the frequency of episodes may increase and the onset of each episode may be more abrupt.

Precipitants

Some theories on the pathogenesis of affective disorders assign primary causal relevance to the psychosocial environment, but it is now generally accepted that psychosocial or physical events contribute more to the timing of an episode than to causing it. Causality is likely to be largely biological and especially genetic (Goodwin & Jamison 1990). Precipitating events seem to be important in the onset of the first episode but not in subsequent ones. One study found that approximately 53% of unipolar patients and 47% of bipolar patients had stressful life events prior to the onset of an episode (Marneros et al 1990). The kind of life event seems to be unspecific, and the only common factor in all life events appears to be sleep reduction.

Rapid cycling

Although the cycling nature of bipolar disorder (*la folie circulaire*) was described by Falret in 1851, it was not until the 1970s that researchers began to identify and investigate the subpopulation of patients with bipolar disorder who experienced a high frequency of mood changes. During the past decade, the phenomenon of rapid cycling bipolar disorder has been widely accepted and its significance as a course modifier, particularly with respect to pharmacological intervention, has attracted considerable research interest. 'Normal cycling' in the context of bipolar disorder has not been defined, but the definition of rapid cycling most frequently cited in the literature is that of Dunner and Fieve (1974): four major depressive, manic, hypomanic or mixed states are required to have occurred within a 12-month period.

Approximately 13–20% of individuals will develop rapid cycling bipolar disorder during the course of their illness. Those who develop rapid cycling are greatly over-represented in the bipolar II group, with a large female preponderance. Hypothyroidism (which is more prevalent in females) and menstrual cycle irregularities have been suggested as causal factors in the switch to rapid cycling. An alternative explanation cites the observation that rapid cycling is greatly over-represented in those individuals with bipolar II disorder, the hallmark of which is depression. The well-documented female predisposition to depressive recurrence may thus account for the unequal sex distribution of rapid cycling.

The differing pharmacological response profile of patients with rapid cycling is intriguing, and raises the question of whether rapid cycling should be classified as a distinct subtype of bipolar illness. Current data do not, however, support this view. To date, studies have recognized few genetic or phenotypic differences between rapid cycling and non-rapid cycling bipolar patients. For example, several family studies have reported a similar family history of bipolar disorder in rapid and non-rapid cycling probands, and suggest that rapid cycling does not breed true. A recent study has investigated the prospective course of illness and potential risk factors for rapid cycling (Kupka et al 2003). The factors that were most strongly associated with rapid cycling gradually increased with episode frequency, failing to indicate a non-linearity at four episodes per year, or at any other time point. Thus, the concept of rapid cycling as a distinct subtype of bipolar disorder does not gain support from the literature.

Antidepressant-induced cycling

The role of antidepressant medication in the induction of mania and cycle acceleration is controversial. Historical studies have attempted to correlate switching rate with increasing use of antidepressant drugs. A retrospective study examining mood fluctuation patterns in patients with affective disorders hospitalized over three decades revealed that rapid mood fluctuations were absent among bipolar patients in 1960, but were evident in 1975 and 1985, suggesting an association with prescribing practices (Wolpert et al 1990). Not all studies, however, support this view.

There is a considerable body of literature that implicates antidepressants in the induction of mania, and a number of studies have shown an association between rapid cycling and antidepressant use. Moreover, certain classes of antidepressants have been suggested to be associated with a higher risk of mania induction and/or cycle acceleration. A meta-analysis by Peet (1994) concluded that a manic switch was less likely to occur with selective serotonin reuptake inhibitors (SSRIs) than with tricyclic antidepressants. A recent study has examined the influence of antidepressant use and gender in the genesis of rapid cycling (Yildiz & Sachs 2003). A significant association was found between rapid cycling and antidepressant use prior to the first episode of (hypo)mania for women, but not for men.

Outcome

Kraepelin's assertion that affective psychoses have a 'good' outcome was over-optimistic. Long-term studies have shown that a significant proportion of patients with affective disorders have an unfavourable outcome, although individuals with affective disorders have a generally more favourable outcome than those with schizophrenic or schizoaffective disorders.

Studies of outcome in affective disorders are limited by heterogeneous definitions of 'unfavourable outcome', and the findings of these studies differ. However, studies focusing on the disability and disturbances of social functioning report that approximately one-third of bipolar patients do not have a 'social full remission', and approximately 25% of patients have persisting alterations to psychosocial functioning (Goodwin & Jamison 1990).

Suicide

The problem of suicide in patients with unipolar and bipolar affective disorders is one of the greatest problems in medicine. Patients with unipolar and bipolar disorders are far more likely to commit suicide than individuals in any other psychiatric risk group. The mortality rate for untreated bipolar patients is higher than that of most types of heart disease and many types of cancer (Goodwin & Jamison 1990). Approximately 15% of patients with bipolar disorder will commit suicide, and the rate of suicidal ideas is much greater. The risk of suicide appears to be greater during the first few years after onset of illness, with rates of completed suicide diminishing over time.

Recent evidence has strongly suggested that lithium reduces the rate of suicide among bipolar patients (Baldessarini et al 2006) and, additionally, lithium has been shown to have anti-viral and immunomodulatory action, which may explain the reduction of mortality in bipolar patients, beyond its anti-suicidal and mood-stabilizing effects (Lieb 2002). A recent study has also demonstrated that risk of suicide attempt and completed suicide is lower during treatment with lithium than during treatment with divalproex (Goodwin et al 2003).

Co-morbidity

A large proportion of individuals with bipolar disorder also abuse drugs and alcohol. Around 35% of patients with bipolar disorder may drink alcohol excessively, and studies have found that women with bipolar II disorder are much more likely to abuse alcohol than their bipolar I counterparts, whereas among the men, bipolar I and bipolar II patients were equally likely to drink alcohol excessively (Goodwin & Jamison 1990).

The data on drug abuse are much less extensive than those on alcohol abuse, but there is convincing data that shows that the rate of misuse of illicit substances such as cocaine and marijuana is greater in bipolar patients than in the general population. These drugs may destabilize the illness and trigger (hypo)mania. Early detection and treatment of drug or alcohol misuse is an essential part of the clinical management of those with bipolar disorders.

The problem of physical co-morbidity in bipolar disorder is now firmly established. Numerous studies have reported an excess of physical co-morbidity in patients with bipolar disorder compared to the general population. Cardiometabolic disease appears to be particularly prevalent in individuals with bipolar disorder, and recent research from the UK has shown that patients with severe mental illness (including bipolar disorder) had a hazard ratio of 3.22 for coronary heart disease mortality for people 18–49 years old (Osborn et al 2007). Obesity, type 2 diabetes mellitus and the metabolic syndrome, all established cardiovascular risk factors, are more prevalent in patients with bipolar disorder (Mackin & Ruttledge 2007). The precise causes of this excess of physical morbidity and premature mortality and not fully understood. Patients with bipolar disorder have a higher prevalence of tobacco smoking, and dietary intake together with reduced levels of physical activity may also contribute. Psychotropic medication, and in particular some of the atypical antipsychotic drugs which are being increasingly used in the management of bipolar disorder, are known to cause significant weight gain, disorders of glucose homeostasis and dyslipidaemias. It is important that healthcare professionals undertake regular monitoring of the physical health status of all individuals with severe mental illness, and offer appropriate primary and secondary interventions.

Neuropsychology

Kraepelin's proposed separation of the psychoses into dementia praecox and manic-depressive insanity, the latter being characterized by an episodic course and benign prognosis, is further undermined by emerging data revealing cognitive dysfunction not only in acute episodes but also in the euthymic phase of bipolar disorder. This intriguing field of research has recently been reviewed by Chowdhury et al (2003).

A number of studies have reported a wide spectrum of cognitive impairments in patients with bipolar disorders in both the manic and the depressive phases of the illness. Abnormalities have been found in tests of frontal lobe function, verbal fluency, verbal memory and sustained attention. More recently, cognitive assessment of euthymic bipolar patients have been undertaken in order to identify trait-dependent rather than state-dependent neuropsychological deficits. A recent study has demonstrated impairment of executive function, which entails a variety of processes responsible for the control of cognition and the regulation of behaviour and thought, in a cohort of patients prospectively verified as euthymic (Thompson et al 2003). Other studies have also demonstrated impairment in verbal recall, verbal and visual declarative memory, recognition and general learning in euthymic bipolar patients.

It is currently unclear when, in relation to the natural history of the illness, cognitive deficits develop. Neuropsychological deficits may represent a progressive disease process, possibly mediated by hypercortisolaemia, resulting in hippocampal cell toxicity, decreased glucocorticoid receptors, and eventual cell death. The balance of evidence supports the view that even during periods of euthymia there remain residual, and possibly progressive, cognitive deficits. Long-term prospective studies are awaited to elucidate further the neuropathophysiological relevance of these early findings.

Management

Early identification and relapse signatures

Emerging studies in schizophrenia suggest that early intervention is important in improving outcome. Accumulating evidence supports the notion that the psychotic process may have a 'toxic' effect upon the brain with long-term sequelae. Such

or carbamazepine may benefit from valproate either alone or in combination. The time to onset of action is similar to that of lithium. Valproate may also be useful in prophylaxis of bipolar disorder, and it may have a particular role in the management of rapid cycling. A recent Cochrane review examined the role of valproate in the maintenance treatment of bipolar disorder and summarized the efficacy and acceptability of valproate (Macritchie et al 2001).

Valproate semisodium (Depakote) is an equimolar combination of sodium valproate and valproic acid, and this formulation has recently been granted a licence in the UK for the treatment of manic episodes associated with bipolar disorder. The National Institute for Clinical Excellence (NICE) has also recently recommended the use of valproate semisodium for the control of the acute symptoms associated with the manic phase of bipolar I disorder (NICE 2003a).

Valproate is generally well tolerated, but side-effects include vomiting, tremor, ataxia, weight gain, rash, hair loss and potentially acute liver damage. In children and patients with a history of liver disease, liver function tests should be performed before treatment, and subsequently monitored.

Carbamazepine

Carbamazepine is a dibenzazepine derivative with a tricyclic structure. Trials show that 50–60% of patients with mania show a favourable response to carbamazepine. There is less evidence to support the role of carbamazepine in the prophylaxis of bipolar disorder, and there is a suggestion that despite the initial response rate, its effectiveness may diminish over 2–3 years.

The most common side-effects are nausea, dizziness, ataxia and diplopia. Other side-effects include headache, drowsiness and nystagmus. Occasionally, serious toxic side-effects may develop, such as agranulocytosis, aplastic anaemia or Stevens–Johnson syndrome. Leucopenia may develop in 1–2% of patients, and this is most frequently transient occurring at the initiation of treatment.

Other mood-stabilizing agents

A number of other anticonvulsant drugs have recently been shown to have efficacy in the management of bipolar disorders. This is unlikely to be a class effect, as not all anticonvulsants have therapeutic effects in the management of depression or mania. Lamotrigine has been shown to have antidepressant effects in bipolar depression, but it appears only to have a weak antimanic effect. It may be particularly useful in the management of bipolar II disorder and rapid cycling bipolar disorder. Gabapentin, used in treatment-resistant temporal lobe epilepsy, may also have a role as adjunctive therapy in bipolar disorder, but recent trials have failed to show any clear benefit in the management of either mania or depression.

Antipsychotics

Antipsychotic drugs are conventionally divided into 'typical' and the newer 'atypical' agents, and both groups have played a role in the management of bipolar disorders. Of the typical antipsychotics, haloperidol (a butyrophenone) is frequently used in the treatment of mania, but phenothiazines and thioxanthenes are also effective. In acutely disturbed patients who refuse oral medication intramuscular preparations may be used. Improvement in manic symptoms usually begins 1–3 days after commencing treatment, and more gradual improvement occurs over the following 2 weeks. Apart from the drowsiness which is associated with treatment with antipsychotic agents, particularly in high dose, extrapyramidal side-effects, particularly acute dystonia, may be troublesome. Anti-parkinsonian medication, such as procyclidine given orally or parenterally, should be used if these side-effects emerge. Typical antipsychotic depot preparations currently retain a role in the management of bipolar disorder, but it is possible they will be supplanted by the newer atypical depot agents in the future. More detailed description of the side-effects associated with antipsychotic drugs is given in Chapter 39.

The currently available atypical agents are amisulpride, aripiprazole, clozapine, olanzapine, quetiapine, risperidone. NICE guidelines recommend the use of olanzapine for control of the acute symptoms associated with the manic phase of bipolar I disorder (NICE 2003a), but subsequent evidence has shown that all atypical agents are efficacious in treating the manic phase of bipolar disorder. Similarly, recent evidence has also demonstrated that some atypical antipsychotics can effectively treat bipolar depression and are effective as mood-stabilizers. Atypical antipsychotics may be better tolerated in terms of neurological side-effects, but there is now clear evidence that many of the atypical agents cause metabolic perturbations such as weight gain and insulin resistance which may lead to increased cardiovascular risk.

The anti-manic effects of antipsychotic drugs are likely to be mediated through blockade of the dopamine (D2) receptor, but other pharmacological mechanisms cannot be excluded.

Antidepressants

The treatment of depression and a description of the various classes of antidepressant drugs are discussed elsewhere in this volume. The management of depression in bipolar disorder can be particularly challenging given the risk of precipitating a switch to (hypo)mania and rapid cycling. As discussed above, tricyclic antidepressants may be associated with a greater risk of destabilizing the illness and causing cycle acceleration.

Benzodiazepines

Benzodiazepines may have a role in the management of acute episodes of affective illness in bipolar disorder, particularly in manic patients who are overactive and require night sedation. The use of benzodiazepines, however, should be limited to the lowest possible dose for the shortest possible time, because of their potential for dependence.

Electroconvulsive therapy (ECT)

ECT is an effective treatment for mood disorders despite the negative public perception. The effectiveness of ECT has recently been demonstrated in a meta-analysis of the efficacy and safety in depressive disorders (UK ECT Review Group 2003). NICE has recently published guidelines on the use of ECT. These recommendations state that ECT should be used only in patients with severe depressive illness, catatonia or a prolonged or severe manic episode, and only then after an adequate trial of other treatment has proven ineffective and/or when the condition is considered to be potentially life-threatening (NICE 2003b).

Treatment of different phases of bipolar illness

The treatment of bipolar disorder can be divided into the following different phases:

* Acute manic or mixed episode
* Acute depressive episode
* Prophylactic treatment
* Treatment in special situations.

Drug management of acute mania or mixed episodes

A summary of the efficacy of commonly used drugs in the treatment of bipolar disorder is given in Table 21.3.

For patients not already established on long-term treatment for bipolar disorder, severe manic or mixed states should be treated with an antipsychotic or valproate because of their rapid antimanic effect. Parenteral medication (antipsychotic or benzodiazepine drugs) may be required in the more disturbed patient refusing oral medication. Less severe forms of mania may be treated with lithium or carbamazepine. If the patient is receiving antidepressant medication this should be tapered and stopped.

If the patient is already receiving long-term treatment for bipolar disorder, it is likely that a mood-stabilizing agent(s) will have been prescribed. Compliance with prescribed medication should be ascertained, and measuring serum levels of lithium, carbamazepine or valproate may be helpful. If poor compliance is an issue, this should prompt a careful enquiry into any side-effects from prescribed medication. Increasing the dose to ensure that the highest well-tolerated dose is offered may control symptoms. If symptoms are inadequately controlled then a combination of lithium or valproate with an antipsychotic should be considered. Clozapine may be considered in refractory illness. Psychotic symptoms during a manic or mixed episode should be treated with an antipsychotic drug, and preferably an atypical agent because of their more favourable side-effect profile.

When full remission of symptoms occurs, drugs used for the treatment of the acute episode may be tapered over a 2-week period and discontinued. Drugs which have been shown to be effective in preventing relapse (especially lithium and valproate) may be continued when long-term treatment is planned (see below).

Drug management of acute depression

Antidepressant monotherapy is not recommended for patients with a diagnosis of bipolar disorder. An antidepressant and an antimanic agent (e.g. lithium, valproate or an antipsychotic) should be considered for the treatment of an acute depressive episode. An antipsychotic should generally be used if there are psychotic symptoms present. However, the atypical antipsychotic quetiapine has been shown to be antidepressant in both bipolar I and bipolar II disorder, and to prevent new episodes (Young et al 2010). If depressive symptoms are less severe, then initial treatment with lamotrigine, lithium or valproate may be effective. If the patient fails to respond to these strategies, then augmentation or switching the antidepressant drug may be effective. ECT should be considered for patients with high suicidal risk, psychosis or severe depression during pregnancy (see above).

The choice of antidepressant for the treatment of bipolar depression should be guided by the risks of precipitating a switch to (hypo)mania. SSRIs are probably safer than tricyclic antidepressants in this regard, but tricyclics may have a role in treatment-resistant depression.

Episodes of bipolar depression which remit tend to be shorter than unipolar depression, and antidepressant treatment should be tapered and discontinued when symptoms have fully resolved. This may occur after as little as 12 weeks of treatment.

Maintenance treatment

Long-term treatment should be considered in a patient who presents following a single manic episode. Patient education is crucial to inform the individual of the importance of maintenance therapy in reducing the risks or relapse, and to encourage compliance with medication. Even in patients established on long-term treatment who have remained well for a number of years, the risks of relapse remain high following discontinuation of

Table 21.3 Summary of the efficacy of commonly used drugs in the treatment of bipolar disorder

	Mania	Depression	Rapid cycling	Prophylaxis
Lithium	+++	+	+	+++
Semisodium valproate	+++	+	++	+
Carbamazepine	+++	+	++	+
Lamotrigine	+	+++	+++	++
Typical antipsychotics	+++	−	+	+
Atypical antipsychotics	+++	++	++	++

+++, good evidence; ++, some evidence; +, limited evidence; −, no evidence.

mood-stabilizing agents, and encouragement to remain on treatment indefinitely should be offered.

Lithium monotherapy should be considered initially, as it has been shown to have efficacy in preventing both manic and depressive relapse, although it is more effective in preventing mania. Lithium is also associated with a reduced risk of suicide in bipolar illness. If lithium is poorly tolerated or ineffective, then valproate or carbamazepine may be considered. Other options include olanzapine and lamotrigine. Olanzapine has been shown to have mood-stabilizing properties and prevents manic more than depressive relapse. Lamotrigine prevents depressive more than manic relapse. If monotherapy fails, then a combination of mood-stabilizing agents should be considered. If the main burden of illness is (hypo)mania, then two antimanic drugs (lithium, valproate or an antipsychotic) should be considered, and where the burden is depression, lamotrigine or an antidepressant in combination with an antimanic agent may be effective.

Drug treatment of rapid cycling

The treatment of rapid cycling bipolar disorder presents a significant challenge. It is important to identify and treat co-morbid conditions (such as hypothyroidism or substance misuse) that may be contributing to cycling. Antidepressants should be tapered and discontinued. Lithium may not be as effective in treating rapid cycling, but several recent studies have provided compelling evidence to support the use of anticonvulsants, particularly lamotrigine.

Drug treatment during pregnancy

Some psychotropic drugs used in the maintenance phase of bipolar illness have teratogenic potential. The risk does not appear to be as great with antipsychotic agents, lamotrigine and antidepressants. Lithium, carbamazepine and valproate are all associated with higher risk of fetal abnormalities. With regard to breast-feeding, there is no absolute contraindication with any of the drugs used in bipolar disorder, but women taking lithium should be advised not to breast-feed.

Experimental drug treatments

Omega-3 fatty acids

The role of omega-3 fatty acids (derived mainly from fish oil) has been investigated in cardiovascular disease with encouraging results, but more recently a link has been suggested between omega-3 fatty acid consumption and depression. One small study has shown that adjunctive eicosapentaenoic acid (EPA) and docosahexanoic acid supplements, used as maintenance therapy, improve symptoms in patients with bipolar disorder (Stoll et al 1999). A recent randomized 4-month, placebo-controlled trial of EPA in bipolar depression showed significant improvements in 'Global Assessment of Function' and improvement on the 'Inventory of Depressive Symptoms' in patients who remained on treatment for >10 weeks, but no differences between placebo and EPA-treated patients at endpoint (Keck et al 2003). Additional trials are needed to clarify these findings, and further investigation into their possible mode of action is awaited.

Antiglucocorticoids

As referred to above, abnormalities of HPA axis function characterize both unipolar and bipolar affective disorders, and elevated corticosteroid levels are found. Such abnormalities may cause or exacerbate both neurocognitive and depressive symptoms, and reduction of cortisol levels may have therapeutic value. Preliminary data suggest that cortisol synthesis inhibitors may have antidepressant effects, and the role of glucocorticoid receptor antagonists in affective disorders has attracted recent research interest. At high doses, the progesterone receptor antagonist mifepristone (RU-486) becomes an antagonist of the glucocorticoid receptor subtype of the corticosteroid receptor, and a recent preliminary study in patients with bipolar disorder has shown that treatment with mifepristone resulted in selective improvement in neurocognitive functioning and mood (Young et al 2004). Further studies are needed to establish the therapeutic value of these agents.

Non-physical management

Although pharmacological treatment is the cornerstone in the management of bipolar disorder, the past several decades have witnessed a growing interest in the role of psychological approaches to alleviate symptoms, restore psychosocial functioning and prevent relapse and recurrence. Some of these developments are considered below.

Psychoeducation

There is a paucity of data on the effects of psychological interventions in bipolar disorder. The psychoeducative approach has been investigated by researchers for many years, but the first studies of its efficacy have only recently been published. Many of the published studies have reported only data on indirect measures of efficacy such as a change in patients' attitudes to medication. The 'Life Goals Programme' is a form of group psychoeducation, which when used as a part of a multimodal programme, has been shown to reduce emergency department use and costs and was one of the first well-structured group interventions specifically designed for bipolar patients.

The first randomized blinded clinical trial comparing the efficacy of group psychoeducation with standard treatment of bipolar I and bipolar II disorder has been published (Colom et al 2003). The treatment tested in this study combined three interventions which have shown some efficacy individually: early detection of relapse signatures, enhancement of treatment compliance, and induction of lifestyle regularity. Group psychoeducation significantly reduced the number of relapsed patients and the number of recurrences per patient, and increased the time to depression, manic, hypomanic and mixed occurrences. The number and length of hospitalizations per patient were also lower. Although these results are encouraging, the nature of the efficacy of psychoeducation is unknown, and future studies are needed to examine the specific content of the programme which is associated with a better outcome.

Interpersonal and social rhythms therapy

Bipolar disorder is associated with persistent deficits in functioning over time, and for many patients, psychosocial functioning remains markedly impaired. Until recently, psychotherapy was considered to be superfluous in the treatment of this patient group, but within the last decade, serious attempts have been made to develop and study manual-based psychological treatments for patients with bipolar I disorder. *Interpersonal and social rhythm therapy* (IPSRT) is a present-focused interpersonal treatment that views the core deficit in bipolar disorder as one of instability and that disturbed biological rhythms may arise from disruptions in social routine. IPSRT appears to be beneficial in terms of reducing the time to recovery from bipolar depressive episodes, but this form of psychotherapy has not proved to be useful in preventing relapse.

Cognitive therapy

The place of cognitive therapy in the management of bipolar disorder has been reviewed by Scott (2001). Beck's original cognitive model of depression and mania has been adapted to provide a framework for understanding the psycho-pathology of bipolar disorders. Cognitive therapy using this model is designed to facilitate acceptance of the disorder and the need for treatment; to help the individual recognize and manage psychosocial stressors and interpersonal problems; to improve medication adherence; to teach strategies to cope with depression and hypomania; to teach early recognition of relapse signatures; and to identify and modify negative automatic thoughts, and underlying maladaptive assumptions and beliefs.

Preliminary findings indicate that cognitive therapy may be beneficial for patients with bipolar disorder, and may be particularly suitable for patients who wish to take an equal and active role in their therapy. Randomized, controlled trials are needed, however, to establish the short-term and long-term benefits of cognitive therapy in bipolar disorder, and whether any reported health gain exceeds that of standard treatment.

Conclusions

It is clear that in recent years the concept of bipolar disorder has expanded, and the inclusion of more subtle variations of mood within the bipolar spectrum has challenged the often quoted lifetime incidence rate of ~1%. The increasing recognition of the importance of accurate diagnosis and treatment of individuals with bipolar disorders has significant public health and funding implications. Sadly, compared with schizophrenia, for example, the bipolar disorders remain the poor relation, and it is only in recent years that researchers have turned their attention to the investigation of the pathogenesis and management of these severe mental illnesses. Although still in its infancy, our understanding of these disorders is rapidly increasing. Continued research interest and activity should provide us with further insights into the mechanisms underlying the development of bipolar disorders, which ultimately may have profound consequences for the timing and choice of treatment.

Further reading

Goodwin, F.K., Jamison, K.R., 2007. Manic-depressive illness: bipolar disorders and recurrent depression, second ed. Oxford University Press, New York.

References

Akiskal, H.S., 1996. The prevalent clinical spectrum of bipolar disorders: beyond DSM-IV. J. Clin. Psychiatry 17 (Suppl. 3), 117–122.

Akiskal, H.S., Mallya, G., 1987. Criteria for the 'soft' bipolar spectrum: treatment implications. Psychopharmacol. Bull. 23, 68–73.

Akiskal, H.S., Djenderedjian, A.H., Rosenthal, R.H., et al., 1977. Cyclothymic disorder: validating criteria for inclusion in the bipolar affective group. Am. J. Psychiatry 134, 1227–1233.

Angst, J., 1966. Zur Ätiologie und Nosologie endogener depressiver Psychosen. Eine genetisch, soziologische und klinische Studie. Springer, New York.

Angst, J., 1978. The course of affective disorders. II. Typology of bipolar manic-depressive illness. Arch. Psychiatr. Nervenkr. 226, 65–73.

Angst, J., Gamma, A., Benazzi, F., et al., 2003. Toward a re-definition of subthreshold bipolarity: epidemiology and proposed criteria for bipolar II, minor bipolar disorders and hypomania. J. Affect. Disord. 73, 133–146.

Baldessarini, R.J., Tondo, L., Davis, P., et al., 2006. Decreased risk of suicides and attempts during long-term lithium treatment: a meta-analytic review. Bipolar Disord. 8 (5 Pt 2), 625–639 Erratum: Bipolar Disord. 2007; 9(3):314.

Baumann, B., Bogerts, B., 2001. Neuroanatomical studies on bipolar disorder. Br. J. Psychiatry 178 (Suppl. 41), s142–s147.

Chowdhury, R., Ferrier, I.N., Thompson, J.M., 2003. Cognitive dysfunction in bipolar disorder. Curr. Opin. Psychiatry 16, 7–12.

Colom, F., Vieta, E., Martinez-Aran, A., et al., 2003. A randomized trial on the efficacy of group psychoeducation in the prophylaxis of recurrences in bipolar patients whose disease is in remission. Arch. Gen. Psychiatry 60, 402–407.

Craddock, N., Jones, I., 1999. The genetics of bipolar disorder. J. Med. Genet. 36, 585–594.

Craddock, N., Sklar, P., 2009. Genetics of bipolar disorder: successful start to a long journey. Trends Genet. 25, 99–105.

Dunner, D.L., Fieve, R.R., 1974. Clinical factors in lithium carbonate prophylaxis failure. Arch. Gen. Psychiatry 30, 229–233.

Falret, J.P., 1851. De la folie circulaire ou forme de maladie mentale caractérisée par l'alternative régulière de la manie et de la mélancolie. Bulletin of the Academy of Natural Medicine, Paris.

Goodwin, F.K., Jamison, K.R., 1990. Manic depressive illness. Oxford University Press, New York.

Goodwin, F.K., Fireman, B., Simon, G.E., et al., 2003. Suicide risk in bipolar disorder during treatment with lithium and divalproex. J. Am. Med. Assoc. 290, 1467–1473.

Goodwin, G.M., Consensus Group of the British Association for Psychopharmacology, 2009. Evidence-based guidelines for treating bipolar disorder: revised second edition recommendations from the British Association for Psychopharmacology. J. Psychopharmacol. 23, 346–388.

Griesinger, W., 1845. Die Pathologie und Therapie der psychischen Krankheiten für Ärzte und Studierende. Krabbe, Stuttgart.

Harrison, P.J., 2002. The neuropathology of primary mood disorder. Brain 125, 1428–1449.

Keck, P.E., McElroy, S.L., Freeman, M.P., et al., 2003. Randomized, placebo-controlled trial of eicosapentaenoic acid in bipolar depression. Bipolar Disord. 5 (Suppl. 1), 100.

Kraepelin, E., 1896. Dementia praecox. In: The clinical roots of the schizophrenia concept. Cambridge University Press, Cambridge, pp. 15–24.

Kupka, R.W., Luckenbaugh, D.A., Post, R.M., et al., 2003. Comparison of rapid and non-rapid cycling bipolar disorder based on prospective mood ratings in 539 outpatients. Am. J. Psychiatry 162, 1273–1280.

Lieb, J., 2002. Lithium and antidepressants: inhibiting eicosanoids, stimulating immunity, and defeating microorganisms. Med. Hypotheses 59, 429–432.

Mackin, P., Ruttledge, S., 2007. Physical comorbidity in bipolar disorder. In: Soares, J.C., Young, A.H. (Eds.), Bipolar disorders: basic mechanisms and therapeutic implications. Informa Healthcare, New York, pp. 387–400.

Macritchie, K.A.N., Geddes, J.R., Scott, J., et al., 2001. Valproic acid, valproate and divalproex in the maintenance treatment of bipolar disorder. Cochrane Database Syst. Rev. (3) CD003196.

Marneros, A., 2001. Expanding the group of bipolar disorders. J. Affect. Disord. 62, 39–44.

Marneros, A., Deister, A., Rohde, A., 1990. The concept of distinct but voluminous bipolar and unipolar diseases. Part III: Unipolar and bipolar comparison. Eur. Arch. Psychiatry Clin. Neurosci. 240, 90–95.

McGuffin, P., Rijsdijk, F., Andrwe, M., et al., 2003. The heritability of bipolar affective disorder and the genetic relationship to unipolar depression. Arch. Gen. Psychiatry 60, 497–502.

McQuade, R., Young, A.H., 2000. Future therapeutic targets in mood disorders: the glucocorticoid receptor. Br. J. Psychiatry 177, 390–395.

Moore, P.B., Shepherd, D.J., Eccleston, D., et al., 2001. Cerebral white matter lesions in bipolar disorder: relationship to outcome. Br. J. Psychiatry 178, 172–176.

NICE: National Institute for Clinical Excellence, 2003a. Olanzapine and valproate semisodium in the treatment of acute mania associated with bipolar I disorder. Technology appraisal No. 66. Online. Available: www.nice.org.uk (accessed 12.05.04.).

NICE: National Institute for Clinical Excellence, 2003b. Guidance on the use of electroconvulsive therapy. Technology appraisal No. 59. Online. Available: www.nice.org.uk (accessed 12.05.04.).

Osborn, D.P., Levy, G., Nazareth, I., et al., 2007. Relative risk of cardiovascular and cancer mortality in people with severe mental illness from the United Kingdom's General Practice Research Database. Arch. Gen. Psychiatry 64, 242–249.

Peet, M., 1994. Induction of mania with selective serotonin reuptake inhibitors and tricyclic antidepressants. Br. J. Psychiatry 164, 549–550.

Perris, C., 1966. A study of bipolar (manic-depressive) and unipolar recurrent depressive psychoses. Acta Psychiatr. Scand. 194 (Suppl.), 1–89.

Porter, R., 2002. Madness: a brief history. Oxford University Press, Oxford.

Scott, J., 2001. Cognitive therapy as an adjunct to medication in bipolar disorder. Br. J. Psychiatry 178 (Suppl. 41), s164–s168.

Stoll, A.L., Severus, W., Freeman, M.P., et al., 1999. Omega3 fatty acids in bipolar disorder: a preliminary double-blind, placebo-controlled trial. Arch. Gen. Psychiatry 56, 407–412.

Thompson, J.M., Gray, J.M., Mackin, P., et al., 2003. The executive-visuo-spatial sketchpad interface in euthymic bipolar disorder: implications for visuo-spatial working memory architecture. In: Kokinov, B., Hirst, W. (Eds.), Constructive memory. NBU Series in Cognitive Science. New Bulgarian University, NBU Press, Sofia, p. 305.

UK ECT Review Group, 2003. Electroconvulsive therapy – systematic review and meta-analysis of efficacy and safety in depressive disorders. Lancet 361, 799–808.

Wernicke, C., 1900. Grundriss der psychiatrie. Thième, Leipzig.

Wolpert, E.A., Goldberg, J.F., Harrow, M., 1990. Rapid cycling unipolar and bipolar affective disorders. Am. J. Psychiatry 147, 725–728.

Yildiz, A., Sachs, G.S., 2003. Do antidepressants induce rapid cycling? A gender-specific association. J. Clin. Psychiatry 64, 814–818.

Young, A.H., Gallagher, P., Watson, S., et al., 2004. Improvements in neurocognitive function and mood following adjunctive treatment with mifepristone (RU-486) in bipolar disorder. Neuropsychopharmacology 29, 1538–1545.

Young, A.H., McElroy, S.L., Bauer, M., et al., EMBOLDEN I (Trial 001) Investigators, 2010. A double-blind, placebo-controlled study of quetiapine and lithium monotherapy in adults in the acute phase of bipolar depression (EMBOLDEN I). J. Clin. Psychiatry 71, 150–162.

Appendix 1
Diagnostic criteria: ICD-10

Hypomania

A. The mood is elevated or irritable to a degree that is definitely abnormal for the individual concerned and sustained for at least 4 consecutive days.

B. At least three of the following signs must be present, leading to some interference with personal functioning in daily living:
    1. Increased activity or physical restlessness
    2. Increased talkativeness
    3. Difficulty in concentration or distractibility
    4. Decreased need for sleep
    5. Increased sexual energy
    6. Mild overspending, or other types of reckless or irresponsible behaviour
    7. Increased sociability or overfamiliarity.

C. The episode does not meet criteria for mania, bipolar affective disorder, depressive episode, cyclothymia or anorexia nervosa.

Mania

A. Mood must be predominantly elevated, expansive or irritable, and definitely abnormal for the individual concerned. The mood change must be prominent and sustained for at least 1 week (unless it is severe enough to require hospital admission).

B. At least three of the following signs must be present (four if the mood is merely irritable), leading to severe interference with personal functioning in daily living:
    1. Increased activity or physical restlessness
    2. Increased talkativeness ('pressure of speech')
    3. Flight of ideas or the subjective experience of thoughts racing
    4. Loss of normal social inhibitions, resulting in a behaviour that is inappropriate to the circumstances
    5. Decreased need for sleep
    6. Inflated self-esteem or grandiosity
    7. Distractibility or constant changes in activity or plans
    8. Behaviour that is foolhardy or reckless and whose risks the individual does not recognize, e.g. spending sprees, foolish enterprises, reckless driving
    9. Marked sexual energy or sexual indiscretions.

C. There are no hallucinations or delusions, although perceptual disorders may occur (e.g. subjective hyperacusis, appreciation of colours as especially vivid). (If delusions or hallucinations are present then the episode is specified as 'mania with psychotic symptoms'.)

D. The episode is not attributable to psychoactive substance use or to any organic mental disorder.

Bipolar affective disorder

A. The current episode meets the criteria for hypomania, mania, depression or a mixed state. (If the current episode is classified as mixed, then both manic and depressive symptoms must be prominent most of the time during a period of at least 2 weeks.)

B. There has been at least one other affective episode in the past, meeting the criteria for hypomanic or manic episode, depressive episode or mixed affective episode. (If the current episode is classified as depression, then there must have been at least one authenticated hypomanic or manic episode or mixed affective episode in the past.)

Cyclothymia

A. There must have been a period of at least 2 years of instability of mood involving several periods of both depression and hypomania, with or without intervening periods of normal mood.

B. None of the manifestations of depression or hypomania during such a 2-year period should be sufficiently severe or long-lasting to meet the criteria for manic episode or depressive episode (moderate or severe); however, manic or depressive episode(s) may have occurred before, or may develop after, such a period of persistent mood instability.

C. During at least some of the periods of depression at least three of the following should be present:
    1. Reduced energy or activity
    2. Insomnia
    3. Loss of self-confidence or feelings of inadequacy
    4. Difficulty in concentrating
    5. Social withdrawal
    6. Loss of interest in or enjoyment of sex and other pleasurable activities
    7. Reduced talkativeness
    8. Pessimism about the future or brooding over the past.

D. During at least some of the periods of mood elevation, at least three of the following should be present:
    1. Increased energy or activity
    2. Decreased need for sleep
    3. Inflated self-esteem
    4. Sharpened or unusually creative thinking
    5. Increased gregariousness
    6. Increased talkativeness or wittiness
    7. Increased interest and involvement in sexual and other pleasurable activities
    8. Over-optimism or exaggeration of past achievements.

Appendix 2
Diagnostic criteria: DSM-IV

Hypomania

A. A distinct period of persistently elevated, expansive, or irritable mood, lasting throughout at least 4 days, which is clearly different from the usual non-depressed mood.

B. During the period of mood disturbance, three (or more) of the following symptoms have persisted (four if the mood is only irritable) and have been present to a significant degree:
    1. Inflated self-esteem or grandiosity
    2. Decreased need for sleep

Continued

of 9 years see death as a temporary state (Nagy 1948) and as a reversible, external event – as going away on a journey from which one returns later (Jones 1911; Rochlin 1959; Speece & Brent 1984). Weininger (1979) found that children younger than 4 years did not understand the distinction between animate and inanimate objects and only 20% of children under the age of 9 saw death as final.

Statistical data grossly under-represent the true figures for suicide for several reasons:

- A legal verdict of suicide demands evidence of intent. A rigorous application of this definition excludes a large number of deaths from this category where the intent is not clear or the method renders the intent more ambiguous. For example, only 54% of deaths by drowning are deemed to be suicides, while 98% of deaths by hanging are recorded as such. Many deaths which may appear as accidents may indeed be suicides, such as those who may be viewed as falling out of windows instead of jumping out, and those who are killed in road accidents when they are drunk (Zilbroog 1937).

- Social, cultural and religious attitudes often inhibit disclosure of deaths by suicide. Suicide has evoked greater primitive fear and censure than murder throughout history (Anderson 1998).

- Suicide has been seen as a dishonourable act, a sin or a work of the devil from around 500 BC; an act so terrible that the death would return to haunt the living. Unsuccessful suicides suffered severe retribution. Successful ones were denied a decent burial and their property was confiscated. Their bodies would not be brought out of the house through the door but through a window or hole in the wall. Attempted suicide was a punishable offence in the UK from 1745 until as late as 1961 (Retterstol 1998, 2000).

Suicide rates have fluctuated in the twentieth century. The rate declined significantly during the two World Wars. It rose in the 1930s, possibly because of the economic depression, and again after the Second World War through the 1950s and the early 1960s. It fell in the late 1960s and the early 1970s, but has steadily increased since, especially among young men. The reasons for these changes are not clear.

The most common methods of suicide are hanging, self-poisoning (usually overdoses) and carbon monoxide poisoning through car exhausts. Some 54% of the sample reported by the recent National Confidential Inquiry (Safer Services 1999) used violent methods such as hanging, jumping from a height or in front of a moving vehicle, accounting for two-thirds of male and two-fifths of female suicides. Men took their lives more commonly by physical methods followed by overdoses; women most frequently resorted to overdoses, followed in frequency by hanging. Occasionally, suicide is a result of a suicide pact, a *folie à deux*, and sometimes, it may follow murder.

The drugs most frequently used in overdoses are prescribed psychotropic drugs. People who have previously harmed themselves are more likely to kill themselves with psychotropic drugs. Paracetamol ingestion surprisingly accounts for only 4% of the suicides by overdose.

Patient characteristics associated with suicide

- The male to female ratio is 3:1. Men outnumber women in all age groups (Arto et al 1988; Barraclough & Hughes 1987; Safer Services 1999). This may be because women are freer in expressing their feelings (Gould 1965) and the less aggressive methods, such as drug overdose, that they employ are also less effective. The ratio is higher among teenagers and young people (Burton et al 1990; McClure 1987; Moser et al 1987; Safer Services 1999).

- Nearly half of the suicides will have made an attempt previously (Hawton & Catalan 1987). However, three-fifths of men and two-fifths of women succeed at their first attempt (Isometsa & Lonnqvist 1998).

- Unbearable psychological pain characterizes suicide. Schneidman (1993) terms it as 'psychache'. Feelings of rage, hopelessness and despair predominate. Rage and violence are intimately linked in youth suicide (Hendin 1991). Furman (1984) and Zetzel (1965) highlight the depressed person's incapacity to maintain hope when confronted with loss. Beck (1975) argues that hopelessness is a more accurate indicator of suicide than is depression.

- Severe mental illness is common, especially depression (Arto et al 1988; Barraclough & Hughes 1987), and also schizophrenia, personality disorders, drug and alcohol dependence. About a half have co-morbid illness (Safer Services 1999). Around 38% abuse alcohol, 23% abuse drugs and 17% misuse both. Drug addicts are at a higher risk and prescribed drugs, particularly antidepressants and methadone, make the risk greater (Oyefeso et al 1999). Young men are vulnerable in the early phase of a first major depressive episode (Brent et al 1993). The risk is also pronounced in the phase of recovery from a major depression (Arieti 1959; Kernberg 1984).

- Depression is an important element in those who are suffering from schizophrenia. They more often kill themselves in non-psychotic periods when they have acquired some insight into the devastating consequence of their illness (Roy 1982).

- Women who suffer from postpartum psychiatric disorders are vulnerable to suicide, particularly in the first year (Appleby et al 1998).

- Self-harm and violence are significant associations. Of those who kill themselves, 63% have a history of self-harm and 19% a history of violence (Safer Services 1999).

- Suicides are associated with bereavement and a failure to mourn. A recent loss such as death of a parent or spouse is significantly more common (Barraclough 1987), particularly in the first year (Bunch 1972; McMahon & Pugh 1971). According to Bunch and Barraclough (1971), suicides tend to take their lives around death anniversaries, especially of parents.

- Suicide is linked with chronic and severe physical illness (Harris & Barraclough 1994), particularly in the elderly (Sainsbury 1962). In the younger age group, suicide is four times more common in those suffering from epilepsy (Barraclough 1987; Sainsbury 1986).

- Suicides are more frequent in the spring and summer. The seasonal variations, however, greatly diminished in England and Wales in the last two decades of the twentieth century (Yip et al 2000).

The social characteristics associated with suicide

- Living in over-crowded inner city areas with significant social deprivation and poor economic conditions has a strong association with suicide, especially among young men (Diekstra 1989; et al 1989; Platt 1984; Pritchard 1988, 1992). About two-thirds of suicides are unemployed (Safer Services 1999). The association with unemployment is stronger in the younger age group both among men and women (Gunnell et al 1999). Poor physical health and reactive depression commonly accompany unemployment.
- Social isolation (Sainsbury 1955) and absence of an intimate relationship are also linked with a higher incidence of suicide. Two-thirds live alone and nearly three-quarters are without a partner (Safer Services 1999). Suicide is thus more common among those who have remained single, are divorced or widowed.
- Suicide is more frequent among prisoners compared with the general population (Gunn & Taylor 1993). Death from abuse of opioids is 10 times more common in prisons (Harris & Barraclough 1998, Gore 1999).

The National Confidential Inquiry into Suicide and Homicide, which monitored suicides by people with mental illness over a 2-year period between 1996 and 1998 (Safer Services 1999), while confirming the above patient characteristics, adds:

- The risk is greater in the first year of mental illness, especially after a major affective disorder. Some 22% of the suicides reported occurred in the first year of illness and 15% had more than five admissions prior to the suicide.
- Of all suicides, 4% were psychiatric inpatients and one-third of these killed themselves on the ward, usually by hanging in the evening or at night; 25% of the wards reported that the ward design made it difficult to observe seriously-at-risk patients and another 27% reported nurse shortages at the time of the suicide.
- Of all suicides, 3% were homeless and these were more often young men with a history of depression, schizophrenia or drug and/or alcohol dependence; 28% of the patients were disengaged with the mental health services, having discharged themselves against medical advice or having been discharged at their own request. They were usually non-compliant with medication.
- Patients who killed themselves were particularly vulnerable in the first few months after discharge. A quarter of post-discharge suicides happened within 3 months of discharge from the hospital, usually within the first week and commonly on the day after discharge. About two-fifths of the post-discharge suicides happened before the first follow-up appointment.

Contact with services and communication of risk

The recognition of suicidal thoughts in patients arouses anxiety in the professionals. Doctors often do not recognize the risk and fail to ask suicidal patients about suicide plans or previous suicide attempts (Michel & Valach 1992; Murphy 1975; Richman & Rosenbaum 1970).

Nearly a quarter of all suicides will have been in contact with mental health services in the year before death (Barraclough et al 1974; Murphy 1975). In the sample monitored by the National Confidential Inquiry, half had been in contact with the mental health services in the week before death and a fifth in the previous 24 hours.

According to the findings of the Inquiry, at final contact, the risk of suicide was estimated to be low or absent in 85% of cases. When the risk was estimated to be moderate or high, the information was not communicated to other members of the mental health team in 14% of cases. When patients were seen by two services prior to suicide, important information known by one service was frequently unknown to the other. Only in just over half the suicides, the mental health services had contact with the family of the deceased.

Characteristics of adolescent suicides

Suicide is the most common cause of death after road traffic accidents among male adolescents. Some 50% of adolescents who have attempted suicide before re-attempt (Pfeffer et al 1994) and 1–11% of these eventually kill themselves. Suicidal male adolescents and young men are less likely than older adults to maintain contact with their GPs or seek alternative help (Vassilas & Morgan 1993). Sexual and physical abuse are frequently associated with adolescents who take their lives (Romans et al 1995). There is often a history of bullying. Pregnant teenage girls (Gabrielson et al 1970) and children who have run away from home (Shaffer & Caton 1984) are particularly vulnerable to suicide. Dysfunctional family background, mental illness and/or suicide of a parent and mental illness of a sibling contribute significantly to suicides in young people (Agerbo et al 2002). Adolescents, depending on their personality, development and family circumstances, may find a melancholic solution (depression, suicidal behaviour) or a manic solution (alcohol, drugs, reckless driving) to their problems (Polmear 2004).

Deliberate self-harm

Definitions

Non-fatal self-harm has been defined variously in the last 50 years as 'attempted suicide', 'parasuicide', 'deliberate self-harm' (which is classified further as 'deliberate self-poisoning' and 'deliberate self-injury'), and 'suicidal act'. Stengel (1952) believed that this behaviour, although not fatal, carried a measure of suicidal intent and called it 'attempted suicide'. Kreitman (1977) described it as 'parasuicide' and Morgan (1979) as 'deliberate self-harm', suggesting that the actions, although volitional, did not reflect a wish to die. Critics (Asch 1980) argue that the term 'deliberate self-harm' has a punitive connotation and underplays the emotional intensity characterizing the act. The distinction between suicidal behaviour and deliberate self-harm is often a matter of degree. Campbell and Hale (1991), highlighting the ambivalence inherent in the behaviour, propose the term 'suicidal act', defining it 'as the conscious or unconscious intention at the time of the act to kill the self's body'.

Epidemiology

The prevalence of self-harm has risen significantly in the West since the 1960s (Hawton & Catalan 1987). The rate fell briefly in the 1980s and has returned to its rising trend in the 1990s.

The prevalence of self-harm in the general population is reckoned to be between 14 and 600 persons per 100 000 population per year in different parts of the world (Raleigh 1996). It is common in Europe, especially in young people. An estimated 140 000 hospital referrals for deliberate self-harm are made in England and Wales each year (Hawton et al 1998). The prevalence for self-harm, like the suicide data, is an underestimation because the source of this information is mainly hospital records, and a large proportion of self-harmers may not report the incident, may only see their family physician or may seek help from an agency that is not linked to a hospital, e.g. the Samaritans. Self-destructive behaviour also takes many forms other than overt attacks on the body, e.g. addiction, reckless driving, dangerous sexual behaviour, repeated accidents and provoking others to attack. These behaviours are not necessarily conscious and do not fit within the narrow definition of 'deliberate self-harm'.

Overdoses are the most common method of self-harm requiring acute admission to hospital, especially among women. Self-poisoning constitutes 90% of self-harming behaviour, and self-injury, mainly in the form of cutting of forearm and wrist, contributes largely to the rest. Frequently the self-harm includes both cutting and overdose. There is often concomitant heavy drinking and/or drug abuse.

The drugs used for overdoses follow the pattern described with completed suicides and mirror the prevalent prescribing trends and availability of drugs. Psychotropic drugs are more commonly used by those being treated for mental illness, and non-opiate analgesics such as paracetamol and aspirin are more frequently used by young people because of their easy access. The use of minor tranquillizers and sedatives in overdoses has diminished reflecting the changes in prescribing habits (Hawton 1996a).

Patient characteristics

- Deliberate self-harm is commoner in women and the female to male ratio is 1.3:1. It is more frequent in the younger age group, mainly between the ages of 15 and 24. However, the incidence of self-harm in adolescent boys is low.

- Self-harm is usually impulsive, especially among adolescents. It is frequently accompanied by alcohol and drug abuse, more so in male teenagers (Fombonne 1998).

- Patients who cut habitually may be highly aroused prior to the self-harm and may experience feelings of depersonalization. The cutting may relieve the tension.

- A sense of hopelessness, difficulty in controlling feelings of anger and hostility, and a tendency to aggression are frequently associated with self-harm (Brent 1997). Individuals who harm themselves are self-critical and over-sensitive to criticism. They oscillate between thick-skinned and thin-skinned states of mind, being sometimes inaccessible and defensively aggressive (thick-skinned) and being fragile and vulnerable (thin-skinned) at other times (Bateman 1998; Rosenfeld 1987).

- Patients who self-harm have problems in relationships. A charged incident or event, such as an argument with parents or a break-up of a relationship, may trigger the self-injury.

- There is often a history of loss of a parent in early life either by separation or by death. Emotional neglect, physical and sexual abuse during development are strongly associated with self-injury (Cohen-Sandler et al 1982; Links 1990; Romans et al 1995; Shearer et al 1990). Victims of sexual abuse are most likely to cut themselves. The earlier the origin of such abuse in childhood development, the greater is the propensity to cut and the severity of such behaviour. The families of self-harmers are often dysfunctional with unresolved conflicts and limited support. There is frequently a family history of depression, alcohol and/or drug abuse, violence and life-threatening behaviour. Parents who self-harm have a poor relationship with their children.

- There may be a history of mental illness, most commonly personality disorder or depression, which may of course coexist. Self-injurious behaviour is also seen in other psychiatric conditions such as bipolar affective disorder, schizophrenia (e.g. amputation when in a psychotic state), eating disorders, obsessive–compulsive disorder, post-traumatic stress disorder, dissociative disorder and anxiety and panic disorders. Favazza (1987) argues for a separate diagnostic entity called deliberate self-harm syndrome because of the heterogeneity of the condition. About 5–8% of self-harming patients may require hospital admission for treatment of the mental illness (Hawton 1996b).

- Chronic physical illness, as with suicide, is associated with self-harm. Men suffering from epilepsy are more prone to harm themselves.

Social characteristics associated with deliberate self-harm

The social characteristics associated with deliberate self-harm are similar to those found with suicides and include poor socio-economic conditions, over-crowded inner city areas with considerable social deprivation, homelessness, unemployment, social isolation, and remaining single or having been divorced. Self-harm is more common in young people who have run away from home (Rotheram-Borus 1993). It is also more frequent in those with a previous criminal record and in those who are held in custody (Feldman 1988; Gunn & Taylor 1993).

The family and the suicidal person

The family environment is of vital importance in the origin of suicidal behaviour (Marsh 1998). A child's development is influenced by the dynamic organization of the family, how his/her parents assume their responsibilities and relate to each other, and by their responses to his/her development. The process is inevitably affected by traumatic experiences such as loss of a parent or sibling, exposure to violence, seduction and deprivation, and physical and mental illness in the family. How a child is marked by these events will depend on how his/her family reacts to them, the availability of other significant people in the child's life, and his/her age (Ackerman 1958; Schafer 1968).

Suicidal patients have a strong family history of affective disorders, alcohol and drug abuse (Brent et al 1994). Shaffer (1974) found that 55% of families that had suffered suicides of children had a family member who had consulted a general practitioner or a psychiatrist previously. The families of suicidal individuals also display significant marital conflict, family disharmony, domestic violence and suicidal behaviour. Carroll et al (1980) note that self-harming patients have a higher family prevalence of separation, violence, physical abuse and sexual abuse compared with other psychiatric populations. A high proportion of suicidal patients report their parents as cold, distant, secretive, resistant to change and intolerant of crisis (Shaffer & Piacentini 1994; Simpson 1976). Early exposure to family violence has been linked with uncontrolled rage and aggression in children who later kill themselves (Hendin 1991). Children of parents who have committed suicide are afraid that they may be overwhelmed by their potential for self-destruction (Schwartz et al 1974).

Sometimes suicide may be attempted as a solution to a conflict if the family fails to address it for fear of confrontation. Children frequently act as receptacles for family tensions and help to maintain a precarious equilibrium within the family. They become the focus for family hostility and the scapegoating is often a contributory factor in the suicidal behaviour (Sabbath 1969).

Richman and Rosenbaum (1970) found in their family studies that aggression was a striking feature in the behaviour of all family members involved with the suicidal person. The families saw themselves as victims of the suicidal person's difficult behaviour and he/she was frequently the repository of aggression within the family. Families, reacting to their anger, often withdraw from the suicidal or self-mutilating patient.

Suicide is a catastrophic event and may buckle even the most resilient family. It leaves behind many damaged lives and broken relationships. It creates enormous personal suffering and provokes a gamut of feelings: shock, perplexity, anger, despair, blame, guilt, shame and abandonment. The family is seized by a sense of failure that it had not ensured the safety or survival of its family member. The grief may persist for a lifetime. There is also a loss of hope invested by the family in the person who has killed him/herself.

The death may also cause considerable family disruption and shift in responsibilities. For example, children may be forced to assume adult responsibilities in the wake of a parent's suicide. The family may be forced into economic difficulties. The suicide may leave the family with little emotional reserve to comfort each other. Many families disintegrate after a suicide. In Shaffer's study, 25% of families had broken up 1–4 years after a child's suicide.

The impact of suicide on the family members is determined by their roles and responsibilities within the family (e.g. of parents, spouses and siblings), their developmental stages (e.g. of children) and histories, and the cultural and religious beliefs within the family. The various members of the family mutually affect one another by their reactions to the violent and untimely death.

The impact of suicide on mental health professionals

The reaction of mental health professionals to the suicide of their patients is not commonly discussed (Gitlin 1999). In a survey of Scottish consultants in psychiatry, a third of them reported depressive symptoms in response to the most distressing suicide of their patients (Alexander et al 2000). Themes that emerged included guilt, lack of support, feeling blamed and unrealistic expectations from within and outside the profession that the suicide was preventable.

Psychoanalytic theories of suicide and suicidal behaviour

Suicide is a tragic end to an inner turmoil. It derives from a complex interplay of internal and external factors determined by the individual's psychic development and his conscious and unconscious attitudes to life and death.

The psychic meaning given to death by suicidal patients can be conceived overall as reactions to separation, loss and abandonment (Hendin 1991). These may be triggered not only by a real person, but also by indignities, disappointments and loss of significant parts of oneself (e.g. health). Freud (1917), in his seminal paper 'Mourning and Melancholia', observed that the ambivalent feelings of love and hatred for what was lost were inherent in pathological depression. Anger and aggression, as reactions to loss, are so unacceptable to the depressed individual that they are repressed and turned upon himself. Indeed the term 'melancholia' has its roots in the Greek words *menos* and *cholos*, meaning black bile or black fury (Rycroft 1968). There is an unconscious feeling of damage and destruction, and to quote Padel (1995), 'Melancholic depression is pathological mourning, not necessarily of a real person, but of an internal object you feel you have destroyed'.

Campbell and Hale (1991), drawing on Freud's formulation, highlight the role that ambivalence and violence play in a suicidal act. They suggest that suicide is a form of 'acting out', whereby the unconscious conflict generating unbearable psychic tension finds relief in the physical action of killing oneself.

Violence in suicide is underestimated. *The Oxford English Dictionary* defines suicide as an act of taking one's life, a self-murder – a self that submits to murder by itself (derived from Latin *sui* meaning self, *caedere* meaning to kill). Suicide and homicide indeed have a common unconscious origin. The outcome depends on whether the victim is located inside oneself as in suicide or outside as in homicide (Asch 1980). Suicide thus has two components: an aggressive wish to kill and a submissive wish to be killed (Menninger 1933), with an accompanying confusion between the self and the other (Maltsberger 1993; Pollock 1975).

Internal motives and suicide phantasies

Campbell and Hale (1991) argue that suicidal behaviour is driven by suicidal phantasies and these are rooted in childhood. Their argument is based on 500 interviews over a 4-year period, with patients seen within 24 h of a suicide attempt in the accident and emergency (A&E) department of a large metropolitan hospital and on comments made by suicidal patients in psychoanalytic psychotherapy before and after suicide attempts.

Laplanche and Pontalis (1973) define 'phantasy' as 'an imaginary scene in which the subject is a protagonist, representing the fulfillment of a wish in a manner that is distorted to a greater or lesser extent by defensive processes'. It is distinguished in Britain from the word 'fantasy', which is used in the sense of 'caprice, whim and fanciful invention' (Rycroft 1968). Phantasies are primarily about the body and express the instinctual aims and the defences in relation to people and what they represent (termed 'objects' in psychoanalysis) (Hinshelwood 1989).

A suicide phantasy involves a disturbed relationship between two people (Asch 1980). It carries sets of opposing elements: a passive victim and an intolerable persecutor, an idealized good self and a bad body, a conscious wish to die and a less conscious desire to survive (Campbell & Hale 1991). An alarming state of confusion, chaos and loss of control result when the suicidal patient, who had hitherto kept the conflicting elements apart, is not able to maintain the split. The body is identified with the intolerable persecutor. The patient repudiates the body, and thus attacks the internal persecutor, with the hope that the core part of the self will remain alive – what Campbell and Hale call the 'surviving self' – even when the body is being killed (Maltsberger & Buie 1980).

Several suicide phantasies may be at play. The phantasies are not mutually exclusive, although a particular phantasy may be dominant in a particular individual. The wish to die and the attendant suicidal phantasies may fluctuate in the patient's mind.

The most common suicide phantasy is of merging. The wish to kill oneself may be driven by a desire to reside in a world beyond where all that is lost or denied in this life would be restored. Death may be seen as a return to the heaven where we were born, i.e. to the mother's womb (Jones 1911), to sleep in order to wake up to a better life. The gods of sleep and death in Greek mythology, *Hypnos* and *Thanatos*, are indeed brothers (Friedlander 1940).

The aim of suicide may also be a desire for fusion with another person (Sandler 1960; Meissner 1981). The suicidal person may identify him/herself with a significant other who has died, for example a parent, a sibling or a partner. He or she may be driven to kill him/herself by a wish to join the dead, thereby regaining in his/her mind the loved person who is lost. The identification is particularly strong if the death has occurred in the person's childhood or adolescence, predisposing him to depression when beset with a loss in later life (Bowlby 1973; Zilbroog 1937). The experience of good family relationships before the loss, the family's ability to mourn and the availability of other carers will of course modify this outcome (Birtchnell 1980).

The act of dying together (e.g. as in a suicide pact) may result from a similar yearning for fusion and a belief in sharing life as well as death. The wish may also find expression in religious beliefs with phantasies of fusion with God (Asch 1966). Suicide in the wake of a murder also may follow such belief, at least in the mind of the murderer-suicide, but is more often a result of extreme jealousy. Suicide phantasy may also involve the notion of punishment, either as revenge against others or as self-punishment.

The phantasy of revenge is aimed at people who are important to the suicidal person, such as parents or other loved ones. The person, seeking retribution for perceived neglect or wrongdoing, is preoccupied with the impact of his or her death on others. The 'surviving self', in the role of the invisible observer, enjoys the anguish, guilt and remorse that would be evoked by his or her death (Campbell & Hale 1991). As Menninger (1933) observes, the greatest hurt a child could inflict on his/her parents is to attack what is most precious to them, i.e. him/herself. 'A rejection of life usually includes a rejection of the parents from whom the life originated' (Hendin 1991).

The wish for self-punishment is driven by a severe sense of guilt. Freud (1916) notes: 'The sense of guilt was present before the misdeed, … it did not rise from it, but conversely the misdeed arose from the sense of guilt'. The guilt may be associated with unconscious feelings of hostility and forbidden impulses, particularly in adolescents. Freud also links guilt with a sense of failure in matching the expectations of one's ideal self. Sometimes the guilt may be over real events, as observed in combat soldiers. The suicidal person, in his/her desperate attempts to placate the oppressive conscience, may seek punishment by submitting him/herself to dangerous situations or by enlisting others to punish him/her.

Suicide is sometimes impelled by a fear of punishment or retaliation, real or imaginary, especially in children. They may be afraid of being chastised for what they perceive as their transgression of parental rules. Suicide may also be an attempt to escape unbearable feelings of shame, humiliation and loneliness.

Another suicide phantasy is of elimination (Campbell & Hale 1991), which is seen predominantly in adolescents with disturbances of body image. Adolescence demands negotiating bodily changes and developing a sense of ownership of the body. A teenager who is frightened by his growing body and is unable to master his urges sees his body as alien and a danger to himself. 'It was as if puberty had suddenly changed the body into an enemy' (Laufer 1968). He is acutely persecuted by his body and wishes to be rid of it in self-defence. The phantasy of elimination may also be dominant in elderly people who are frightened of growing old or of dying badly.

A suicide phantasy may carry an irresistible fascination with death and the act of killing oneself, an addiction to near-death (Joseph 1982). It offers an illusion of mastery over a situation and compensates for feelings of helplessness and loss of control over one's life (Hendin 1991). The phantasy harbours a grandiose wish to triumph over death by actively seeking it. The individual gambles with his/her life and risks his/her body in various ways, such as drink-driving, delinquency and reckless sexual behaviour.

Another phantasy seen in suicidal individuals is the rescue phantasy. The individual sees him/herself as a victim in a submissive relationship with death. He/she plays a game of Russian roulette with fate as the executioner who will decide if he/she lives or dies, thus expressing his ambivalence about living (Asch 1980). Similarly he forces others, e.g. a parent or a wife, by manipulation or blackmail, to be responsible for his survival. The threat of suicide is used to control the behaviour of others by evoking guilt feelings in them (Hendin 1991; Kernberg 1984). Behind the wish to be rescued may also lie a panic that he is no longer safe in his own hands.

Behavioural and cognitive theories

Behavioural and cognitive theories mainly examine processes underlying anxiety and depression. According to learning theories, an individual becomes vulnerable to depression if adequate reinforcements are not available in the environment, either because of changes in the environment or because of the person's limited capacity to generate reinforcers, as, for example, when a child loses a parent (Ferster et al 1997; Shaffer & Piacentini 1994).

Families of suicidal patients have a greater tendency for suicidal behaviour compared with other psychiatric patients (Kreitman et al 1970; Shaffer & Piacentini 1994). Learning theories posit that such behaviour is a learned currency of communication within this 'subculture'. The self-harm also elicits attention from others and this reinforces the behaviour through operant conditioning. The behaviour may be reinforced through a similar mechanism if the self-harm generates pleasurable sensory stimulation.

The focus of cognitive theories is on thought processes. Ellis (1962) observed that irrational thinking led to emotionally destructive states of mind. Beck (1974) proposed that depression was a result of negative attributions to experience, for example, seeing oneself as wholly responsible for one's misfortunes (internalized attributions), generalizing experiences that were particular (global attributes), and expecting negative experiences to repeat themselves (stable attributes). Beck and co-workers (1987), differentiating between anxiety and depression, state that a depressed patient 'takes his interpretations and predictions as facts. In anxiety, they are simply possibilities'.

Seligman (1975) introduced the notion of 'learned helplessness'. He and his colleagues, while studying the relationship between fear and learning, found that dogs subjected to electric shocks each time they tried to leave their cage, later made no effort to escape even when it was possible. Brown et al (1977), extending Seligman's theme, suggest that the loss of

a parent in early life sensitized a child, through learned helplessness, to respond to a future loss with depression. Beck (1974, 1975) has argued that hopelessness is a catalyst for suicide and is a more sensitive marker than depression. Fawcett et al (1987), followed up 954 patients with major affective disorder in a prospective study over a 4-year period and found similarly a strong relationship between hopelessness and suicide in the 25 patients who killed themselves.

Klerman (1986), advocating interpersonal therapy, emphasized the difficulties that a depressed individual encounters in his interactions with others because of conflicts and criticism.

Social theories

Emile Durkheim, an influential sociologist of the late nineteenth and early twentieth centuries, was concerned with the pathological states of society that provoked individuals to suicide (Harre et al 1986). He argued that suicide was caused by a breakdown in the relationship between society and the individual, and that it resulted from a failure in man's integration into society and in the regulation of his relationship with it.

Durkheim classified suicide into several types based on the nature of the disturbance between the individual and society. Over-integration into society with an under-developed sense of one's individuality makes man susceptible to an *altruistic* suicide. The socially accepted suicide of early Christians who sought martyrdom to reach God, the immolation of Buddhist priests in protest against social oppression and persecution, and the suicide of whole troops of soldiers in the face of the conquering enemy may be seen as examples of altruistic suicide (Asch 1966). Conversely, under-integration and an overdeveloped sense of individuality impel man to an *egoistic* suicide because of a loss of meaningful life with people and social isolation.

Over-regulation of a man's relationship with society restricts his freedom and may drive him into a *fatalistic* suicide. Under-regulation results in breakdown of social rules of behaviour and leads to a state of hopelessness – *anomie* – and thus provokes an *anomic* suicide. Anomie can be economic or domestic and can take both acute and chronic forms. Acute economic anomie is caused by sudden changes in a person's financial fortunes, either by an economic disaster or a sudden fortune, the individual in either situation failing to adjust to the change. Chronic economic anomie stems from greed and endless pursuit of novelty. Acute domestic anomie follows divorce and in its chronic form is a result of man's marital discontent.

Durkheim's theories have several flaws (Harre et al 1986). They imply that psychological equilibrium is possible only under certain social conditions. They underplay the individual's psychological structure that contributes to his/her self-destruction. They also ignore the cultural differences in reactions to social situations.

Phillips (1974), elaborating on Durkheim's hypothesis that anomic individuals are vulnerable to suicide, suggests that these individuals are more at risk when the notion of suicide has been heavily publicized. He argues that suggestion, contrary to Durkheim's assertion, has a significant impact on suicide rates through imitation. He calls it the 'Werther effect' after Goethe's semi-autobiographical novel, *The Sorrows of Young*

Werther, describing the suicide of its young grief-stricken hero. The publication of the book in 1774, towards the height of the Romantic Movement, was followed by an alarming swell of suicides in Europe. Phillips found in his study, comparing the numbers of suicides before and after publicized suicides, that national rates increased in the month after a highly publicized suicide. For example, there was a 12% rise in the USA and a 10% rise in the UK following the death of Marilyn Monroe, and a 10% increase in the USA and a 17% increase in the UK after the suicide of Stephen Ward, the osteopath involved in the Profumo affair. Presentations for deliberate self-harm by women rose by 44% in England and Wales in the week after the death of Diana, Princess of Wales, and suicides rose by 17% after the funeral. The latter was particularly marked in women between the ages of 25 and 44 years (Hawton et al 2000). Phillips suggests that the size of the Werther effect varies with the strength of the publicity and the regional importance of the death.

The adverse media influence on suicidal behaviour, especially of adolescents, through coverage of news and television dramas has been much debated. The studies are beset with methodological problems and the findings are conflicting (Simkin et al 1995). Schmidtke and Häfner (1988) described a significant rise in suicides in Germany in the wake of a television film depicting a young man's suicide. Platt (1987), investigating the impact of a suicidal attempt in a British soap opera, found the result inconclusive.

Conversely, a more recent study (Salib 2003) argues that a brief but significant reduction in suicides in England and Wales found after the terrorist attacks in America on 11 September 2001 supports Durkheim's theory that periods of external threat create group integration within society and lower the suicide rate through greater social cohesion.

Ethological theories

Jones and Daniels (1996) report that several non-human mammals such as primates (macaques, marmosets, squirrel monkeys), carnivores (leopards, lions, jackals, hyenas), rodents and marsupials (opossums) resort to self-harm when they are in high states of arousal and the usual modes for expression of aggression are denied to them. Self-harming behaviour in animals, according to Chamove et al (1984), is displaced social aggression. Physical isolation provokes self-directed aggression, as it does in incarcerated human populations. Jones and Daniels suggest that the developmental, biochemical and genetic constituents of such behaviour may be common in man and these animals.

Harlow (1959) found that an infant monkey sought physical contact from its carers. It formed an attachment to a soft fluffy 'mother' in preference to a metal wire 'mother' with a rubber nipple. Anderson and Chamove (1985), in experiments with macaques, found that maternal deprivation and insecure early attachment, for example separation of the baby from its mother, predispose these primates to self-aggression later in life. Reuniting the baby with its mother, however, may mitigate this behaviour. Rosenblum (1998), in his experimental studies of the macaque's susceptibility to panic, show that insecure social attachments result in inadequate social and cognitive skills to master unexpected triggers and may lead to 'acute endogenous distress' similar to human panic disorder.

Suicide bombing

A suicide bomber may be defined as a person who kills him/herself deliberately while detonating a bomb. The phrase 'suicide bomb' was used by *The Times* newspaper in London in August 1945 to refer to a Japanese kamikaze plane.

Suicide bombing, which has serious social, political and economic consequences, has become common news in the last 20 years. In more modern times, it began with the Hezbollah in Lebanon in 1982 and has been used with telling effect by Palestinian organizations in the Middle East, by the Tamil Tigers in Sri Lanka, and more recently in Iraq. The most obvious example is the attack on the World Trade Centre in New York and the Pentagon outside Washington DC, on 11 September 2001, which resulted in nearly 3000 deaths.

Suicide attacks have been common in war throughout history, as a desperate measure to prevent capture, as self-sacrifice and as offensive action. The Japanese used their men as bomb-laden human missiles when they attacked American ships and aircraft carriers from the sky (in the form of kamikaze pilots) and in the water (through midget submarines) in the Second World War. These actions had political and social support, and had precedents in the country's history and culture. Suicide bombings have been targeted not only on military installations, but also on civilian populations in the last decade.

The psychology behind suicide bombing is complex and appears to have its own logic. Nasra Hassan, a Pakistani journalist, interviewed nearly 250 recruit and training bombers in the Middle East and found that they are usually young unmarried men between the ages of 17 and 28 years, educated, religiously devout and fiercely loyal to their group. They are not depressed, nor are they impulsive, lonely, helpless or driven by economic despair, although the despair of their community may explain the support for them (Margalit 2003).

The motives for suicide bombing are varied. It is sustained by a fiery mixture of nationalism and religious and revolutionary ideology. It is seen not only as defiance against oppressive occupation, but also as an act of religious martyrdom. The bombers are encouraged by their organizations to 'greet death as an old friend' and not to fear it. Suicide bombing is frequently an act of revenge for a specific event, or for the killing of a close relative or friend.

Suicide bombing evokes visceral fear and horror in the targeted population. It also provokes rage and hatred. The bombers, by making themselves the victims of their own act, also aim to claim the moral ground for their cause.

Physician-assisted suicide

In 2001, Diane Pretty, a 43-year-old woman who was paralysed from motor neuron disease, petitioned the UK High Court asking that she should be allowed to commit suicide with the help of her husband because she suffered from the terminal stage of the illness. The Court, while sympathetic to her cause, refused her request, stating that the law had a duty to protect the weak and vulnerable. She appealed to the Law Lords and the European Courts, but they refused to overturn the decision of the High Court. Diane Pretty's case rekindled the debate on euthanasia and assisted suicide. It highlighted the legal, moral, ethical and religious dilemmas surrounding the issue.

Ward and Tate (1994) state that nearly 30% of British doctors are confronted with requests for euthanasia by patients with severe disability or terminal illness. Pain, humiliation and futility are cited as the most common reasons (Van der Mass et al 1991).

A distinction should be made between voluntary and involuntary euthanasia, and assisted suicide. Euthanasia refers to intentional killing or shortening of life of a seriously ill person by an act of omission or commission, seemingly for the benefit of the person. It is voluntary if it is at the individual's request, and involuntary if no request is made nor any consent given.

Euthanasia became a public debate for the first time in the late nineteenth century when it was argued that it was necessary to achieve a good death by allowing the patient to die with less pain. The Nazi regime made euthanasia a pernicious state policy in the 1930s and the 1940s to eliminate the sick, the disabled, the mentally ill and those deemed 'unworthy of life'.

The preoccupation of medicine in the 1950s to the 1970s was to extend life at all costs (Van Delden 1998). However, the twin concept of patient rights and patient autonomy have brought to the forefront the seriously ill person's right to decide how and when he or she should die (Heintz 1994).

Only a handful of states in the world have endorsed the practice of physician-assisted suicide. Switzerland has allowed it with stringent guidelines since 1941. The state of Oregon (USA) made it lawful in 1997, the Netherlands in 2001 and Belgium in 2002. The Northern Territory of Australia legalized it in 1997, but the Federal Parliament repealed it 7 months later.

The advocates of assisted suicide contend that if doctors could withdraw life-sustaining treatment to relieve suffering and accelerate death at the request of a mentally competent patient, assisted suicide could be justified on similar moral grounds (Doyal & Doyal 2001).

A moral argument against assisted suicide is the double effect – that an action while arguably good in itself has an unintended but foreseen negative consequence (Jeffrey 1994). Another moral argument against it is 'the slippery slope'. It is feared that regulations cannot be adequately enforced and vulnerable sections of society such as the poor, elderly and mentally ill may be seen as burdens to society or their families and 'seduced to death' (Hendin 1997). Hendin argues that palliative care has become a casualty of the Dutch euthanasia policies.

Factors that increase the risk of suicide attempts

- **The tendency to deal with internal conflict with physical action** (Campbell & Hale 1991). Suicidal patients who are withdrawn and manifestly neglectful of their physical state are more likely to act out conflicts with their bodies.
- **A suicide plan.** A premeditated and planned attempt with a suicide note, secrecy, precautions against discovery and preparations in anticipation of death, such as giving away one's possessions and making a will, makes the patient more vulnerable to repetition (Hawton & Catalan 1987).
- **A previous suicide attempt**, especially if planned, carries a risk that is 27 times greater than in the general population (Hawton & Fagg 1988). The risk is higher in the first year after an attempt. The use of a dangerous method, such as hanging, jumping from a height or in front of a moving vehicle, shooting and carbon monoxide poisoning in a previous attempt heightens the risk (Brent 1997).
- **Young men with a history of several previous narcotic overdoses** are also at greater risk (De Moore & Robertson 1996; Hawton & Fagg 1988; Nordentoft et al 1993; Suokas & Lönnqvist 1991).
- **A recent experience** of failure or of loss through death, separation or divorce.
- **Chronic unresolved grief.** Patients who have not mourned their losses adequately are particularly at risk, especially around death anniversaries.
- **Family history of suicide or deliberate self-harm.** These patients are twice as likely to attempt suicide as those without the history (Roy 1984).
- **A lack of concern in the suicidal patient for him/herself and for others, and in others for him/her** (Campbell & Hale 1991). A patient who is cut off from him/herself fails to evoke concern in others. Professionals should be alert to experiences of loss of empathy for an actively suicidal patient.
- **Hopelessness**, which is a more accurate indicator of suicide than depression (Beck 1975; Fawcett et al 1987). Patients who feel hopeless are more likely to drop out of treatment (Brent et al 1995).

Of course, social characteristics such as unemployment, poverty, social isolation and absence of a close relationship, as described earlier, predispose an individual to suicide and self-harm.

Management of suicidal behaviour

Assessment

Assessment should be prompt and should be made before the crisis is dissipated, especially in teenagers. The impetus for assessment and treatment may be lost if the adolescent's family and/or caretakers are not involved from the beginning (Sprague 1997).

The assessment should be detailed and should include interviewing the patient, his partner and family members and other helping agencies involved. The behaviour of the patient should be closely observed. It is important to note that the patient's mental state may be clouded by the drugs used in the overdose and by alcohol. Psychotropic drugs in large doses impair the

Barraclough, B.M., 1987. The suicide rate of epilepsy. Acta Psychiatr. Scand. 76, 339–345.

Barraclough, B.M., Hughes, J., 1987. Suicide: clinical and epidemiological studies. Croom Helm, Beckenham.

Barraclough, B.M., Bunch, J., Nelson, B., et al., 1974. A hundred cases of suicide: clinical aspects. Br. J. Psychiatry 125, 355–373.

Bateman, A., 1998. Narcissism and its relation to violence and suicide. Int. J. Psychoanal. 79, 13–25.

Beck, A.T., 1974. The development of depression: a cognitive model. In: Freidman, R., Katz, M. (Eds.), The psychology of depression – contemporary theory and research. Winston-Wiley, Washington DC, pp. 3–27.

Beck, A.T., 1975. Cognitive Therapy and the Emotional Disorders. International Universities Press, New York.

Beck, A.T., Weissman, A., Lester, D., et al., 1974. The measurement of pessimism: the hopelessness scale. J. Consult. Clin. Psychol. 42, 861–865.

Beck, A.T., Kovacs, M., Weissman, A., 1975. Hopelessness and suicidal behaviour. J. Am. Med. Assoc. 234, 1146–1149.

Beck, A.T., Brown, G., Steer, R.A., et al., 1987. Differentiating anxiety and depression: a test of cognitive content-specificity hypothesis. J. Abnorm. Psychol. 96, 179–183.

Bertolote, J.M., Fleischmann, A., De Leo, D., et al., 2003. Suicide and mental disorders: do we know enough? Br. J. Psychiatry 183, 382–383.

Birtchnell, J., 1980. Women whose mothers died in childhood: an outcome study. Psychol. Med. 10, 699–713.

Bowlby, J., 1973. Separation: attachment and loss, vol. 2. Basic Books, New York.

Brent, D.A., 1997. The aftercare of adolescents with deliberate self-harm. J. Child Psychol. Psychiatry 38, 277–286.

Brent, D.A., Johnson, B., Bartle, S., et al., 1993. Personality disorder, tendency to impulsive violence, and suicidal behaviour in adolescents. J. Am. Acad. Child Adolesc. Psychiatry 32, 69–75.

Brent, D.A., Perper, J.A., Moritz, G., et al., 1994. Suicide in affectively ill adolescents: a case control study. J. Affect. Disord. 31, 193–202.

Brent, D.A., Birmaher, B., Holder, D., et al., 1995. A clinical psychotherapy trial for adolescent major depression. Symposium conducted at the 42nd Annual Meeting of the American Academy of Child and Adolescent Psychiatry, New Orleans, LA.

Brown, G., Harris, T., Copeland, J., 1977. Depression and loss. Br. J. Psychiatry 130, 1–18.

Bunch, 1972. Recent bereavement in relation to suicide. J. Psychosom. Res. 16, 316–326.

Bunch, J., Barraclough, B.M., 1971. The influence of parental death anniversaries on suicide dates. Br. J. Psychiatry 118, 621–626.

Burton, P., Low, A., Briggs, A., 1990. Increasing suicide rates among young men in England and Wales. Br. Med. J. 300, 1695–1696.

Campbell, D., Hale, R., 1991. Suicidal acts. In: Holmes, J. (Ed.), Textbook of psychotherapy in psychiatric practice. Churchill Livingstone, London.

Carroll, J., Schaffer, C.B., Spensley, J., et al., 1980. Family experiences of self-mutilating patients. Am. J. Psychiatry 137, 852–853.

Chamove, A.S., Anderson, J.R., Nash, V.J., 1984. Social and environmental influences on self-aggression in monkeys. Primates 25, 319–325.

Cohen-Sandler, R., Berman, A.L., King, R.A., 1982. Life stress and symptomatology: determinants of suicidal behavior in children. J. Am. Acad. Child Psychiatry 21, 178–186.

Commonwealth Department of Human Services and Health, 1995. Youth suicide in Australia: a background monograph. Australian Government Publishing Service, Canberra.

De Moore, G.M., Robertson, A.R., 1996. Suicide in the eighteen years after deliberate self-harm. Br. J. Psychiatry 169, 489–494.

Department of Health, 1992. The health of the nation: a strategy for health in England. HMSO, London.

Diekstra, R.F., 1989. Suicide and attempted suicide: an international perspective. Acta Psychiatr. Scand. 80, 1–24.

Dooley, D., Catalan, R., Rook, K., et al., 1989. Economic stress and suicide: multi-variate analysis of economic stress and suicidal ideation. Part 2. Suicide Life Threat. Behav. 19, 337–351.

Doyal, L., Doyal, L., 2001. Why active euthanasia and physician assisted suicide should be legalised. Br. Med. J. 323, 1079–1080.

Ellis, A., 1962. Reason and emotion in psychotherapy. Lyle Stuart, New York.

Favazza, A.R., 1987. Bodies under siege: self-mutilation in culture and psychiatry. John Hopkins University Press, Baltimore and London.

Fawcett, J., Scheftner, W.A., Clark, D., et al., 1987. Clinical predictors of suicide in patients with major affective disorders: a controlled prospective study. Am. J. Psychiatry 144, 35–40.

Feldman, M.D., 1988. The challenge of self-mutilation: a review. Compr. Psychiatry 29, 252–269.

Ferster, C.B., Skinner, B.F., Cheney, C.D., et al., 1997. Schedules of reinforcement. Appleton-Century-Crofts, New York.

Fombonne, E., 1998. Suicidal behaviours in vulnerable adolescents. Br. J. Psychiatry 173, 154–159.

Freud, S., 1916. Some character-types met within psycho-analytic work. Standard Edition of the Complete Works of Sigmund Freud, Vol. XIV. Papers on Metapsychology and Other Works 14, 309–333.

Freud, S., 1917. Mourning and melancholia. Standard Edition of the Complete Works of Sigmund Freud, Vol. XIV. Papers on Metapsychology and Other Works 14, 237–258.

Friedlander, K., 1940. On the longing to die. Int. J. Psychoanal. 21, 416–426.

Furman, E., 1984. Some difficulties in assessing depression and suicide in childhood. In: Sudak, H., Ford, A.B., Rushforth, B. (Eds.), Suicide in the young. John Wright/PSG Inc, Boston, pp. 245–258.

Gabrielson, L.W., Gabrielson, I.W., Klerman, L.W., et al., 1970. Suicide attempts in a population pregnant as teenagers. Am. J. Public Health 60, 2289–2301.

Gitlin, M.J., 1999. A psychiatrist's reaction to a patient's suicide. Am. J. Psychiatry 156, 1630–1634.

Gore, S.M., 1999. Suicide in prisons: reflection of the communities served or exacerbated risk? Br. J. Psychiatry 175, 50–55.

Gould, R.E., 1965. Suicide problems in children and adolescents. Am. J. Psychother. 21, 228–245.

Gunn, J., Taylor, P.J., 1993. Forensic psychiatry. Butterworth-Heinemann, Oxford.

Gunnell, D., Lopatatzidis, A., Dorling, D., et al., 1999. Suicide and unemployment in young people. Analysis of trends in England and Wales, 1921–1995. Br. J. Psychiatry 175, 263–270.

Harlow, H.F., 1959. Love in infant monkeys. Sci. Am. 200, 68–74.

Harre, R., Lamb, R. (Eds.), 1986. The dictionary of personality and social change. Blackwell, London.

Harris, E.C., Barraclough, B.M., 1994. Suicide as an outcome for medical disorders. Medicine 73, 281–296.

Harris, E.C., Barraclough, B.M., 1998. Excess mortality of mental disorder. Br. J. Psychiatry 173, 11–53.

Hawton, K., 1996a. Self-poisoning and the general hospital. Q. J. Med. 89, 879–880.

Hawton, K., 1996b. Deliberate self-harm. Medicine 75, 77–80.

Hawton, K.E., Catalan, J., 1987. Attempted suicide: a practical guide to its management, second ed. Oxford University Press, Oxford.

Hawton, K.E., Fagg, J., 1988. Suicide and other causes of death, following attempted suicide. Br. J. Psychiatry 152, 359–366.

Hawton, K.E., Arensman, E., Townsend, E., et al., 1998. Deliberate self-harm: systematic review of efficacy of psychosocial and pharmacological treatments in preventing repetition. Br. Med. J. 317, 441–447.

Hawton, K.E., Harriss, L., Appleby, L., et al., 2000. Effect of death of Diana, Princess of Wales, on suicide and deliberate self-harm. Br. J. Psychiatry 177, 463–466.

Heimann, P., 1950. On counter-transference. Int. J. Psychoanal. 31, 81–84.

Heintz, A.P.M., 1994. Euthanasia: can be part of good terminal care. Br. Med. J. 308, 1656.

Hendin, H., 1991. Psychodynamics of suicide with particular reference to the young. Am. J. Psychiatry 148, 1150–1158.

Hendin, H., 1997. Seduced by death: doctors, patients, and the Dutch cure. Norton, New York.

Hinshelwood, R.D., 1989. A dictionary of Kleinian thought. Free Association Books, London.

Hinshelwood, R.D., 1999. The difficult patient: the role of 'scientific psychiatry' in understanding patients with chronic schizophrenia or severe personality disorder. Br. J. Psychiatry 174, 187–190.

Isometsa, E.T., Lonnqvist, J.K., 1998. Suicide attempts preceding completed suicides. Br. J. Psychiatry 173, 531–535.

Jeffrey, D., 1994. Active euthanasia: time for a decision. Br. J. Gen. Pract. 44, 136–138.

Jones, E., 1911. On dying together. In: Jones, E. (Ed.), Essays in applied psychoanalysis, vol. I. Hogarth Press, London, pp. 9–21.

Jones, I.H., Daniels, B.A., 1996. An ethological approach to self-injury. Br. J. Psychiatry 169, 263–267.

Joseph, B., 1982. Addiction to near-death. Int. J. Psychoanal. 63, 449–456.

Kernberg, O.F., 1984. Diagnosis and clinical management of patients with suicide potential. In: Kernberg, O.F. (Ed.), Severe personality disorders: psychotherapeutic strategies. Yale University Press, Yale, pp. 254–263.

Klerman, G.L., 1986. Evidence for increase in rates of depression in North America and Western Europe in recent decades. In: Hippius, H., Klerman, G.L., Matussek, N. (Eds.), New results in depression research. Springer-Verlag, Berlin.

Kreitman, N., 1977. Parasuicide. Wiley, London.

Kreitman, N., Smith, P., Tan, E.S., 1970. Attempted suicide as language: an empirical study. Br. J. Psychiatry 116, 465–473.

Laplanche, J., Pontalis, J.B., 1973. The language of psycho-analysis. Hogarth Press, London.

Laufer, M., 1968. The body image, the function of masturbation and adolescence. Psychoanal. Study Child 23, 114–137.

Lewinsohn, P.M., Rohde, P., Seeley, J.R., 1994. Psychosocial risk factors for future adolescent suicide attempts. J. Consult. Clin. Psychol. 62, 297–305.

Links, P.S., 1990. Family environment and borderline personality disorder. American Psychiatric Press, Washington DC.

Maltsberger, J.T., 1993. Confusions of the body, self and others in suicidal states. In: Leenaars, A. (Ed.), Suicidology: essays in honour of Edwin Schneidman. Jason Aronson, Northvale NJ.

Maltsberger, J.T., Buie Jr., D.H., 1974. Countertransference hate in the treatment of suicidal patients. Arch. Gen. Psychiatry 30, 625–633.

Maltsberger, J.T., Buie Jr., D.H., 1980. The devices of suicide: revenge, riddance and rebirth. Int. Rev. Psychoanal. 7, 61–72.

Margalit, A., 2003. The suicide bombers. New York Rev. Books 50, 16 January.

Marsh, D.T., 1998. Serious mental illness in the family. Wiley, Chichester.

McClure, G.M., 1987. Suicide in England and Wales. Br. J. Psychiatry 150, 309–314.

McMahon, B., Pugh, T.F., 1971. Suicide in the widowed. Am. J. Epidemiol. 81, 23–31.

Meissner, W.W., 1981. Internalization in psychoanalysis. International University Press, New York.

Menninger, K.A., 1933. Psychoanalytic aspects of suicide. Int. J. Psychoanal. 14, 376–390.

Michel, K., Valach, L., 1992. Suicide prevention: spreading the gospel to general practitioners. Br. J. Psychiatry 160, 757–760.

Morgan, H.G., 1979. Death wishes: the understanding and management of DSH. Wiley, Chichester.

Morgan, H.G., Priest, 1991. Suicide and other unexpected deaths among psychiatric in-patients. The Bristol confidential inquiry. Br. J. Psychiatry 158, 368–374.

Morgan, H.G., Jones, E.M., Owen, J.H., 1993. Secondary prevention of non-fatal self-harm: the green card study. Br. J. Psychiatry 163, 111–112.

Moser, K.A., Goldblatt, P.Q., Fox, A.J., et al., 1987. Unemployment and mortality: comparison of the 1971 and 1981 longitudinal study census samples. Br. Med. J. 294, 86–89.

Murphy, G.E., 1975. The physician's responsibility for suicide. II Errors of omission. Ann. Intern. Med. 82, 305–309.

Nagy, M., 1948. The child's theories concerning death. J. Genet. Psychol. 73, 3–27.

Nordentoft, M., Breum, L., Munck, L.K., 1993. High mortality by natural and unnatural causes: a 10 year follow-up study of patients admitted to a poisoning treatment centre after suicide attempts. Br. Med. J. 306, 1637–1641.

Ogden, T.H., 1979. On projective identification. Int. J. Psychoanal. 60, 357–373.

Oliver, R.G., Hetzel, B.S., 1973. An analysis of recent trends in suicide rates in Australia. Int. J. Epidemiol. 2, 91–101.

Oyefeso, A., Ghodse, H., Clancy, C., et al., 1999. Suicide among drug addicts in the UK. Br. J. Psychiatry 175, 277–282.

Padel, R., 1995. Whom Gods destroy – elements of Greek and tragic madness. Princeton University Press, Princeton NJ.

Pfeffer, C.R., Klerman, G.L., Hurt, S.W., et al., 1991. Suicidal children grow up: demographic and clinical risk factors for adolescent suicide attempts. J. Am. Acad. Child Adolesc. Psychiatry 30, 609–616.

Pfeffer, C.R., Hurt, S.W., Kakuma, T., et al., 1994. Suicidal children grow up: suicidal episodes and effects of treatment during follow-up. J. Am. Acad. Child Adolesc. Psychiatry 33, 225–230.

Phillips, D.P., 1974. The influence of suggestion on suicide: substantive and theoretical implications of the Werther effect. Am. Sociol. Rev. 39, 340–354.

Pierce, D.W., 1981. The predictive validation of a suicide intent scale: a five year follow up. Br. J. Psych. 139, 391–396.

Platt, S., 1984. Unemployment and suicidal behaviour: a review of the literature. Soc. Sci. Med. 19, 93–115.

Platt, S., 1987. The aftermath of Angie's overdose. Is soap opera damaging your health? Br. Med. J. 294, 954–957.

Pollock, G.H., 1975. On mourning, immortality and utopia. J. Am. Psychoanal. Assoc. 23, 334–362.

Polmear, C., 2004. Dying to live: mourning, melancholia and the adolescent process. J. Child Psychother. 30, 263–274.

Pritchard, C., 1988. Suicide, unemployment and gender in the British Isles and European Economic Community (1974–1985). A hidden epidemic? Soc. Psychiatry Psychiatr. Epidemiol. 23, 85–89.

Pritchard, C., 1992. Is there a link between suicide in young men and unemployment? A comparison of the UK with other European Community Countries. Br. J. Psychiatry 160, 750–756.

Raleigh, V.S., 1996. Suicide patterns and trends in people of Indian subcontinent and Caribbean origin in England and Wales. Ethn. Health 1, 55–63.

Reinherz, H.Z., Giaconia, R.M., Silverman, A.B., et al., 1995. Early psychosocial risks for adolescent suicidal ideation and attempts. J. Am. Acad. Child Adolesc. Psychiatry 34, 599–611.

Retterstol, N., 1998. Suicide in a cultural history perspective Part 1. Suicidologi 2.

Retterstol, N., 2000. Suicide in a cultural history perspective Part 2. Suicidologi 3.

Richman, J., Rosenbaum, M., 1970. A clinical study of the role of hostility and death wishes by the family and society in suicide attempts. Isr. Ann. Psychiatry Relat. Discip. 8, 213–231.

Rochlin, G.R., 1959. The loss complex: a contribution to the aetiology of depression. J. Am. Psychoanal. Assoc. 7, 299–316.

Romans, S.E., Martin, J.L., Anderson, J.C., et al., 1995. Sexual abuse in childhood and deliberate self-harm. Am. J. Psychiatry 152, 1336–1342.

Rosenblum, L.A., 1998. Experimental studies of susceptibility to panic. NIMH Grant Award MH-42545, New York State Psychiatric Institute, Columbia University, New York.

Rosenfeld, H., 1987. Afterthought: changing theories and changing techniques in psychoanalysis. Impasse and interpretation. Tavistock, New Library of Psychoanalysis, London.

Rotheram-Borus, M.J., 1993. Suicidal behavior and risk factors among runaway youths. Am. J. Psychiatry 150, 103–107.

Roy, A., 1982. Suicide in chronic schizophrenia. Br. J. Psychiatry 141, 171–177.

Roy, A., 1984. Family history of suicide. Arch. Gen. Psychiatry 40, 971–974.

Rycroft, C., 1968. A critical dictionary of psychoanalysis. Nelson, London.

Sabbath, 1969. The suicidal adolescent – the expendable child. J. Am. Acad. Child Psychiatry 8, 272–289.

Safer Services, 1999. National Confidential Inquiry into Suicide and Homicide by People with Mental Illness – Report. Department of Health, London.

Sainsbury, P., 1955. Suicide in London. Maudsley Monograph no 1. Chapman and Hall, London.

Sainsbury, P., 1962. Suicide in later life. Gerantologia Clinica 4, 161–170.

Sainsbury, P., 1986. Epidemiology of suicide. In: Roy, A. (Ed.), Suicide. Williams and Wilkins, Baltimore MD.

Salib, E., 2003. Effect of 11 September 2001 on suicide and homicide in England and Wales. Br. J. Psychiatry 183, 207–212.

Sandler, J., 1960. On the concept of the super-ego. Psychoanal. Study Child 15, 128–162.

Schafer, R., 1968. Aspects of internalization. International University Press, New York.

Schmidtke, A., Häfner, H., 1988. The Werther after television films: new evidence for an old hypothesis. Psychol. Med. 18, 665–676.

Schneidman, E.S., 1993. Suicide as psychache. J. Nerv. Ment. Dis. 181, 147–149.

Schwartz, D.A., Flinn, D.E., Slawson, P.F., 1974. Treatment of the suicidal character. Am. J. Psychother. 28, 194–207.

Seligman, M.E.P., 1975. Helplessness: on depression, development and death. WH Freeman, San Francisco.

Shaffer, D., 1974. Suicide in childhood and early adolescence. J. Child Psychol. Psychiatry 45, 406–451.

Shaffer, D., 1985. Notes on developmental issues in the study of suicide. In: Rutter, M., Izard, C., Read, P. (Eds.), Depression in childhood: developmental issues. Guildford Press, New York.

Shaffer, D., Caton, C., 1984. Runaway and homeless youth in New York city. A report to the Ittleson Foundation, New York.

Shaffer, D., Piacentini, 1994. Suicide and attempted suicide. In: Rutter, M., Taylor, E., Hersov, L. (Eds.), Child and adolescent psychiatry, modern approaches. Blackwell, Oxford, pp. 407–424.

Shearer, S.L., Peters, C.P., Quaytman, M.S., et al., 1990. Frequency and correlates of childhood sexual and physical abuse histories in adult female borderline inpatients. Am. J. Psychiatry 145, 1424–1427.

Simkin, S., Hawton, K., Whitehead, L., et al., 1995. Media influence on parasuicide: a study of the effects of a television drama portrayal of paracetamol self-poisoning. Br. J. Psychiatry 167, 754–759.

Simpson, M.A., 1976. Self-mutilation and suicide. In: Schneidman, E.S. (Ed.), Suicidology: contemporary developments. Grune and Stratton, New York, pp. 281–315.

Speece, M.W., Brent, S.B., 1984. Children's understanding of death: a review of three components of a death concept. Child Dev. 55, 1671–1686.

Sprague, T., 1997. Clinical management of suicidal behaviour in children and adolescents. Clin. Child Psychol. Psychiatry 2, 113–123.

Stengel, E., 1952. Enquiries into attempted suicides. Proc. R. Soc. Med. 45, 613–620.

Suokas, J., Lönnqvist, J., 1991. Outcome of attempted suicide and psychiatric consultation: risk factors and suicide mortality during a five-year follow-up. Acta Psychiatr. Scand. 84, 545–549.

Van Delden, J.M., 1998. Physician-assisted suicide. A review. Br. Med. J. 316, 1543.

Van der Mass, P.J., Van Delden, J.J., et al., 1991. Euthanasia and other medical decisions concerning the end of life. Lancet 338, 669–674.

Van Praag, H.M., Plutchik, R., 1985. An empirical study of the 'cathartic effect' of attempted suicide. Psychiatry Res. 16, 123–130.

Vassilas, C.A., Morgan, H.G., 1993. General practitioners' contact with victims of suicide. Br. Med. J. 307, 300–301.

Ward, B.J., Tate, B.A., 1994. Attitudes among NHS doctors to request for euthanasia. Br. Med. J. 308, 1332–1334.

Watts, D., Morgan, G., 1994. Malignant alienation: dangers for patients who are hard to like. Br. J. Psychiatry 164, 11–15.

Weininger, O., 1979. Young children's concept of the dying and dead. Psychol. Rep. 44, 395–407.

Wheat, W., 1960. Motivational aspects of suicide in patients during and after psychiatric treatment. South. Med. J. 53, 273.

WHO, 2001. World Health Report 2001: mental health – new understanding, new hope. World Health Organization, Geneva.

Winnicott, D.W., 1949. Hate in the countertransference. Int. J. Psychoanal. 30, 69–74.

Yip, P.S.F., Chao, A., Chiu, C.W.F., 2000. Seasonal variation in suicide: diminished or vanished. Experience from England and Wales, 1982–1996. Br. J. Psychiatry 177, 366–369.

Zetzel, E., 1965. On the incapacity to bear depression. In: Schur, M. (Ed.), Drives, affects and behaviour, vol. 2. International University Press, New York.

Zilbroog, G., 1937. Considerations on suicide with particular reference to that of the young. Am. J. Orthopsychiatry 7, 15–31.

Unusual psychiatric syndromes

23

Sadgun Bhandari

CHAPTER CONTENTS

Introduction

The unusual psychiatric syndromes are a collection of largely eponymous symptom complexes and conditions, which are relatively rare and are unusual in their presentations. The first six syndromes described are delusions or delusional disorders and most may be diagnosed using contemporary classificatory systems. Othello syndrome, De Clerambault syndrome, Ekbom syndrome and *folie à deux* are diagnosed as delusional disorders in the ICD-10 (WHO 1992) and DSM-IV (APA 1994), where they present as pure syndromes. Munchausen syndrome is classified under somatoform disorders as factitious disorder and Munchausen by proxy is a form of child abuse and does not feature in contemporary classifications. The culture-bound syndromes will be discussed separately.

Capgras syndrome

Capgras syndrome was first described by Capgras and Reboul-Lachaux in 1923. The main characteristic of the syndrome is the delusion that a person, usually a close relative, has been replaced by a double or an imposter (Box 23.1). Christodoulou (1991) suggests that Capgras syndrome is one of a group of four syndromes known collectively as the *delusional misidentification syndromes*:

Diagnostic significance

Delusional jealousy can occur as a monodelusional disorder and is then diagnosed as a delusional disorder. It can also occur as a symptom of other disorders most commonly schizophrenia, and affective disorders (especially depression, which may enhance feelings of inadequacy). Alcohol abuse is present in 6–20% with morbid jealousy. According to Soyka et al (1991), this association holds good for male alcoholics only.

Morbid jealousy has also been described in a number of organic conditions including infections, endocrine disorders and dementia.

Enoch and Trethowan (1991) also suggest that psychiatric disorders such as depression are often quite common in relatives of patients suffering from delusional jealousy.

Management

Treatment is primarily with antipsychotics. As with schizophrenia, currently atypical antipsychotics would be an important aspect of pharmacological management. If the delusions are part of another disorder then the underlying disorder should be treated. Compliance with medication may be poor due to the nature of the delusion and in such cases compulsory treatment may be necessary.

Psychotherapy for morbid jealousy has included:

• Behavioural psychotherapy employing treatments for obsessions
• Cognitive behaviour therapy that focuses on addressing factors that precipitate and maintain the jealousy and factors in the individual's personality that predispose to jealousy
• Marital therapy
• Conjoint therapy.

Dangerousness

Delusional jealousy carries a high risk for violence. It is a major contributor to domestic violence and in a recent study, jealousy/possessiveness was a factor in about 30% of spousal homicide by male perpetrators (Dobash et al 2009). Delusional jealousy has a high rate of recurrence and can reoccur when a new partner replaces a former partner. Instances of repeat homicides following release from hospital or prison have been reported (Scott 1977). For the safety of partners of patients with morbid jealousy, temporary or permanent separation may be necessary.

Folie à deux

Folie à deux is also known as communicated insanity, contagious insanity, infectious insanity, psychosis of association and induced psychosis. In DSM-IV it is called *shared psychotic disorder*. The term was first coined by Lasegue and Falret in 1877. It refers to several syndromes in which mental symptoms, particularly paranoid delusions, are transmitted from one person to one or more others with whom the apparent instigator is in some way intimately associated; thus two or more individuals come

Box 23.4

Folie à deux

• Characterized by two persons, usually closely related, sharing the same delusion
• The dominant partner has the primary illness and induces the delusion in the submissive partner
• Separation often resolves the delusion in the secondarily affected person.

to share the same delusional ideas (Enoch & Trethowan 1991) (Box 23.4). In rare cases, whole families are affected (*folie à famille*). Various subtypes of this rare syndrome have been described; the commonest is *folie imposée* where the patient who suffers from the primary psychosis is dominant and imposes the delusion on the second individual, who is both submissive and suggestible. Delusions are usually persecutory.

Clinical aspects

This condition is rare and information is mainly obtained from case reports. Three essential criteria have been proposed for the diagnosis of true *folie à deux* (Dewhurst & Todd 1956):

• Marked similarity in the general and sometimes specific content of the partner's psychosis
• Unequivocal evidence that the partners accept, support and share each other's delusions
• Evidence that the partners have been intimately associated over a long period of time.

About 90% of relationships described are within the nuclear family, sister–sister dyads being the most common.

The duration of association between the two persons is long but the duration of exposure to the psychosis is variable. One of the most consistent findings is that of social isolation; this refers not to physical isolation but the impairment of the extent and/or nature of communication with others.

Explanatory theories

The psychological mechanism of identification is considered to be most important. Hereditary factors have also been postulated as the condition tends to occur in close relatives, although it does occur in husband–wife dyads as well.

Diagnostic significance

In the primarily affected individual, schizophrenia is the commonest diagnosis but delusional disorder and affective disorder can also occur. The cases secondarily affected might also suffer from schizophrenia or other psychiatric disorders.

Management

The first step in treatment is separation of the two persons suffering from the delusions because about 40% of the cases who are secondarily affected respond to this treatment. Primary cases need treatment of the underlying condition, usually schizophrenia, and secondary cases who do not improve with separation may require antipsychotic medication.

To prevent recurrence, social isolation needs to be addressed. Social support is important and family therapy may also be appropriate.

Cotard syndrome

Cotard syndrome is characterized by nihilistic delusions, which at their most extreme, are manifested by the person denying his own existence or that of the external world (Box 23.5). Cotard described his case in 1880, and in 1897 Seglas first used the eponym. It has been suggested that in his original description Cotard had described a syndrome with related symptoms but over time the name applied to nihilistic delusions (Berrios & Luque 1995). There is a considerable amount of debate as to whether Cotard syndrome is a distinct clinical entity.

Clinical aspects

The condition is characterized by delusions of negation (beliefs that specific body parts do not exist, that the person is dead or that the world does not exist). Accompanying features include delusions of guilt and immortality, anxiety, depression, suicidal behaviour, hypochondriacal delusions and auditory hallucinations with depressive content. The commonest delusions reported are those involving the body followed by those about existence. Cotard syndrome occurs more commonly in late middle age.

Diagnostic significance

In their review of 100 cases reported in the literature, Berrios and Luque (1995) found co-morbid depression reported in 89% of the cases. Cotard syndrome has also been reported with schizophrenia and organic disorders.

Management

The treatment of Cotard syndrome is essentially that of the underlying condition, most often depression. Since psychotic symptoms are present, ECT may be indicated. Risk of suicide is high.

Ekbom syndrome

Synonyms for Ekbom syndrome include delusions of infestation, delusional parasitosis and delusional infestation (Box 23.6). Ekbom (1938) described eight patients with the delusional

Box 23.5

Cotard syndrome
- Characterized by nihilistic delusions ranging from denial of the integrity of body organs to denial of internal and external existence
- Syndromal presentation is rare; Cotard syndrome usually accompanies depressive illness.

Box 23.6

Ekbom syndrome
- Characterized by a delusion of infestation with small organisms
- Condition rarely presents to psychiatrists; more commonly to dermatologists
- Can present as a delusional disorder, or as a symptom of schizophrenia or depression, especially in the elderly.

conviction that they were infested with small organisms such as mites or insects, a condition he called *Dermatozoewahn* or 'delusion of animal life in skin'. Patients with this uncommon condition, the subject of sporadic case reports, most often present to dermatologists. Delusional infestation is the preferred term, as Ekbom syndrome also refers to the restless legs syndrome.

Clinical aspects

The condition occurs more frequently with advancing age and the female to male ratio is 2:1. Patients tend to delay clinical consultation. Insects such as spiders, dragonflies and fleas are among the commonest complained of and patients may show 'the matchbox sign' by bringing specimens of the alleged organisms. Cleaning rituals are common and patients may fear contaminating others.

Since 2002, there has been a growth in the number of cases of 'Morgellons' in which people believe themselves to be infested with inanimate matter such as fibres and threads. The spread has been fast due to the internet. Patients believe that they have skin problems and unspecific neuropsychiatric symptoms (Freudenmann & Lepping 2009).

Diagnostic significance

Primary delusional infestation is diagnosed as a delusional disorder, somatic type. Secondary delusional infestation has been described in association with organic disorders, schizophrenia and affective disorders. *Folie à deux* may be associated in 5–15% of these cases (Enoch & Trethowan 1991). Delusional infestation with tactile hallucinations may occur in cocaine users – 'cocaine bug'.

Management

Whether presenting as a delusional disorder or as a schizophrenic symptom, treatment is with antipsychotics. Pimozide was often used in the past although there is no conclusive evidence that it is more effective than any other antipsychotic agent and moreover, owing to cardiac side-effects, it would no longer be recommended. As the evidence base is limited, treatment with antipsychotics is best informed by treatment for schizophrenia (Freudenmann & Lepping 2009).

Munchausen syndrome

Otherwise known as hospital hobos, peregrinating problem patients, hospital addiction syndrome or factitious disorder, this syndrome was first described by Asher in 1951. It is classically

Box 23.7

Munchausen syndrome

- Characterized by recurrent, feigned dramatic presentation of a medical condition in order to obtain investigations and treatment
- Not much is understood about underlying aetiological factors
- Management is difficult due to lack of engagement in treatment.

characterized by a patient presenting to hospital with dramatic symptoms suggesting a medical emergency, and necessitating investigations and treatment including surgery (Box 23.7). Patients have a history of wandering from one hospital to another with a similar presentation, with no obvious gain. The term may be applied to other presentations, not necessarily dramatic, where physical signs or abnormal laboratory results are fabricated, all these conditions subsumed under the rubric of factitious disorders. Asher originally described three sub-types (acute abdominal, haemorrhagic and neurological), but over time, a much wider variety of presentations have been described. Munchausen has been also used to describe factitious presentations of psychiatric symptoms but diagnostic criteria are not clear (Enoch & Trethowan 1991).

Clinical aspects

The disorder is commoner in males. The patients are well-informed about medical conditions and may be members of the medical or allied professions. A criminal record is common. The course varies from episodic to a chronic unremitting one. Presentation is often late at night or at weekends, patients are demanding and attention-seeking, often 'break the rules', and have no visitors.

Association with a range of physical and psychiatric conditions (eating disorders, depression, borderline personality disorder, diabetes, asthma and brain damage) has been described (Robertson & Hossain 1997).

Explanatory theories

Many psychological mechanisms have been postulated to explain this behaviour but not enough is known about the condition to understand the aetiological factors completely. Sussman et al (1987) suggest that Munchausen syndrome is a result of complex interaction of personality factors and psychosocial stressors.

Diagnostic significance

The condition must be differentiated from those in which patients adopt a patient role in order to obtain drugs or shelter, or in response to an acute psychosocial crisis. Malingering should be ruled out, although it is unlikely to present recurrently.

Management

Management is difficult as the patients are reluctant to engage in treatment. Early detection is important. Treatment is primarily psychotherapeutic and should aim to promote social integration

and reduce inappropriate behaviour (Robertson & Cervilla 1997). Prognosis is regarded as generally poor.

Munchausen syndrome by proxy

The syndrome was first described by Meadow in 1977 and is also known as Munchausen by proxy syndrome, Meadow syndrome or Polle syndrome (Box 23.8). Munchausen syndrome by proxy consists of the induction of an appearance, or a state, of physical ill health in a child, by a parent (or someone *in loco parentis*), where the child is subsequently presented to health professionals for diagnosis and/or treatment, usually persistently. The perpetrator denies the aetiology of the child's illness and the acute symptoms and signs of the illness decrease after separation from the perpetrator (Bools et al 1992). The harm to the child results from the direct production of physical signs and diseases in the child and indirectly through medical intervention.

Clinical aspects

The most common presentations involve seizures, failure to thrive, vomiting and diarrhoea, asthma/allergies and infections. Abuse usually involves young children, starting from the first year of life, with the average age just over 3 years at diagnosis, and the mortality is estimated at 9% (Rosenberg 1987). Average length of time to establish a diagnosis of Munchausen syndrome by proxy generally exceeds 6 months, and often there is a history of a sibling having died of undiagnosed causes, suggesting that cases may go undetected (Schreier & Libow 1994).

In nearly every case, the perpetrator is the biological mother (Rosenberg 1987). They usually have a background of having worked in the health sector and/or are medically knowledgeable. They usually appear caring and doctors and other professionals are reluctant to believe that the mothers are responsible for the cruelty to the child (Schreier & Libow 1994). In 30–35% of cases returning home, the fabrication of illness is repeated. The long-term psychological outcome is poor, regardless of the child returning home or going into care outside the home (Bools et al 1993).

Diagnostic significance

Little is known about the relation between psychiatric disorders and Munchausen syndrome by proxy. Depression and personality disorder have been diagnosed in patients assessed by psychiatrists.

Box 23.8

Munchausen syndrome by proxy

- Characterized by repeated fabrication of an illness in a child, in order to obtain medical intervention for the child, resulting in harm to the child
- Almost all cases are perpetrated by the biological mother
- Not enough is known about the characteristics of the perpetrators
- Requires a high index of suspicion to facilitate early identification and intervention.

Management

The key to management is early identification. Clues include the nature of presentation of the illness and attitude of mother. Covert video surveillance has also been used (Samuels et al 1992). Once identified, the management is aimed at protecting the child (and other siblings). Treatment of the perpetrator may be through family therapy or psychiatrists.

Ganser syndrome

This syndrome was first described by Ganser in 1898. It is characterized by a patient giving approximate answers to simple and familiar questions, in a setting of disturbed and clouded consciousness (Box 23.9). The other two features of the complete syndrome include hysterical conversion symptoms and hallucinations. Associated features include psychogenic amnesia. It is thought to be a hysterical dissociative state that occurs as a result of an unconscious effort by the subject to escape from an intolerable situation (Enoch & Trethowan 1991). The symptom that has attracted the most attention is that of approximate answers or talking past the point (*vorbeireden*).

The complete syndrome is very rare. Scott (1965) suggested that it is useful to distinguish between the Ganser *symptom* (approximate answers) and Ganser *syndrome*, the symptom being more common. Lishman (1987) discusses the difficulty with the concept of the symptom as it requires an element of subjective interpretation on the part of the examiner and it is unclear how approximate the answer should be before the symptom is considered to be present.

Diagnostic significance

This condition needs to be distinguished from true dementia, pseudodementia (in depression or schizophrenia) and conscious simulation of symptoms (malingering).

Management

Hospitalization may be necessary for investigation and in order to remove the patient from the stressful environment. Underlying depression should be treated. Improvement is the most likely outcome.

Box 23.9

Ganser syndrome

- A rare syndrome characterized by approximate answers, clouded consciousness, hallucinations and hysterical conversion symptoms
- Symptom of approximate answers is more common than the other symptoms
- Resolution is the likely outcome.

Culture-bound syndromes

The term 'culture-bound syndromes' conjures up images of rare and exotic psychiatric disorders, and indeed many disorders are described as culture-bound syndromes. However, there are difficulties with the term because the disorders it is applied to are often not distinct disease entities and are not strictly culture-bound, occurring in multiple cultures. The culture-bound syndromes therefore include a heterogenous group of phenomena, some of which are true syndromes, some culturally based aetiologic explanations for psychiatric disorders, and others, folk terms for common behaviours or emotions, otherwise known as 'idioms of distress' (Levine & Gaw 1995). According to Littlewood (1990), the term 'culture-bound' was applied to local patterns of behaviour that did not fit into the Western psychiatric classifications. Littlewood also suggests that the term is redundant because all reactions are to an extent culturally determined. Patterns characteristic of Western societies, such as overdoses and anorexia nervosa, are as culture-bound as any others.

The following are some of the common conditions described under this heading:

- Koro
- Amok
- Latah
- Wendigo (Windigo, Wihtigo, Witiko)
- Possession states
- Others.

Koro

This occurs in South-East Asia and affects Chinese people. Patients are usually males, who believe that the penis is withdrawing inside the abdomen. This results in a panic as the person also believes that once the penis has completely retracted he will die. Remedial action is taken by tying the penis with strings and getting help from relatives and friends. It can affect females as well and may occur individually or in epidemics. Koro responds to reassurance and education. In psychiatric terms, koro is an anxiety state and is not delusional.

Koro epidemics have been described in other cultures including Thailand (*rok joo*) and Assam in India (*jinjina bemar*).

Koro-like states characterized by fear of the penis shrinking have been described in individuals from outside South-East Asia, but these patients do not show the other features of koro and have a history of psychiatric conditions including anxiety, depression and schizophrenia (Berrios & Morley 1984).

Amok

This occurs in the Philippines and Malaysia and is confined to males who, after a real or imagined insult, brood for several days and then return in a blind fury during which they attempt to kill everyone encountered. The frenzy is halted only when the person himself is killed or is caught and bound. There is amnesia for the behaviour. The essence of amok is blind, murderous

Gender and sexuality in psychiatry

Gender and sexuality in psychiatry

24

Shubuladè Smith   Susannah Whitwell

Introduction

Prior to the 1960s, women were seen as the weaker more emotional sex, lacking robustness and prone to nervous disorder. After the sexual revolution, feminism stamped out the differences between men and women insisting that males and females be treated in the same way in all walks of life. Around the same time, legal restrictions on sexuality were removed allowing fuller participation in society of a hitherto marginalized group. This is more acceptable, but ignoring differences between individuals may result in inappropriate comparisons and inappropriate treatments. This chapter attempts to redress the balance; we look at some of the most important aspects of the fundamental differences in people and how they might affect the presentation and management of the psychiatric disorder.

Epidemiology of psychiatric disorders

The National Morbidity Survey provides a snapshot of the prevalence of mental disorder in the UK population. Since 1993, the three surveys demonstrate that women are more likely to suffer from all mental disorders than men, other than psychotic disorders and alcohol and drug dependence. This trend has not changed over time. Despite concerns that rates of alcohol and substance misuse have increased, it appears that since 2000, the prevalence of substance dependence has reduced in men while it has remained the same for women.

Disorders specifically associated with gender identity

Gender identity disorders

Gender identity disorders are described in both ICD-10 (including the categories of transsexualism, dual-role transvestism and gender identity disorder of childhood) and DSM-IV (gender identity disorder classified as occurring either in childhood or in adults). They are characterized by a persistent or recurrent discomfort about assigned gender and identification with the opposite gender and may be associated with cross-dressing. Dual role transvestism describes cross-dressing as in order to enjoy the temporary experience of membership of the opposite gender but without sexual arousal and without transsexualism. In contrast, fetishistic transvestism is characterized by sexual arousal by cross-dressing (which can be categorized as a disorder of sexual preference).

While it is less likely that an individual with dual role transvestism or fetishistic transvestism would come into contact with mental health services or even see themselves as experiencing a psychiatric disorder, psychiatrists are sometimes asked to see transsexual individuals. This is characterized by the belief that one is the gender opposite that assigned at birth. It often starts before puberty, is associated with cross-dressing (without sexual arousal) and it is often associated with considerable distress, which can result in self mutilation and suicidality. Recent studies based on men seeking gender reassignment surgery estimate a prevalence of 1:10 000. The ratio of men and women seeking treatment of transsexualism is 3:1.

The management of transsexualism incorporates extensive psychological evaluation and psychotherapy to help ensure the psychological stability of an individual who wishes to undertake endocrine therapy and in some cases, gender reassignment surgery following a period of a 'real life test', where an individual lives in the preferred gender role by means of clothing, name and cross-gender socialization. Guidelines for treatment of individuals are the internationally recognized Standards of Care of the World Professional Association for Transgender Health. If a person's request for gender reassignment surgery is due to primary transsexualism and not secondary to a co-morbid psychiatric condition such as affective disorder, personality disorder or psychosis, gender reassignment surgery appears to alleviate distress with 86% being stable or showing an improvement in global function post-surgery (Johansson et al 2009).

Disorders specifically associated with sexual orientation

Until the 1950s, many in the medical profession regarded homosexuality as evidence of mental illness and it was only removed from DSM-III in 1973. In the past, there has been controversy about psychoanalytic attitudes towards homosexuality and a small minority of clinicians have suggested that homosexuality should be considered a psychiatric disorder, often in light of their religious views. However, in mainstream psychiatry, homosexuality is not regarded as a mental illness.

A number of recent studies, using both clinic and community samples, have examined the rates of psychiatric illness in homosexual individuals. Gay men and lesbians appear to be at higher risk than their heterosexual counterparts for a number of stress-related disorders including anxiety, drug and alcohol abuse and depression. Lesbian and bisexual women are particularly at risk of substance dependence. In gay men, there is an excess of suicidality, particularly in adolescence, and gay men vastly outnumber their heterosexual peers in eating disorder services (King et al 2008). Recent research has focused on the role of social stigmatization, prejudice and the stress of coping with the AIDS epidemic as possible causal factors to account for this increased prevalence of psychiatric disorders in this population. The psychiatrist has an important role in helping people feel comfortable with their sexuality.

Disorders specifically associated with being female

Menarche

There are no specific disorders associated with menarche. Theories that early psychological stress results in earlier age of reproductive maturation have not been upheld. Unpreparedness/early menarche tends to be associated with more negative emotional reactions but is not as traumatic an event as portrayed in the literature. Early menarche has been associated with a greater incidence of conduct disorder, later psychosocial difficulties and lifetime history of mental disorder. In particular, early maturers, especially those with conduct disorder, were more likely to experience depressive symptoms as adults. In contrast, Bisaga et al (2002) found that adolescent females who had a later onset of menarche were more likely to report depressive symptoms. However, the most robust findings are that early menarche is associated with a greater incidence of mental distress and higher rates of conduct disorder (Copeland et al 2010).

The main importance of puberty to psychiatrists is that it heralds the onset of the reproductive period of a woman's life and this coincides with a greater risk of psychiatric illness, particularly depression.

Menstrual cycle

Cyclical changes in mood and other symptoms may be associated with the menstrual cycle. Frank (1931) described this as premenstrual tension, now commonly called 'premenstrual syndrome' (PMS).

Clinical features

- Anxiety
- Irritability
- Depression
- Lethargy

- Headache
- Abdominal distension/bloatedness
- Breast swelling and tenderness
- Fluid retention and weight gain.

Most women having ovulatory cycles experience some cyclical symptoms, but for 3%, these symptoms are severe and result in a marked disturbance of their everyday functioning.

In the WHO International Classification of Disease, premenstrual symptoms are classified under genitourinary diseases, and in Britain, few psychiatrists will be confronted by women complaining specifically of premenstrual syndrome, this being more commonly seen by gynaecologists. In America, however, the symptoms associated with the premenstrual phase have made their way into DSM-IV and are classified as a mood disorder, not otherwise specified – Premenstrual Dysphoric Disorder (PMDD). This represents the severe end of PMS. Until now, there has been little consensus with regard to diagnosis; there has been frequent use of unstandardized rating scales and retrospective self-reporting. It thus comes as no surprise that the prevalence of the disorder ranges from 3% in some studies to 90% in others. A recent study found prevalences of PMS in 10.3% and PMDD in 3.1% of women. Despite the acceptance of the diagnosis into the American psychiatric classification system, there remains controversy regarding the disorder. For DSM-V, there is a PMDD subwork group accumulating evidence as to whether PMDD can be deemed a valid diagnosis.

For a diagnosis of PMDD:

- Symptoms should recur cyclically during the luteal phase of the cycle
- Symptoms should remit after the onset of menses and remain absent for at least 1 week during the follicular phase
- Symptoms cause marked interference with usual activities of life
- Symptoms should have been documented by prospective daily ratings during at least two consecutive cycles.

Aetiology

PMS is only associated with ovulatory cycles: hysterectomy and ovariectomy eliminate PMS, whereas symptoms persist after a hysterectomy if the ovaries remain, implying that ovulation causes changes in mood.

Progesterone deficiency, progesterone excess, raised prolactin levels, raised and decreased levels of oestrogen have been postulated as causal, as have changes in oestradiol/progesterone ratio, although no difference in hormonal levels has been found between PMDD sufferers vs non-sufferers.

Serotonin may play a role as 5HT uptake in platelets and levels of 5HT in whole blood are reduced during the late luteal phase in women with PMS compared to non-sufferers, and SSRIs appear to be effective in women with PMS.

Women who report PMS have a higher prevalence of co-existing depressive disorder, anxiety disorder and substance misuse, tend to be unemployed and have poor marital relationships, and are more likely to experience psychological disturbance related to reproductive events. This latter finding may indicate an inherent abnormality of steroidal hormone metabolism/response in these women.

Box 24.1

Premenstrual syndrome

PMS is unlikely to be the sole complaint of a patient attending a psychiatrist. The main importance of PMS to most psychiatrists is that patients with major mental illness such as schizophrenia and bipolar disorder might have pre-menstrual exacerbations of their illness. This may in part be related to changes in fluid balance, especially for drugs such as lithium. The control of levels in certain patients may be extremely difficult at this time. There is also a possibility that there is a change in receptor sensitivity which coincides with the marked hormonal changes that occur particularly in the late luteal phase.

Treatment

- Progesterone vaginal suppositories were found to have no better effect than placebo.
- Oestrogen has had little success, the fears about endometrial hyperplasia severely curtailing widespread use of this method.
- Oral contraceptive pill has not been very effective and its use is implicated in the onset of depression in certain women.

Other treatments range from changing diet, exercise, vitamin B_6 and evening primrose oil, to more drastic interventions such as GnRH agonists, danazol and even surgical ablation. The SSRIs have been found to significantly relieve symptoms of PMS in women and are first-line treatment for PMDD, with fluoxetine and sertraline being licensed by the FDA in America for this purpose (Box 24.1) (Jarvis et al 2008).

Disorders associated with childbirth

Pregnancy

Major depressive disorders affect 10% of women of childbearing age. When they become pregnant, this situation does not improve. Evans et al (2001) found that a higher percentage of women reached the threshold for depressive disorder antenatally than postnatally (13.5% at 32 weeks of pregnancy vs 8.9% at 8 weeks postpartum). A greater number of women reached the threshold during the early stages of pregnancy (18–32 weeks) than in later stages of pregnancy (32 weeks postpartum). They concluded that symptoms of depression are no less common or severe postnatally than antenatally. Depression in pregnancy is more common in those who are economically poorest and this finding has been replicated around the world. In addition to depression, the most common psychiatric disturbance seen in pregnancy is mild anxiety.

When seen, psychiatric symptoms tend to occur in early pregnancy and are often a reaction to an unplanned pregnancy in the context of a poor marital relationship. These problems are best helped with counselling, education and reassurance. A psychotherapeutic approach addressing the issues of impending motherhood, the meaning of this to the woman and exploration of her own parenting may reveal important concerns about her own ability to mother (Raphael-Leff 1986).

development of increased sensitivity of hypothalamic dopamine D2 receptors may predict the onset of depressive disorder. The consensus, however, is that psychosocial factors are more important in the aetiology of this disorder than biological factors.

Treatment

Psychological treatments have been found to improve outcome in the short term, although they are not superior to spontaneous remission in the long term (Cooper et al 2003).

- Full psychiatric history, with particular reference to DSH or harm to baby
- Counselling/psychotherapy/cognitive behaviour therapy
- Antidepressants can be given even if breast-feeding (see below). Lithium should be avoided when breast-feeding
- Admit (preferably to specialist mother and baby unit), if illness is severe and there is risk of DSH or harm to the baby.

Prevention

Preventative measures include staff training, especially for midwives and GPs. Antenatal education may help mothers distinguish between the blues and more severe mood symptoms which may require professional help. Antenatal detection, close follow-up and prophylaxis in high risk patients. Early detection: monitor mothers with severe postnatal blues, as there is a high risk of depression later. Screening, e.g. Edinburgh Postnatal Depression Scale.

Prognosis

Most postnatal depression will have resolved by 6 months after birth. Unfortunately, the depression may have serious detrimental effects on the marital relationship and the mother–infant relationship.

Postnatal depression and child development

Severe mood disturbance during the postnatal period may affect child development by interfering with usual mother–child bonding process. Depressed mothers are less responsive to infant cries, and usually more withdrawn or hostile than non-depressed mothers (Murray et al 1996). The infant's way of relating to others may be negatively influenced by this early relationship to a depressed mother. Children, especially males, whose mothers are depressed 3 months postpartum appear to have lower IQ scores, more attentional problems, more difficulty with mathematical reasoning and are more likely to have special educational needs (Hay et al 2001). Boys whose fathers are depressed in the postnatal period have higher rates of conduct disorder later in life, even when maternal postnatal depression is controlled for (Ramchandani et al 2005).

Puerperal (postnatal) psychosis

Epidemiology

In 0.1–0.2% of live births, the mother experiences a psychotic illness. These postnatal psychoses are mainly affective, but can be schizophrenic or organic. There is a substantially increased risk in women with a previous history of psychiatric hospitalization. Risk of admission increases in the first 3 months postpartum, with days 10–19 being the crucial risk period for women with previous psychiatric history (Munk-Olsen et al 2009).

Hippocrates described puerperal psychoses in the fifth century BC, thinking they were the result of breast-milk erroneously entering the brain. Much later, in 1858, Marcé's study of 310 women with mental illness associated with childbirth seemed to confirm a distinct clinical syndrome consisting of a predominance of delirium and lability of mood occurring 4–5 days postpartum. Today, researchers continue to search for the humoral mechanism that might underlie the aetiology of this disease, but the distinction of postnatal psychosis from other major psychotic illness remains in doubt. This is because the clinical features of puerperal psychoses closely resemble those of psychoses occurring at other times and no differences have been found between the subsequent psychiatric morbidity or hormone levels of psychotic mothers compared with mothers with non-psychotic illness or mothers who remain well postpartum. However, the clinical picture shows these women with puerperal psychosis to be more deluded, hallucinated, labile and more likely to be disorientated than in non-puerperal psychosis, and onset is usually within 2 weeks after delivery, suggestive of some biological trigger to the disorder.

Aetiology

Kendell et al (1987) found that there is an increased risk of psychiatric admission if the mother is unmarried, if it is her first baby and if delivery is by caesarean section. These all indicate that psychological stress may be the important factor. However, depressive/manic presentations are commoner; a past history of manic-depression or postnatal psychosis leads to a one in five chance of an affective disorder after childbirth, i.e. much higher risk of relapse, and in high risk women who do relapse after childbirth, it has been shown that the onset of psychotic symptoms are preceded by increased dopamine receptor sensitivity (Wieck et al 1991). These findings support a biological basis to the illness.

Clinical features

- Severe insomnia in the absence of a crying baby
- Confusion and memory impairment
- Markedly changeable behaviour with rapid shifts from elation to profound sadness or rage, from inappropriate laughter to tearfulness
- Paranoid delusions re: hospital staff or family
- Thought interference
- Periods of florid psychosis may be interspersed with intervals of lucidity
- Marked guilt, depression, anxiety, irritability

- Suicidal and/or infanticidal thoughts
- Often, the initial stages of mood lability may be difficult to distinguish from postnatal blues.

Management

Risk of postnatal psychosis is 100 times greater in first-time mothers with previous psychiatric hospitalization compared with all other mothers. Clearly women with psychiatric histories should be identified early and carefully monitored postpartum. The first 30 days postpartum are an especially risky period and this can be readily predicted. However, close monitoring should continue for up to 1 year postpartum.

Inpatient treatment is often needed, preferably with the baby but not if the mother is too disturbed or infanticidal. Mother and baby units are specialist wards where the baby is cared for by nurses and the mother's care of the child can be monitored over time. Midwife and health visitor involvement should be maintained.

Observe the mother for up to 1 week prior to discharge to ensure she is coping adequately with the baby. Treat any coexisting illness. Do not forget the postnatal examination just because the person is in a psychiatric unit, and do not forget the father. He may be confused, upset and may even be the subject of a delusion. Lovestone and Kumar (1993) identified that fathers whose partners become postnatally unwell have much higher rates of psychiatric disorders, compared with fathers whose partners remain well after birth. Information, education and reassurance about his partner's illness, together with involving him in the care of his child, will help to alleviate some of his concerns, at the same time as facilitating the bonding process.

Treatment

- Antipsychotics (choice of drug will depend on whether the mother is breast-feeding or not)
- Antidepressants (usually given in conjunction with an antipsychotic as the illnesses are often affective in nature)
- ECT
- Lithium has been used prophylactically in patients at high risk of relapse, but there are concerns about teratogenicity. The changes in fluid balance that occur after birth can make it very difficult to control blood levels of lithium and therefore toxicity is always a risk
- Lithium should not be given to breast-feeding women
- Oestrogen prophylaxis has not been found to reduce risk of relapse, but Kumar et al (2003) found its use was associated with lower doses of psychotropic medication and earlier discharge.

Breast-feeding

Many women will wish to breast-feed, but all psychotropic medications enter the breast milk and may affect the neonate (Burt et al 2001).

- Generally it is advisable to keep doses to a minimum and use shorter-acting drugs if psychotropic medications are given to a breast-feeding woman.

- Time feeds to avoid peak drug levels, e.g. giving the dose after the last breast-feed at night in older infants may help to reduce exposure to the drug.
- The infant should be monitored for adverse drug effects as well as close attention being paid to their feeding, growth and development.

Psychotropic medications are excreted in breast milk in differing amounts and this will play a part in determining the risks to the baby. Sodium valproate and carbamazepine are excreted in relatively small amounts in breast milk; in contrast large amounts of lamotrigine and lithium are found. The risk to the neonate, however, is also determined by the risks posed by even small amounts of the drug. Although only small amounts of clozapine are excreted in breast milk the neonate has the same risk as adults of life-threatening agranulocytosis. It is recommended that clinicians determine management on a case-by-case basis, weighing up the risk/benefit of breast-feeding in that individual and ensuring that the woman and her partner are fully aware and understand the potential risks to their child. In women who choose to breast-feed while taking psychotropic medication, there should be very careful monitoring of the baby.

Prognosis

For the acute illness, the prognosis is very good, but the risk of relapse after further births is very high (up to 50%).

Other disorders associated with childbirth

Phobias, OCD and anxiety states may interfere markedly with child-care and are common in the perinatal period (Ross & McLean 2006). Wijma et al (1997) found PTSD in 1.7% of women following traumatic childbirth.

Menopause

The menopause is defined as 12 months after the last menses; the average age in Britain is 51. This time in a woman's life is associated with many changes, including children leaving home, death of parents and the loss of reproductive capability. This is a time of reappraisal of roles, particularly the maternal one.

The menopause is another time in the reproductive cycle which is anecdotally associated with psychiatric symptoms. Recently, a large epidemiological study found a correlation between transition into the menopause and depression which appeared to be mediated by a combination of hormonal and psychosocial factors including hot flushes, PMS, employment and marital status (Freeman et al 2006). However, synthesizing findings from a number of studies found conflicting evidence of mood disorder associated with menopausal transition itself (Vesco et al 2007).

The role of hormone replacement therapy (HRT)

HRT has been said by many women not only to improve their physical symptoms, but also their mood. Evidence of improvement in psychological symptoms has been found only in those women who have undergone surgical menopause, but this improvement is not sufficient to help those who are clinically depressed. When sexual symptoms are the main complaint, HRT seems to be more effective.

Women presenting with psychiatric symptoms should be treated with psychological/psychiatric interventions, as the response to HRT has been found to be no better than placebo. More recently, there have been concerns about the risk of certain cancers and cardiovascular disease in women taking HRT in the long term and therefore, given the lack of evidence for their efficacy in psychiatric disorder, their use for mood improvement is not recommended.

Hormonal aspects of psychiatric illness

Women who suffer from affective disorders following one reproductive event are more vulnerable to recurrences associated with others. A proportion of women may have increased sensitivity or an abnormal response to the neuromodulatory effects of hormones, which result in them being more vulnerable to psychiatric disorder during times of hormonal flux. This would be supported by previous findings that the excess of depression in women disappears in the postmenopausal years. On the other hand, the later onset of schizophrenia in women may be a result of protective effects of oestrogen.

Disorders showing a higher prevalence in women

Eating disorders, depression, anxiety and phobic disorders, dementia and somatization disorder, borderline personality disorder and deliberate self-harm all show a higher prevalence in women than men. They are discussed in the relevant chapters.

Disorders showing a higher prevalence in men

While there are gender differences in a wide range of psychiatric disorders, there are very few disorders that can be said to be specifically associated with being male. An exception is the semen loss anxiety disorder such as Dhat, described in non-Western cultures and which is classified as a culture bound syndrome. Related to this is Koro, the belief that the penis will retract into the body and cause death. These disorders are best classified as neurotic disorders.

There is a higher prevalence of developmental disorders such as attention deficit hyperactivity disorder (ADHD), autistic spectrum disorders (ASD) and conduct disorders, drug and alcohol problems and a rising suicide rate in males. In addition, mental illness is associated with higher levels of violence and aggression, particularly in the context of antisocial personality disorder and psychopathy. The higher rates of suicide in the context of lower prevalence of depression when compared with women gives rise to the possibility that illness in men may present in an atypical way that goes

unrecognized, for example presenting with anger management problems or drug and alcohol addiction which masks underlying affective disorder. Initial presentations in males are more likely to be via the police or criminal justice system and men are less likely than women to present to primary care with mental health concerns. This may be due to perceived stigma, lack of awareness and practical issues about accessing help during working hours as well as unrecognized masked depression.

Psychopathy/aggression/violent crime

In the general population, the most serious violent crime is carried out by males. There is a slightly smaller gender difference in a mentally disordered population (Hodgins et al 2008). The aetiology of violence is heterogenous and complex but a cause of spousal violence of note is pathological, delusional or morbid jealousy (also known as Othello syndrome). In a sample of 20 individuals with delusional jealousy, 19 were male and 12 had harmed their spouse, three of them using a weapon. The risk was found to be increased by command hallucinations, paranoid delusions and alcohol use (Silva et al. 1998).

Suicide

Suicide accounts for 1–2% of total global mortality and is a leading cause of premature death. Worldwide, the rate of completed suicide is four times higher for men than for women (with the exception of China, which has a high rate of female suicide). In the UK, overall rates of suicide in both men and women fell from 1963 to 1973. The rates in women have continued to fall since then; however, the rates in men increased from 1975 to 1990, by 23%. The increase was particularly seen in young men as well as the traditional peak in the elderly. Factors associated with the increasing rates of suicide in males were thought to include psychosocial stresses of unemployment and increasing substance abuse and alcohol consumption. From 1990, rates of suicide in both men and women have fallen in the UK, coinciding with government policy focusing on suicide, increasing prescription of antidepressant medication and car exhaust emission legislation. The Office of National Statistics reported that 12 men per 100 000 and 5 women per 100 000 completed suicide in 2007.

Addiction

Alcohol dependence and drug addiction are more common in men and this increase is an important risk factor in the increased rates of violence, suicide and antisocial behaviour described above. The increase in addictions is partly due to the 'male role' in society with particularly alcohol seen as a socially acceptable coping mechanism for men.

Disorders presenting differently in women compared to men

Schizophrenia

Recently, it has become clear that schizophrenia occurs more often in men than women, and presents differently in men and women. In women, it starts later and typically has a less severe course. Women with schizophrenia tend to have more affective symptoms; have fewer and shorter hospitalizations; achieve a higher educational level; are more likely to be in a marital relationship and to be employed. Men have a greater vulnerability to negative symptoms. Women have a better treatment response. However, women are more prone to the side-effects of antipsychotic medication, in particular weight gain, hyperprolactinaemia and cardiac arrhythmias. They are possibly less likely to respond to treatment than men, if the disease is chronic. Women may be protected by the neuromodulatory effects of oestrogen on dopamine receptors in the brain.

Bipolar illness

This illness has an equal prevalence in men and women, but bipolar disorder tends to occur later in women than men. Women experience depressive episodes, mixed mania and rapid cycling more often than men, and more often have a seasonal pattern of mood disturbance. Bipolar II disorder, which is predominated by depressive episodes, appears to be more common in women than men (Arnold 2003).

Gender differences in treatment

For the most part, male sex is the reference point for treating psychiatric illness, thus treatment of women is often extrapolated from findings in men. However, there are physiological and psychosocial factors which should be taken into account during treatment. Physiological mechanisms showing gender differences include total blood volume, absolute percent body fat, gastric emptying, hepatic metabolism and renal clearance. These all tend towards increased blood levels of a drug after ingestion and decreased renal clearance in women compared with men. Psychosocial factors also influence treatment with men being less likely to present to services of their own volition than women and women who present being more likely to request talking therapies. However, women (especially those living in deprived areas) are more likely to be prescribed psychotropic medication than other groups.

Finally, sexual and physical abuse are commonplace in people with psychiatric disorders, with women being three times more likely than men to have experienced sexual abuse. Sexual abuse is particularly associated with low self-esteem, suicidal behaviour, borderline personality disorder, eating disorder, sexual dysfunction, somatization disorder and substance misuse. It is often underreported, yet the severity of the abuse is linked to greater psychopathology in later life. Women with severe mental illness are more at risk of sexual abuse than other groups over their life course and although there is no evidence of causality, sexual abuse worsens the outcome in these women.

Service provision

A 'one size fits all' model of mental health service provision can fail to meet the needs of all the different individuals who require mental health input. Women are major users of psychiatric services. Recent government directives encouraging single sex provision have had some impact on inpatient services; also, the Improving Access to Psychological Therapies (IAPTs) scheme may reduce hospital admissions. This is likely to benefit women as they are more likely to seek talking therapies. However, access to mental healthcare for men remains an issue. Public health campaigns, e.g. Time for Change, may help to reduce the stigma that prevents men presenting to services. Creative ways to engage men are needed, just as providing crèche facilities has improved women's access to health services. Men may, for example, be more likely to access a group in which the emphasis is on overall wellbeing rather than a specific discussion of mental health. If psychiatric services are able to target the different needs of different groups more effectively, the benefits will be felt in terms of parenting, family life, costs to the health service caused by repeated morbidity and indeed the recovery of working hours lost to psychiatric illness. The return to better functioning of a sizeable group can only be of advantage to society as a whole.

References

Arnold, L.M., 2003. Gender differences in bipolar disorder. Psychiatr. Clin. North Am. 26, 595–620.

Bisaga, K., Petkova, E., Cheng, J., et al., 2002. Menstrual functioning and psychopathology in a county-wide population of high school girls. J. Am. Acad. Child Adolesc. Psychiatry 41, 1197–1204.

Burt, V.K., Suri, R., Altshuler, L., et al., 2001. The use of psychotropic medications during breast-feeding. Am. J. Psychiatry 158, 1001–1009.

Cohen, L.S., Altshuler, L.L., Harlow, B.L., et al., 2006. Relapse of major depression during pregnancy in women who maintain or discontinue antidepressant treatment. J. Am. Med. Assoc. 295, 499–507.

Cooper, P.J., Murray, L., Wilson, A., et al., 2003. Controlled trial of the short- and long-term effect of psychological treatment of post-partum depression. I. Impact on maternal mood. Br. J. Psychiatry 182, 412–419.

Copeland, W., Shanahan, L., Miller, S., et al., 2010. Outcomes of early pubertal timing in young women: a prospective population-based study. Am. J. Psychiatry 167, 1218–1225.

Evans, J., Heron, J., Francomb, H., et al., 2001. Cohort study of depressed mood during pregnancy and after childbirth. Br. Med. J. 323, 257–260.

Frank, R., 1931. The hormonal causes of premenstrual tension. Arch. Neurol. Psychiatry 26, 1053.

Freeman, E.W., Sammel, M.D., Lin, H., et al., 2006. Associations of hormones and menopausal status with depressed mood in women with no history of depression. Arch. Gen. Psychiatry 63, 375–382.

Harris, B., Othman, S., Davies, J., et al., 1992. Association between postpartum thyroid

Nevertheless, the full extent of the problem of childhood sexual abuse only began to be acknowledged in the 1970s, largely as a result of feminist writers who drew attention to the frequency of childhood victimization. Researchers started to try to measure the extent of the problem. Finkelhor's (1979) study of college students revealed that one-fifth of females and one in 11 males had been sexually abused as children. This, and other similar studies, led to a gradual acceptance by healthcare professionals in the 1980s that childhood sexual abuse was an important and relevant problem. In contrast, in the 1990s there was a highly polarized debate, originating in the USA, about the status of memories of sexual abuse recovered as a consequence of therapy and the plausibility, or not, of the so-called false memory syndrome. There is little doubt that at least some of this has arisen as a consequence of over-zealous therapists, believing that repression of memories of childhood abuse lies at the root of much psychiatric morbidity and seeking to uncover it in therapy. Brandon et al (1998) review this debate and discuss implications for clinical practice. It would be a pity if these issues were to detract from the progress that has been made in the recognition and treatment of the effects of childhood sexual abuse, when for the majority of sufferers the problem is not a difficulty in remembering, but rather not being able to forget or shake off its impact, in all the many spheres described below. Childhood sexual abuse remains a highly emotive subject and one on which it can be hard to retain an appropriate perspective without falling into the trap of either over- or underemphasizing its significance.

Definition

There is no universal definition of child sexual abuse, although Schechter and Roberge's (1976) definition is widely accepted. This refers to the sexual exploitation of children as:

> The involvement of dependent, developmentally immature children and adolescents in sexual activities that they do not fully comprehend, are unable to give informed consent to, and that violate the social taboos of family roles.

This is a broad definition. The area can be further conceptualized according to the following description of the acts involved (after Sheldrick 1991):

- Exposure: the viewing of sexual acts, pornography and exhibitionism
- Molestation: fondling the genitals of the child or asking the child to touch the adult's genitals
- Sexual intercourse: vaginal, anal or oral intercourse, without use of excessive force
- Rape: strictly speaking, this is vaginal intercourse without consent, but other forms of intercourse may also involve the threat of violence or actual violence.

The term 'child sexual abuse' thus covers a wide range of experiences. In addition, it includes experiences with other children as well as with adults, ranging from strangers to close members of the family. The abuse may take the form of a single incident or, at the other extreme, consist of repeated, sadistic sexual assaults.

'Sadistic sexual abuse' involves the terrorization of children, and its aim is total domination of the child. It has much in common with acts of torture. Certain features may alert a clinician that sadistic abuse has been involved, including: descriptions of ritualistic punishments; abuse requiring hospitalization or surgical repair; and bizarre acts including bondage, the use of excreta or the use of confinement or sensory deprivation (Sinason 1994). Following the allegations of ritualistic abuse on the UK island Orkney in 1991, there remains controversy about the extent of so-called satanic abuse. In this form of abuse, children may be subject to sexual abuse as part of 'satanic' or 'black magic' ceremonies. To date, seven cases of ritualistic abuse have successfully been brought to prosecution in the UK.

Methodological difficulties

Since the early 1980s, the number of research studies being carried out has increased rapidly, so there is now a substantial amount of literature on the psychological sequelae of childhood sexual abuse. However, the quality of these studies is variable and there remain a number of methodological problems to be addressed. The most important of these are outlined below:

- **Lack of a universally accepted definition:** as a result of this, studies vary in the definitions they use. Some confine themselves to abuse involving physical contact only, while others use a much broader definition. In addition, a number of studies employ a measure of age discrepancy between perpetrator and victim. Where this is applied, an age difference of at least 5 years is usually required for an experience to count as abuse. Some research is limited solely to abuse within the family, while other research includes any unwanted sexual experiences. There is also a wide variation in the upper age limit applied to victims, ranging from 12 to 18 years. Because of the diverse definitions used, it is hard to make valid comparisons between many of the studies. Furthermore, the range of definitions used has led to a wide variation in estimates of incidence and prevalence (see below).

- **Retrospective nature of most studies:** the majority of studies that have been carried out are retrospective, cross-sectional and correlational, rather than longitudinal. Subjects of sex abuse research are often questioned simultaneously about abusive events in the past and their current level of psychological functioning. Childhood abuse reports are then treated as independent variables whereas psychological functioning is considered a dependent variable. However, cause and effect may not be so straightforward; for example, it is possible for current psychological distress to influence retrospective reports of abuse. Some subjects may not report abuse that they have experienced for a number of different reasons, including amnesia, distress, embarrassment and a desire to forget. If these subjects are then included in 'no abuse' comparison groups, the between-group differences will be obscured. It is also possible that some subjects will make false claims of abuse and there is no satisfactory way to ensure the validity of responses. There are a small number of prospective studies, e.g. Calam et al (1998), Noll et al

(2003) and Spataro et al (2004), which follow up verified cases such as those on social service registers. While this approach has the advantage of making use of externally validated cases, the results may not generalize to all instances of childhood sexual abuse because such a small proportion of cases (about 5%) are reported to the authorities. Such cases are also likely to be more severe in nature and in addition have lost the shroud of secrecy that encompasses most instances of abuse.

- **Nature of the population studied:** the subjects chosen for many studies include specific 'problem populations', for example, prostitutes, drug addicts and psychiatric patients. While these studies confirm a high prevalence of childhood sexual abuse in these particular populations, it is not clear what percentage of all sexually abused children go on to develop these problems. Many studies have been carried out on college students (e.g. Finkelhor 1979), but this is not a group representative of the general population in terms of intelligence and social class. The majority of studies have also been on Caucasian subjects, but at least one (Russell et al 1988) has suggested that African American incest victims report greater degrees of trauma than white victims. Most studies have only looked at effects on female victims. This means that there is a comparative lack of data on the long-term effects of childhood sexual abuse on men. King et al (2002), have published a study of the child and adult sexual molestation of men, in an attempt to redress the balance.

- **Confounding effects of other forms of abuse:** there has been a tendency for research in this area to examine sexual abuse in relative isolation, in spite of the fact that it frequently occurs in the context of physical and psychological abuse. If other forms of abuse are not taken into account, it is difficult to infer any specific causality to sexual abuse alone. Studies vary in the extent to which they examine other forms of abuse. Briere (1992) suggests that future research should encompass all three forms of abuse and use multivariate procedures in the analysis in order to try to overcome this problem.

- **Data collection methods:** there are many different methods used to elicit information about sexual abuse, including face-to-face or telephone interviews, symptom rating scales, case note studies and questionnaires. Childhood sexual abuse is a sensitive subject and, not surprisingly, the method used will influence the results obtained. Wyatt and Peters (1986) conclude, for example, that face-to-face interviews yield higher prevalence rates than self-administered questionnaires. It is generally accepted that female interviewers are most appropriate for both female and male victims. A validated, structured sexual trauma interview has been used in many general population studies (Russell 1983), but a number of other studies use measures of unknown reliability.

Prevalence

The variation in the definition of sexual abuse has led to wide discrepancies in prevalence rates, which range from less than 10% to over 30%. In addition, many studies focus only on women. The rates depend on whether an age difference between the individuals involved is taken as a defining factor, what the upper age limit is, whether encounters involving no physical contact are included and whether multiple or single episodes are considered. If the most rigorous definition of unwanted sexual assaults involving attempted or actual penetration is applied, then it is estimated that approximately 5–10% of children will have been sexually abused by the age of 16 (Fergusson & Mullen 1999). The majority of abusers of girls are male, but up to 20% of the abusers of boys may be female. Girls are most often abused by a family member and boys by someone outside their immediate family. The risk of abuse by a stepfather is almost five times the risk of abuse by a biological father. In an important study, Baker and Duncan (1985) interviewed a representative sample of 2000 British men and women. Twelve percent of the women and nearly 9% of the men reported having been sexually abused before the age of 16 years. Some 46% of the incidents involved physical contact and 5% consisted of full sexual intercourse. The authors estimate that there are 4.5 million adults in the UK who were sexually abused as children. Some 49% of the abusers were known to the child, and girls were at greater risk of incestuous abuse. Boys (44%) were more likely than girls (33%) to experience abuse by someone known to them but not related to them. A total of 63% had experienced one incident but 23% were abused repeatedly by one person, and 14% by a number of people. Girls were more likely than boys to experience revictimization. Some 54% of the sample reported a damaging effect on their lives. This study indicates that social class is not a factor in the risk of abuse, although some North American studies have found an association with lower social class.

Russell (1983) surveyed a community sample of 900 women in San Francisco and found much higher rates, with 28% having been sexually abused before the age of 14 years and 38% before the age of 18 years. Only 2% of the intrafamilial cases and 6% of the extrafamilial cases had been reported to the police. A total of 23% of the intrafamilial abuse was classified as very serious. The data suggest that where stepfathers abuse their stepdaughters, they are much more likely than any other relative to abuse at the most serious level: 47% of all abuse carried out by stepfathers was classified as very serious. In New Zealand, Anderson et al (1993) found, in a general population study of women, an overall prevalence of abuse before the age of 16 years of 32%. Nearly 20% reported unwanted contact with their genitalia and in 12% the abuse involved attempted or completed intercourse. Clearly, sexual abuse is a significant international problem. There may be many reasons for the variation in prevalence rates between countries, including methodological differences, but equally it is possible that sexual abuse is more common in some countries than in others.

There is generally less information available about the prevalence of sexual abuse of boys. Much of the attention paid to the problem of sexual abuse arose from the activity of the women's movement and many studies have focused only on women. Finkelhor (1984) reviews the literature on sexual abuse in boys and estimates that the prevalence rates for abusive experiences under the age of 13 or before puberty lie between 2.5% and 5%. A survey of over 2000 men in primary care in England (Coxell et al 1999) found a prevalence rate of 5%. In 81% of these the perpetrator was male and the mean age at the first episode was 11 years.

The consequences of childhood sexual abuse

The initial and short-term effects are reported in a number of studies which are reviewed by Browne and Finkelhor (1986). These include states of fear, anxiety, depression, anger and hostility as well as inappropriate sexual behaviour, somatic symptoms, truancy and delinquency (Box 25.1). Calam et al (1998) found that two-thirds of children in abuse cases undergoing investigation exhibited such symptoms. The short- and long-term effects of sexual abuse are not necessarily the same. Along with maturity comes a more complex understanding of what has taken place so that powerful emotions such as guilt and shame may take effect at a later stage. The debate about 'recovered memory' aside, clinical experience suggests that it is possible in some cases for memories of sexual abuse to be suppressed, only for them to re-emerge later in life in response to specific triggers.

More common is the phenomenon of so-called sleeper effects, which are silent during childhood but emerge with considerable impact in adulthood. This is particularly the case with sexual dysfunction but applies to other symptoms as well. There are no specific or unique adult outcomes of childhood sexual abuse and not all children subjected to it will go on to develop problems. It is estimated that about one-third of victims report no long-term adverse effects. Some features of sexual abuse are consistently associated with a poor outcome (Box 25.2).

Long-term effects

Emotional/psychological

The long-term consequences of childhood sexual abuse are not specific or unique. Rather, it has potential to give rise to a number of inter-related negative outcomes which can continue to have an effect throughout the lifespan. Mullen et al (1993) found that women who had experienced penetrative abuse were significantly more likely to suffer from eating disorders, anxiety, depression, suicidal behaviour and substance misuse than those

Box 25.2

Abuse characteristics that predict adverse outcome

- Abuse by father or stepfather
- Associated violence and/or threats
- Penetrative sexual acts
- Multiple abusers
- Bizarre abuse.

who had experienced other forms of abuse. The high rates of psychopathology were associated with psychiatric admission rates, between 5 and 16 times the rates in the non-abused control groups. Seriously abused women were more likely to come from families where emotional and/or physical abuse had also taken place. A prospective study of both men and women found that both sexes were significantly more likely to have received psychiatric treatment (Spataro et al 2004).

Depression, low self-esteem and suicidal behaviour

Depression is the most commonly reported symptom in women who have been sexually abused as children, and the association has been demonstrated in many studies (Bagley & Ramsay 1986; Hill et al 2001; Spataro et al 2004). Both childhood abuse and lack of parental care increase the risk of depression in later life. In a North London community sample, Bifulco et al (1991) found that 64% of women who had a history of childhood sexual abuse were clinically depressed at some point during their 2-year study, compared to 26% of those who had not been sexually abused. The highest rates of depression were seen in those who had experienced intercourse. Lack of parental care, separation from a parent and physical abuse all also had significant links with depression, and these appeared to interact additively. Only 5% of the sample had experienced sexual abuse in isolation from these factors. A wide range of depressive symptoms are reported by women who had been sexually abused, including feelings of guilt, inferiority, low self-esteem and impaired feelings of interrelatedness (Mullen et al 1993). A further study has

Box 25.1

Psychological effects of sexual abuse

Nature of trauma	Acute responses	Modifiers	Outcomes
Type of abuse	Fear	Family and peer support	Direct
Duration	Anxiety	Temperament	Feelings of guilt, shame, anger and hostility
Frequency	Depression	Attachment	Flashbacks
Relationship to abuser	Anger		Sleep disturbance
Use of force	Hostility		Sexual dysfunction
Age of onset	Sexualization		Dissociation
			Difficulty with close relationships
			Revictimization
			Becoming an abuser
			Indirect
			Depression and low self-esteem
			Anxiety
			Self-harm and suicidal behaviour
			Eating disorder
			Somatization
			Substance misuse
			Personality disorder, especially borderline states

examined the role of adult relationships in moderating the link between childhood abuse, neglect and depression. The authors found that the risk for depression associated with childhood sexual abuse was unaffected by the quality of intimate adult relationships, while the risk associated with poor parental care was substantially altered (Hill et al 2001).

Another study has attempted to unravel some of the complex interactions between self-esteem in adulthood and childhood adversity (Romans et al 1996). It was found that women who report childhood sexual abuse have a greater expectation that unpleasant things will happen to them and are less sure that they can affect their own destiny than other women. Banyard et al (2004) suggest that the experience of powerlessness in childhood sexual abuse can act as a long term stressor.

Many studies have found a link between past sexual abuse and self-harm (Browne & Finkelhor 1986). Rates of suicide attempts in women with a history of childhood sexual abuse have been found to be 2–3 times the rates in control groups (Green 1993). A large UK study on a non-clinical population found that the proportion of suicide attempts linked to having a history of childhood sexual abuse was 28% in women and 7% in men (Bebbington et al 2009). Mullen et al (1993) found very high levels of suicidal behaviour (70 times that in the control group) in a group of women who had been subjected to severe abuse, many of whom had been subjected to physical abuse as well. It may well be that where physical force has been involved in the abuse, victims are at much greater risk of self-harm than was previously thought. Most of the studies in this area have focused on the mental health consequences in women. It has been hypothesized that there may be differences between the sexes, with women more likely to internalize their feelings of anger, which are then expressed in self-destructive behaviours, whereas men are more likely to project their anger outwards (Hilton & Mezey 1996). However, the study by King et al (2002) found that men who reported childhood sexual abuse were 2.4 times more likely to report any type of psychological disturbance and 3.7 times more likely to have self harmed than those in the comparison group.

Anxiety, post-traumatic stress and dissociation

Anxiety, tension, insomnia and nightmares are all commonly reported by adults who suffered childhood sexual abuse (Bagley & Ramsay 1986; Browne & Finkelhor 1986). It appears that anxiety is most likely to be a consequence where force or threat of force has been used. Some authors regard these symptoms as manifestations of delayed or chronic post-traumatic stress disorder (PTSD). In some cases, symptoms of anxiety and intrusive memories of the trauma seem to be elicited by exposure to events that evoke memories of the original abuse (Lindberg & Distad 1985). Spataro et al (2004) found that both men and women were three times more likely than controls to have been diagnosed with an anxiety disorder. Women who have been sexually abused also report a higher incidence of dissociation experiences than do non-abused comparison groups. It has been hypothesized that dissociation, which has originally been used as a coping mechanism during abuse, later becomes a symptom in its own right (Briere & Runtz 1988).

Eating disorders and somatization

Mullen et al (1993) found a strong link between a history of childhood sexual abuse and both anorexia and bulimia (Ch. 18). It appears that about 30% of patients with eating disorders have experienced previous sexual abuse. There has been much recent debate about whether childhood sexual abuse is a specific risk factor for eating disorders, and in particular it has been suggested that this may be the case in bulimia nervosa. A community study found a rate of 26% for contact sexual abuse in subjects with bulimia. This rate was significantly higher than the rate in the control group but not significantly higher than figures for patients with other psychiatric diagnoses (Welch & Fairburn 1994). In a study comparing patients with bulimia and depression with controls, it was found that childhood sexual abuse appears to be a vulnerability factor for psychiatric disorder in general but not for eating disorder in particular. There was some evidence that eating-disordered patients who had been sexually abused were also more likely to have a history of taking overdoses and shoplifting (Vize & Cooper 1995). Another study has confirmed findings of increased co-morbidity in similar patients, including an increased risk of suicide attempts and substance abuse (Sullivan et al 1995).

Patients who suffer from somatization disorder have been shown to be more likely to have been sexually abused than a control group (Morrison 1989). An association has also been shown, in a number of studies, between childhood sexual abuse and gynaecological symptoms, especially unexplained chronic pelvic pain (Lampe et al 2003). Walker et al (1988) have shown that the rate of sexual abuse in sufferers of pelvic pain is twice that found in a general population survey. They also found that chronic pelvic pain was strongly associated with a lifetime history of depression. Pelvic pain may be a metaphorical way of describing chronic psychological pain and could also confer secondary gain, such as the avoidance of sexual contact. There is also an association with other forms of abdominal pain, in particular irritable bowel syndrome and functional constipation. A study of psychiatric patients over the age of 50 found that the impact of sexual abuse on illness burden was equivalent to adding 8 years of age, and for bodily pain and activities of daily living the effect was even higher, being comparable to adding 20 years of age (Talbot et al 2009).

Emotionally unstable/borderline personality disorder, multiple personality disorder and psychotic symptoms

The diagnosis of borderline personality disorder and its differentiation from other personality disorders is highly variable in clinical practice. The diagnosis of multiple personality disorder is even more controversial and it is one that is rarely made outside North America. It has been renamed dissociative identity disorder in DSM-IV. A number of studies have detected high rates of childhood sexual abuse in patients with borderline personality disorder. Figures range from 40% up to 80%. Rates of personality disorder diagnosis are raised in both men and women according to recent findings (Spataro et al 2004). Although the higher incidence of borderline personality disorder in women has been linked to increased incidence of childhood sexual abuse in girls (Herman et al 1989), certain features of borderline personality disorder, such as suicidal or self-harming

Factors that influence outcome

About one-third of adults who have been sexually abused as children consistently report no long-term effects. The impact of the abuse will vary according not only to the severity of the abuse but also to the phase of the child's development when it occurs, the resilience and temperament of the individual child and the nature of the family environment. The damaging effect of early abuse reflects not just the increased vulnerability of young children but also the fact that perpetrators of such abuse are generally more disturbed.

It has been hypothesized that individual differences in resilience and temperament may partly explain the variation in outcome. Binder et al (1996) have studied a group of women who were functioning well following experiences of childhood sexual abuse. While the severity of the abuse explained this to some extent, lower levels of symptomatology were also seen in women who had special talents or abilities and who had not felt responsible for the abuse. Having a supportive relative in the background had also helped a number of them.

The child's family environment is extremely important. In particular, a good relationship with the mother can protect a child from the more severe consequences of the abuse. Peters (1988) found that lack of maternal warmth was the strongest predictor of difficulties in adulthood. If a child discloses sexual abuse, the support of other family members is essential for a benign outcome. If the child is not supported but is disbelieved or blamed for breaking up the family, then an adverse outcome is much more likely. Only about 5% of children disclose their sexual abuse during childhood. Some only disclose as adults because they fear that a younger relative may be at risk from the same perpetrator. This latter situation can place clinicians in a difficult position with the issue of confidentiality, on the one hand, and the requirement to report to social services any child who is currently at significant risk of abuse, on the other. (See Crowe and Dare 1998, for a discussion of this predicament.)

Recently, attachment theory has been applied to the study of outcome. Many of the family dynamics associated with childhood sexual abuse, such as role reversal and rejection, are consistent with a model of insecure attachments. Alexander (1993) has studied the differential effects of abuse characteristics and attachment as predictors of the long-term effects of childhood sexual abuse. This work suggests that symptoms such as depression, distress, intrusive thoughts and avoidance are best predicted by characteristics of abuse severity. Personality functioning such as borderline and avoidant personality disorders appear to be better predicted by attachment measures. The weakness of this work is that it is retrospective in nature, and there is a real need for prospective studies in this area.

Factors outside the family may also be important in determining outcome. Russell et al (1988) showed that African American incest victims suffered from worse sequelae than white American victims. This was partly explained by their being subject to more severe abuse, but this did not account for all of the variance. The authors suggest that being raised as an African American female in a racist and sexist society may compound the effects of abuse.

Box 25.5

Factors placing a child at risk of sexual abuse (Finkelhor 1984)

- Having a stepfather
- Having lived without the mother
- Not being close to mother
- Mother never having finished secondary school
- Having a mother who is punitive about sexual matters (e.g. masturbation)
- No physical affection from mother
- Low family income
- Having two friends or fewer in childhood.

Children most at risk

Emotional and physical abuse and disorders of family interaction often precede and accompany child sexual abuse and exacerbate its effects. Growing up in a dysfunctional family increases the risk, not only of intrafamilial sexual abuse, but also of extrafamilial sexual abuse. Children who are neglected and unloved are more vulnerable to approaches from those with paedophilic intentions. Certain family characteristics are linked to an increased risk of child sexual abuse (Box 25.5).

Theories of childhood sex abuse effects

Post-traumatic stress disorder

Researchers in the area of child sexual abuse have noted that the constellation of symptoms described by many adult childhood abuse victims resembles the diagnostic criteria for PTSD (Herman 1994) (Ch. 16). In this model, psychological trauma occurs when human coping mechanisms are overwhelmed by a force in the face of which the individual is powerless. This leads to symptoms such as anxiety, sleep disorders, hypervigilance, intrusive memories or flashbacks and dissociative reactions. While many victims of childhood sexual abuse continue to describe such symptoms long after the abuse took place, this model is limited in that it does not take into account the wider interpersonal and social problems that many victims experience. In addition, it focuses on force and powerlessness as the main threat to the child, which is not always the case. In the more seductive forms of abuse, there may not be much force involved and the child may even enjoy some aspects of the attention at the time, only realizing later the significance of what happened to him or her. Guilt, shame and feelings of being responsible for the abuse are common consequences of childhood sexual abuse. It can damage a child's developing capacity for trust, intimacy, sexuality and self-esteem, and these are not readily accounted for in the PTSD model.

Box 25.6

Finkelhor and Browne's (1986) 'traumagenic' factors

Traumatic sexualization

This results from reinforcement of the child's sexual responses, such that the child learns to use sexual behaviour to gratify non-sexual needs. Gives rise to inappropriate and premature sexual activity, confused sexual identity, and aversion to sex and intimacy, as well as deviant patterns of sexual arousal.

Stigmatization

The child's sense of being damaged by and blamed for the abuse. This may be reinforced by the abuser, by peers or other family members. Leads to shame, guilt and low self-esteem.

Betrayal

The child's wellbeing is disregarded and the abuser exploits the child's trust and vulnerability. Leads to depression, mistrust, anger and fear of intimate relationships.

Powerlessness

The child is unable to protect him- or herself. Leads to anxiety, fear, perception of self as victim and identification with the aggressor.

Finkelhor's traumagenic factors

Finkelhor and Browne (1986) have proposed an alternative model of four traumagenic dynamics (Box 25.6). This model encompasses many features of PTSD but also goes beyond it and allows sexual abuse to be conceptualized as a situation or a process rather than an event.

Psychodynamics and attachment theory

Childhood sexual abuse often takes place in the context of emotional neglect and in some cases physical abuse as well, and tends to occur in families that are characterized by insecure and disorganized patterns of attachment. Within such environments, many features that are known to facilitate healthy psychological development may be lacking. The central focus of the psychodynamic view of early infant development is the attachment to the mother. This two-person stage of development involves the formation of 'affectional bonds' (Bowlby 1988). A nurturing and secure base is established from which the infant is able to explore both the inner and outer worlds. An infant needs to be helped to deal with separations and other painful and threatening experiences as well as with the powerful internal feelings that these give rise to. If the parent feels threatened by the infant's protests and is unable to help the infant to contain his or her feelings, then the infant has no model on which to base the regulation of his or her own affect. Instability of affect, an unstable sense of the self and a view of intimate relationships as threatening may all result. The importance of the early environment is borne out in research that indicates that an adverse outcome is much more likely where there is a disturbed relationship with the mother. In many families, childhood sexual abuse takes place as a result of a 'cycle of deprivation', in which one or both parents experienced some form of abuse as a child.

Following on from the two-person stage of development is the three-person or 'Oedipal' stage of development. A normal child is able to play with the 'fantasy' of marrying his or her opposite-sex parent and learns that this wish cannot be fulfilled in reality. However, in incest, the child actually takes the place of the mother or father. This rupture of the normal barrier between fantasy and reality is both traumatic and psychologically damaging. The child's ability to fantasize and deal with internal and external reality in a symbolic way is jeopardized. (See Garland 1991, for further discussion of this theory of trauma.)

Another important contribution of psychodynamic theory to the understanding of childhood sexual abuse is the concept of unconscious defence mechanisms. Powerful intrapsychic defence mechanisms may come into play in order to help the child to survive the trauma. These in turn can contribute to later psychopathology. If emotions are too painful to be borne, the victim may resort to using earlier, infantile defence mechanisms such as splitting, projection and denial. The split-off and denied experience is then not integrated with the rest of the victim's internal world. Other unconscious defence mechanisms that are often seen in sexually abused patients include: the compulsion to repeat the trauma; turning passive into active; somatization; and identification with the aggressor (Rosen 1996). All these can contribute to personality disorders and distorted object relations.

Therapeutic approaches

When taking a history from a patient, it is important that a history of childhood sexual abuse is inquired about in a sensitive way (see also Chs 37 and 38.) Many psychiatric patients who have been abused do not spontaneously give a history of sexual abuse and may not be aware of its relevance to their symptoms. Jacobson and Herald (1990) studied psychiatric inpatients and found that 44% of them had experienced serious sexual abuse which had not, until then, been disclosed to any of their therapists or doctors. Their study suggests that this important aspect of the history is often neglected. It is up to clinicians to routinely ask about sexual abuse in a manner that is not intrusive and which respects the patient's threshold for discussing aspects of the abuse further. Without awareness of the underlying trauma, sexually abused patients suffering from depression, substance abuse, eating disorders and so on, can come to be regarded as 'treatment-resistant patients'.

The selection of psychotherapy for patients who have experienced childhood sexual abuse must be guided above all by what the patient feels able to cope with. It is also important to assess what areas of healthy functioning the patient possesses and the degree of familial and social support he or she has access to. The therapeutic process can be disturbing and distressing for a patient who has been sexually abused, and it may well have an impact on his or her family as well. Some patients will need supportive therapy over a considerable period of time before being able to acknowledge their traumatized feelings. Many patients will prefer to see a female therapist.

The initial task in any of the therapeutic approaches described below is to develop a sense of trust between the patient and the therapist. If this is established, the patient may idealize the therapist as a longed-for, caring parent and may find separations such as the therapist's holidays difficult to cope with, necessitating additional arrangements at these times. Equally, the dynamic of abuser and abused will almost inevitably enter the therapeutic relationship at some stage and the therapist should be alert for this in the transference. It is important that the abuse itself is not focused on exclusively, as this may reinforce a patient's self-image as a victim. The whole person needs to be taken into account and, given the disturbed and deprived family backgrounds that often accompany sexual abuse, there are inevitably significant other dimensions to the therapy. Work with patients who have been severely sexually abused often needs to be long-term in nature. Where resources exist, the various modes of therapy can offer victims of childhood sexual abuse different therapeutic opportunities, and it is not uncommon for patients to move from one type of treatment to another, e.g. individual therapy may precede group treatments. However, brief psychotherapy can have a beneficial effect, as shown in a randomized trial of treatment for severe irritable bowel syndrome (Creed et al 2005). This study found that a reported history of abuse was associated with marked improvement following psychological treatment.

Cognitive and solution-focused therapy

This type of therapy aims to identify and modify the patient's cognitive distortions. Many victims of sexual abuse believe that they are bad themselves and were responsible for the abuse. An attributional style of self-blame is often combined with low self-esteem and feelings of powerlessness in intimate relationships. Distorted beliefs are challenged in the therapy with more accurate alternatives. Jehu (1988) gives a detailed account of cognitive therapy with childhood sexual abuse victims.

Psychodynamic therapy

This focuses on enabling patients to work through, or psychologically process, the complex mixture of feelings that inevitably arise from sexual abuse. The therapist needs to help patients to foster a more positive sense of self, while creating an environment in which the patient feels safe enough to disclose the most painful aspects of their experience. Initially a patient may fear that the therapist will not be able to bear hearing about the worst aspects of the abuse. These patients often need to explore feelings of intense anger, not only towards the abuser but also towards those who failed to protect them. There may be disturbing fantasies of revenge as well as shame and guilt. The patient will unconsciously transfer onto the therapist expectations of seduction, exploitation, abandonment or neglect. The therapist's focus on the patient's internal world may at times be felt to be intrusive and even abusive. As with all psychodynamic therapy, the working through of the transference forms the cornerstone of the work. (See Grant 1991, for a case study and discussion of long-term, individual psychotherapy with a childhood sexual abuse survivor.)

Couple therapy

The relationships of previously sexually abused men and women are often characterized by discord, overdependence, dissatisfaction and distress. It is not uncommon for sexual abuse to be disclosed in the context of a relationship problem or in the treatment of sexual difficulties. Sometimes a combination of couple therapy and individual therapy for the victim is required (Douglas et al 1989). Jehu (1988) gives an account of couple therapy and treatment for sexual dysfunction.

Family therapy

Family therapy is more often used in the treatment of children and their families, but it can have a place in the treatment of adolescents or adults within the family context. In particular, family therapy is useful for focusing on the role reversals and the loss of boundaries that tend to occur in abusive and dysfunctional families. The collusion of the non-abusing parent and the secondary gain achieved by scapegoating the victim will often need to be addressed. Bentovim et al (1988) give a full account of assessment and treatment using family therapy.

Group therapy

The treatment of childhood sex abuse survivors in therapeutic groups can be particularly effective at reducing the sense of isolation that many victims suffer from (Ch. 37). Discovering that others have also been abused can help patients to talk about experiences that they have not previously been able to share. A sense of trust develops such that feelings of hostility, shame and guilt can be worked through. In a group environment, the secrecy that has surrounded the abuse is inevitably challenged and this in itself can be therapeutic. Patients vary in their capacity to make use of groups and careful assessment of this is needed. Possible group treatments include long-term, analytic group therapy, either in a group of childhood sexual abuse survivors or in a heterogeneous group. A more informal setting may be provided by self-help groups in the community, who aim to offer support. Welldon (1998) gives an account of group therapy within a specialist forensic psychotherapy service. In this service, perpetrators and victims of incestuous sexual abuse (not previously known to each other) are treated together, in the same group. She argues that this is a powerful therapeutic milieu in which the intergenerational nature of the abuse can be addressed and in which perpetrators have to face the damage they have inflicted. She also highlights the careful assessment process required in considering treatments for both victims and perpetrators.

Conclusion

Psychotherapy is an important part of treatment for survivors of childhood sexual abuse but their other treatment needs should not be overlooked. Depression, eating disorders, substance abuse and other co-morbid psychiatric disorders will often require treatment in their own right. In this respect, the treatment of childhood sexual abuse victims is similar to that of other patients suffering from these disorders.

References

Alexander, P.C., 1993. The differential effects of abuse characteristics and attachment in the prediction of long-term effects of sexual abuse. J. Interpers. Violence 8, 346–362.

Anderson, J., Martin, J., Mullen, P., et al., 1993. Prevalence of childhood sexual abuse experiences in a community sample of women. J. Am. Acad. Child Adolesc. Psychiatry 32, 911–919.

Aristotle, 1976. Ethics (J.A. Thomson, Trans.). Penguin, London.

Bagley, C., Ramsay, R., 1986. Sexual abuse in childhood: psychosocial outcomes and implications for social work practice. J. Soc. Work Hum. Sex. 4, 33–47.

Bagley, C., Thurston, W.E., 1996. Understanding and preventing child sexual abuse, vol. 2. Arena, Aldershot.

Bagley, C., Young, L., 1995. Juvenile prostitution and child sexual abuse: a controlled study. In: Bagley, C. (Ed.), Child sexual abuse and mental health in adolescents and adults. Avebury, Aldershot, pp. 70–76.

Baker, A.W., Duncan, S.P., 1985. Child sexual abuse: a study of prevalence in Great Britain. Child Abuse Negl. 9, 457–467.

Banyard, V.L., Williams, L.M., Siegel, J.A., 2004. Childhood sexual abuse: a gender perspective on context and consequences. Child Maltreat. 9, 223–238.

Bebbington, P.E., Cooper, C., Minot, S., et al., 2009. Suicide attempts gender and sexual abuse: data from the 2000 British Psychiatric Morbidity Survey. Am. J. Psychiatry 166, 1135–1140.

Beitchman, J.H., Zucker, K.J., Hood, J.E., et al., 1992. A review of the long term effects of child sexual abuse. Child Abuse Negl. 16, 101–118.

Bentovim, A., Elton, A., Hildebrand, J. et al., (Eds.), 1988. Sexual abuse in the family: assessment and treatment. Wright, London.

Bifulco, A., Brown, G., Adler, Z., 1991. Early sexual abuse and clinical depression in adult life. Br. J. Psychiatry 159, 115–122.

Binder, R.L., McNiel, D.E., Goldstone, R.L., 1996. Is adaptive coping possible for adult survivors of childhood sexual abuse? Psychiatr. Serv. 47, 186–188.

Bowlby, J., 1988. A secure base: clinical applications of attachment theory. Routledge, London.

Brandon, S., Boakes, J., Glaser, D., et al., 1998. Recovered memories of childhood sexual abuse. Implications for clinical practice. Br. J. Psychiatry 172, 296–307.

Briere, J., 1992. Methodological issues in the study of sexual abuse effects. J. Consult. Clin. Psychol. 60, 196–203.

Briere, J., Runtz, M., 1988. Post sex abuse trauma. In: Wyatt, G., Powell, G. (Eds.), Lasting effects of child sexual abuse. Sage, Newbury Park, pp. 85–99.

Browne, A., Finkelhor, D., 1986. Initial and long-term effects: a review of the research. In: Finkelhor, D. (Ed.), A sourcebook on child

sexual abuse. Sage, Newbury Park, pp. 143–179.

Calam, R., Horne, L., Glasgow, D., et al., 1998. Psychological disturbance and child sexual abuse: a follow-up study. Child Abuse Negl. 22, 901–913.

Coid, J., Petruckevitch, A., Feder, G., et al., 2001. Relation between childhood sexual and physical abuse and risk of revictimisation in women: a cross-sectional survey. Lancet 358, 450–454.

Coxell, A., King, M., Mezey, G., et al., 1999. Lifetime prevalence, characteristics, and associated problems of non-consensual sex in men: cross sectional survey. Br. Med. J. 318, 846–850.

Creed, F., Guthrie, E., Ratcliffe, J., et al., 2005. Reported sexual abuse predicts impaired functioning but a good response to psychological treatments in patients with severe irritable bowel syndrome. Psychosom. Med. 67, 490–499.

Crowe, M., Dare, C., 1998. Survivors of childhood sexual abuse: approaches to therapy. Advances in Psychiatric Treatment 4, 96–100.

Dhaliwal, G.K., Gauzas, L., Antonowicz, D.H., et al., 1996. Adult male survivors of childhood sexual abuse; prevalence sexual abuse characteristics and long term effects. Clin. Psychol. Rev. 16, 619–639.

Douglas, A., Matson, I.C., Hunter, S., 1989. Sex therapy for women incestuously abused as children. Sex. Marital Ther. 4, 143–160.

Fergusson, D.M., Mullen, P.E., 1999. Childhood sexual abuse: an evidence based perspective. Sage, Thousand Oaks.

Figueroa, E., Silk, K.R., 1997. Biological implications of childhood sexual abuse in borderline personality disorder. J. Personal. Disord. 11, 71–92.

Finkelhor, D., 1979. Sexually victimized children. Free Press, New York.

Finkelhor, D., 1984. Child sex abuse: new theory and research. Free Press, New York.

Finkelhor, D., Browne, A., 1986. Initial and long term effects: a conceptual framework. In: Finkelhor, (Ed.), A sourcebook on child sexual abuse. Sage, Newbury Park, pp. 180–198.

Finkelhor, D., Russell, D., 1984. Women as perpetrators: review of the evidence. In: Finkelhor, D. (Ed.), Child sex abuse: new theory and research. Free Press, New York, pp. 171–187.

Freud, S., 1896. The aetiology of hysteria, standard edition, vol. 3. Hogarth, London.

Freud, S., 1905. Three essays on the theory of sexuality, standard edition, vol. 7. Hogarth, London.

Garland, C.B., 1991. External disasters and the internal world: an approach to psychotherapeutic understanding of survivors. In: Holmes, J. (Ed.), Textbook of psychotherapy in psychiatric practice. Churchill Livingstone, London, pp. 507–532.

Glasser, M., Kolvin, I., Campbell, et al., 2001. Cycle of child sexual abuse: links between being a victim and becoming a perpetrator. Br. J. Psychiatry 179, 482–494.

Goff, D.C., Brotman, A.W., Kindlon, D., et al., 1991. Self-reports of childhood abuse in chronically psychotic patients. Psychiatry Res. 37, 73–80.

Grant, S., 1991. Psychotherapy with people who have been sexually abused. In: Holmes, J. (Ed.), Textbook of psychotherapy in psychiatric practice. Churchill Livingstone, London, pp. 489–505.

Green, A.H., 1993. Child sexual abuse: immediate and long term effects and intervention. J. Am. Acad. Child Adolesc. Psychiatry 32, 890–902.

Greenfield, S.F., Strakowski, S.M., Tohen, M., et al., 1994. Child abuse in first episode psychosis. Br. J. Psychiatry 164, 831–834.

Herman, J.L., 1994. A new discovery. In: Herman, J.L. (Ed.), Trauma and recovery. Pandora, London, pp. 115–129.

Herman, J.L., Perry, J.C., van der Kolk, B.A., 1989. Childhood trauma in borderline personality disorder. Am. J. Psychiatry 146, 490–495.

Hill, J., Pickles, A., Burnside, E., et al., 2001. Child sexual abuse, poor parental care and adult depression: evidence for different mechanisms. Br. J. Psychiatry 179, 104–109.

Hilton, M.R., Mezey, G.C., 1996. Victims and perpetrators of child sexual abuse. Br. J. Psychiatry 169, 408–415.

Jacobson, M.D., Herald, C., 1990. The relevance of childhood sexual abuse to adult psychiatric inpatient care. Hosp. Community Psychiatry 41, 154–158.

Jehu, D., 1988. Beyond sexual abuse. Therapy with women who were childhood victims. Wiley, Bath.

King, M., Coxell, A., Mezey, G., 2002. Sexual molestation of males: association with psychological disturbance. Br. J. Psychiatry 181, 153–157.

Lampe, A., Doering, S., Rumpold, G., et al., 2003. Chronic pain syndromes and their relation to childhood abuse and stressful life events. J. Psychosom. Res. 54, 361–367.

Lindberg, F.H., Distad, L.J., 1985. Post-traumatic stress disorders in women who have experienced childhood incest. Child Abuse Negl. 9, 329–334.

Moncrieff, D.C., Drummond, B., Candy, K., et al., 1996. Sexual abuse in people with alcohol problems. A study of the prevalence of sexual abuse and its relationship to drinking behaviour. Br. J. Psychiatry 169, 355–360.

Morrison, J., 1989. Childhood sexual histories of women with somatization disorder. Am. J. Psychiatry 146, 239–241.

Mullen, P.E., Martin, J.L., Anderson, J.C., 1993. Childhood sexual abuse and mental health in adult life. Br. J. Psychiatry 163, 721–732.

Mullen, P.E., Martin, J.L., Anderson, J.C., et al., 1994. The effect of child sexual abuse on social, interpersonal and sexual function in adult life. Br. J. Psychiatry 165, 35–47.

A history of sexual disorders

- Havelock Ellis began a scientific enquiry into sexuality in 1910.
- Up until the 1940s, only psychoanalysts discussed sex as the central pivot in the neurotic conflict.
- Kinsey et al (1948, 1953) published two books leading to a wider appreciation of sexual relationships and their problems. But, due to non-random sampling, and the over-representation of American white, middle-class sex offenders and criminals in the sample, their studies are flawed. However, they remain a cornerstone of the literature and have been widely generalized to the population.
- Between 1940 and 1970, specific behavioural techniques were proposed for premature ejaculation (stop–start technique, Semans 1956), vaginismus and anorgasmia (self-stimulation, attributed to Hastings).
- In 1970, Masters and Johnson published *Human Sexual Inadequacy*, which became the template for the development of modern approaches to sexual therapy. It emphasizes the importance of the relationship as an integral part of the sexual problem, predicting outcome. Therapy targeted the 'marital unit' and behavioural techniques were superimposed. Masters and Johnson's published work has never been replicated in subsequent studies (Hawton 1986).
- AIDS/HIV infection was first described in 1981 and it has since transpired that it is associated with significant psychological morbidity, as are all chronic medical conditions (Jones et al 1994).
- In 1992, the British government made sexual health (and psychiatric wellbeing) a priority in the Health of the Nation strategy (DoH 1994). With the establishment of the Faculty of Family Planning and Reproductive Health Care of the Royal College of Obstetricians and Gynaecologists in 1993, they supported both closer links and liaison between family planning and genitourinary medicine with input from psychiatric and psychological services (RCOG 1993). The government proposed a module as part of higher specialist training, which expects trainees to acquire skills in reproductive medicine and the ability to recognize and refer patients with psychosexual problems. The expectations of

the Royal College of Psychiatrists are that training schemes give the opportunity to experience psychosexual and marital therapy. Some physicians are clearly concerned at the lack of expertise for such a large problem, and have suggested that genitourinary clinics are the obvious place to develop integrated services. Yet specialist clinics are not generalized or well-established within the National Health Service (NHS) in the UK and many individuals feel uncomfortable about discussing their sexual health needs with their general practitioners (GPs).
- In 1994, Johnson et al (1994) published a major survey of British sexual attitudes, the most comprehensive to date. For a summary, see Puri and Hall (1998).

The epidemiology of sexual disorders

The most common sexual problems reported are loss of sexual drive and erectile failure (which increases markedly with age: 0.8% at age 30; 6.7% at age 50; 55% at age 74), but less is known about the specific prevalence of other disorders. Premature ejaculation has been reported as occurring in at least 20% of married men, and anorgasmia during intercourse in 42% of women. Up to 38% of women report anxiety and inhibition during sexual activity and 16% complain of lack of pleasure (Rosen et al 1993). Although the dysfunction may be purely organic or psychological, it is usually a mixture of both (Crowe & Jones 1992).

The classification of sexual disorders

The general classification of sexual disorders

Kaplan (1974) and Hawton (1986) both arrived at the following distinctions, essentially growing out of the work of Masters and Johnson: sexual problems can be broadly divided into problems of motivation (sexual desire), problems of arousal (erection, lubrication and penetration) and problems of orgasm (Table 26.1).

Masters and Johnson found the subcategories of *primary vs secondary* and *total vs situational* useful in assessment. Primary

Table 26.1 Categories of sexual dysfunction

Aspect of sexuality affected	Women	Men
Interest	Impaired sexual interest	Impaired sexual interest
Arousal	Impaired sexual arousal or poor lubrication	Erectile dysfunction (impotence)
Orgasm	Orgasmic dysfunction	Premature ejaculation Delayed ejaculation Ejaculatory pain
Other types of dysfunction	Vaginismus Dyspareunia (pain during intercourse) Sexual phobias	Dyspareunia Sexual phobias

dysfunction is present since the first attempt at intercourse, and secondary follows a period of successful function, whereas total dysfunction is present under all circumstances, compared with situational, which appears only under certain circumstances.

Clearly in many cases, there are combinations of problems; e.g. a male partner may experience both impotence and impaired sexual interest, while premature ejaculation in a man may be associated with lack of interest on the partner's side. The other frequently quoted, but less helpful, classification is that of *functional vs organic*. Using the example of impotence caused in part by diabetic neuropathy, a man may experience *performance anxiety* leading to an expectation that he will fail to achieve an erection. Equally, where no specific physical cause can be found for impotence in an ageing male, there may be some, as yet, undiscovered physical change occurring; the frequency of this problem throws doubt on the *psychogenic* label.

There is a range of behaviours not yet discussed but which were described as far back as 1877 by Lasegue, who coined the term *l'exhibitionisme* (exhibitionism). Such behaviours are often linked with other similar behaviours, and the term *paraphilias* or *parasexual* has been assigned to them. Some have suggested that they be labelled *antisocial sexual behaviours*. The risk here is that we are approaching the interface with legal aspects of sexuality, and society's general misinterpretation of sexual orientation or preference and gender identity. The question of deviation often comes to light because of distress caused to others, such as partners or the general public, and public disorder offences, and only rarely by self-referral.

ICD-10 and DSM-IV classification of sexual disorders

Both ICD-10 (WHO 1992) and DSM-IV (APA 1994) provide operational systems for the diagnosis and classification of sexual disorders. The following disorders are recognized within a single section of ICD-10:

- Lack or loss of sexual desire
- Sexual aversion and lack of sexual enjoyment
- Failure of genital response
- Orgasmic dysfunction
- Premature ejaculation
- Non-organic vaginismus
- Non-organic dyspareunia
- Excessive sexual drive
- Other sexual dysfunction, not caused by organic disorder or disease
- Unspecified sexual dysfunction, not caused by organic disorder or disease.

In addition to the above sexual disorders, gender identity disorders, disorders of sexual preference (paraphilias), and psychological and behavioural disorders associated with sexual development (sexual maturation disorder, ego-dystonic sexual orientation, sexual relationship disorder and unspecified others) are recognized within other sections of ICD-10.

In contrast to ICD-10, DSM-IV includes all sexual disorders within one section entitled, 'Sexual and Gender Identity

Box 26.1

Normal sexual response cycle

- Desire
- Arousal, mediated by parasympathetic and central nervous system
- Plateau
- Orgasm, mediated by sympathetic and central nervous system
- Resolution, longer in men and increases with age.

Disorders'. Thus, the sexual dysfunctions as listed in ICD-10 are coupled with:

- Sexual dysfunction due to a general medical condition: characterized by a disturbance in the processes that characterizes the sexual response cycle (Box 26.1) or by pain associated with sexual intercourse
- Substance-induced sexual dysfunction: characterized by disturbance in sexual desire and in the psychophysiological changes that characterize the sexual response cycle and causes marked distress and interpersonal difficulty
- Paraphilias: characterized by recurrent, intense sexual urges, fantasies or behaviours that involve unusual objects, activities or situations and cause significant distress or impairment in social, occupational or other important areas of functioning. The paraphilias include:
  - **A.** Exhibitionism
  - **B.** Fetishism
  - **C.** Frotteurism
  - **D.** Paedophilia
  - **E.** Sexual masochism
  - **F.** Sexual sadism
  - **G.** Transvestic fetishism
  - **H.** Voyeurism
  - **I.** Paraphilia not otherwise specified (e.g. telephone scatology)
- Gender identity disorders: characterized by a strong and persistent cross-gender identification accompanied by persistent discomfort with one's biologically assigned sex
- Sexual disorder not otherwise specified: one's personal judgements must also take into account society's notions of deviance and concepts of gender role, with some (accepted) activities varying from culture to culture.

At the turn of the twenty-first century, reproductive endocrinologists and neuroanatomists began to question the whole psychological emphasis that had been placed on sexual disorders and dysfunction, suggesting through experimental work with rats, that there was a much greater role than previously thought for central and peripheral neurotransmitters at each stage of the sexual cycle. The advent of first-generation phosphodiesterase type 5 (PDE-5) inhibitors and the success of sildenafil in male erectile dysfunction has fuelled interest in pharmacological treatment of female sexual dysfunction. The emphasis has changed (much to the dismay of many sex therapists) from the psychosocial to the organic, with the possibility that these partially effective treatments might soon allow a greater organic understanding and therefore potential for pharmacological solutions.

Particular attention has been paid to the: (1) amygdala, periventricular nucleus of the hypothalamus and median preoptic area centrally and peripherally; (2) effects of dopamine, noradrenaline (norepinephrine) and acetylcholine; (3) vasoactive intestinal peptide responses mediated by parasympathetic fibres; (4) sympathetic and parasympathetic spinal cord chain and nuclei responses.

First, although psychological and physical factors interact in sexual dysfunction, the experimental evidence so far indicates that *female sexual arousal* is a neuromuscular and vasocongestive event controlled by parasympathetic and *inhibitory* sympathetic inputs. Autonomic preganglionic parasympathetic and inhibitory sympathetic fibres to the vagina and clitoris originate in the spinal cord in the sacral parasympathetic nucleus at the sacral level and in the dorsal grey commissure/intermediolateral cell column at the thoracolumbar level, respectively (see Ch. 2).

Parasympathetic fibres are conveyed by the pelvic nerve and sympathetic fibres by the hypogastric nerve and the paravertebral sympathetic chain. The activity of these spinal nuclei is controlled by descending projections from the brain and sensory afferents (conveyed in the pudendal, pelvic and vagus nerves) *from* the genitalia.

A key but unresolved issue concerns the neurotransmitters involved in the control of vaginal smooth muscle contractions. It appears that vasoactive intestinal peptide and nitric oxide may be responsible for the increase in vaginal blood flow during sexual arousal, whereas noradrenaline is inhibitory. Acetylcholine, previously thought to be crucial, now appears to play only a minor role compared to noradrenaline and acetylcholine in the regulation of vaginal blood flow.

Within the central nervous system, serotonergic projections from the brain to the spinal cord are inhibitory to the induction of genital arousal via a spinal reflex. Dopamine seems the most likely candidate (with as yet other unidentified transmitters) regulating the display of sexual behaviour. Anatomists and electrophysiologists point to a contribution from the paraventricular nucleus of the hypothalamus and the median preoptic area, respectively, as key elements in genital arousal. These recent animal models should assist in deciphering the neurochemical pathways controlling vaginal sexual arousal and the development of suitable pharmacological treatments for female sexual dysfunctions.

It should be noted that classification of female sexual dysfunction has been criticized, particularly where it has involved dependence on analogies of the male sexual response cycle, and the importance of age-related physiological transitions has been emphasized (Basson et al 2003; Aslan & Fynes 2008).

As an elaboration on DSM-IV and ICD-10, one paper in particular merits a re-examination of long-held beliefs relating to the physiology of erectile function and dysfunction (Sachs 2000), including the idea that there is a *singular physiology of erection*. Sachs claims that there appear to be pleural neural, neurochemical and endocrine mechanisms at work, on which erectile function depends. He argues for a behavioural context in which erection occurs founded on a context-dependent physiology researched using laboratory rats. The medial amygdala is essential for *non-contact* erection in response to inaccessible oestrous females, but not for erection during copulation. Even the specific dopamine receptors important to erection may differ, depending on context. It follows that if there is not a singular physiology of erectile dysfunction, the general physiology of erectile dysfunction may vary from context to context. Thus, some disorders of the central nervous system may not be manifested in sleep related erection and consequently labelled 'psychogenic' erectile dysfunction. Like Freud and later Francis Crick ('The Amazing Hypothesis'), this concept supports the axiom that all psychological processes have a somatic basis and therefore there can be no psychogenic dysfunction that does not involve organic processes, which may respond to drug treatment.

A revised classification is suggested for erectile dysfunction based on this idea and closer attention should be paid to male sexual arousal and its relationship to sexual motivation. Indeed the former term has so many meanings in the literature that it is impeding research into the physiology of sexual arousal, where so much depends upon comparisons between animals and humans. It is a logical progression of this research that attention should now be paid to two variables: whether or not erection occurs and whether the context is sexual. Currently, the occurrence of penile erection *within* a sexual context is viewed as the only case in which sexual arousal may be inferred unambiguously.

Sex therapy

There are three steps in the provision of sex therapy: referral, assessment and treatment.

Referral

The 'ticket' of entry to the GP can be a casual, incidental or disguised problem. Identification can be problematic, since with the time constraints of an average GP, once the patient's history has been taken and a physical examination performed, more time is needed for further listening, non-judgemental reassurance and possibly counselling. The neutrality of a GP is not felt by all attenders, but talking about a sexual problem can dispel fears and reduce anxiety. Simple behavioural techniques (stop–start for premature ejaculation or a sensate focus approach, see below) are rarely beyond most practitioners' abilities, yet their lack of basic training makes many feel disempowered to offer straightforward, sensible advice. Referral often ensues, despite the fact that primary care will remain the first point of contact for many patients and successful treatment can be effected in the community.

In Canada in 1985, Maurice (1985) called for sexual medicine to be advanced as a new medical subspecialty. The development to date has been fragmented and haphazard. Joint clinics providing collaborative academic and clinical integration is the probable way forward, attractive to both providers and purchasers alike. The training opportunities that should be available to all higher trainees will then be more widespread in availability. At present, joint multidisciplinary clinics are a rarity. To where a GP refers a patient will depend upon local relationships with providers of secondary care and knowledge of specialist services. At present, specialized services exist because of the dedication of a few consultant psychiatrists, urologists and gynaecologists, who frequently work without extra staff or resources. The family GP is often consulted for help and this trend will probably continue as Trusts squeeze this perceived patient luxury out of their service.

Note that the past decade (2000–2010) has seen a marked increase in the output and availability of online resources for medical practitioners. Awareness of the content of these and their role in the referral process is recommended, as is an awareness of the range of online materials (both responsible and irresponsible) which patients may have consulted before coming to a medical professional. A selection of important resources is included at the end of this chapter.

Assessment

The components of the assessment of patients and couples referred for sex therapy are as follows:

- Assessment: history from both partners, separately and together. Remember to ask about:
  a. Physical pathologies, especially diabetes, hypertension, neurological disorders (especially multiple sclerosis) and endocrine disorders (e.g. hypogonadism, hyperprolactinaemia)
  b. Sexually transmitted diseases, including HIV serostatus
  c. Alcohol and illicit drug use
  d. Prescribed medications and contraception if appropriate
  e. Physical disabilities
  f. Genital deformities
  g. Marital disharmony/relationship difficulties
  h. Stress or problems in other areas of the patient's lives, e.g. financial worries
  i. Psychiatric morbidity, especially anxiety and depression, psychoses
  j. Sexual preferences
  k. Social and cultural assumptions or expectations regarding sexual roles and behaviours.
- Physical examination: coupled with reassurance
- Education: explain simple functional anatomy and physiology to develop common ground for discussion. Allow free expression of language and identify areas of confusion
- Screening: routine haematological and biochemical screening, and proceed to hormonal studies if indicated.

Taking the history alone can take two or three sessions, and it is useful to send the patient/couple a self-assessment questionnaire prior to their initial visit. Patients sometimes find it easier to write down their problems and return them so that an appropriate member of the multidisciplinary team can do an initial assessment based on the answers received. It may be that what transpires at the interview is very different from what the patient(s) initially identified as the problem, in which case feedback and discussion can be very helpful in formulating a management plan, which may involve a number of health professionals.

Treatment

Sex therapy draws its treatment options from several areas of psychological and physical medicine. Techniques include:

- Counselling with or without behavioural programmes (e.g. Masters & Johnson 1970)
- Cognitive therapy (Beck et al 1979)
- Psychodynamic psychotherapy
- Systemic couple therapy (Crowe & Ridley 1990)
- Hypnosis (Fromm et al 1970)
- Drug treatments, e.g. sildenafil, yohimbine, anti-androgens and hormonal replacement
- A combination of psychodynamic and behavioural techniques (Kaplan 1974)
- Mechanical sex aids, e.g. vibrators, dilators and vacuum tumescence pumps with penile ring constriction
- Local drug treatments, e.g. intracavernosal injections of papaverine, phentolamine and prostaglandins (Virag 1982a)
- Vascular surgery for correction of a venous 'leak' and proximal vessel reconstruction for arteriosclerosis (usually unsuccessful because distal disease usually coexists) (Virag 1982b)
- Penile prosthetic implants (Loeffler 1960).

Practitioners vary considerably in the emphasis they place on physical, psychological and relationship factors in sex therapy. However, it is preferable, and the general consensus is moving in this direction, to treat sexual disorders as far as possible in the context of a relationship, married or unmarried, heterosexual or homosexual. Extremely sensitive individuals can be treated alone, at least initially, and if a patient has no partner, therapy along individual lines is still possible.

Whatever the outcome of the assessment, psychological factors are most likely to be responsible for sexual dysfunction unless a patient is clearly physically ill and a treatable organic cause is present. Psychological/behavioural techniques should generally be tried first, and only if these fail or the patient refuses to engage after persistent encouragement to do so, should pharmacological or surgical solutions be resorted to. Psychological/behavioural techniques, relationship issues and their impact on sexuality and mechanical and pharmacological treatments are now discussed.

Psychological/behavioural techniques

The Masters and Johnson (1970) *sensate focus approach* aims to reduce anxiety and improve non-verbal, tactile communication between partners. Essentially, it is a set of homework exercises designed to help couples become more comfortable with physical contact and closeness. Patients are encouraged to communicate using touching, although speaking is not forbidden. However, this is a graded approach to re-establishing a sexual dialogue, and initially breast and genital touching is not allowed; this has two purposes, it:

- Reduces anxiety
- Can liberate sexual urges.

Box 26.4

Categories of erectile impotence treatment

Intracavernosal injections

- α1-adrenoreceptor antagonists (phenoxybenzamine
- and phentolamine)
- Smooth muscle relaxants (papaverine)
- Prostaglandins.

Orally administered drugs

- Sildenafil citrate (Viagra)
- Second generation PDE-5 inhibitors–tadalafil (Cialis), vardenafil (Levitra)
- α2-adrenoreceptor antagonists (yohimbine).

Sex hormones

- Testosterone
- Luteinizing hormone-releasing hormone
- Bromocriptine.

Surgical

- Penile prostheses
- Vascular surgery.

Erectile dysfunction (failure of genital response)

Erectile dysfunction (ED) has multiple causes and accounts for around 50% of all men attending psychosexual clinics. Erection is a neurovascular phenomenon which can be interfered with at the conscious/unconscious interface with its cognitive accompaniments, e.g. negative self-image and depression. Fears and phobias, non-sexual stress, and the state of the patient's relationship can contribute to erectile dysfunction.

Normal erection is dependent upon an intact arterial supply and is mediated via the autonomic nervous system via S2, 3 and 4, and intact venous valves. Centrally mediated α2 effects have been noted by Wagner and Brindley (1980) using the α2 antagonist, idazoxan, which is similar to yohimbine, administered orally. It is known that there is an age-related increase in impotence that is in part a result of unknown physiological/anatomical changes occurring. The contribution of androgens is uncertain, but they do affect nocturnal erections via the limbic system. Two types of erection are known: *psychic* (mediated via thoracic sympathetic outflow) and *reflex* (mediated via sacral parasympathetic outflow). Clearly, anatomical defects may interfere with erections, but endocrine, neurological and vascular pathologies are the most prevalent and important causes of impotence:

- **Endocrine:** diabetes via arteriopathy and neuropathy; hypothalamic–pituitary dysfunction (hyperprolactinaemia – phenothiazines and alcohol); hypogonadism (reported in HIV infection); endorphins – naltrexone improves impotence in apparent 'psychogenic' impotence
- **Neurological:** peripheral and autonomic neuropathy, pelvic surgery/irradiation and multiple sclerosis

- **Vascular:** arteriopathy of pelvic vascular bed and proximal supply. Incompetent venous valves.

Management

Advanced investigations

The patient's history is elicited as previously mentioned. Investigations in addition to laboratory blood tests can include:

- Nocturnal penile tumescence: indicates the presence of nocturnal erections and may distinguish 'organic' from 'functional' causes. Total absence of early morning and nocturnal erections is strongly suggestive of an organic cause for the impotence
- Dynamic cavernometry: detects venous incompetence by infusing normal saline into the corpus cavernosum
- Penile-brachial penile pressure index: indicates local arterial disease to penis. Proceed to angiography if necessary
- Diagnostic intracavernosal injection of papaverine or phentolamine: indicates 'capacity' for erection (if successful, arterial disease less likely).

Management

Treatment options

Phosphodiesterase-5 inhibitors

A number of chemical pathways are implicated in the erectile response. The most important mechanism involves cyclic guanosine monophosphate (GMP), the formation of which is mediated by nitric oxide. Sildenafil inhibits phosphodiesterase (PDE), increases levels of cyclic guanosine monophosphate (GMP), and thus relaxes smooth muscle in the penis and effects erection. The drug acts through neural mechanisms to restore erectile function in response to sexual stimulation. It is not an aphrodisiac. The dose is 25–100 mg and it has been proven to be effective in patients with depression, diabetes, spinal cord injury, hypertension, and neural damage due to surgery. It is safe for use in patients over the age of 65, but is contraindicated with concomitant use of nitrates. It is fast-acting, with an efficacy window of 25 min to 4 h. The most common adverse events in clinical studies were headache, flushing and dyspepsia – these were usually transient and mild. Discontinuation due to adverse events was shown to be 2.5% in flexible-dose studies (compared with 2.3% on placebo).

The cascade of neurotransmitter and physiological events that leads to the production of the chemical messenger cyclic guanosine monophosphate (cGMP) causes the blood vessels in the penis to relax, thus increasing blood flow. The enzyme PDE-5 breaks down cGMP, reducing blood flow, which in turn reduces the erection. There are 11 isoforms of PDE, but in the penis the predominant isoform is number 5. The PDE-5 inhibitors reinforce the erectile process and help maintain erections. In addition to sildenafil and the newer tadalafil there is another compound not available in the UK, vardenafil. All three have a similar chemical structure with three to five benzene rings and various side chains of methane, hydrogen and oxygen. Tadalafil is a reversible, potent and efficacious inhibitor of PDE-5. Furthermore, tadalafil's 36 h duration of action (longer half-life) and faster onset coupled with its low side-effect profile compared with its competitors suggests that it has the edge over them. It is solely excreted by the liver, but alcohol and food have no influence over this drug's pharmacokinetics (see Ch. 39).

Some PDE inhibitors appear to be less effective in patients with diabetes mellitus types 1 and 2. Sildenafil potentiates the potency of organic nitrates and is associated with significant reductions in blood pressure; there have been case reports of both infarction and ischaemia associated with the use of sildenafil. The use of this drug in patients with pre-existing cardiac disease and those using organic phosphates is discouraged if not contraindicated. In randomized controlled trials with 80 healthy volunteers tadalafil produced no statistically significant differences in blood pressure or heart rate compared with placebo. The incidence of myocardial infarction and cardiac death was the same as placebo. Furthermore, tadalafil has been used safely in over 1300 men with stable cardiovascular conditions complicated by hypertension, diabetes mellitus and hyperlipidaemia.

All drugs have side-effects related to the distribution of the drug and the mode of action. PDE-5 is located in neurons and the gut, so the commonest side-effects are headache, back pain and dyspepsia, with nasal congestion, myalgia and flushing being less prominent. Yet only around 2.1% of patients in trials discontinued the drug because of these effects. As with most medication continued usage reduces side-effects over time.

Intracavernosal injections

Pharmacologically induced penile erection (PIPE) was pioneered by Wagner and Brindley (1980) using α1-adrenoreceptor blocking drugs. Virag (1982a) used the smooth muscle relaxant papaverine to similar effect. A combination of papaverine and phentolamine, or papaverine alone, can be injected into the base of the corpora cavernosa to produce an erection for intercourse. The dose is usually 120 mg, and the patient or his partner are taught to inject using a sterile technique. An optimal dose produces an erection for between 30 min and 2 h. Although early results showed an impressive response, it is not a treatment acceptable to all (Hollander & Diokno 1984), and is not without risk of priapism or penile fibrosis. Injections should not be used more than twice weekly. Erections that last longer than 6 h are potentially dangerous and can cause necrosis; the treatment is to withdraw around 60 ml of blood from the penis and inject phenylephrine 1–5 mg (an α-adrenergic agonist), which will allow the erection to subside. Patients must be advised of the risks and given written instructions about what to do if an emergency arises.

Yohimbine

This orally administered drug remains popular with many therapists. Having been available for more than 30 years, its use is on the increase. Being a derivative of the yohimbine tree, it has a mixed pharmacological identity, but the main component is an α2-adrenoreceptor antagonist with central neural effects, whose main therapeutic influence has been on the 'psychogenic' impotent male. Yohimbine has also been used to treat the anorgasmic male – 20–40 mg 45 min prior to applying an erotic stimulus (usually a vibrator), which increases the likelihood of orgasm.

Hormonal treatment

Testosterone plays a small part in the erectile mechanism, being more important for sexual interest and drive. However, lowered testosterone levels can produce impaired sexual interest and ejaculatory failure. Replacement using testosterone or bromocriptine can resolve this, but since testosterone is extensively metabolized by the liver, parenterally administered testosterone esters are preferred. Negative feedback mechanisms do unfortunately produce diminished effects after prolonged usage.

Luteinizing hormone releasing hormone is given to men with hypogonadism, and some women with postmenopausal atrophic vaginitis benefit from the rejuvenating effects of hormone replacement therapy.

Surgical treatments

Surgery does have a place in the treatment of erectile failure of organic origin and psychogenic impotence resistant to other forms of treatment. Loeffler (1960) first described the use of implanted surgical plastic splints into the penis. Since then, flexible/hinged and inflatable implants have been developed. Both types are inserted into the corpora cavernosa bilaterally, but this is a complicated procedure often complicated by technical failure, local infection and wound dehiscence and an unaesthetic outcome. Although they have a place in the treatment of impotence, counselling of both partners should precede the treatment, and in particular it should be made clear to the couple that the procedure is irreversible.

Revascularization of the larger arteries supplying the penile vascular bed affected by peripheral vascular disease is sometimes attempted, but the distal vessels are usually also affected and the results variable and short-lived. Surgical plugging of dysfunctional venous valves within the penis has been successful in some cases.

Future developments in treatment

The future of the treatment of sexual disorders lies partly with the psychosexual behavioural programmes, which remain the best option for female problems, premature ejaculation and motivational difficulties, coupled with pharmacological treatments for impotence unresponsive to first-line therapies. It should be noted that female sexual dysfunction is the subject of considerable discussion and research due to the complexity of the issues involved. Pharmacological treatments for both erectile dysfunction and female anorgasmia are likely to become increasingly available. The problem to date is the lack of dedicated centres offering a comprehensive service with an eclectic approach to assessment and treatment. With the extent of the problem now more widely acknowledged by various professionals and the public it must be hoped that trainees will gain greater exposure to departments that offer a valuable and rewarding resource.

References

APA, 1994. Diagnostic and statistical manual of mental disorders, fourth ed. American Psychiatric Association, Washington DC.

Aslan, E., Fynes, M., 2008. Female sexual dysfunction. Int. Urogynecol. J. 19, 293–305.

Bancroft, J., 1989. Human sexuality and its problems. Churchill Livingstone, Edinburgh.

Basson, R., Leiblum, S., Brotto, L., et al., 2003. Definitions of women's sexual dysfunction reconsidered: advocating expansion and revision. J. Psychosom. Obstet. Gynaecol. 24, 221–229.

Beck, A.T., Rush, A.J., Shaw, B.F., et al., 1979. Cognitive theory of depression. A treatment manual. Guilford, New York.

Crowe, M., Jones, M., 1992. Sex therapy: the successes, the failures, the future. Br. J. Hosp. Med. 48, 474–482.

Crowe, M., Ridley, J., 1986. The negotiated timetable: a new approach to marital conflicts involving male demands and female reluctance for sex. Sexual Marital Ther. 1, 157–173.

Crowe, M., Ridley, J., 1990. Therapy with couples. A behavioural-systems approach to marital and sexual problems. Blackwell Scientific, Oxford.

DoH, 1994. Health of the nation. HMSO, Department of Health, London.

Fromm, E., Oberlander, M.I., Gruenwald, D., 1970. Perceptual and cognitive process in different states of consciousness: the waking state and hypnosis. J. Project. Techn. Personal. Assess. 34, 375–387.

Hawton, K., 1986. Sex therapy: a practical guide. Oxford University Press, Oxford.

Hollander, J.B., Diokno, A.C., 1984. Successes with penile prostheses from patients' viewpoint. Urology 23, 141.

Johnson, A.M., Wadsworth, J., Wellings, K., et al., 1994. Sexual attitudes and lifestyles. Blackwell Scientific, Oxford.

Jones, M.B., Klimes, I., Catalan, J., 1994. Psychosexual problems in people with HIV infection: controlled study of gay men and men with haemophilia. AIDS Care 6, 587–593.

Kaplan, H., 1974. The new sex therapy. Brunner/Mazel, New York.

Kinsey, A.C., Pomeroy, W.B., Martin, C.F., 1948. Sexual behaviour in the human male. WB Saunders, Philadelphia.

Kinsey, A.C., Pomeroy, W.B., Martin, C.F., Gebhard, P.H., 1953. Sexual behaviour in the human female. WB Saunders, Philadelphia.

Loeffler, R.A., 1960. Perforated acrylic implant in the management of organic impotence. J. Urol. 97, 716.

Masters, W.H., Johnson, V.E., 1970. Human sexual inadequacy. Churchill, London.

Maurice, W.L., 1985. Sexual medicine. J. Canad. Med. Assoc. 132, 1123–1125.

Puri, B.K., Hall, A.D., 1998. Revision notes in psychiatry. Arnold, London.

Rosen, R.C., Taylor, J.F., Leiblum, S.R., et al., 1993. Prevalence of sexual dysfunction in women: results of a survey study of 329 women in an out-patient gynaecological clinic. J. Sex Marital Ther. 19, 171–188.

RCOG, 1993. Report of the RCOG Working Party on Structured Training. Chameleon Press for Royal College of Obstetricians and Gynaecologists, London.

Sachs, B.D., 2000. Contextual approaches to the physiology and classification of erectile function, erectile dysfunction, and sexual arousal. Neurosci. Behav. Rev. 24, 541–560.

Saunders, D., 1985. The woman book of love and sex. Sphere, London.

Saunders, D., 1987. The woman report on men. Sphere, London.

Semans, S., 1956. Premature ejaculation: a new approach. South. Med. J. 49, 3–8.

Virag, R., 1982a. Intracavernous injection of papaverine for erectile failure. Lancet ii, 938.

Virag, R., 1982b. Revascularisation of the penis. In: Bennet, A. (Ed.), Management of male impotence. Williams & Wilkins, Baltimore, pp. 219–233.

Wagner, G., Brindley, G.S., 1980. The effect of atropine and alpha blockers on human penile erection. In: Zorgniotti, A.W., Rossi, G. (Eds.), Vasculitic impotence. CC Thomas, Springfield, pp. 77–81.

Waldinger, M.D., Hengeveld, M.W., Zwinderman, A.H., 1994. Paroxetine: treatment of premature ejaculation – a double-blind, randomised, placebo controlled study. Am. J. Psychiatry 151, 1377–1379.

WHO, 1992. ICD-10 Classification of mental and behavioural disorders. World Health Organization, Geneva.

Online resources

www.library.nhs.uk/mentalHealth/SearchResults.aspx?catID=8617
NHS Evidence – Mental Health – Sexual Disorders subsection.

www.basrt.org.uk
British Association for Sexual and Relationship Therapy.

www.relate.org.uk/sex-therapy/index.html
Relate – Sex Therapy subsection.

www.rcpsych.ac.uk/training/curriculum2009.aspx
Royal College of Psychiatry Curricula.

Organic psychiatry and epilepsy

Pádraig Wright   Marina Zvartau-Hind

CHAPTER CONTENTS

calcium, iron, folic acid and vitamin B_{12} levels, serum tests for syphilis, HIV serology, plasma levels of therapeutic drugs and tests for illicit drugs. Further tests may be appropriate to rule out specific illnesses.

Electroencephalography

An electroencephalogram (EEG) is regarded as a routine investigation in patients with neuropsychiatric disorders. It is certainly indicated if epilepsy is suspected or to rule out organic causes for behavioural abnormalities. EEG is useful in ruling out non-convulsive status epilepticus, metabolic encephalopathies and prion diseases in patients with acute confusional states and dementia.

A standard EEG or sleep EEG may suffice, or an EEG with additional electrodes (in the foramen ovale, nasopharynx and intracranially, for example) or with activating procedures (hyperventilation, stroboscopic retinal stimulation and sleep), may be appropriate if there is high suspicion of epilepsy. A 24-hour EEG recording is also helpful in diagnosing epilepsy and in evaluating possible non-epileptic seizures (see below and Ch. 35).

Neuroimaging

The skull X-ray is occasionally useful but has largely been replaced by computed tomography (CT) and magnetic resonance imaging (MRI), which effectively visualize space-occupying brain lesions, infarcts and white matter lesions, show brain atrophy and allow for visualization of the ventricular system. CT is often used in emergency settings to rule out haemorrhage, skull fractures and space-occupying lesions. Magnetic resonance imaging (MRI) is used more commonly as it has higher resolution and allows for more effective visualization of brain structure and detection of abnormalities near the base of the skull. Enhancement of the images by infusion of contrast material demonstrates regions of blood–brain barrier breakdown, smaller size lesions and vascular structures that may not be seen on a non-enhanced scan. Positron emission tomography (PET), single photon emission computed tomography (SPECT), functional magnetic resonance imaging (fMRI) and magnetic resonance spectroscopy (MRS) are increasingly used in clinical practice (see Ch. 35).

Focal organic psychiatric syndromes

The psychiatric syndromes associated with lesions of specific cortical lobes will now be described (see also Ch. 2).

Lesions of the frontal lobe

The frontal lobe is conventionally divided into the motor cortex anterior to the central sulcus and the prefrontal cortex anterior to the motor cortex. Lesions in the motor area of the frontal cortex may cause Broca aphasia if the dominant hemisphere is involved and executive aprosodia (difficulty recognizing emotional content and expression of speech) if the non-dominant hemisphere is involved.

The prefrontal cortex represents approximately 30% of the total human cortex. Despite this, it has been called 'the silent

region, because even relatively large lesions may not produce significant neurological signs or cognitive impairment. In contrast, however, modest lesions may cause marked change in personality, cognition and behaviour. These are often so stereotyped that the term frontal lobe syndrome has been applied. The clinical features of the frontal lobe syndrome are given below.

Personality changes

Disinhibition with overfamiliarity, tactlessness, over-talkativeness and sometimes childish excitement. Lack of concern for the future and the consequences of actions. Lack of social and ethical control. Lack of judgement and insight. Irritability and aggression or indifference and apathy. Lack of motivation and initiative with slowing of thought and motor activity.

Cognitive dysfunction

Deficits in sequencing or temporal ordering of behaviour, with difficulties in problem-solving, planning and mental flexibility. Memory dysfunction with poor recall and recognition.

Behavioural changes

Three relatively distinct behavioural syndromes may occur, depending on the cortical region damaged, as follows:

- Dorsolateral prefrontal lesions: executive dysfunction, loss of initiative, slowing of thought and behaviour, perseveration, poor memory recall (as evidenced by poor verbal fluency) and changes in mood, especially depression (dysexecutive syndrome)
- Medial frontal lobe lesions: apathy, mutism and poor performance on tasks that require suppression of inappropriate responses (amotivational syndrome)
- Orbitofrontal lesions: disinhibition, impulsiveness, distractibility, loss of emotional and social control, lability and irritability.

These behavioural syndromes rarely occur in isolation in clinical practice, but because the dorsolateral prefrontal, medial frontal and orbitofrontal regions are components of specific frontal-subcortical-thalamic circuits (Cummings 1993), lesions (especially bilateral lesions) of the striatum may produce frontal lobe syndrome by disruption of such circuits.

Lesions of the temporal lobe

The major symptoms of temporal lobe damage are disorders of memory and language. It is important to realize that both of these functions depend on brain regions other than the temporal lobe, most notably the frontal lobe.

Disorders of memory (the amnestic syndrome)

The amnestic syndrome is present when organic memory impairment is out of proportion to other cognitive impairments. It is caused by bilateral damage to medial temporal lobe (hippocampus, amygdala and fornix) and certain mid-line structures (mammillary bodies and medial parts of thalamus). Major causes of the amnestic syndrome are as follows:

- Wernicke encephalopathy: the clinical picture is usually of acute onset of clouding of consciousness/delirium with nystagmus, external rectus paralysis, paralysis of conjugate gaze, ataxia and peripheral polyneuropathy
- Wernicke–Korsakoff syndrome: the delirium of Wernicke encephalopathy resolves and is followed by anterograde memory disturbance in the presence of intact short-term or working memory. A retrograde amnesia of a variable degree is also common, as is confabulation (Kopelman 1995). Wernicke–Korsakoff syndrome is caused by thiamine deficiency, which in turn is usually caused by malnutrition in chronic alcohol dependence (see Ch. 2) but may also be caused by malabsorption syndromes associated with carcinoma of the stomach or by hyperemesis gravidarum
- Head injuries (see below)
- Herpes simplex encephalitis (see below)
- Infarction in posterior cerebral arteries
- Hypoxia (see below).

Amnesia is also a feature of the Kluver–Bucy syndrome (hyperorality, over-attention to external stimuli, agnosia, hypersexuality and loss of fear) which is caused by bilateral damage to the medial temporal lobe as a result of tumour or infection, most commonly herpes simplex encephalitis.

Transient global amnesia consists of attacks of sudden global amnesia lasting several hours and followed by complete recovery. Patients are typically men in their middle years, attacks are sudden and there is usually no clouding of consciousness. Anterograde memory loss is profound but short-term memory remains intact. There is complete amnesia for the attack on recovery. The aetiology of transient global amnesia is unclear but transient ischaemic attacks, epilepsy and migraine have been implicated. The differential diagnosis includes dissociative disorders, hypoglycaemia and temporal lobe epilepsy (Hodges 1994).

Disorders of language

Technical terms used in describing disorders of language include:

- Aphasia or dysphasia (impaired ability to formulate and/or comprehend speech)
- Dysarthria (impaired ability to articulate words caused by inadequate control of the muscles necessary for speech)
- Mutism (failure to produce any speech or sounds)
- Alexia (loss of the ability to read)
- Agraphia (loss of the ability to write).

The structures subserving speech are largely located in the left hemisphere and include the anterior or Broca's area in the frontal lobe and the posterior or Wernicke's auditory association area in the posterio-superior temporal lobe. The most important aphasias may be differentiated on the basis of patients' abilities to comprehend speech (including reading and writing), speak fluently and repeat words or phrases as follows:

- Comprehension resides in Wernicke's area and lesions there produce sensory (or receptive or anterior) aphasia in which comprehension and the ability to repeat words is greatly impaired but speech is fluent albeit with paraphasias, jargon and neologisms.
- Lesions involving Broca's area produce expressive (or motor or posterior) aphasia in which comprehension is intact but speech is non-fluent or telegraphic and the ability to repeat words is impaired.
- Lesions involving the arcuate fasciculus which connects Wernicke's and Broca's areas produce conductive aphasias with intact comprehension and fluent speech but with a strikingly impaired ability to repeat words.
- Global aphasia, the most common and severe aphasia, is characterized by an almost complete absence of both speech and comprehension. It is usually caused by large lesions of both Wernicke's and Broca's areas, often following occlusion of the left internal carotid or middle cerebral artery, and almost always accompanied by a right hemiplegia.

Lesions of the parietal and occipital lobes

Lesions of the parietal and occipital lobes may cause a wide variety of symptoms including visuospatial difficulties, dyspraxias, agnosias, disturbances of body image and a specific syndrome, Gerstmann syndrome. These are described in detail in Chapter 2.

Lesions of the diencephalon and other brain regions

Lesions of the deep midline structures may cause disorders of memory and hypersomnia, while lesions involving the hypothalamus commonly cause hyperphagia (although anorexia nervosa has also been described). Tumours in this region can cause an obstructive hydrocephalus with diffuse cognitive impairment.

Lesions of the basal ganglia may be associated with a wide variety of psychiatric symptoms in addition to motor abnormalities. Bilateral lesions of the putamen and caudate, for example, can cause a syndrome identical to frontal lobe syndrome, symptoms identical to the negative symptoms of schizophrenia and obsessive–compulsive symptoms (Laplane et al 1989). Lesions of the basal ganglia can also produce an atypical aphasia, dysarthria and aprosodia.

Thalamic lesions may cause language disorders and executive dysfunction in addition to a disturbance in memory if the dorsomedial nuclei are involved.

Generalized organic psychiatric syndromes

Both acute and chronic organic psychiatric syndromes – delirium and dementia (which will be discussed separately below), respectively cause generalized neuropsychological deficits.

Delirium

Delirium is also called acute organic reaction, acute confusional state, acute brain syndrome, organic psychosis and ICU psychosis. Impairment of consciousness ranging from mild impairment in concentration and attention to deep coma, and typically worsening at night, is the universal feature of delirium but disturbances of perception, thinking and psychomotor behaviour are also common. Delirium has been defined as impaired consciousness with intrusive abnormalities of perception and affect (Lishman 1987), causes significant morbidity and mortality and is probably the commonest psychiatric syndrome. Delirium is common among older adults in acute care setting with prevalence estimates ranging from 10% to 60% (Rockwood & Lindesay 2002) and is associated with poor outcomes (McCusker et al 2002).

The following terms have been used to describe the various impairments of consciousness observed in patients with delirium:

- **Clouding of consciousness:** the mildest stage of impairment characterized by slight deterioration in thinking, attention, perception and memory
- **Drowsiness:** the patient falls asleep in the absence of sensory stimulation and exhibits slowness of action, slurred speech, reduced muscle tone and reduced reflexes
- **Stupor:** the patient is unconscious and responds only to noxious stimuli
- **Coma:** the patient is deeply unconscious and cannot be roused
- **Confusion:** an imprecise term usually referring to unclear and incoherent thought processes, its use is best avoided
- **Twilight state:** this term is used to describe an organic condition usually associated with epilepsy and characterized by abrupt onset/termination, variable duration and unexpected violent acts or emotional outbursts during otherwise apparently normal behaviour
- **Oneroid state (dream-like state):** the patient appears disorganized and confused and often experiences elaborate visual hallucinations. Oneroid states are not clearly differentiated from delirium and may be associated with dissociative disorders
- **Fugue state:** characterized by amnesia for personal knowledge, memories and personality. Fugue states are rare, are usually caused by acute stress, are transient (hours) and resolve fully. Very infrequently, a fugue state may persist and the sufferer may develop a new personality and travel extensively.

There are many causes of delirium (Box 27.2) but the clinical picture is remarkably similar in all cases (see Box 27.3 for ICD-10 diagnostic criteria). Patients exhibit clouding of consciousness, disturbances of memory (poor registration, retention and recall and amnesia for the duration of the delirium), distractibility, slowed thinking and impaired reasoning progressing to disorganization and fragmentation of thought and ultimately to incoherence. Illusions are frequent and vivid visual hallucinations are common (visual hallucinations indicate an organic lesion until proven otherwise). Delusions – often fleeting and

Box 27.2

Common causes of delirium (with or without focal lateralizing signs)

Cardiovascular disorders
- Myocardial infarction
- Pulmonary embolism
- Heart failure

Endocrine/metabolic disorders
- Diabetes
- Hypothyroidism
- Hyperthyroidism
- Electrolyte disturbances
- Hypoxia

Gastrointestinal disorders
- Hepatic failure
- Pancreatitis

Genitourinary disorders
- Renal failure
- Urinary tract infection

Infections and Intoxications
- Alcohol
- Prescribed and illicit drugs
- Carbon monoxide poisoning

Neurological disorders
- Intracranial bleeding
- Subdural haematoma
- Sepsis
- Head injury
- Meningitis
- Encephalitis
- Tumours
- Postconvulsive.

Box 27.3

The ICD-10 diagnostic criteria for delirium not induced by alcohol or other psychoactive substances

- Symptoms should be present from each of the following areas for a definite diagnosis:
  - Impairment of consciousness and attention
  - Global disturbance of cognition
  - Psychomotor disturbance
  - Emotional disturbances, e.g. depression, anxiety or fear, irritability, euphoria, apathy or wondering perplexity.

persecutory in content – are also common. Initial fear and anxiety is eventually replaced by apathy and indifference while arousal, agitation and hypervigilance are followed by listlessness and hypoactivity (fluctuation between hyperactivity and hypoactivity is frequent). Disorientation in time and in place is common. Apraxia, dysnomia and dysgraphia are common but are not specific to delirium and also occur in dementia.

The individual clinical picture is coloured by the patient's pre-morbid personality and the primary illness.

In patients who are admitted with delirium, mortality rates are 10–26% (McCusker et al 2002). Patients who develop delirium during hospitalization have a mortality rate of 22–76% (APA 1999). Early diagnosis and aggressive investigation is therefore essential in order to determine the primary cause and initiate appropriate treatment. Delirium associated with alcohol withdrawal is usually treated with vitamins (B) and reducing doses of benzodiazepines (although these should be used with caution, especially in elderly patients, because they may alter mental status) (see Ch. 16). Small doses of antipsychotics are also useful (although antipsychotics with anticholinergic properties are best avoided because they may worsen delirium). Even though case reports showed evidence that cholinesterase inhibitors may play a role in the management of delirium, larger trials and systematic review did not support this use (Overshott et al 2008). Delirium and its treatment have been reviewed by Meagher (2001).

The dementias

The diagnosis of dementia is clinical and requires the presence of acquired, persisting, usually progressive, global impairments of multiple higher cortical functions (especially memory and intellect) and of personality (emotional lability, socially inappropriate behaviour, impaired judgement and avolition) in clear consciousness. Functional impairment is a necessary prerequisite for the clinical diagnosis of dementia, which may be further supported by neuroimaging. While the clinical diagnosis of dementia depends on psychiatric, neuropsychological and neuroimaging evaluations, a precise neuropathological diagnosis can only be made postmortem. The traditional classification of dementia into presenile (onset before the age of 65 years) and senile (onset after that age), or cortical (Alzheimer, vascular, Lewy body, Pick, frontal lobe and alcoholic dementias and prion diseases) and subcortical (Parkinson disease, Huntington disease, progressive supranuclear palsy, dementia associated with the acquired immune deficiency syndrome, dementia associated with multiple lacunar infarcts and Binswanger disease) is referred to in this discussion, but is gradually falling into disuse.

Alzheimer disease

The clinical features, pathology and treatment of Alzheimer disease (AD) are described in Chapter 32. It is important for the psychiatrist to realize that AD is not a disorder of specific brain regions or of specific neurotransmitter systems. Thus, while senile plaques and neurofibrillary tangles are characteristically accompanied by loss of neurons in frontal and temporal cortex and of cholinergic neurons in the nucleus of Meynert and other basal nuclei, neuronal loss and neurotransmitter dysfunction occurs throughout the brain. Neurotransmitter abnormalities are thought to follow neuronal loss and may be summarized as follows:

- **Acetylcholine:** cholinergic neuronal loss occurs in the nucleus of Meynert, the largest cholinergic nucleus, and other basal nuclei. This is associated with reduced choline

acetyltransferase activity which correlates with both cognitive impairment and neuropathological findings. Treatments directed at improving cholinergic function may reduce cognitive impairment in some patients with AD (see Ch. 39). It is also worth noting that oestrogens modulate hippocampal choline acetyltransferase activity and that oestrogen replacement therapy delays the onset of AD. Thus women's increased vulnerability to Alzheimer disease may be attributable to postmenopausal hypo-oestrogenaemia.

- **Serotonin:** cortical and hippocampal concentrations of serotonin and its metabolites are reduced, as are the numbers of serotonin $5HT_2$ receptors.
- **Dopamine:** cortical and basal ganglia concentrations of dopamine are reduced, and the latter is probably responsible for the parkinsonism that patients with AD may experience.
- **Noradrenaline (norepinephrine):** cortical concentrations of dopamine hydroxylase and subsequently of noradrenaline (norepinephrine) are reduced.
- **Excitatory and inhibitory amino acids:** concentrations of the excitatory amino acid glutamate, and of its N-methyl-D-aspartate receptors, are reduced, as are cortical levels of inhibitory gamma-aminobutyric acid and glutamic acid decarboxylase.

Patients with AD almost always suffer from weight loss. It is unclear whether this is because they are unable to care for themselves and become malnourished, or because AD is a systemic disorder and not central nervous system-specific. It is also unclear whether incontinence is secondary to cognitive impairment or follows neuronal deterioration. Alzheimer disease is inevitably fatal and patients with it have a mortality rate several-fold greater than that of age-matched controls. Death occurs earlier in male patients and in those with a younger age of onset (Burns et al 1991) and is more frequently due to bronchopneumonia than any other cause.

Vascular dementia and Binswanger disease

The clinical features, pathology and treatment of vascular dementia are described in Chapter 32. Cerebrovascular disease is the second leading cause of dementia after AD. The incidence of dementia associated with acute stroke may be high, with 10–35% of patients developing dementia within 5 years following a hemispheric stroke. It is more common in men than women and hypertension is the most significant risk factor. The clinical course is often stepwise, with sudden cognitive decline and/or focal signs (primitive reflexes, dysphasias and amnesias, for example) and syndromes (e.g. Gerstmann syndrome) developing after cerebral infarcts or haemorrhages. Treatment directed at hypertension and at the prevention of cerebrovascular disease may slow the progress of vascular dementia. Vascular dementia is associated with a higher mortality rate than AD, the 5-year survival rate is 39% for patients with vascular dementia compared with 75% for age-matched controls (Brodaty et al 1993).

Binswanger disease causes subcortical dementia (see below) and is a severe form of subcortical cerebrovascular disease (sometimes referred to as progressive subcortical arteriosclerotic – or vascular – encephalopathy) with periventricular white

Disease Surveillance Unit (www.cjd.ed.ac.uk). Bearing in mind the typical presentation, psychiatrists should exercise a high degree of vigilance for new variant Creutzfeldt–Jakob disease.

Subcortical dementias

Subcortical dementias are said to differ from cortical dementias in that psychomotor retardation and depression are prominent, memory may be improved by effort, and apraxia, agnosia and aphasia are mild or absent. However, recent neuropathological investigations which reveal neuronal loss in subcortical regions in Alzheimer disease and in the cortex in Parkinson disease cast doubt upon the existence of subcortical dementia as a separate clinicopathological entity. The subcortical dementia associated with multiple lacunar infarcts has many symptoms in common with the subcortical dementias described below and will not be discussed further.

Parkinson disease

Parkinson disease affects at least 1% of people over the age of 70 years. The dominant symptoms of akinesia, tremor and rigidity are caused by neuronal loss in the substantia nigra and related brainstem nuclei, which in turn causes almost complete dopamine depletion in the striatum, nucleus accumbens, hippocampus and frontal cortex. Treatment is with dopaminergic and/or antimuscarinic/anticholinergic drugs (see Ch. 39).

Depression occurs in almost 50% of patients with Parkinson disease and psychotic symptoms secondary to dopaminergic medication are not uncommon. However, the relationship between dementia and Parkinson disease is unclear. Symptoms of dementia in patients with Parkinson disease, most of whom are elderly, may be caused by:

- Difficulties in undertaking cognitive evaluations in patients with bradykinesia and other motor symptoms
- Cognitive impairment associated with antiparkinsonian medications
- Cognitive impairment associated with normal ageing concurrent Alzheimer or other dementia.

However, even when all of these potential causes are controlled for, 20–40% of patients with Parkinson disease have an unexplained dementia which most often manifests late in the course of the illness (Biggins et al 1992). It is generally accepted that this is an intrinsic part of Parkinson disease, although reports of reduced choline acetyl-transferase activity and of cortical Lewy bodies in the brains of patients with Parkinson disease raise other possibilities.

Dementia in patients with Parkinson disease should be treated in the same manner as any other dementia but caution should be exercised when prescribing anticholinergic/antimuscarinic and dopaminergic medications, the former of which may impair cognition and both of which may cause confusion. The treatment of psychosis caused by dopaminergic medication presents clinicians with a problem – reducing the dosage of dopaminergic medication risks losing control of the Parkinson disease, while antipsychotic medication may cause extrapyramidal symptoms.

Huntington disease

Huntington disease, described by George Huntington in 1872, is now known to affect about 5 per 100 000 of the world population, males and females equally.

Aetiology:

Huntington disease is inherited in an autosomal dominant manner with complete penetrance. The Huntingtin gene on chromosome 4 at 4p16.3 normally encodes the protein Huntingtin. This gene includes a trinucleotide repeat of CAG which encodes glutamine. Expansion of this trinucleotide repeat beyond 35 encodes a mutated Huntington protein, which is toxic to specific neurons. The precise pathophysiology is not yet understood.

Pathology:

Huntington disease is characterized by marked neuronal loss and gliosis in the striatum, particularly the head of the caudate nucleus, and in the frontal lobes. This is accompanied by a reduced concentration of gamma aminobutyric acid in the striatum and an increased concentration of dopamine and somatostatin in other components of the basal ganglia.

Clinical aspects and outcome:

Onset is usually in the fifth decade of life but may be as early as 10 years of age. Clumsiness is usually the first symptom, followed by uncontrollable twitching of the face, shoulders and fingers. Patients often try to conceal these movements by pretending that they are voluntary, for example by scratching the head following an uncontrolled upward movement of the arm. Symptoms progress to generalized chorea with ataxia, dysarthria, difficulty in swallowing and, ultimately, gross writhing and seizures.

Personality changes predate the onset of chorea by several years in about 40% of patients and range from moodiness and irritability to violence and criminal behaviour. Depression is the commonest psychiatric disorder but affective and paranoid psychosis are not uncommon. A subcortical dementia, often characterized by a prolonged course with relative sparing of memory and insight, may precede the onset of chorea.

The diagnosis of Huntington disease depended on clinical evaluation, EEG and neuroimaging prior to the development of genetic testing. The EEG reveals low amplitude waves while CT and MRI show caudate, and perhaps frontal, atrophy. Reduced basal ganglia metabolism may be evident on functional neuroimaging prior to the onset of chorea.

The treatment of patients with Huntington disease is symptomatic. Thus, the dementia should be treated as with any other dementia, psychiatric disorder should be treated as appropriate and consideration should be given to treatment of chorea with antipsychotic medication. Planning for the long-term care of an increasingly dependent individual is extremely important. Death typically occurs 10–15 years after diagnosis. Patients with Huntington disease, and their relatives, have an increased risk of suicide.

Genetic testing for Huntington disease:

It is possible to confirm the diagnosis of Huntington disease in patients, to identify the gene in relatives of patients, and to undertake prenatal testing. Such testing is associated with significant ethical implications and should only be undertaken at appropriate centres and by experienced individuals.

Perhaps somewhat surprisingly, a Canadian study of almost 150 asymptomatic individuals found that testing enhanced psychological wellbeing, irrespective of whether results indicated the presence or absence of the gene for Huntington disease (Wiggins et al 1992).

Progressive supranuclear palsy

Progressive supranuclear palsy or Steele–Richardson syndrome is a subcortical dementia caused by neuronal loss and gliosis in the brainstem, cerebellum and basal ganglia and accumulation of neurofibrillary tangles. Onset is commonest in the sixth decade and the clinical features include paralysis of the extraocular muscles, postural instability, dysarthria, cervical and truncal dystonia and ataxia. There is no effective treatment.

Human immunodeficiency virus (HIV)-associated dementia

AIDS dementia complex (ADC) is a term that describes a unique constellation of HIV-related neuropsychiatric findings. The cumulative incidence of the disorder in patients with HIV is 25–38% and the prevalence is around 37% (McArthur 2004). Milder forms of ADC affect an additional 30–40% of patients. Its prevalence will increase as a consequence of increased life expectancy in patients who are HIV-positive or have developed acquired immunodeficiency syndrome (AIDS). HIV-associated dementia will therefore represent an increasing cause of personal morbidity and mortality and of public healthcare resource utilization in the future.

Neuropathology:

It is thought that HIV-infected peripheral macrophages carry the HIV virus into the brain where it damages neurons indirectly, disease onset and progression depending on:

- Viral properties (high levels of immunological nitric oxide synthase and of the gp41 protein are particularly associated with severe and/or rapidly progressive dementia)
- Host properties (extensive immune activation is associated with severe and/or rapidly progressive dementia)
- Concurrent non-HIV infection (cytomegalovirus and other infections are associated with severe and/or rapidly progressive dementia) (Adamson et al 1999).

Clinical features, treatment and outcome:

About 10% of all HIV-positive patients who develop AIDS present with dementia. The onset is generally insidious, but once established disease progression may be either rapid or modest, death occurring in weeks or years, respectively. Clinical features include cognitive impairment, psychomotor retardation, tremor, ataxia, dysarthria and incontinence. Death is usually caused by concurrent opportunistic infection and may be preceded by akinetic mutism and seizures. Mean survival from diagnosis of HIV-associated dementia is about 6 months (McGuire 1996).

The treatment of HIV-associated dementia is largely symptomatic. However, there is evidence that treatment with multiple antiretroviral agents is superior to either no treatment or monotherapy in patients with AIDS dementia complex. It is important to exclude reversible causes of dementia which in patients with AIDS will include concurrent infection and side-effects of anti-HIV and other treatments in addition to those discussed below.

Other dementias

Patients with a number of other relatively rare dementias may occasionally present to the psychiatrist. The causes of these dementias include the leucodystrophies, the commonest of which are metachromatic and adrenocortical leucodystrophy, and Gaucher and Kuf diseases.

Metachromatic leucodystrophy

The term leucodystrophy refers to abnormality of the cerebral white matter. Metachromatic leucodystrophy is an autosomal recessive disease that is caused by deficiency of aryl sulphatase A which results in deposition of sphingolipid in neurons and their demyelination (sphingolipid is also deposited in other cells). The activity of aryl sulphatase A may be measured in leukocytes. Infantile and adult forms occur, the latter characterized by psychiatric (personality change, behavioural disturbance, psychosis and dementia) and neurological (cerebellar and pyramidal symptoms, rigidity and seizures) symptoms. Treatment is largely symptomatic but gene therapy and bone marrow transplantation show promise.

Adrenocortical leucodystrophy

The precise pathophysiology of this X-linked disorder is unknown. Symptoms include personality change, dementia, pyramidal features, aphasia, apraxia, dysarthria and blindness. Subclinical or clinical adrenal insufficiency is invariably present. Hematopoietic stem cell transplantation in eligible patients is beneficial.

Gaucher disease

Gaucher disease (cerebroside lipoidosis or glucocerebrosidase deficiency) is an autosomal recessive, inborn error of metabolism in which glucocerebroside is deposited in the brain and reticuloendothelial system, and Gaucher cells are present in bone marrow. The infant form causes impaired neurodevelopment while the juvenile form is characterized by systemic manifestations (splenomegaly, hepatomegaly and erosion of limb and pelvic bones) with relative sparing of the brain. These latter features also occur in the adult form and may be accompanied by dementia, psychosis, behavioural disturbance, ataxia, anaemia and jaundice.

Gaucher disease may be treated by imiglucerase (enzyme replacement) or miglustat (glucosylceramide synthetase inhibition). Enzyme replacement improves hematological abnormalities, reduces hepatosplenomegaly and increases quality of life in a few months.

Kuf disease

Kuf disease is the juvenile or adult form of cerebral sphingolipidosis. Lipofuscin is deposited in the brain and causes dementia, ataxia and myoclonus.

Box 27.4

Causes of potentially reversible dementia

Psychiatric causes (pseudodementia)

- Depressive pseudodementia
- Schizophrenic pseudodementia
- Dissociative pseudodementia

Systemic causes

- Drug toxicity
- Electrolyte imbalance
- Infection (including concurrent infection in patients with AIDS)
- Hypoxia
- Poisoning
- Hypothyroidism
- Hypoglycaemia
- Vitamin deficiency
- Alcohol
- Renal failure and dialysis dementia
- Hepatic failure including Wilson disease

Intracranial causes

- Normal pressure hydrocephalus
- Subdural haematoma
- Tumours
- Neurosyphilis.

Potentially reversible dementias and pseudodementia

Dementia is potentially reversible in a small proportion of patients. Psychiatrists should be aware of the causes of such apparent dementias (Box 27.4) and should undertake suitable investigations and initiate appropriate treatment when applicable. Of the many causes of potentially reversible dementia, normal pressure hydrocephalus and pseudodementia are discussed further below.

Normal pressure hydrocephalus

Normal pressure or obstructive-communicating hydrocephalus is caused by obstruction within the subarachnoid space rather than within the ventricular system and is therefore potentially reversible. It may be associated with subarachnoid haemorrhage, Alzheimer disease, head injury, posterior fossa tumour or meningitis. The clinical features include dementia, psychomotor retardation, ataxic gait and urinary incontinence which, in contrast to Alzheimer disease, occurs early in the course of illness. Psychotic symptoms rarely occur. Neuroimaging reveals dilated ventricles with little or no evidence of cortical atrophy while cerebrospinal fluid (CSF) pressure is normal or low at lumbar puncture.

Treatment most commonly requires the insertion of a shunt between the lateral ventricles and the inferior vena cava and it is important to realize that this may effectively alleviate even severe degrees of dementia (Bekkelund et al 1999). However, even with a high level of suspicion, early detection and immediate treatment, outcome is uncertain and the dementia often progresses.

Pseudodementia

Pseudodementia may be defined as dementia diagnosed in patients who have psychiatric disorders that are associated with apparent cognitive decline. Depression in elderly patients is especially associated with such cognitive decline, but it may also be present in patients with schizophrenia or with dissociative disorders. A diagnosis of pseudodementia is suggested by the following findings:

- A family history of depression or schizophrenia
- A personal history of depression, schizophrenia or dissociative disorder
- Other depressive, schizophrenic or dissociative symptoms are present
- Depressive, schizophrenic or dissociative symptoms precede cognitive impairment
- Acute onset of cognitive impairment
- Retention of normal cognitive function in some domains (patients may be able to learn new information, for example)
- Cognitive impairment may be reversed by effort or by taking more time than is usual to complete a task
- Cognitive impairment may be reversed by treatment of the underlying depression, schizophrenia or dissociative disorder.

A trial of treatment – usually antidepressant medication or electroconvulsive therapy – is appropriate if there is any doubt about the diagnosis of dementia.

Specific movement disorders

The term specific movement disorders is used to signify a group of syndromes that primarily fall within the clinical practice of neurology, but which may either initially present with psychiatric symptoms, or which are frequently associated with significant psychiatric morbidity. These disorders, which must be considered in the psychiatric differential diagnosis, may be conveniently classified as eponymous and non-eponymous specific movement disorders (Parkinson and Huntington diseases have been described above).

Eponymous specific movement disorders

Friedreich ataxia

Friedreich ataxia is an inherited spinocerebellar degeneration caused by an expanded triplet repeat (Ch. 3). Sclerosis of the dorsal and lateral columns of the spinal cord causes clumsiness, nystagmus, ataxia, dysarthria, dysphagia, scoliosis, unusual swaying and irregular movements, paralysis of the muscles of the lower limbs and impaired proprioception. Disease onset is usually during adolescence. Many patients develop cardiomyopathy, arrhythmia and/or diabetes mellitus. Dementia does not occur but depression is common and a small proportion of patients have learning disability.

Sydenham chorea

Sydenham chorea is an autoimmune disorder of the basal ganglia that follows rheumatic fever. Psychiatric symptoms including irritability, obsessions, compulsions, tics and psychosis accompany the chorea in most patients. Penicillin prevents further attacks while valproate and antipsychotic drugs provide symptomatic treatment. There is some evidence that chorea gravidarum, some cases of obsessive–compulsive disorder and Tourette syndrome and possibly some cases of schizophrenia represent adult neuropsychiatric sequelae of Sydenham chorea.

PANDAS, or Pediatric Autoimmune Neuropsychiatric Disorders Associated with Streptococcal infections, is a diagnostic term used in children who have a rapid onset of obsessive–compulsive disorder and/or tic disorders, following group A streptococcal infections. An autoimmune pathology is proposed.

Gilles de la Tourette syndrome

The Gilles de la Tourette (1885) eponymous syndrome affects 1/2000 of the population and consists of multiple tics (rapidly repeated involuntary muscle movements such as grimacing or blinking) with onset before 16 years and which precede vocal tics, coprolalia, echolalia and echopraxia. Associated features include attention deficit hyperactivity disorder, learning difficulty and obsessive–compulsive disorder. In one study, generalized tics affecting the entire body were found in 64% of patients, coprolalia in 50%, obsessive–compulsive symptoms in 63%, and attention deficit hyperactivity disorder in 17% of patients (Kano et al 1998).

Concordance for Gilles de la Tourette syndrome in monozygotic twins is 53% (Pauls & Leckman 1988) and both the syndrome and its associated features are commoner in the first degree relatives of patients. The partial efficacy of dopamine receptor antagonists implicates dopaminergic dysfunction in this disorder, while Anderson et al (1992) have reported reduced serotonin levels in postmortem brain tissue. Treatment with haloperidol (or pimozide or clonidine less often) is effective in about 50% of patients.

Wilson disease

Wilson disease (hepatolenticular degeneration) is a rare, recessively inherited defect in a copper transporter protein which causes defective incorporation of copper into apo-caeruloplasmin and failure to excrete copper in bile. Copper is deposited in the liver (jaundice, cirrhosis, hepatosplenomegaly, ascites and oesophageal varices), basal ganglia (tremor, rigidity, athetosis and dystonia), cerebral cortex (personality change, behavioural disorder, psychosis with delusions and hallucinations, clouding of consciousness, epilepsy and dementia; bulbar symptoms may also occur) and eye (brown/green Kayser–Fleischer rings at the corneal edge). Up to 66% of patients first present to a psychiatrist, while 50% have psychiatric symptoms and receive treatment, including hospitalization, for schizophrenia, depression and anxiety before final diagnosis (Rathbun 1996).

Investigations reveal low serum caeruloplasmin and copper, and high urinary copper. Structural neuroimaging may show basal ganglia cavitation and cortical atrophy. Neurological features are more responsive than hepatic or psychiatric symptoms to treatment with chelating agents such as D-penicillamine.

Non-eponymous specific movement disorders

Benign essential tremor

Benign essential tremor is a fine to moderate, slowly progressive tremor affecting the hands, head and voice. This disorder is dominantly inherited in some patients, is exacerbated by movement or anxiety and alleviated by alcohol, and may be associated with social phobia (George & Lydiard 1994). Propranolol and primidone are effective treatments.

Focal dystonias

Focal dystonias consist of tonic spasm of localized (hence focal) muscle groups. The cause of these disorders is unknown (and patients may present to neurologists or psychiatrists) but they cause significant disability and include:

- Blepharospasm (tonic spasm of the orbicularis oculi muscles producing closure of the eye and preventing vision)
- Oromandibular dystonia (tonic spasm of the muscles around the mouth preventing speech)
- Spasmodic torticollis (tonic spasm of the sternocleidomastoid muscle producing flexion of the neck and rotating the head to the contralateral side)
- Writer's cramp (tonic spasm of the muscles of the hand and forearm such that a pen is held and applied to paper with excessive force, preventing writing).

Anxiety exacerbates these disorders and comorbid depression is common. Botulinum toxin injected into the affected orbicularis oculi provides prolonged relief from blepharospasm, while oromandibular dystonia may respond to anticholinergic/antimuscarinic drugs. Spasmodic torticollis generally resolves with time but nerve transection may occasionally be necessary. Writer's cramp may be relieved by altering the way a pen is held (pencil grips designed for children may be useful).

Epilepsy

Definition

Epilepsy may be defined simply as a tendency to suffer recurrent seizures or more comprehensively as a recurrent abnormality of the electrical activity of the brain, which causes changes in motor, sensory or autonomic function and/or in behaviour or consciousness. A practical clinical definition of epilepsy is of two or more seizures occurring within a year of each other.

Classification

Epilepsy may be classified by clinical description of the seizures (e.g. petit mal, grand mal, or tonic–clonic seizures) or by specification of the anatomical location of the epileptic focus

Interictal psychiatric illness

It was formerly believed that epilepsy was associated with a specific personality type described as pedantic, egocentric, religiose and 'socially adhesive', and patients with complex partial epilepsy have been described as dependent, circumstantial and excessively metaphysical (Tizard 1962). Recent research does not support these reports (Treiman 1993). The effects of the social, domestic, occupational and treatment implications of epilepsy on patients' lives and behaviour are clearly very significant.

Slater et al (1963) described a schizophreniform psychosis in patients with epilepsy, almost all of whom had temporal lobe complex partial epilepsy, which differed from schizophrenia as follows:

- The pre-morbid personality was usually normal
- There was usually no family history of schizophrenia
- There was preservation of affective response
- The psychosis began 10–15 years after the onset of the epilepsy.

Flor Henry (1969) found that this syndrome was commoner in temporal lobe complex partial epilepsy, especially when the focus was in the dominant hemisphere. Whether this psychosis and epilepsy have a common cause or the epileptic discharges cause the schizophreniform symptoms is unclear.

Neuroses and sexual dysfunction are commoner in patients with epilepsy and may be related to the disease and the limitations it imposes, and to the side-effects of AEDs. Depression, deliberate self-harm and suicide also occur more frequently than in the general population.

The episodic dyscontrol syndrome is a somewhat controversial clinical syndrome consisting of unprovoked and senseless violence, personality disorder and EEG abnormalities mapped to the temporal lobes. It may develop following head injury and carbamazepine may be an effective treatment.

The treatment of epilepsy

Medical treatment

The treatment of epilepsy is almost always symptomatic, but if a cause is apparent, for example a tumour, this should be removed. The goal of AED treatment should be monotherapy, and if a second or third AED provides control, the withdrawal of previously added AEDs should be considered. Barbiturates should be avoided in contemporary AED treatment.

A summary of the AED treatment of epilepsy is provided in Table 27.3. However, the treatment of epilepsy is advancing rapidly and the reader is referred to an appropriate source, for example the British National Formulary in the UK, for the most recent advice (see also Ch. 39).

The plasma levels of AEDs should be monitored (especially with combination therapy, because of the risk of AED–AED interactions such as valproate or phenytoin induction of enzymes that metabolize carbamazepine) but the 'rule' is that the patient, not the laboratory value, should be treated. Equally, the dosage should not be increased if it is effective, despite AED levels below the advised range. In addition to monitoring AED plasma levels, regular full blood counts and evaluations of thyroid, renal and hepatic function are advised with some AEDs (see Ch. 39).

AEDs induce the metabolism of ethinyloestradiol and a dosage of 50 µg is necessary if the contraceptive pill is prescribed. Women with epilepsy should plan their pregnancies and should consider withdrawing AEDs before conception and during pregnancy, although it is almost certainly safer to take AEDs than to have seizures while pregnant. If these occur, patients can be reassured that seizures that do not lead to cyanosis probably do not affect the fetus. Folate supplements are advised for women taking AEDs (and are now advised for all women) before and during pregnancy, and vitamin K supplements are advised for pregnant women taking carbamazepine or phenytoin.

Status epilepticus consists of recurrent seizures without recovery of consciousness between them. Treatment requires immediate intravenous lorazepam, diazepam, midazolam or clonazepam. This should be followed by an intravenous loading dose of phenytoin and a subsequent phenytoin infusion. Patients with status epilepticus should be transferred immediately to an intensive care unit.

Patients who have not had seizures for a prolonged period may wish to consider AED withdrawal. This must be an individualized decision based on:

- The length of time the patient has been seizure-free (a 2-year minimum is recommended)
- The normality of the EEG with current AED treatment (it would be unwise to withdraw treatment from a patient whose EEG exhibits significant epileptic activity)
- The side-effects of current AEDs

Table 27.3 A summary of the AED treatment of epilepsy

	First-line treatment	Second-line treatment
Generalized		
Tonic–clonic	Carbamazepine Lamotrigine Phenytoin Valproate[a]	Clobazam
Absence	Ethosuximide Valproate[a] Ethosuximide Acetazolamide	Clonazepam Clobazam
Partial (focal)		
	Carbamazepine[b] Lamotrigine[b] Phenytoin[b] Valproate[b] Tiagabine Topiramate Vigabatrin	Clonazepam[c] Clobazam[c] Acetazolamide[c] Gabapentin

[a]Valproate is also effective in patients who experience both tonic/clonic and absence seizures.

[b]If none of these AEDs are effective, two of them may be prescribed in combination.
[c]One or other of these AEDs may be added to the most effective monotherapy identified.

- Social factors such as the patient's work, hobbies and need for a driving licence.

If AEDs are to be withdrawn, a careful record of seizure type and frequency must be made and an EEG recorded before reducing dosage, again when dosage is reduced to half the initial dosage, and finally when AEDs are stopped. Any increase in seizure frequency or severity, or deterioration in the EEG, should lead to the planned withdrawal being reconsidered or abandoned or deferred.

Surgical treatment

The surgical treatment of epilepsy has advanced significantly in recent years and is directed at either removal of the cause of the epilepsy (for example a tumour or sclerotic temporal lobe) or prevention of seizure spread by tractotomy, callosotomy or sub-pial resection. Preoperatively, AED treatment must be optimized, the epileptic focus must be defined (scalp and depth EEG, CT and MRI) and the risk and/or extent of postoperative cognitive and/or motor impairment evaluated. Outcome is best in younger patients, but overall about 50% of patients become seizure-free (most continue to require AEDs). Mortality is less than 1% and morbidity between 5% and 20%, depending on the neurosurgical centre and the site of the lesion.

Legal aspects of epilepsy

All countries impose driving restrictions on people with epilepsy. In the UK, for example, a driving licence may only be obtained if a patient has had no seizures while awake during the previous year, or has had seizures only when asleep during the previous 3 years.

Aggressive behaviour is probably no more common in patients with epilepsy than in the general population and is usually related to peri-ictal confusion when it does occur. Violence due directly to epilepsy is extremely rare, and is characterized by being unprovoked, sudden, short-lived, undirected, purposeless, and associated with evidence of a seizure such as confusion and absence of recall (Gunn & Fenton 1971). UK law enshrines the concept of *mens rea* or guilty mind. The mind is said to be absent during ictal or peri-ictal automatisms, and thus *mens rea* is not possible. In law, automatisms may be sane and due to an external factor such as head injury, or insane and due to an internal factor such as epilepsy. In general, if found not guilty due to sane automatism, the accused goes free; if found not guilty due to insane automatism the accused is detained in a secure hospital (although judges now have discretion in sentencing). Epileptic automatism is only likely to succeed as a defence when:

- Epilepsy has been diagnosed prior to the offence
- There was no evidence of premeditation
- There was no attempt to conceal the crime or escape (which would imply awareness)
- The accused was objectively confused
- There is no evidence of recall of the offence.

Non-epileptic seizures

Non-epileptic seizures (NES) are also referred to as pseudoseizures, a term best avoided, and as non-epileptic attack disorder. NES is a dissociative disorder which may be defined as a tendency to suffer recurrent seizures which cannot be diagnosed as epilepsy and which occur in association with psychologically stressful events.

It is thought that deep psychological conflicts are responsible for NES but previous learning plays a role. NES is commoner in patients with personality disorder and among health professionals and the relatives of epileptic patients. A significant proportion of patients with NES also have epilepsy (Wada 1985) and research evidence suggests that many patients with NES have been abused during childhood (Betts 1990). Some of the features that help to differentiate between NES and epilepsy are listed in Table 27.4 and EEG telemetry is also helpful in making the diagnosis.

Table 27.4 Differences between epileptic and non-epileptic seizures (NES)

	NES	Epilepsy
Location	In safety, rarely in public	Anywhere
Seizure type	Asymmetrical, non-stereotyped, prolonged, frequent	Symmetrical, stereotyped, brief, infrequent
Consciousness	Normal	Impaired
Response to stimulus	Present, e.g. resists attempts to open eyes	Absent
Corneal reflex	Normal	May be absent
Plantar reflex	Normal	May be extensor
Injury	Rare	Frequent
Incontinence	Usually absent	May be present
Precipitant	Usually present	Usually absent
EEG/telemetry	Usually normal	Usually abnormal
Prolactin	Usually normal	May be elevated

Once diagnosed, behaviour therapy aimed at rewarding seizure-free periods and not rewarding seizures is effective in about 50% of patients. It is absolutely essential that this is accompanied by psychological support and instruction in appropriate functional behaviour (Betts 1998). Many patients with NES take AEDs because of comorbid epilepsy or through misdiagnosis. AEDs should be discontinued in the latter group, both because of their side-effects and because they may disinhibit the patient and promote NES. However, this is not always possible.

Sleep disorders (parasomnias)

Sleep is a recurrent behaviour consisting of inactivity and loss of awareness and of responsivity. Sleep differs from coma in that a sleeping individual either awakens spontaneously or can be roused. The physiology of sleep and the EEG changes associated with it are described in Chapter 35, while disorders associated with sleep (parasomnias) and their evaluation and treatment are discussed here.

Insomnia

Insomnia is subjective dissatisfaction with the quantity or quality of sleep. It is commoner with increasing age and may be primary or secondary. Primary insomnia requires training in sleep hygiene (avoid drinks and stimulants for up to 6 hours before retiring, retire at the same time each night to a comfortable bed in a warm dark room, remain in bed whether sleeping or not, set alarm for the same time each day and always get up at that time, avoid sleeping when not in bed) but a brief period of treatment with hypnotics may be appropriate (see Ch. 39 for further advice). Secondary insomnia usually resolves when the primary disorder, for example depression, is treated.

Nightmares and night terrors

Nightmares, unpleasant dreams that awaken the individual from rapid eye movement (REM) sleep, are very common during childhood but decrease in frequency thereafter. Night terrors are uncommon and familial, occur almost exclusively during childhood, and are unpleasant dreams occurring during non-REM (stages III and IV) sleep, which awaken the child. Although initially terrified, the child usually returns to sleep and has little subsequent recall of the episode. Training in sleep hygiene is helpful and night terrors almost always resolve with age.

Sleep walking, sleep paralysis and Kleine–Levin syndrome

Sleep walking (somnambulism) is a common familial disorder that occurs during non-REM (stages III and IV) sleep and is largely confined to childhood. More or less purposeful actions may be carried out but the patient has no recall of these when awakened. Sleep walkers may harm themselves and should be protected from stairs, windows, knives and machinery.

Sleep walking is an automatism and has been used as a defence against criminal prosecution.

Sleep paralysis affects approximately 10% of the population (Penn et al 1981) and causes patients to awaken while paralysed during REM sleep. Training in sleep hygiene is helpful.

The Kleine–Levin syndrome is rare and consists of periods of compulsive eating, clouded consciousness, visual or auditory hallucinations, and hypersomnia. These last up to 72 h and are accompanied by bursts of high-voltage δ-waves on the EEG.

Narcolepsy

The cardinal symptom of narcolepsy (the narcoleptic syndrome) is excessive daytime drowsiness with the sudden onset of REM sleep, often in unusual circumstances. This must be accompanied by either cataplexy (sudden atonia with resultant collapse, often triggered by an emotional event such as laughter) or frequent (several times per year) sleep paralysis. No consistent neuropathological features have been found. Narcolepsy is virtually always familial and 99.5% of patients have the HLA antigen DR2 (DR15/DQ6), making narcolepsy the disease that most strongly exhibits HLA association and implying a susceptibility gene on the short arm of chromosome 6. Hypnagogic and hypnopompic hallucinations occur in about 25% of narcoleptic patients. The hypersomnia of narcolepsy may be treated with mazindol, dexamphetamine or methylphenidate. Cataplexy responds to selective serotonin reuptake inhibitors, which have fewer side-effects than older treatments such as clomipramine or imipramine.

Sequelae of cerebral insults

The sequelae of cerebral insults may be minimal and short-lived or severe and permanent. Their extent depends on whether the insult is focal or generalized, as well as on its severity and duration. Focal and generalized cerebral insults will now be discussed.

Focal cerebral insult

Focal cerebral insults are the result of intracranial or pericranial pathologies affecting a specific region of the brain.

Head injury

Any trauma to the head that is associated with a skull fracture, loss of consciousness, amnesia and/or headache (as distinct from local pain from the injury) with vomiting constitutes a head injury (HI). About 3/100 population suffer HIs each year in developed countries and up to 30% of these HIs are moderate or severe (Powell 1994). At least 50% of all HIs are caused by road accidents in most countries, the remainder being caused by other accidents (30%), sporting injuries (10%) and assaults (10%). Young adults and elderly individuals are at greatest risk of HI and the risk for males is three times that for females.

Classification and pathophysiology

Open HI in which the skull is fractured and the brain injured directly is relatively rare and follows road and other accidents and blunt instrument or gunshot assaults. Closed HIs are commoner and follow similar events, which cause brain injury at the site of trauma (coup) and directly opposite it (contrecoup). The frontal, anterior temporal and occipital poles are more susceptible to contrecoup injury because the brain is more mobile in the anteroposterior than in the transverse plane. At a microscopic level, HI causes shearing of nerve fibres, nerve tracts and blood vessels.

General clinical features

Textbooks of neurology or neurosurgery should be consulted for details of the general effects of HI. However, it is important to remember that while HI has obvious direct effects such as skull fracture and loss of consciousness, these are exacerbated by associated events including the following:

- Alcohol and drugs, to which HI is very often related
- Raised intracranial pressure caused by bleeding and/or cerebral oedema
- Cardiovascular and/or metabolic imbalance following damage to vital centres
- Epileptic seizures
- Secondary infections
- Iatrogenic effects of treatment.

Psychiatric features

See Box 27.7 for the psychiatric sequelae of HI.

Whether or not psychiatric sequelae follow HI depends on pre-HI, peri-HI and post-HI factors as presented in Box 27.7.

Box 27.7

The psychiatric sequelae of HI: pre-, peri- and post-HI aetiological factors

Pre-HI factors

- Pre-morbid personality
- Personal history of psychiatric illness, especially alcohol dependence
- Family history of psychiatric illness

Peri-HI factors

- Site of brain injury (temporal lobe injury is especially likely to cause psychiatric sequelae)
- Extent of injury (risk of psychiatric sequelae increases as extent of brain injury increases)

Post-HI factors

- Development of epilepsy (psychiatric sequelae are commoner in patients who develop post-HI epilepsy)
- Emotional response to the HI, its cause and where responsibility lies (e.g. the emotional response to HI sustained in a road accident for which the patient was responsible may differ to that following a serious assault by a stranger)
- Marital, domestic, financial, social and occupational consequences of HI and its physical and psychiatric sequelae
- Medicolegal issues.

HI can cause almost any psychiatric disorder and many post-HI patients will suffer more than one disorder, the disabling effects of which are frequently additive. The commonest sequelae of HIs that are of interest to the psychiatrist are the following:

- Postconcussive syndrome
- Personality disorder
- Cognitive disorder
- Anxiety disorder
- Affective disorder
- Psychotic disorder
- Epilepsy.

Postconcussive syndrome:

This is the commonest psychiatric disorder following HI. Depending on the definitions used and population examined, approximately 50% of patients with minor head injury have symptoms of postconcussive syndrome at 1 month and 15% have symptoms at 1 year (Legome et al 2009). Its aetiology is much debated. An organic genesis with psychologically driven persistence was proposed by Lishman (1988) but more recently it has been suggested that psychosocial, cognitive-behavioural and coping factors may greatly influence post-concussional symptoms, especially during their late phase (Jacobson 1995). Such symptoms include headache, fatigue, dizziness, increased sensitivity to noise, sexual dysfunction, mild cognitive impairment, sleep disturbance and alterations in mood (irritability, anxiety and depression).

Postconcussive symptoms generally resolve following mild or moderate HI (although they frequently last many months and often require specific treatment such as antidepressant drugs, in which context it is worth noting that post-HI patients are especially sensitive to such medications) but persist indefinitely in up to 20% of patients following severe HI.

Personality disorder:

Postconcussive syndrome is the commonest psychiatric disorder following HI, but it is likely that personality disorder causes the greatest amount of distress to patients and their relatives following HI. Almost all patients who suffer severe HI, especially to the frontal lobes, will develop personality disorder, as will a considerable proportion of patients following less-severe HI. Two changes in personality have been described following HI (and there is some evidence that these may represent the release of previously controlled pre-morbid personality characteristics):

- Emotional blunting accompanied by avolition, apathy and indifference, which make rehabilitation extremely difficult
- Emotional irritability accompanied by impaired judgement, egocentric behaviour, rage, verbal and physical aggression and sexual disinhibition, all of which may predispose to criminal behaviour.

Post-HI personality disorder is frequently accompanied by post-HI cognitive disorder, which further compounds the difficulties experienced by patients and those caring for them.

Cognitive disorder:

Cognitive disorder develops in a very significant proportion of patients following HI. Risk increases with increasing post-traumatic amnesia (PTA) (almost all patients with PTA of 24 h or more

- Anxiety (especially concerns about further subarachnoid haemorrhages)
- Minor mood changes (including improvements in mood)
- Psychiatric syndromes associated with hydrocephalus and which may not manifest for months or years following the haemorrhage.

Intracranial haematoma

Relatively trivial HI (such as striking the head on overhead cupboards or when getting into a car) may cause acute intracranial haematomas, which are usually subdural in elderly and extradural in younger patients. Up to 50% of patients with intracranial haematoma are alcohol-dependent. Onset is insidious – often over several months – and clinical features include headache, cognitive impairment, dementia, hyperreflexia, extensor plantar reflexes, pupillary dilation and ptosis (indicating tentorial herniation of the temporal lobe, or coning), hemiparesis, clouding of consciousness and coma. Psychiatrists should maintain a high level of suspicion for intracranial haematoma in elderly and/or alcohol-dependent patients. CT is usually diagnostic and surgical evacuation gives excellent results in at least 50% of patients.

Infection

Most infections that cause significant fever may be associated with delirium, especially in very young or elderly patients. In addition, a considerable number of infectious diseases are associated with intracranial infection and cause illness ranging in severity from headache and anxiety through delirium to dementia and death. A list of the more common infectious processes that are associated with psychiatric symptoms is presented in Box 27.8 and they will be discussed below. The infections listed may exert their effect directly, indirectly via toxins or immunologically via the host's immune response to the infectious organism.

Encephalitis

Encephalitis, or inflammation of the brain, is generally thought to have a viral origin, although it is rarely possible to demonstrate the causative virus. Lyme disease is caused by a bacterium and the cause of encephalitis lethargica is unknown.

The neuropsychiatric features of encephalitis include headache, photophobia, impaired consciousness ranging from clouding to coma, focal neurological signs, seizures, postencephalitic amnesia and death. Symptoms may be subtle and the diagnosis of encephalitis should be considered in all patients with confusion or dementia. Investigations are often inconclusive apart from diffuse slow waves on the EEG, but protein and white cells may be increased in CSF, antibody titres may increase in blood and structural neuroimaging may reveal areas of necrosis.

The commonest causes of viral encephalitis are listed in Box 27.8. The following infections deserve mention:

- Herpes simplex is the commonest cause of clinically significant encephalitis in Europe and warrants aggressive investigation because antiviral medication may attenuate the effects of infection, which include psychiatric symptoms and postencephalitic amnesia.

Box 27.8

Infectious processes and their causative organisms associated with psychiatric symptoms

Encephalitis

- Viral encephalitis caused by herpes simplex, influenza, polio, mumps, measles (including subacute sclerosing panencephalitis), rubella, papovavirus (progressive multifocal leucoencephalopathy), rabies and several other viruses, many of which are transmitted by arthropods
- Bacterial encephalitis caused by *Borrelia burgdorferi* (Lyme disease)
- Encephalitis lethargica (von Economos encephalitis)

Meningitis

- Viral meningitis
- Bacterial including tubercular meningitis
- Fungal meningitis

Neurosyphilis

- Cerebral abscess
- Bacterial (including tubercular) abscess
- Fungal abscess
- Parasitic abscess

Malaria

Acquired immune deficiency syndrome

- Subacute sclerosing panencephalitis is caused by the measles virus, affects adolescents and is associated with myoclonus, epilepsy, dementia and death within a few years of diagnosis.
- JC papovavirus causes progressive multifocal leucoencephalopathy leading to paresis, aphasia, dementia and death in immunocompromised patients.
- Rabies is associated with an acute organic reaction, psychomotor arousal and seizures.
- Arthropod-borne viruses (especially *Ixodes* and *Culex* species) are responsible for several epidemic encephalitides, such as Russian endemic encephalitis, Semliki forest encephalitis and West Nile encephalitis.

First described in a patient from Lyme, Connecticut, USA, Lyme disease is an arthropod-borne infection caused by the spirochaete *Borrelia burgdorferi* that can lead to encephalitis, meningitis and radiculoneuritis. A small proportion of patients, especially those with CSF antibody to *B. burgdorferi*, develop fatigue, depression, amnesia and sleep disorders months or years after the primary infection (Kaplan et al 1999). Treatment is with doxycycline (erythromycin, amoxicillin or ceftriaxone are other alternatives).

Encephalitis lethargica (von Economos encephalitis) is an epidemic encephalitis that was reported from a number of countries during the early decades of the twentieth century. Patients experienced increasing lethargy and ophthalmoplegia initially, followed by parkinsonism, dystonia, oculogyric crisis, tics, personality change, schizophreniform psychosis and marked apathy.

Meningitis

Viral meningitis rarely causes significant psychiatric morbidity. Bacterial meningitis was once a common cause of neuropsychiatric sequelae but modern antibiotic therapy means that it is now rarely encountered. Tubercular meningitis usually involves the basal meninges and is relatively uncommon. Psychiatric features include irritability, apathy and personality disturbance. Tubercular meningitis is exceedingly difficult to diagnose because physical symptoms, including pyrexia, neck stiffness and impaired consciousness, appear late. A high level of suspiciousness should therefore be exercised when evaluating high-risk patients with psychiatric symptoms with a history of tuberculosis or who are immunocompromised by disease or treatment. Fungal meningitis is also increasingly common in this group of patients and is clinically similar to tubercular meningitis.

Neurosyphilis

Caused by the spirochaete *Treponema pallidum*, neurosyphilis is now rare in developed countries. However, it was once a major cause of neuropsychiatric illness and remains so in developing countries. About 50% of patients with neurosyphilis develop general paresis of the insane (GPI), while 25% develop tabes dorsalis and a further 25% develop meningovascular neurosyphilis. Cerebral gummata may also occur. The clinical presentation of patients with these syndromes will now be described.

Patients with GPI may present with classic grandiose delusions but depression, psychosis or dementia are more common. Untreated GPI is fatal. Antibiotic therapy prevents disease progression and allows recovery in about 10% of patients. Fleminger (1992) has provided the following useful mnemonic to assist recall of the clinical features of GPI:

P – Personality (irritability, impaired judgement)

A – Affect (depression, elation)

R – Reflexes (increased, extensor plantar reflex)

E – Eye (Argyll Robertson pupil, which reacts to accommodation but not to light)

S – Sensorium (clouding of consciousness, dementia, seizures)

I – Intellectual deterioration

S – Speech (aphasia) and sensory abnormalities.

Patients with tabes dorsalis present with pain, ataxia, Charcot's joints (painless, swollen, abnormally mobile joints damaged by excessive movement caused by loss of proprioception and sensation), tabetic facies, urinary incontinence and impotence.

Patients with meningovascular neurosyphilis present with headache, insomnia, lassitude, confusion and seizures, and with focal signs and symptoms (aphasia, monoplegia, hemiplegia, cranial nerve palsies and bulbar symptoms) caused by endarteritis (perivascular inflammation of the small intracranial vessels). Response to antibiotic therapy is excellent but relapse may occur.

If suspected, the diagnosis of syphilis should be pursued aggressively. Most psychiatric inpatients have serum tests for syphilis such as the Venereal Disease Research Laboratory (VDRL) and *T. pallidum* haemagglutination (TPHA) tests. The fluorescent treponemal antibody absorption (FTA-ABS) test is more specific and is useful to confirm the diagnosis and exclude false positive results. CSF tests for syphilis are positive in almost all patients with neurosyphilis.

Neurosyphilis is treated with intramuscular procaine penicillin (tetracycline, doxycycline or erythromycin if allergic to penicillin) for 10–21 days. The CSF must be examined regularly for at least 5 years. The psychiatric manifestations of neurosyphilis should be treated symptomatically.

Cerebral abscess

The signs and symptoms of cerebral abscess are those of a space-occupying lesion (see below). The onset is usually rapid (evidence of raised intracranial pressure, focal neurological signs and seizures), in which case diagnosis is relatively straightforward. Abscesses of insidious onset are more often confused with psychiatric disorders and the diagnosis should be considered in psychiatric patients with impaired consciousness and/or fever. Neurological signs may be absent or few and early neuroimaging is warranted. Bacteria derived from the middle ear, mastoid or nasal sinuses, systemic infection or head injury are the commonest cause, but tubercular and fungal abscesses may occur in immunocompromised patients. The treatment of cerebral abscess depends on the causative organism.

Malaria

Malaria caused by *Plasmodium falciparum* is a relatively common cause of neuropsychiatric disorder in malarious regions and may occur in travellers returning from such regions. Symptoms include headache, depression and fever, while drowsiness or an acute organic reaction may herald cerebral malaria, which may be fatal or have lasting neuropsychiatric sequelae such as personality change, depression and partial seizures (Varney et al 1997). Acute organic reactions are less common in patients with *P. vivax* malaria. Chronic malaria may be accompanied by headache, lethargy, anorexia, fatigue and depression. The diagnosis of malaria relies on demonstrating the parasite in a blood film. Treatment depends on the causative organism and requires expert advice because antimalarial-resistant parasites are increasingly common.

Acquired immune deficiency syndrome

HIV-associated dementia is discussed above. HIV-positive patients are frequently anxious or depressed and have an increased risk of suicide. These and other psychiatric symptoms may be caused by reaction to the diagnosis, infection of the brain by HIV or opportunistic pathogens, treatment with anti-HIV and other drugs, and tumours.

Cerebral tumours

Cerebral tumours cause symptoms common to all space-occupying brain lesions and consequent upon raised intracranial pressure (headache, apathy, emotional blunting, impaired cognition, altered consciousness and brain herniation syndromes) and focal effects (see above), the latter including seizures and depending on the site of the tumour. The absolute size of the tumour and its rate of growth also influence its clinical effects. Thus, a small, rapidly growing tumour such as an astrocytoma may cause dramatic symptoms while a slow-growing tumour such as a frontal meningioma may silently reach a very considerable size. A patient's pre-morbid personality is a further and important determinant of the psychiatric sequelae of cerebral tumours. Cerebral metastases cause symptoms and signs similar to those of primary tumours.

At least 50% of patients with cerebral tumours have psychiatric symptoms (Lishman 1987) and perhaps as many as one in every five patients with such tumours, especially if malignant, first present to a psychiatrist. Cerebral tumours are found in 4% of psychiatric patients at autopsy in comparison with 2% of the general population. Psychiatrists should therefore be alert to this diagnosis, especially in patients with atypical or treatment-refractory illness. The neuropsychiatric features of patients with cerebral tumours should be treated symptomatically and, if possible, the tumour should be treated specifically.

Generalized cerebral insult

While focal cerebral insults directly affect a specific region of the brain, generalized cerebral insults are the result of pathologies – often extracranial and also affecting the complete organism – that affect the whole brain.

Metabolic disorders

Almost all metabolic disorders can impair the function of the brain, especially if severe or long-lasting. The most important of these are now discussed.

Hypoxia

The effects of hypoxia depend on its severity, rate of onset and duration. Mild acute hypoxia is readily compensated for by increased respirations and pulse. Moderate acute hypoxia causes apprehension and restlessness (air hunger), followed by clouding of consciousness. Seizures, coma and death occur if it becomes severe or persists for too long. Patients who survive moderate or severe hypoxia may suffer chronic amnesia, temporal lobe epilepsy or dementia, caused by the sensitivity of the hippocampus and temporal lobe specifically, and the brain in general, to low levels of oxygen.

Mild to moderate chronic hypoxia is initially compensated for by increased respirations and pulse, increased haemoglobin concentration and reduced activity. Chronic hypoxia of increasing severity is initially associated with fatigue, impaired concentration and judgement, irritability and memory disturbance. Personality change and dementia occur if it increases in severity and/or persists.

Electrolyte imbalance

The neuropsychiatric effects of electrolyte imbalance depend on the ions involved, the severity of the disturbance and the underlying cause. Extreme imbalance may cause an acute organic reaction, seizures or coma, and may ultimately prove fatal. Less severe disturbances are associated with the following psychiatric presentations:

- **Acidosis:** clouding of consciousness gradually progressing to coma; papilloedema may be evident
- **Alkalosis:** clouding of consciousness, impaired memory, confusion and tetany (overbreathing in patients with anxiety may cause these features as well as perioral and peripheral paraesthesia)
- **Hypocalcaemia and hypercalcaemia:** discussed with parathyroid disorders (see below)
- **Hypokalaemia:** confusion, apathy and lethargy with a flaccid limb paralysis which may be mistaken for a conversion symptom
- **Hypomagnesaemia:** disorientation, depression, acute organic reaction and coma
- **Hyponatraemia:** irritability, apathy and clouding of consciousness progressing to coma.

Uraemia and renal dialysis

Uraemia rarely occurs in isolation, and electrolyte imbalance, the causative disease and its treatment will modify the clinical picture. The commonest psychiatric features of moderate uraemia include apathy, fatigue, impaired cognition and drowsiness, while uraemic encephalopathy classically fluctuates, is associated with impaired cognition and may progress to acute organic reaction, convulsions and coma (Burn & Bates 1998). Chronic uraemia is associated with depression which responds to antidepressant therapy.

End-stage renal failure and renal dialysis impose great demands on patients (reduced energy and work capacity, impaired concentration, psychosexual difficulties, side-effects of dialysis and immunosuppressive or other treatments, and fear of organ rejection or death), their relatives (anxiety, financial and marital problems) and renal unit personnel. Because of this, it is increasingly common for a liaison psychiatrist to work with patients, their relatives and personnel in renal units. Quality of life for patients depends on treatment – transplant patients fare better than patients treated with continuous ambulatory peritoneal dialysis who in turn fare better than haemodialysis patients.

Patients undergoing haemodialysis commonly experience anxiety, lethargy, depression and psychosexual difficulties and may experience psychiatric symptoms consequent upon uraemia and electrolyte imbalance (see above). Two specific neuropsychiatric syndromes have also been described:

- **Dialysis dementia:** progressive dementia and seizures probably caused by the accumulation of aluminium from perfusion fluids in the brain. This has become uncommon since the introduction of aluminium-free dialysates.
- **Dialysis disequilibrium:** confusion, acute organic reaction, seizures or coma probably caused by cerebral oedema following excessively rapid haemodialysis.

Hepatic failure

A fluctuating chronic organic state has been described in which psychiatric (drowsiness, confusion, personality change, visual hallucinations, mania and delirium) and physical (motor retardation, flapping tremor of hands, grimacing, ataxia, hyperreflexia, clonus and coma) symptoms wax and wane in unison. This disorder improves with a low-protein diet.

Neuropsychological findings in patients with cirrhosis include selective deficits in attention and fine motor skills with preservation of general intellect, memory, language and visuospatial perception, suggesting a subcortical – possibly basal ganglia – pathophysiology (McCrea et al 1996).

Polydipsia

Polydipsia may be caused by diabetes insipidus or be associated with schizophrenia or another psychiatric disorder, or its treatment. Diabetes insipidus may be cranial (reduced secretion of antidiuretic hormone or ADH) or nephrogenic (renal insensitivity to ADH, which may be caused by lithium carbonate). Psychogenic polydipsia causes polyuria, which may lead to hyponatraemia (see above). Polydipsia occurs in at least 10% of institutionalized psychiatric patients and may respond to atypical antipsychotics or behaviour therapy (Buckley 1998, Tohen & Grundy 1998).

Porphyria

Three of the six porphyrias may cause psychiatric symptoms. The commonest, acute intermittent porphyria (AIP), may be precipitated by alcohol, drugs (combined oral contraceptives, barbiturates, sulphonamides, methyldopa and griseofulvin), infection or fasting, and may cause anxiety, irritability, confusion, severe depression, a paranoid psychosis with hallucinations and an acute organic reaction and coma. The 'madness' of King George III has been attributed to AIP. Variegate porphyria and coproporphyria are rare causes of psychiatric symptoms.

Carcinoma (non-metastatic psychiatric effects)

The effects of primary and metastatic cerebral tumours have been described above. Cancers, especially bronchogenic carcinoma, may also cause non-metastatic neuropsychiatric syndromes, the psychiatric symptoms of which include anxiety, depression, acute organic reactions, schizophrenia and dementia (limbic encephalopathy). Three may occur independently of neurological symptoms. Furthermore, psychiatric symptoms may precede physical symptoms in pancreatic (McGee et al 1994) and perhaps other cancers. Occult cancer is thus a differential diagnosis in patients with treatment-resistant psychiatric illness or dementia. Hormone secretion by tumours may be responsible for these syndromes and many patients have cortical neuronal loss and gliosis.

Carcinoid syndrome

Carcinoid syndrome is caused by metastatic tumours that secrete vasoactive substances such as serotonin and histamine. The majority of patients with this syndrome experience psychiatric symptoms including anxiety, depression, insomnia and confusion.

Vitamin deficiencies

The psychiatric sequelae of vitamin deficiency have been described in prisoners of war, in individuals from developing countries where famine occurs and in those who are elderly, alcoholic, mentally ill or have gastrointestinal disease. Studies have also been undertaken in volunteers. While panvitamin deficiency causes apathy and impaired cognition and may lead to psychosis, specific symptoms are associated with deficiencies of individual vitamins.

Thiamine (B_1) deficiency (cerebral beri-beri):

Acute thiamine depletion causes Wernicke encephalopathy and Korsakoff psychosis. Replacement therapy generally reverses the confusion, clouding of consciousness and neurological symptoms of the former and will also reverse or reduce memory disturbance in a proportion of patients with the latter, if commenced promptly. Chronic thiamine deficiency causes apathy, fatigue, irritability, depression and cognitive impairment prior to the development of classic beri-beri.

Nicotinic acid (B_3) deficiency (pellagra):

Acute nicotinic acid depletion causes encephalopathy with an acute organic reaction, parkinsonism and primitive reflexes. Chronic deficiency causes apathy and lassitude initially, with confusion, depression, paranoid psychosis with hallucinations and occasional violence as the disease progresses. Established pellagra is characterized by the triad of dermatitis, diarrhoea and dementia. Replacement therapy is generally effective at all stages of disease.

Pyridoxine (B_6) deficiency:

Pyridoxine deficiency may cause depression and, much less frequently, an acute organic reaction.

Cyanocobalamin (B_{12}) deficiency (pernicious anaemia):

Anxiety, depression, psychosis, acute organic reaction and dementia have been attributed to vitamin B_{12} deficiency (in addition to subacute combined degeneration of the spinal cord) and are said to respond to replacement therapy (Shulman 1967).

Folate deficiency (folate dementia):

Folate deficiency is common and may be associated with lassitude, impaired cognition, depression and dementia. However, it is probable that these symptoms occur only following severe, prolonged deficiency.

Endocrine disorders

Psychiatric symptoms occur in a large proportion of patients with a range of different endocrine diseases, may lead to incorrect psychiatric diagnoses (Box 27.9) and may have medicolegal significance. Such symptoms usually resolve upon treatment of the primary endocrine disease.

Psychiatric treatment may be required if acute organic reactions occur or if treatment of the primary disease is prolonged or impossible.

Hypopituitarism:

Hypopituitarism may follow pituitary tumours or hypophysectomy. Weight- and hair-loss and impotence or amenorrhoea develop in addition to the psychiatric symptoms seen in Addison disease – including cognitive impairment – and hypothyroidism. An acute organic reaction leading to coma may occur during pituitary crises.

Replacement therapy for the underlying disease usually ensures resolution of psychiatric symptoms (McGauley 1989) but symptomatic psychotropic treatment may be required in the short term.

Acromegaly:

Fatigue, avolition, emotional lability and apathy may occur and occasionally are so severe as to resemble depression.

Hyperprolactinaemia:

Psychotic symptoms have been described in association with hyperprolactinaemia.

Treatment is problematic because antipsychotic drugs, being dopamine D_2 receptor antagonists, may worsen the non-psychiatric symptoms of hyperprolactinaemia, while bromocriptine, a dopamine D_2 receptor agonist, may worsen

Box 27.9

Endocrine disorders and the psychiatric diagnoses for which they may be mistaken

Hypothyroidism

- Dementia
- Depression
- Psychosis

Hyperthyroidism

- Anxiety disorder
- Depression (agitated)

Addison disease

- Dementia
- Depression
- Psychosis

Cushing syndrome

- Depression
- Psychosis
- (Mania with corticosteroid therapy, see below)
- Anxiety

Hypopituitarism

- Dementia
- Depression
- Anorexia nervosa
- Psychosis

Acromegaly

- Depression

Hypoparathyroidism

- Anxiety disorder
- Depression

Hyperparathyroidism

- Depression
- Dementia

Phaeochromocytoma

- Anxiety disorder
- Panic disorder

Diabetes mellitus

- (see below)

Hypoglycaemia (insulinoma)

- Anxiety
- Intoxication
- Personality disorder
- Automatism
- Temporal lobe epilepsy

psychosis. There is some evidence that atypical antipsychotic drugs maybe effective in combination with bromocriptine (Soygur et al 1997).

Hypothyroidism:

Hypothyroidism is caused by low plasma thyroxine (or tri-iodothyronine) caused by thyroid disease, thyroidectomy or drugs.

Symptoms develop insidiously and include impaired concentration, psychomotor retardation, depression, dementia and 'myxoedematous madness', a paranoid psychosis with hallucinations and delusions first described by Asher (1949). Acute organic reaction, seizures and coma may occur.

Myxoedema has been used successfully as a defence against homicide (Easson 1980).

Psychiatric symptoms usually resolve with thyroxine replacement therapy but symptomatic psychotropic treatment may be required in the short term. Depression associated with hypothyroidism is relatively treatment-resistant (Denicoff et al 1990) and patients with dementia of more than 2 years' duration do not always recover.

Hyperthyroidism:

The psychiatric symptoms of hyperthyroidism include overactivity and irritability resembling anxiety, depression, mild to moderate cognitive impairment and acute organic reaction during thyroid crises. Affective or schizophreniform psychosis occurs occasionally.

Psychiatric symptoms almost invariably resolve with treatment of the thyroid disorder.

Hypoparathyroidism:

The psychiatric features of hypoparathyroidism, which most commonly develops following thyroidectomy, include anxiety, depression, irritability, epilepsy, acute organic reaction and cognitive impairment (if untreated). Psychosis is probably no more common than in the general population.

Psychiatric symptoms increase as hypocalcaemia worsens, but they respond rapidly to treatment with vitamin D.

Hyperparathyroidism:

Hyperparathyroidism is usually caused by a parathyroid adenoma and is frequently associated with depression, anergia and irritability. About one in three patients receive a psychiatric diagnosis prior to the definitive diagnosis being made. Cognitive impairment occurs in a large proportion of patients, as does acute organic reaction during parathyroid crisis.

Psychiatric symptoms are related to plasma calcium and respond to removal of the causative adenoma.

Diabetes mellitus:

There are four psychiatric syndromes associated with diabetes mellitus, as follows:

- Psychological reactions to a lifelong disease that requires treatment with daily injections, imposes limitations on lifestyle and increases risk for disabling (e.g. blindness or impotence) and fatal (e.g. myocardial infarction or stroke) diseases such as anxiety, hypochondriasis and depression
- Psychiatric symptoms caused by metabolic imbalance (hyperglycaemia/ketoacidosis, lactic acidosis and hypoglycaemia), such as anxiety, irritability, aggression, confusion and acute organic reaction
- Psychiatric symptoms associated with the long-term effects of diabetes mellitus including cerebrovascular disease – which may account for the cognitive impairment and dementia described in some diabetic patients (Perlmutter et al 1984) – impaired vision and renal failure
- Co-morbid psychiatric illness in diabetic patients that is unrelated to their diabetes mellitus.

Thus, a proportion of diabetic patients may require general psychiatric treatment (because of their reaction to the diagnosis and treatment of diabetes mellitus or because of co-morbidity) while some will require specific treatment such as antidepressant therapy for pain associated with diabetic neuropathy, psychological and pharmacological treatment of sexual dysfunction and psychoeducation directed towards improved compliance with diabetic treatment regimens.

There is considerable evidence that major depression occurs in at least 20% of diabetic patients and that it is both poorly recognized and poorly treated (Lustman et al 1997).

Hypoglycaemia:

Hypoglycaemia may be caused by excess insulin administration, insulinoma, liver disease or alcohol.

Psychiatric symptoms include anxiety, aggression, behavioural disturbance, mood disorder, clouding of consciousness, amnesia and coma. Automatisms may occur and hypoglycaemic automatism has been used as a defence against criminal conviction. Episodic hypoglycaemia may occur with insulinoma and may present as psychiatric disorder while chronic hypoglycaemia has been associated with dementia.

Addison disease:

Addison disease is caused by adrenal failure and is associated with weakness, apathy, fatigue, depression, irritability and weight-loss.

Marked cognitive impairment may occur (and may lead to a diagnosis of dementia), as may an acute organic reaction during Addisonian crises. Psychosis occurs infrequently. Psychiatric symptoms almost always resolve with replacement therapy for the underlying disease but symptomatic psychotropic treatment may be required in the short term.

Cushing syndrome:

Corticosteroid treatment is the commonest cause of Cushing syndrome, with adrenocorticotrophin secreted by pituitary adenomas (Cushing disease) and other tumours accounting for the remainder.

At least 50% of patients develop psychiatric symptoms which include depression (which is less common with corticosteroid treatment, see below) during which biological and psychotic symptoms may occur and, less often, psychosis, mania, anxiety and cognitive impairment. Impotence and amenorrhoea are common.

Psychiatric symptoms usually resolve with treatment of the underlying disease but psychotropic treatment may be required in the short term.

Phaeochromocytoma:

Phaeochromocytomas are usually benign (90%) tumours of the adrenal (90%) or sympathetic chain chromaffin cells that secrete adrenaline and noradrenaline and, often in response to emotion or excitement, cause episodes of severe panic with palpitations, sweating, tremor, headache, tachycardia, hypertension, pallor and intense fear. Confusion and excitement may also occur. Catecholamines and their metabolites are increased in blood and urine and the tumour may be detected by MRI.

Psychiatric symptoms may suggest a diagnosis of anxiety or panic disorder but they invariably respond to surgical treatment of the tumour.

Poisoning

Poisoning with carbon monoxide, prescribed and illicit drugs, and toluene is relatively common, while poisoning with heavy metals is relatively rare.

Carbon monoxide poisoning

The hippocampus and basal ganglia are particularly sensitive to carbon monoxide (CO) poisoning (and concurrent hypoxia), which most often occurs during suicide attempts with car exhaust fumes. The neuropsychiatric effects of CO poisoning depend on the concentration of the gas and the duration of exposure:

- **Mild CO poisoning:** an acute organic reaction with amnesia and extrapyramidal symptoms is usual upon recovery of consciousness. These features resolve over days or weeks leaving minimal or no long-term sequelae.
- **Moderate CO poisoning:** a prolonged acute organic reaction with severe amnesia and extrapyramidal symptoms is usual upon recovery of consciousness. These features resolve over weeks or months but relapse often occurs a few weeks after an apparently complete recovery. A small proportion of patients die at this stage while persistent severe extrapyramidal symptoms or dementia develop in some survivors.
- **Severe CO poisoning:** persisting coma leading to death.

Follow-up studies suggest that more than 50% of patients suffer permanent personality change or cognitive deficit, while 2% develop permanent extrapyramidal disorders or dementia. It has been suggested that a law requiring catalyst vehicle exhaust systems and automatic idling stop, and exhaust tubes that are incompatible with vacuum cleaner tubes (the commonest means by which CO is transferred from the exhaust pipe to the car interior) would reduce suicides from CO poisoning (Ostrom et al 1996).

Poisoning with drugs

Many drugs, whether available over the counter, by prescription or illicitly, can alter brain function and cause psychiatric symptoms. Indeed it is largely because of this effect that illicit drugs are abused (see Ch. 29). The psychiatric side-effects of commonly prescribed drugs will now be discussed.

Antibacterial and antituberculous drugs:

Intramuscular procaine penicillin may cause anxiety and hallucinations, while a large number of antibiotics including chloramphenicol, cephalexin, gentamicin, nitrofurantoin and the sulphonamides have been reported to cause acute organic reactions.

Isoniazid may cause prolonged psychosis and cycloserine has been associated with confusion, depression and schizophreniform psychosis in patients receiving antituberculous therapy.

Anticholinergic/antimuscarinic and dopaminergic drugs:

Anticholinergic/antimuscarinic drugs may cause confusion, excitement and visual hallucinations, especially in elderly patients, while dopaminergic drugs cause acute organic reactions, affective disorders and psychosis. These side-effects are commoner in patients with a history of psychiatric illness (see Ch. 39).

Anticonvulsant drugs:

Psychiatric side-effects from AEDs may arise directly or may be mediated indirectly by sedation and disinhibition. Carbamazepine, lamotrigine and topiramate are associated with confusion, depression and agitation (especially in elderly patients). Lamotrigine may also cause irritability and aggression. Most other AEDs cause similar side-effects while psychosis may occur with both vigabatrin and topiramate (see Ch. 39).

Barbiturates, benzodiazepines and related drugs:

Barbiturates, prescribed infrequently now in comparison to a few decades ago, may cause euphoria and irritability. In addition to dependency, these drugs and benzodiazepines may cause drowsiness, lethargy, ataxia and depression on the one hand, and disinhibition with excitement and aggression on the other. Elderly patients may become very confused. Withdrawal effects from barbiturates are similar to those of alcohol and delirium and seizures may occur (see Ch. 39).

Cardiovascular drugs:

The neuropsychiatric side-effects of digitalis, the older antihypertensive drugs and diuretics are well recognized, and more recently, similar side-effects have been described for newer cardioactive drugs. Digitalis toxicity is often associated with confusion, disorientation and hallucinations, and depression and excitement have also been reported. Depression or euphoria may be caused by beta-blocking, diuretic, ganglion-blocking (trimetaphan), calcium channel blocking and centrally acting (rauwolfia, methyldopa, clonidine and moxonidine) antihypertensive drugs, and by antihypertensive drugs that affect the renin-angiotensin system. Vasodilator and adrenergic-blocking antihypertensive drugs appear less likely to cause such side-effects.

Corticosteroid drugs:

It has long been recognized that corticosteroid drugs may cause psychosis with paranoia and auditory hallucinations, mild elation or depression in the short term, and mania or more severe depression with an increased risk of suicide in the longer term. The latter may be associated with an acute organic reaction and may persist for several weeks. These side-effects are more common with higher dosages and in patients with a history of psychiatric illness. Recovery is usual upon withdrawal of corticosteroid therapy but prolonged psychotropic treatment – including treatment with antipsychotic drugs or lithium if appropriate – may be required if corticosteroid withdrawal is impossible. Acute organic reaction may be precipitated by rapid corticosteroid withdrawal.

Contraceptive drugs:

Hormonal contraceptive drugs, both combined and progesterone-only formulations, may cause depression. This may resolve with the addition of pyridoxine but if not, discontinuation of hormonal (and initiation of non-hormonal) contraception may be necessary.

Cytotoxic drugs:

Vinca alkaloid and platinum drugs are neurotoxic, but while they may cause neurological disorders including encephalopathy, pure psychiatric symptoms are relatively uncommon. Confusion has been reported with α and β interferons, and affective and sleep disorders with gonadorelin analogues. Cytotoxic antibiotics and antimetabolites are relatively free from neuropsychiatric side-effects.

Opiate drugs:

Although widely abused because they induce mild euphoria and drowsiness, opiates are relatively free from significant psychiatric side-effects. Sedation and depression may occur, especially in elderly patients.

Toluene poisoning

The inhalation of toluene in adhesives ('glue-sniffing) produces dizziness and euphoria in the very short term. Hallucinations, seizures and coma may occasionally evolve. In the longer term, a chronic paranoid psychosis, temporal lobe epilepsy and intellectual impairment have been described (Byrne et al 1991). Suggestions that cortical atrophy may occur are unproven.

Heavy metal poisoning

All heavy metals may cause acute and chronic organic reactions and this and the relative rarity of heavy metal poisoning makes the diagnosis extremely difficult unless a clear account of exposure can be obtained.

Lead poisoning in children causes an encephalopathy that may be associated with permanent intellectual impairment. Adults exhibit anorexia and colic with cognitive impairment and, infrequently and only with chronic exposure, psychosis. Cerebral and cerebellar calcification may occur.

Mercury poisoning causes depression and mild cognitive impairment more frequently than the more famous 'erythism' or Mad Hatter disease (poor attention and concentration with severe anxiety and agitation), and while there have been suggestions that mercury from dental amalgam may have these effects, there is no evidence that this is the case (Foerster & Breyer-Plaff 1996).

Thallium poisoning almost always follows accidental or intentional ingestion of rat poison. Clinical features include severe peripheral neuropathy, abdominal pain, nausea, vomiting, alopecia and acute organic reaction. The vast majority of patients make a complete recovery.

Arsenic poisoning most often occurs during industrial exposure. Psychiatric symptoms include mild impairment of new learning, recent memory and concentration. This may only manifest a few years after exposure. Recovery is usual on cessation of exposure.

Autoimmune and other disorders

Psychiatric symptoms occur in patients with several autoimmune disorders and may be aggravated by treatment with steroids. Autoimmune disorders therefore deserve consideration in the psychiatric differential diagnosis.

Amyotrophic lateral sclerosis (motor neuron disease)

Amyotrophic lateral sclerosis (ALS) develops from the fifth decade of life onwards. Patients initially present with weakness and atrophy of the muscles of the hands. This progresses proximally and some patients have cranial nerve/craniobulbar muscle weakness which may impair breathing, swallowing and speech, and may be associated with pseudobulbar emotional lability. Many patients with ALS are depressed and have chronic pain and there is evidence that these symptoms are frequently unrecognized and untreated (Ganzini et al 1999).

Cerebral sarcoidosis

Neurosarcoidosis usually presents with meningo-encephalitis or cranial nerve palsies caused by cerebral sarcoid granulomata. Less frequently, patients present with clouding of consciousness, hallucinations and aphasia (Hayashi et al 1995). Treatment should be directed at the control of symptoms and at the underlying sarcoidosis.

Systemic lupus erythematosus

Psychiatric symptoms, including anxiety, major depression, affective and schizophreniform psychoses, acute organic reactions and dementia with personality change and emotional lability occur in at least one-third of patients (Rubio et al 1998) with systemic lupus erythematosus (SLE) and may occasionally be the presenting symptom. These symptoms are usually short-lived and are best treated symptomatically and by controlling the underlying SLE. Cerebral SLE detected by structural and functional neuroimaging is as common in patients without psychiatric symptoms as in those with such symptoms (Sabbadini et al 1999).

Multiple sclerosis

A proportion of patients with multiple sclerosis (MS) present to psychiatrists and may receive diagnoses of conversion disorder before MS is identified. Depression is the commonest psychiatric symptom in patients with MS and there is an increased risk of suicide. Patients with bilateral bulbar lesions may exhibit emotional incontinence. Euphoria occurs in less than 10% of patients, being commonest in those with cognitive impairment. Cognitive impairment occurs in 50% of patients and is closely related to the number of cerebral lesions. Dementia may occur. There is some evidence that emotional incontinence is particularly responsive to selective serotonin reuptake inhibitors (Nahas et al 1998). Otherwise, psychiatric illness in patients with MS should be treated symptomatically.

Myasthenia gravis

A proportion of patients with myasthenia gravis (MG) are referred to psychiatrists with fatigue and muscle weakness and may receive a diagnosis of conversion disorder. Patients with MG may suffer from depression and anxiety and there is some evidence that such symptoms exacerbate the MG.

References

Adamson, D.C., McArthur, J.C., Dawson, T.M., et al., 1999. Rate and severity of HIV-associated dementia (HAD): correlations with Gp41 and iNOS. Mol. Med. 5, 98–109.

Anderson, G.M., Pollak, E.S., Chatterjee, D., et al., 1992. Postmortem analysis of subcortical monoamines and amino acids in Tourette syndrome. In: Chase, T.N., Friedhoff, A.J., Cohen, D.J. (Eds.), Tourette syndrome: genetics, neurobiology and treatment advances in neurology. Raven Press, New York, pp. 123–133.

APA: American Psychiatric Association, 1999. Practice guideline for the treatment of patients with delirium. Am. J. Psychiatry 156 (5 Suppl.), 1–20.

Asher, R., 1949. Myxoedematous madness. Br. Med. J. ii, 555–562.

Bekkelund, S.I., Marthinsen, T.A., Harr, T., 1999. Reversible dementia in idiopathic normal pressure hydrocephalus. A case report. Scand. J. Prim. Health Care 17, 22–24.

Besson, J.A., 1993. Structural and functional brain imaging in alcoholism and drug misuse. Curr. Opin. Psychiatry 6, 403–410.

Betts, T., 1990. Pseudoseizures: seizures that are not epilepsy. Lancet ii, 9–10.

Betts, T., 1998. Epilepsy, psychiatry and learning difficulty. Martin Dunitz, London.

Biggins, C.A., Boyd, J.L., Harrop, F.M., et al., 1992. A controlled longitudinal study of dementia in Parkinson's disease. J. Neurol. Neurosurg. Psychiatry 55, 566–571.

Brodaty, H., McGilchrist, C., Harris, L., et al., 1993. Time until institutionalization and death in patients with dementia. Role of caregiver training and risk factors. Arch. Neurol. 50, 643–650.

Brun, A., 1987. Frontal lobe degeneration of the non-Alzheimer type 1 – neuropathology. Arch. Gerontol. Geriatr. 6, 193–208.

Buckley, P.F., 1998. Novel antipsychotics and patient care in state hospitals. Ann. Pharmacother. 32, 906–914.

Burn, D.J., Bates, D.J., 1998. Neurology and the kidney. J. Neurol. Neurosurg. Psychiatry 65, 810–821.

Burns, A., Lewis, G., Jacoby, R., et al., 1991. Survival in Alzheimer's disease. Psychol. Med. 21, 363–370.

Byrne, A., Kirby, B., Zibin, T., et al., 1991. Psychiatric and neurological effects of chronic solvent abuse. Can. J. Psychiatry 36, 735–738.

Cavazos, J.E., Spitz, M., 2009. Seizures and epilepsy, overview and classification: treatment and medication. Online. Available: Emedicine.com.

Collinge, J., Beck, J., Campbell, T., et al., 1996. Prion protein gene analysis in new variant cases of Creutzfeldt-Jacob disease. Lancet 348, 56.

Commission on Classification and Terminology of the International League Against Epilepsy, 1989. Proposal for revised classification of epilepsies and epileptic syndromes. Epilepsia 30, 389–399.

Cummings, J.L., 1993. Frontal-subcortical circuits and human behaviour. Arch. Neurol. 50, 873–878.

Denicoff, K.D., Joffe, R.T., Lakshman, M.C., et al., 1990. Neuropsychiatric manifestations of altered thyroid state. Am. J. Psychiatry 147, 94–99.

Dreifuss, F.E., Bancaud, J., Henricksen, O., et al., 1981. Proposal for a revised clinical and electroencephalographic classification of epileptic seizures. Epilepsia 22, 489–503.

Eames, P., 1997. Traumatic brain injury. Curr. Opin. Psychiatry 10, 49–52.

Easson, W.M., 1980. Myxedema psychosis – insanity defense in homicide. J. Clin. Psychiatry 41, 316–318.

Fleminger, S., 1992. Organic psychiatry. In: Appleby, L., Forshaw, D.M. (Eds.), Postgraduate psychiatry, clinical and scientific foundations. Butterworth-Heinemann, Oxford.

Fleminger, S., Curtis, D., 1997. Prion diseases. Br. J. Psychiatry 170, 103–105.

Flor Henry, P., 1969. Psychosis and temporal lobe epilepsy: a controlled investigation. Epilepsia 10, 363–395.

Foerster, K., Breyer-Plaff, U., 1996. Amalgam – etiology of psychiatric disorders? Versicherungsmedizin 48, 62–64.

Ganzini, L., Johnston, W.S., Hoffman, W.F., 1999. Correlates of suffering in amyotrophic lateral sclerosis. Neurology 52, 1434–1440.

George, M.S., Lydiard, R.B., 1994. Social phobia secondary to physical disability. A review of benign essential tremor (BET) and stuttering. Psychosomatics 35, 520–523.

Goldstein, L.B., 1993. Prescribing of potentially harmful drugs to patients admitted to hospital after head injury. J. Neurol. Neurosurg. Psychiatry 58, 753–755.

Graff-Radford, N.R., Woodruff, B.K., 2007. Frontotemporal dementia. Semin. Neurol. 27, 48–57.

Gunn, J., Fenton, G.W., 1971. Epilepsy, automatism and crime. Lancet i, 1173–1176.

Hayashi, T., Onodera, J., Nagata, T., et al., 1995. A case of biopsy-proven sarcoid meningoencephalitis presented with

Introduction

Alcohol is the most commonly used mood altering substance in Western society, used by over 90% of the UK population. Psychiatrists are usually involved with dependent drinkers – those at greatest risk of alcohol complications. The overall cost to society is largely related to the incidence of problems in the far larger *normal drinking* population. This has been termed the 'prevention paradox', as reducing alcohol consumption among people who drink marginally more than the recommended levels, through public education and brief interventions, may be more cost- and health-effective than treating the smaller number of dependent users. Current recommendations for safe drinking are for men not to exceed 3–4 units per day and for women not to exceed 2–3 units per day. A *unit of alcohol* is equivalent to 10 mL or 8 g of absolute alcohol, approximately half a pint; 284 mL, of normal strength lager, a glass (125 mL) of average strength wine or a single measure (25 mL) of spirits). A third of the UK working population drink more than is recommended.

Metabolism

Alcohol is hydrophilic and rapid absorption occurs from all parts of the gastrointestinal tract with peak levels being reached 30–60 min after ingestion. This is enhanced by the absence of food in the stomach or the presence of carbon dioxide bubbles (note the effect of Champagne and 'tequila slammers'). The primary route of metabolism (Fig. 28.1) is hepatic oxidation by the rate-limiting enzyme alcohol dehydrogenase (ADH) to acetaldehyde, which is subsequently oxidized by aldehyde dehydrogenase (ALDH). There is a racial distribution

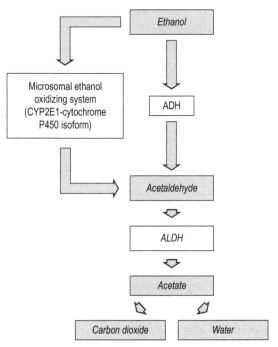

Figure 28.1 • Metabolism of ethanol.

of ALDH2 (responsible for most of the second oxidative process). Lack of activity in the South-East Asian population is responsible for the 'flushing reaction' (tachycardia, hypertension, a facial flush and weakness), which many experience from small amounts of alcohol. A deficit occurs in half of 'normal' Chinese and Japanese subjects but only 2% of Japanese alcoholics. With increased alcohol consumption the cytochrome P450 system starts contributing to the metabolism, enhancing the microsomal ethanol-oxidizing system and contributing to the tolerance seen in chronic consumption.

Dependency

The disease concept of alcoholism originated with the writings of Benjamin Rush in the USA and Thomas Totter, who viewed alcoholism as 'a disease of the will'. The clinical syndrome, described by Edwards and Gross (1976), forms the basis for most modern-day operationalized definitions of dependence syndromes (Box 28.1).

Identification and assessment

Effective secondary prevention can only be implemented, if harmful drinking levels are detected. Several questionnaires have been developed, such as the 25-item MAST (Michigan Alcohol Screening Test) and the 4-item CAGE questions (Cutdown, Angry, Guilt and Eye opener). These are effective at identifying severe alcohol problems but may not detect hazardous patterns of consumption. The WHO 10-item AUDIT (Alcohol Use Disorders Identification Test) was designed for use by primary care workers, (Box 28.2), and detects 92% of harmful drinkers and 94% of those who drink above recommended levels. Screening tools in primary care improve the identification of alcohol problems (Wallace & Haines 1985). Useful measures of alcohol-related problems (which correlate with severity of dependence) include the self-reporting Alcohol Problems Questionnaire (APQ) and the Severity of Alcohol Dependence (SADQ).

Physical examination and laboratory investigations may also help identification. Investigations include:

- LFTs especially γ-GT (sensitivity 20–90%, specificity 55–90%). Levels fall quickly with abstinence, with moderate levels (300–500 mmol/L) returning to normal within 1–2 months of abstinence

Box 28.1

Edwards and Gross alcohol dependency syndrome

- Narrowing of drinking repertoire (loss of variation in pattern of intake)
- Salience (primacy) of drink-seeking behaviour
- Increased tolerance to alcohol
- Repeated attempts at withdrawal from alcohol
- Relief or avoidance of withdrawal symptoms by further drinking
- Reinstatement of dependent drinking after a period of abstinence
- Subjective awareness of compulsion to drink.

10-item AUDIT questionnaire (WHO)

1. How often do you have a drink containing alcohol?

   0 = Never; 1 = Monthly or less; 2 = 2–4 times/month; 3 = 2–3 times/week; 4 = 4 or more times/week

2. How many units of alcohol do you drink on a typical day when you are drinking?

   0 = 1 or 2; 1 = 3 or 4; 2 = 5 or 6; 3 = 7–9; 4 = 10 or more

3. How often have you had 6 or more units if female, or 8 or more if male, on a single occasion in the last year?

4. How often during the last year have you found that you were not able to stop drinking once you had started?

   0 = Never; 1 = Less than monthly; 2 = Monthly; 3 = Weekly; 4 = Daily or almost daily

5. How often during the past year have you failed to do what was expected of you because of drinking?

   0 = Never; 1 = Less than monthly; 2 = Monthly; 3 = Weekly; 4 = Daily or almost daily

6. How often during the last year have you needed an alcoholic drink in the morning to get yourself going after a heavy drinking session?

   0 = Never; 1 = Less than monthly; 2 = Monthly; 3 = Weekly; 4 = Daily or almost daily

7. How often during the last year have you had a feeling of guilt or remorse after drinking?

   0 = Never; 1 = Less than monthly; 2 = Monthly; 3 = Weekly; 4 = Daily or almost daily

8. How often during the last year have you been unable to remember what happened the night before because you had been drinking?

   0 = Never; 1 = Less than monthly; 2 = Monthly; 3 = Weekly; 4 = Daily or almost daily

9. Have you or somebody else been injured as a result of your drinking?

   0 = No; 1 = Yes, but not in the past year; 4 = Yes, during the past year

10. Has a relative or friend or doctor or other health worker been concerned about your drinking or suggested you cut down?

    0 = No; 1 = Yes, but not in the past year; 4 = Yes, during the past year

Scoring: 0–7 Lower risk, 8–15 Increasing risk, 16–19 Higher risk, 20+ Possible dependence

- MCV (sensitivity 20–50%, specificity 55–100%)
- Carbohydrate deficient transferrin (an iron transport protein variant) has been used with a sensitivity for heavy drinking of 60–70% and a specificity of 95%.

Epidemiology of alcohol use

Prevalence

The average UK *per capita* level of consumption is just over 10 units a week, with peak mean consumption occurring in 16–24 year olds (males, 18 units/week; females, just under 11 units/week). Recent data from the UK indicates that 41% of men and 34% of women drink over the recommended limits on at least 1 day per week; 25% of men and 16% of women binge

at least once a week (defined as over 8 units for men, and over 6 units for women). In the same survey, 20% of children aged 11–15 reported drinking alcohol in the week prior to interview, with 17% believing it was 'OK to get drunk at least once a week' (NHS 2009). Other data suggests that 6% of men and 2% of women are harmful or higher risk drinkers (defined as scoring 16 or more on the AUDIT (Box 28.2), with dependence rates of 9.3% of men and 3.6% of women (NHS 2009). Since 2000, dependence has decreased in men from 11.5%, but increased in women from 2.8%. Lifetime rates of alcohol use disorders are higher in men, with approximately one-quarter of men being classified as problem drinkers at some time in their lives (Institute of Alcohol Studies 2004). The Epidemiological and Catchment Area (ECA) study in the USA reported a 14% lifetime prevalence of alcohol dependency with a male to female ratio of 2:1 (Reiger et al 1991).

Patterns of use

In vino-cultural countries, 80% of alcohol is consumed at moderate levels, with food, on a daily basis. In the UK, food related consumption is 50%, with a significant proportion consumed during binge-drinking episodes. Binge-drinking is variously defined as consumption of half or more of the recommended maximum weekly amount during a single session or the consumption of more than 6 units for women and 8 units for men during a drinking session. The motive for such consumption patterns is clearly drunkenness. Binge-drinking is a normal mode of alcohol consumption among 18–24-year-olds (40% of men and 22% of women reported binge consumption in the last year). People in the UK binge-drink more than any other Western country, exceptions being Germany and Finland. Recent changes to opening hours in the UK were aimed at reducing such drinking patterns.

Age

Adults drink less with advancing age. The heaviest drinking occurs in the late teens and early 20s, when the sex differences in consumption are least evident. Although the marketing of flavoured alcoholic beverages ('alcopops') to young consumers is of concern, most alcohol consumed by the young is in the form of traditional alcoholic beverages. The peak age for dependence is between 30 and 44 years.

Gender

Men drink about three times as much as women in the UK, and experience the onset of dependency at an earlier age. In Asian and Hispanic cultures the male/female ratio of consumption is nearer 10:1. Recent studies from many countries suggest that young women are now drinking at levels comparable with young men, with binge consumption posing a significant risk for health and wellbeing.

Harmful patterns of alcohol consumption in women are often compounded by other risky behaviours such as unprotected sex and illicit drug use. Women appear more sensitive to the harmful effects of alcohol and experience a greater degree of intoxication for a given amount of alcohol. Reasons for this increased vulnerability include a higher proportion of body fat, a lower

Conditioning theory

Classic and operant learning theories with relief drinking and cued response/relapse, are two commonly cited mechanisms. The two main dimensions of the condition within this framework are seen as withdrawal avoidance and reward, with the latter seemingly the more important. Such explanations have an important role in directing some therapeutic interventions, such as relapse prevention. Modelling (vicarious learning) and social learning theory also propose aetiological theories.

Personality traits

Half a century of research has failed to identify the alcoholic or addictive personality, however attractive the idea may sound. Several personality traits have been shown to have an association with alcoholism (Box 28.5) but only dissocial ones are consistent.

Life events and stress

The 'tension reduction' hypothesis views alcohol's anxiolytic effects as primary, while other studies show an increased frequency of life events preceding the onset of alcohol misuse. The onset of alcohol use during adolescence leads to a higher susceptibility to stress-induced alcohol consumption (Siegmund et al. 2005) and a greater risk of developing alcohol addiction in adulthood (Grant & Dawson 1997).

Sociological

The wider sociocultural context determines both the availability of alcohol and the attitude to drinking and intoxication. Price and other legislative controls have a significant impact on *per capita* consumption.

Neurobiology of ethanol, tolerance, dependence and withdrawal

Alcohol acts by disrupting distinct receptor or effector proteins, via direct or indirect interactions. Psychoactive effects are mediated through modulation at a number of neurotransmitters systems; primarily upon glutamate and GABA receptor-gated channels to which alcohol binds directly. Its anxiolytic activity is probably mediated through the acute potentiation of the inhibitory neurotransmitters including GABA at GABA-A receptors and taurine (Littleton & Little 1994). Alcohol also inhibits the function of the receptor for excitatory neurotransmitters

such as glutamate and aspartate. The attenuating effect of alcohol on the N-methyl-D-aspartate (NMDA) glutamate receptor is thought to contribute to intoxication, impaired cognition and blackouts. Chronic alcohol consumption results in upregulation of the NMDA-type glutamate receptor. Acute withdrawal of ethanol leads to increased glutamate synaptic release with the excitotoxic effects resulting in neuronal cell death (e.g. cerebellar degeneration), seizures and cognitive dysfunction (blackouts).

Ion channels also constitute a primary target of alcohol (Vengeliene et al 2008). Alcohol inhibits dihydropyridine-sensitive L-type Ca2+ channels (Wang et al 1994) and opens G-protein-activated inwardly rectifying K+ channels (Kobayashi et al 1999; Lewohl et al 1999). This activity can precipitate a cascade of synaptic events involving multiple neurotransmitters, i.e. 5HT3 on inhibitory GABAergic interneurons, with activation of 5-HT3 receptors, which in turn increase release of dopamine and glutamate (Lovinger 1999). Chronic alcohol use leads to adaptive, long-lasting changes (Vengeliene et al 2008).

Thus, alcohol, an agonist at neuroinhibitory GABA receptors and an antagonist at neuroexcitatory glutamate/NMDA receptors, causes glutamate/NMDA receptor upregulation and GABA receptor downregulation, with a decrease in the brain GABA-A receptor density and brain region specific up- or downregulation of a and b subunit gene expression (Golovko et al 2002). Alcohol cessation leads to unopposed and excessive neuroexcitation mediated by upregulated glutamate/NMDA receptors (Fig. 28.2). Benzodiazepines treat the symptoms of alcohol withdrawal due to cross-tolerance with alcohol at the GABA-A receptors. Carbamazepine, also effective in withdrawal, probably acts through this mechanism. Future pharmacological interventions may focus on NMDA antagonism as a means of reducing both withdrawal and the neuronal toxicity associated with exposure to repeated episodes of withdrawal. The management of alcohol withdrawal is discussed below.

Other effects

Alcohol releases dopamine from the nucleus accumbens within the limbic VTA DA system as well as impacting on serotonin pathways involved in priming and reinforcing effects. Alcohol also increases endogenous opioids, which contribute to the euphoria associated with its consumption and this is why naltrexone helps maintain abstinence in some dependent drinkers.

Alcohol may cause stimulation and euphoria, especially when there is a rapid increase in blood alcohol levels and these effects may also be highly reinforcing.

Alcohol-related physical problems

Moderate consumption of alcohol (1–3 units/day) is associated with reduced mortality compared with either life-long abstention or heavy use. This is probably due to its increasing levels of HDL and subsequent reducing rates of coronary heart disease. These interactions call for further research before any public health messages about the positive aspects of drinking alcohol are conveyed (Grønbæk 2006). Regular drinking above the

---

Box 28.5

Predisposing personality traits and alcoholism

- **Childhood:** aggression, inattention, hyperactivity, antisocial behaviours
- **Locus of control:** external
- **Emotional:** dependency, anxiety and alexithymia. Higher neuroticism scores on Eysenck Personality Questionnaire

---

Figure 28.2 • Treatment pathway for patients presenting with alcoholism and depression. (Adapted from CanDo Comorbidity training, AGPN, Winstock, 2006.)

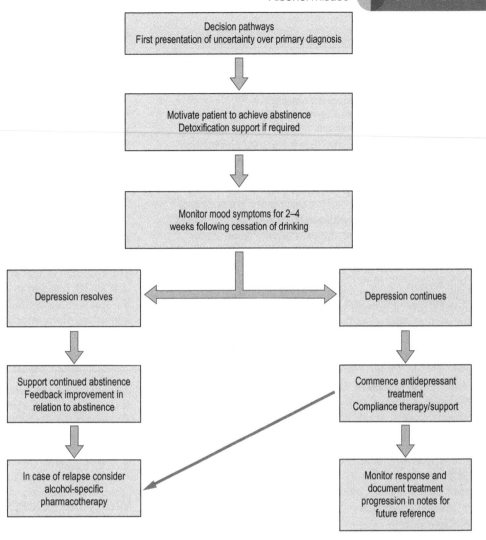

recommended daily limits (2–3 units for women and 3–4 units for men) significantly increases the risk of ill health. Damage may be seen in every physiological system, most commonly the gastrointestinal and nervous systems. Vulnerability to the toxic effects increase with age, female sex, total consumption and pattern of use (constant heavy drinking/binge-drinking). The possible damaging consequences of the now high rates of adolescent binge-drinking on organ dysfunction and damage in this population are largely unknown at present (Spanagel 2009), although the young adolescent brain has been shown to display higher sensitivity to alcohol-induced brain damage and cognitive impairment than the adult brain (Spear & Varlinskaya 2005).

Gastrointestinal tract

- Oesophagitis and reflux
- Gastritis and ulceration anywhere in tract
- Mallory–Weiss tears
- Oesophageal varices
- Pancreatitis

- Portal hypertension
- Carcinoma of tongue, pharynx, larynx, oesophagus, rectum and liver.

Liver

- Acute inflammation consequent upon heavy drinking but reversible with abstinence
- Fatty infiltration which disappears on stopping alcohol
- Alcoholic hepatitis with hepatocellular necrosis and risk of cirrhosis with continued drinking
- Alcoholic cirrhosis
- Haemachromatosis in those with genetic susceptibility
- Hepatic encephalopathy.

Cardiovascular

- Arrhythmias – atrial fibrillation and ventricular extrasystoles
- Dilated cardiomyopathy, beri-beri with high output failure
- Coronary and cerebrovascular disease
- Hypertension, especially in young males.

Prognosis

In Victor's classic 1971 study of 245 patients (Victor et al 1971), only 16% of WE patients inadequately treated recovered fully, with a mortality rate of 17%; 84% developed Korsakoff psychosis. Of these, one-quarter had complete recovery, half had partial recovery and one-quarter had no recovery.

Other neurological consequences of alcohol

Cerebellar degeneration

The anterior lobe and superior vermis demonstrate Purkinje cell loss leading to ataxia of stance and gait.

Amblyopia

With an onset over a matter of weeks, this retrobulbar neuritis rarely leads to blindness. However, it is associated with loss of central vision, especially in the red/green bands and is associated with peripheral neuropathy.

Marchiafava Bignami syndrome

Characterized by ataxia, epilepsy, dysarthria and severely impaired consciousness. A slowly progressive form with dementia and spastic paresis also occurs. The neuropathology is demyelination of the corpus callosum, optic tract and cerebellar peduncles.

Central pontine myelinosis

Acutely there may be nausea, vomiting, confusion and coma. Pseudobulbar palsy, quadriplegia and loss of pain sensation in the limbs and trunk may occur. Neuropathologically there is demyelination of pyramidal neurons in the pons.

Epilepsy

Alcohol lowers the seizure threshold, and may also cause seizures due head injury, hypoglycaemia, subdural haematoma or from direct neurotoxicity, as alcohol is epileptogenic.

Dementia

Mild to moderate cognitive deficits are common in alcoholics, particularly visuospatial, frontal (impulse control) and memory impairment. Damage may be due to direct neurotoxicity, head trauma or nutritional deficiency. Women appear more susceptible than men. It is likely that prevalence rates of alcohol-related brain damage maybe currently underestimated and will rise in future (Kopelman et al. 2009). CT and MRI studies demonstrate ventricular enlargement (Besson 1993) and cortical atrophy (Harper et al 1985) in about two-thirds of alcoholics. Atrophy of the cerebellar vermis is seen in about 30%. Functional imaging shows decreased glucose metabolism and blood flow in cortical areas. Abstinence may be associated with some reversibility in these structural cerebral changes, especially in younger drinkers and women (see Ch. 27).

Amnesia

Alcoholic blackouts are periods of retrograde amnesia arising during a period of intoxication while fully conscious. Occurring more commonly in the binge-drinker, blackouts are not a defence nor a reason for being unfit to plead in court.

Fetal alcohol syndrome

The NICE clinical guidelines on antenatal care advise pregnant women to avoid alcohol in the first 3 months of pregnancy, as it may increase the risk of miscarriage, and to limit alcohol to 1–2 units once or twice a week for the rest of the pregnancy. At this low level, there is no evidence of harm to the unborn baby (NICE 2008). Alcohol fetal damage was first described in the English scientific literature by Jones and Smith (1973). Fetal alcohol syndrome (FAS) is characterized by pre- and postnatal growth retardation, CNS involvement with developmental delay and a characteristic pattern of craniofacial dysmorphism, with the degree of dysmorphism correlating with the decrement in IQ (Steinhausen et al 1993). Its incidence is between 0.5 and 2/1000 live births, although since FAS is a spectrum disorder, the incomplete syndrome maybe overlooked. Alcohol-related brain infant neurotoxicity is the most preventable form of intellectual retardation in children.

Features of fetal alcohol syndrome are:

* Intrauterine growth retardation
* Failure to thrive
* Short stature
* Developmental delay
* Micro-ophthalmia
* Short palpebral fissure
* Short nasal bridge
* Microcephaly with prominent forehead
* Thin upper lip
* Small philtrum
* Cleft palate
* Maxillary hypoplasia
* Gait abnormalities
* Irritable, mood disorder and hyperactivity
* Cardiac abnormalities
* Some show persistent cognitive impairment.

Alcohol-related psychological disorders

The co-morbidity of alcohol misuse and other psychiatric syndromes is common, present in over two-thirds of alcohol dependants.

Alcoholic hallucinosis

Alcoholic hallucinosis is characterized by auditory hallucinations, paranoid symptoms and fear. Hallucinations are usually third person auditory hallucinations, often derogatory or command, occurring in clear consciousness. They may take the form of fragments of conversation or music and there may be secondary delusions or perseveration. The symptoms may be highly distressing and may result in violent suicide. The onset is often associated with a reduction in dose or the precipitation of withdrawal and hallucinosis must be differentiated from delirium tremens, although they may appear as a continuation of hallucinations first experienced during this state. They may, however, arise in the current drinker. Assessment for the presence of other psychotic symptoms is mandatory to exclude other possible functional and organic pathologies, especially Wernicke encephalopathy. Visual hallucinations, although not typical, may occur. The prognosis is usually good, especially in abstinent drinkers, although in some 10–20% hallucinosis persist for more than 6 months. The reinstatement of drinking often results in a recrudescence of symptoms. Hospitalization and treatment with antipsychotic medication may be required. A total of 5–20% of cases subsequently develop schizophrenia, and have an increased family history of psychosis.

Psychiatric co-morbidity

The ECA study reported that having a psychiatric diagnosis triples the likelihood of an individual having a lifetime alcohol disorder. The most common co-morbid conditions are drug-use disorders, mood and anxiety disorders and dissocial personality disorder (Kranzler & Rosenthal 2003). In community-based studies, people dependent on alcohol were seven times more likely to have a drug disorder and two to three times more likely to have a mental disorder compared with others in the community. Rates tend to be higher in clinical samples, reflecting the increased rates of treatment-seeking by dual disorder patients (Berkson's bias). Alcohol dependence is also associated with heavy smoking. Relatives of alcoholic probands have higher rates of depression and drug abuse than controls. Common or closely linked genes may produce a general increase in vulnerability to both mental and substance misuse disorders consistent with the hypothesis of pleiotropy. Shared environmental factors such as poverty or childhood abuse may also jointly predispose. High rates of co-morbid psychiatric disorders have a detrimental impact on prognosis. Identifying the temporal onset of co-morbid disorders is important when planning treatment and considering prognosis, with the primary illness steering the clinical picture.

Affective disorder

Up to 70% of alcoholics complain of dysphoria during heavy drinking. Immediately after detoxification, the rate of depression is 50%, and after 1 month, between 15–20%. In the ECA study, 13.4% of alcoholics reported a mood disorder, while conversely, 22% of those with mood disorder reported alcohol use disorder. Rates of co-morbidity are even higher in those with bipolar disorder (>40%), where the result is higher rates of hospitalizations, shorter remissions, more dysphoria and a poorer clinical outcome. During manic episodes, alcohol consumption can be very high, and contribute to increased risks.

Some 30 years ago, 80–90% of depression in heavy drinkers was assumed to be secondary to alcohol use, but large epidemiological studies now suggest that a diagnosis of alcohol misuse is as likely to pre- as post-date the onset of affective disorders (Merikangas et al 1996). In women, major depression tends to precede drinking, while in men, depression follows on from drinking. Similarly, anxiety disorders tend to precede the onset of alcohol-use disorders more commonly in women than men. The incidence of depressive symptoms falls with abstinence,

but careful assessment is required and treatment must be instituted as untreated depression may precipitate relapse. SSRIs are usually preferable to older antidepressants as they are safer. Dysphoria in the weeks following withdrawal is common and it takes time for appetite and sleep to return to normal. Alcohol may interfere with treatment efficacy and compliance with other psychotropic medication and may lead to a pharmacological nihilism in some current drinkers who are upset at remaining depressed while taking their medication. The commencement of their prescription can be contingent upon achieving a period of abstinence to permit accurate assessment and diagnosis, which can form part of a motivational contract. Clinicians and patients should wait for 2–4 weeks, after withdrawal completion, before commencing antidepressant medication, to see if depressive symptoms resolve spontaneously. Patients should be encouraged to keep a mood diary to highlight the association between abstinence and mood improvement. If abstinence is not followed by an improvement in mood then antidepressant medication should be commenced in conjunction with appropriate counselling (Winstock 2006). Monitoring of mood through diaries, rating scales and regular clinical review should form part of routine relapse prevention and ongoing counselling for these patients. This treatment pathway is illustrated in Figure 28.2.

Although the most widely available and accessible treatment for depression in those with alcohol dependence is antidepressant medication, psychological treatments for depression (CBT) have been shown to be effective both in improving depression and in reducing alcohol consumption.

The degree to which the co-morbidity of affective disorders and alcohol dependence is genetically mediated is unclear and may vary with gender. The US National Comorbidity Study (Kessler et al 1997) reported that among women with alcohol dependence, 86% and 72% had a co-morbid lifetime psychiatric or drug use disorder, respectively, compared with 78% and 57%, respectively for men. Recent twin studies assessing co-morbidity between major depression and alcoholism in women suggest that the co-occurrence of the disorders may be largely genetic (Kendler et al 1993), although in men, the nature of the association is less clear. Such gender differences also exist in the relative prevalence of different disorders. For example, in men, drug disorders and dissocial psychological disorder are the most co-morbid conditions compared to mood and anxiety among women. Depression may also occur as a direct result of the pharmacological effects of alcohol as well as in response to the complications of alcohol use. Other explanations for the association may include shared family environment, poverty, social isolation and unemployment, or both conditions may develop as secondary features of other disorders such as personality disorder, polysubstance abuse and Briquet syndrome.

Suicide

About one-quarter of people dependent on alcohol attempt suicide, and lifetime risk of suicide is estimated at 3–4% (Edwards et al 1997). Depression is implicated in at least half of the suicides and the attempt is often preceded by an increase in very heavy drinking. Risk factors for suicide in alcoholics are similar to those in the general population.

Dissocial personality disorder

In keeping with the Cloniger subtyping of alcohol dependence, those with dissocial personality disorder have an earlier onset of alcohol use disorders, higher rates of drug use and poorer treatment retention and outcome. Risk assessment and a forensic history should routinely be sought.

Pathological jealousy (Othello syndrome)

This is characterized by the abnormal belief (delusion or over-valued idea) of infidelity of the sexual partner, although the actual fact of infidelity may or may not be true. In those with alcohol problems the male:female ratio is 2:1. The predominant characteristic is the abnormal quality of the belief and the accompanying behavioural constellation, such as the inspection of underwear or sheets for staining, searching of clothes and inspection of diaries, in an attempt to prove the infidelity. Repetitive demand for proof may lead to severe aggression and murder and therefore specific enquiry into past and threatened violence is mandatory and the partner should be advised of any risk. In a high-security hospital study, 14% of convicted murderers had this diagnosis (Mowat 1966). The syndrome is not unique to alcohol, with other causes including organic disorders, paranoid personality and the bipolar and schizophrenic psychoses. Abstinence and possibly hospitalization with treatment with antipsychotics may be indicated. In some, however, geographical separation is the only effective means of intervention (see Chs 19 and 23).

Anxiety states

According to the 'anxiety reduction' theory, alcoholics self-medicate what otherwise might be disabling anxiety. Although a review by Cook et al (1998) concludes 'anxiety traits do not appear to be an *important* (my italics) causal factor in alcoholism', in combination with learning theory it may be regarded as one route to alcohol abuse. Conflicting evidence demonstrating that alcohol may increase, decrease or not effect anxiety levels further complicates the picture. However, clinical studies (Allan 1995) consistently report an association between alcohol problems with rates of co-morbidity of between 20% and 30%. The most common anxiety state is panic disorder (3F:M), followed by obsessive–compulsive disorder (OCD) and phobias. Social phobia tends to precede drinking problems, the later presumably self-medicating anxiety. The relative risk for alcohol disorders among those with social phobia is about twice that of the general population (Marshall 1994). There is evidence that buspirone may be helpful in managing persistent anxiety and may increase retention in treatment.

PTSD

Alcohol use disorder is the most common co-morbid diagnosis of men with PTSD, though PTSD is more common in women (25% vs 10%). CNS depressants are a means of dampening the pathological state of hyperarousal associated with PTSD. It has been suggested that the sympathetic hyperactivity that occurs on withdrawal from alcohol can precipitate symptoms of PTSD and be a negative reinforcer for continued consumption.

Eating disorders

Up to 30% of young women with a serious drinking problem have had a significant eating disorder (most commonly bulimia) at some time (Lacey & Moureli 1986), and prevalence rates of alcohol misuse in people with bulimia are between 9% and 49% (Goldbloom 1993).

Other drug use

Dependence upon another drug is the most frequent co-morbid disorder in someone with an existing dependence syndrome; most commonly used are sedatives, such as benzodiazepines and clomethiazole.

Social consequences of excessive alcohol use

Employment

Turning up late for work may be the first indicator of an alcohol problem. Acute and chronic consumption is associated with both accidental injury and reduced productivity. Alcohol has been implicated in 40% of fatal industrial accidents and 35% of non-fatal work-related accidents.

Family

Heavy drinking imposes considerable strain on finances and is associated with increased rates of physical and sexual abuse. Children are at increased risk of conduct disorder and juvenile delinquency as well as developing alcohol misuse themselves. Children of problem drinkers have been called the 'forgotten children' and have to contend not only with the disruption to their own lives but often also having to care for their parents.

Crime and violence

About 66% of male and 15% of female prisoners have serious drinking problems, with higher rates for illicit drug use. Alcohol is strongly associated with violence (including domestic) and public affray. A Scottish study (Gillies 1976) of 400 people accused of murder showed over half were intoxicated at the time of the alleged attack (as were a third of their victims). Alcohol is also associated with rape (40–70%) and paedophile offences.

Drinking and driving

The peak age for drink-driving convictions is 21, with a third of convictions arising in those aged under 26. Over three-quarters of fatal road traffic accidents involve alcohol, and alcohol-related road traffic accidents are more severe than those in which alcohol does not play a role. About one-third of pedestrians killed by day and two-thirds killed at night have measurable blood alcohol levels. The UK legal maximum limit is 80 mg alcohol per 100 mL blood.

Alcohol withdrawal

On the cessation of alcohol, the previously adaptive changes in neurotransmitter function that contribute (along with hepatic metabolic changes) to the development of tolerance become maladaptive, resulting in an excitatory state arising from unopposed glutaminergic activity. It exists in a spectrum of severity, onset and duration and outcomes.

Withdrawal often commences before the blood alcohol level reaches zero following cessation (or marked reduction) of use in the dependant drinker. The symptoms and severity vary between individuals and usually commence 6–24 h after last use, peaking at day 2–3, with the highest risk of fits in the first 24–36 h. Some dependent drinkers may experience no or only minimal withdrawal, with just a few days of insomnia and irritability a couple of days after their last drink. More severely dependent drinkers are woken by withdrawal symptoms within a few hours of their last drink as the blood plasma levels fall, necessitating the immediate consumption of alcohol to relieve the symptoms.

Repeated alcohol withdrawal episodes may be associated with a kindling effect, such that subsequent episodes of withdrawal become more severe. Other factors implicated in the severity of withdrawal include amount and duration of drinking, the use of other sedative drugs such as benzodiazepines and intercurrent medical illnesses.

Alcohol withdrawal features

- **Early (12–24 h):** sweating, tachycardia, increased blood pressure, tremor, nausea, anorexia and vomiting, agitation, anxiety and panic, insomnia and restlessness, transient auditory hallucinations
- **Middle (24–72 h):** temperature elevation, dehydration, grand mal seizures (associated with low K^+ and Mg^{++}), delirium tremens with misperception, loss of insight and visual and/or auditory hallucinations. Tactile disturbances such as pins and needles, burning, crawling and numbness, 'electric flea' tactile hallucinations
- **Late (72+ h):** persistent insomnia and nightmares, tremor and confusion, hallucinosis.

Detoxification and withdrawal management

All patients withdrawing from alcohol will benefit from support; a proportion will require pharmacotherapy (Taylor et al 2009). Medically-assisted detoxification is not a standalone treatment. Its function lies on a spectrum from an elective admission as part of a planned attempt at abstinence with well considered aftercare plans to a crisis harm-reduction admission, prompted by a severe withdrawal or physical frailty. Detoxification should ideally only be undertaken after a full assessment with a treatment plan that outlines not only immediate treatment but also considers broader psychosocial issues that may be risk factors for relapse on discharge. The relapse rate following treatment is high. Some 60% return to problem drinking within a year. Incomplete attempts at detoxification can lead to nihilism in the patient. Liaison between referrer, general practitioner (GP), specialist, aftercare providers and client should begin before treatment and continue after detoxification.

In most cases, withdrawal can be safely managed in the community with the support of a GP or community drug team. Stable accommodation and the commitment of a responsible carer are essential components for any community-based detoxification attempt. In the absence of such supports or in the presence of contraindications to outpatient detoxification, such as a history of delirium tremens (Box 28.8), the patient should be admitted to hospital.

Treatment regimen for medically assisted withdrawal from alcohol

After a full history and examination, treatment of withdrawal should be implemented at the earliest point to minimize the risk of fits. The choice of benzodiazepine should be contingent upon the circumstances, e.g. diazepam may be preferred for medically assisted withdrawal in those with a previous history of seizures, and oxazepam in those with impaired liver function (Taylor et al 2009). In uncomplicated withdrawal, chlordiazepoxide is the benzodiazepine of choice, as it has an intermediate half-life, rapid onset of action and low dependence-forming potential.

Clomethiazole (Heminevrin) should be avoided because of the risk of severe interactions (respiratory depression in overdose) and risk of abuse. Carbamazepine and barbiturates are also effective detoxification agents, but are rarely used. Although not licensed for use in the UK, GHB (γ-hydroxybutyrate) is an effective agent for alcohol withdrawal and has been used in parts of Europe (Beghè & Campanini 2000).

Explanation of symptoms, their progress and how medication helps should be given to all clients, preferably before the commencement of detox. Patients will often be agitated throughout withdrawal and explanations and information may need to be repeated.

Box 28.8

Indications for inpatient detoxification

- Past history of withdrawal seizures or epilepsy
- Co-morbid severe mental illness
- Elderly/frail patients
- Homeless or without a carer
- Intercurrent acute illness
- Repeated failed outpatient attempts.

to do something their doctors tell them to do; people change their behaviours when they perceive that they are able to and that they will benefit. The results of the Project MATCH study in America showed little difference in outcome between MET, CBT and the 12-step facilitation psychological treatments and suggested little was gained from matching patient attributes to therapies (Project MATCH 1997).

Brief interventions

Randomized controlled trials have consistently demonstrated the efficacy of brief interventions, showing positive benefits for patients who are not dependent on alcohol. Consisting of an assessment of alcohol intake, information on harmful drinking and clear advice for the individual, brief interventions have consistently been shown to reduce intake by about 25% (see also Box 28.10 and Babor et al 2001). Further evidence suggests that brief interventions are as effective as more expensive specialist treatments. Tiered care delivery with the sequential delivery of increasingly intensive care is an appropriate treatment pathway for many, while attempts at remaining in contact with clients through extended case monitoring can also be useful. A recent Cochrane review (McQueen et al 2009) reported that following brief interventions delivered to heavy alcohol users admitted to general hospital, their alcohol consumption may be reduced at the 1-year follow-up.

Alcoholics Anonymous

Founded by recovering alcoholics 'Dr Bob' and 'Bill W' in 1935, AA now represents the largest self-help group in the world, with 5–10% of treatment enlisted alcoholics attending. For some it is a panacea, for others another failed therapy. Based on 12 steps (see: www.aa.org/en_pdfs/smf-121_en.pdf), the premise is that alcoholism is a disease without cure that can only be held at bay one day at a time. The fellowship provides friendship, advice and support and takes place at meetings with both diverse clientele and location. Clients admit their powerlessness over the disease and look to a higher power to return their sanity. AA remains a cheap, widely available form of support and all alcoholics should be encouraged to attend at least a dozen or so different meetings to see if the format suits them. Al-Anon and Al-Teen provide support for family members of alcohol dependent individuals.

Residential rehabilitation

These houses are a popular though expensive means of consolidating upon initial abstinence. Often based on the 'Minnesota model' (the first five steps of the 12 AA steps), additional

---

Box 28.10

Elements of brief interventions

- Present screening results
- Identify risks and discuss consequences
- Provide medical advice
- Solicit patient commitment
- Identify goal – reduced drinking or abstinence
- Give advice and encouragement.

See Babor et al (2001).

---

interventions include social skills training, relaxation techniques and structured relapse prevention programmes. They vary greatly in outcome but can be effective for some patients at a particular stage in their drinking careers.

Provision of service

Primary care is a highly suitable environment for the early detection and treatment of alcohol disorders. Support from specialist services should extend to general hospital services, especially emergency departments and trauma wards. Community alcohol teams should liaise between the hospital and GP-based services and where possible, support treatment within the community. Specialized assessments may be needed for pregnant women and patients being considered for liver transplant.

Prognosis

Recovery is a process, not an event. Outcome should be assessed by psychosocial functioning and health as well as actual alcohol intake. A poor prognosis is associated with alcoholic brain damage, co-morbid psychiatric disorder, divorced status, criminal record, low IQ, poor support and motivation.

The Rand report (Armor et al 1976), a multicentre trial with an 18-month follow-up, showed only one-quarter of patients remained abstinent for 6 months, with less than 10% at 18 months. However, there were persistent reductions in levels of consumption in over 70% at follow-up.

Edwards' follow-up of alcoholics over 10 years found that 25% had continued troubled drinking and 12% were abstinent (Edwards et al 1988). The remainder had a patchwork of abstinence and troubled drinking.

A 60-year follow-up of two American groups of socially divergent drinkers (Harvard graduates and socially disadvantaged Boston adolescents) demonstrates the varied outcomes of those with drinking problems (Valiant 2003). At some point, about one-quarter of both groups met the criteria for alcohol abuse. In general, the death rate among those with an alcohol dependence is two to three times higher than the normal population, with the excess deaths attributable to cirrhosis, unnatural causes, lung and oropharyngeal cancers, and cardiovascular disease. The increase in mortality was twice as great for those under 60 than over 60; indeed alcohol dependence was rare after 70 (half had died and one-fifth had achieved long-term abstinence). Other than severity of dependence, the predictors of a positive outcome were: (1) finding a non-pharmacological substitute for alcohol; (2) new relationships; and (3) compulsory contingency supervision (immediate adverse consequence on consumption) or membership of a spiritual group. Men who achieved abstinence had attended on average 20 times more AA meetings than men who continued to drink. Finally, the study suggested that those severely dependent drinkers, with early onset and genetic loading for dependence from socially disadvantaged backgrounds, were more likely to achieve stable abstinence than other men. In summary, Valiant (2003) suggests, '… the most and the least severe alcoholics appeared to enjoy the best, long term chance of remission'.

Further reading

Spanagel, R., 2009. Alcoholism: a systems approach from molecular physiology to addictive behavior. Physiol. Rev. 89, 649–705.

Vengeliene, V., Bilbao, A., Molander, A., et al., 2008. Neuropharmacology of alcohol addiction. Br. J. Pharmacol. 154, 299–315.

References

Addolorato, G., Leggio, L., Anna Ferrulli, A., et al., 2007. Effectiveness and safety of baclofen for maintenance of alcohol abstinence in alcohol-dependent patients with liver cirrhosis: randomised, double-blind controlled study. Lancet 370, 1915–1922.

Allan, C.A., 1995. Alcohol problems and anxiety disorders: a critical review. Alcohol Alcohol. 30, 145–151.

Armor, D.J., Polich, J.M., Stambul, H.B., 1976. Alcoholism and treatment. Rand Corporation and Interscience, Santa Monica.

Babor, T.F., Higgins-Biddle, J.L., Saunders, J.B., et al., 2001. The alcohol use disorders identification test – guidelines for use in primary care, second ed. World Health Organization, Geneva.

Beghè, F., Campanini, M.T., 2000. Safety and tolerability of gamma-hydroxybutyric acid in the treatment of alcohol-dependent patients. Alcohol 20, 223–225.

Besson, J.A., 1993. Structural and functional brain imaging in alcoholism and drug use. Curr. Opin. Psychiatry 6, 403–410.

Cloninger, C.R., Bohman, M., Sigvardsson, S., 1981. Inheritance of alcohol abuse cross fostering: analysis of adopted men. Arch. Gen. Psychiatry 38, 861–868.

Cook, C.H.C., Hallwood, P.M., Thomson, A.D., 1998. B vitamin deficiency and neuropsychiatric syndromes in alcohol misuse. Alcohol Alcohol. 33, 317–336.

Crabbe, J.C., Phillips, T.J., Harris, R.A., et al., 2006. Alcohol-related genes: contributions from studies with genetically engineered mice. Addict. Biol. 11, 195–269.

Dimeff, L., Marlatt, G., 1995. Relapse prevention. In: Hester, R.K., Miller, W.R. (Eds.), The handbook of alcoholism treatment approaches: effective alternatives. Allyn & Bacon, Boston MA, pp. 174–196.

DoH, 2008a. Safe, sensible, social – consultation on further action. Department of Health, London.

DoH, 2008b. The cost of alcohol harm to the NHS in England: an update to the Cabinet Office study 2003. HIAT. Department of Health, London.

Edwards, G., Gross, M., 1976. Alcohol dependence: provisional description of a clinical syndrome. Br. Med. J. 1, 1058.

Edwards, G., Brown, D., Oppenheimer, E., et al., 1988. Long term outcome for patients with alcohol problems: the search for predictors. Br. J. Addict. 82, 801–811.

Edwards, G., Marshall, E.J., Cook, C.C., 1997. The treatment of drinking problems: a guide for the helping professions. Cambridge University Press, Cambridge, p. 95.

Furieri, F.A., Nakamura-Palacios, E.M., 2007. Gabapentin reduces alcohol consumption and craving: a randomized, double-blind, placebo-controlled trial. J. Clin. Psychiatry 68, 1691–1700.

Gilboa, A., Alain, C., Stuss, D.T., et al., 2006. Mechanisms of spontaneous confabulations: a strategic retrieval account. Brain 129, 1399–1414.

Gillies, H., 1976. Homicide in the west of Scotland. Br. J. Psychiatry 128, 105–127.

Goldbloom, D.S., 1993. Alcohol misuse and eating disorders: aspects of an association. Alcohol Alcohol. 28, 375–381.

Golovko, I., Golovko, S.I., Leontieva, L.V., et al., 2002. The influence of ethanol on the functional status of GABAA receptors. Biochemistry 67, 719–729.

Goodwin, D.W., Hermansen, L., Guze, S.B., et al., 1973. Alcohol problems in adoptees raised apart from alcoholic biological parents. Arch. Gen. Psychiatry 28, 238–243.

Grant, B.F., Dawson, D.A., 1997. Age at onset of alcohol use and its association with DSM-IV alcohol abuse and dependence: results from the National Longitudinal Alcohol Epidemiologic Survey. J. Subst. Abuse 9, 103–110.

Grønbæk, M., 2006. Factors influencing the relation between alcohol and cardiovascular disease. Curr. Opin. Lipidol. 17, 17–21.

Harper, C.G., Kril, J.J., Hollowat, R.L., 1985. Brain shrinkage in chronic alcoholics: a pathological study. Br. Med. J. 290, 501–504.

Hodgins, D.C., el-Guebaly, N., Addington, J., 1997. Treatment of substance abusers: single or mixed gender programmes? Addiction 92, 805–812.

Hrubec, Z., Omenn, G.S., 1981. Evidence of genetic predisposition to alcoholic psychosis and cirrhosis: twin concordances for alcoholism and its biological end points by zygosity among male veterans. Alcohol. Clin. Exp. Res. 5, 207–215.

Institute of Alcohol Studies, 2004. Excessive and problem drinking in Great Britain. Online. Available: www.ias.org.ukwww.ias.org.uk.

Johnson, B.A., Rosenthal, N., Capece, J.A., et al., 2007. Topiramate for treating alcohol dependence: a randomized controlled trial. J. Am. Med. Assoc. 298, 1641.

Jones, K.L., Smith, D.W., 1973. Recognition of the fetal alcohol syndrome in infancy. Lancet ii, 999–1001.

Kendler, K.S., Heath, A.C., Neale, M.C., et al., 1992. A population-based twin study of alcoholism in women. J. Am. Med. Assoc. 268, 1877–1882.

Kendler, K.S., Heath, A.C., Neale, M.C., et al., 1993. Alcoholism and major depression in women: a twin study of the causes of comorbidity. Arch. Gen. Psychiatry 50, 690–698.

Kessler, R.C., Crum, R.M., Warner, L.A., et al., 1997. Lifetime co-occurrence of DSM-IIIR alcohol abuse and dependence with other psychiatric disorders in the National Comorbidity Study. Archives of General Psychology 54, 313–321.

Kobayashi, T., Ikeda, K., Kojima, H., et al., 1999. Ethanol opens G-protein activated inwardly rectifying K+ channels. Nat. Neurosci. 2, 1091–1097.

Kopelman, M.D., Thomson, A.D., Guerrini, I., et al., 2009. The Korsakoff syndrome: clinical aspects, psychology and treatment. Alcohol Alcohol. 44, 148–154.

Kranzler, H.R., Rosenthal, R.N., 2003. Dual diagnosis: alcoholism and co-morbid psychiatric disorders. Am. J. Addict. 12, S26–S40.

Lacey, J.H., Moureli, E., 1986. Bulimic alcoholics: some features of a clinical sub-group. Br. J. Addict. 81, 389–393.

Lewohl, J.M., Wilson, W.R., Mayfield, R.D., et al., 1999. G protein-coupled inwardly rectifying potassium channels are targets of alcohol action. Nat. Neurosci. 2, 1084–1090.

Littleton, J., Little, H., 1994. Current concepts of ethanol dependence. Addiction 89, 1397–1412.

Lovinger, D.M., 1999. 5-HT3 receptors and the neural actions of alcohols: an increasingly exciting topic. Neurochem. Int. 35, 125–130.

Marlatt, G., Gordon, J., 1985. Relapse prevention: maintenance strategies in the treatment of addictive behaviours. Guildford Press, New York.

Marshall, J.R., 1994. The diagnosis and treatment of social phobia and alcohol abuse. Bull. Menninger Clin. 58, 58–66.

Mayfield, R.D., Harris, R.A., Schuckit, M.A., 2008. Genetic factors influencing alcohol dependence. Br. J. Pharmacol. 154, 275–287.

McKee, S., Harrison, E., O' Malley, S., et al., 2009. Varenicline reduces alcohol self-administration in heavy-drinking smokers. Biol. Psychiatry 66, 185–190.

McQueen, J., Howe, T.E., Allan, L., et al., 2009. Brief Interventions for heavy alcohol users admitted to general hospital wards. Cochrane Database Syst. Rev. (3), CD005191.

Merikangas, K.R., Angst, J., Eaton, W., et al., 1996. Comorbidity and boundaries of affective disorders with anxiety disorders and substance misuse; results of an international task force. Br. J. Psychiatry 168 (Suppl.), 58–67.

Miller, W.R., 1992. Effectiveness of treatment for substance abuse: reasons for optimism. J. Subst. Abuse Treat. 9, 93–102.

Miller, W.R., Rollnick, S., 1991. Motivational interviewing: preparing people to change addictive behaviour. Guilford Press, New York.

Mowat, R.R., 1966. Morbid jealousy and murder. Tavistock, London.

NHS, 2009. Statistics on Alcohol. The Health and Information centre, NHS, England. Online. Available: www.ic.nhs.uk/webfiles/ publications/alcoholeng2009/Final% 20Format%20draft%202009%20v7.pdf.

NICE National Institute for Clinical Excellence, 2008. Antenatal care: routine care for the healthy pregnant woman. NICE clinical guideline 62. Office of Population, Census and Statistics 1996 report. Her Majesty's Stationery Office, London.

Paille, F.M., Guelfi, J.D., Perkins, A.C., et al., 1995. Double blind multicentre trial

of acamprosate in maintaining abstinence from alcohol. Alcohol Alcohol. 30, 239–247.

Pickens, R.W., Svikis, D.S., McGue, M., et al., 1991. Heterogeneity in the inheritance of alcoholism: a study of male and female twins. Arch. Gen. Psychiatry 48, 19–28.

Polycarpou, A., Papanikolaou, P., Ioannidis, J.P., et al., 2005. Anticonvulsants for alcohol withdrawal. Cochrane Database Syst. Rev. (3) CD005064.

Project MATCH, 1997. Matching alcoholism treatments to client heterogeneity: Project MATCH posttreatment drinking outcomes. J. Stud. Alcohol 58, 7–29.

Reiger, D.A., Farmer, M.E., Rae, D.S., et al., 1991. Comorbidity of mental disorders with alcohol and other drug abuse results from the epidemiological and catchment area (ECA) study. J. Am. Med. Assoc. 264, 2511.

Siegmund, S., Vengeliene, V., Singer, M.V., et al., 2005. Influence of age at drinking onset on long-term ethanol self administration with deprivation and stress phases. Alcohol.Clin. Exp. Res. 29, 1139–1145.

Spanagel, R., 2009. Alcoholism: a systems approach from molecular physiology to addictive behavior. Physiol. Rev. 89, 649–705.

Spear, L.P., Varlinskaya, E.I., 2005. Adolescence. Alcohol sensitivity, tolerance and intake. Recent Dev. Alcohol. 17, 143–159.

Steinhausen, H.C., Willms, J., Spohr, H.L., 1993. Correlates of psychopathology and

intelligence in children with fetal alcohol syndrome. J. Clin. Psychiatry 35, 323–331.

Taylor, D., Paton, C., Kapur, S., 2009. The Maudsley prescribing guidelines, tenth ed. Informa Healthcare, London.

Thomson, A.D., 2000. Mechanisms of vitamin deficiency in chronic alcohol misusers and the development of the Wernicke Korsakoff syndrome. Alcohol Alcohol. 35, 2–7.

Valiant, G.E., 2003. A 60 year follow up of alcoholic men. Addiction 98, 1043–1051.

Vengeliene, V., Bilbao, A., Molander, A., et al., 2008. Neuropharmacology of alcohol addiction. Br. J. Pharmacol. 154, 299–315.

Victor, M., Adams, R.D., Collins, G.H., 1971. Wernicke–Korsakoff syndrome. FA Davis, Philadelphia.

Wallace, P., Haines, A., 1985. The use of a questionnaire in general practice to increase the recognition of patients with excessive alcohol use. Br. Med. J. 290, 1949–1953.

Wang, X., Wang, G., Lemos, J.R., et al., 1994. Ethanol directly modulates gating of a dihydropyridine-sensitive Ca2+ channel in neurohypophysial terminals. J. Neurosci. 14, 5453–5460.

Winstock, A.R., 2006. CanDo: Australian General Practice Network. Online. Available: www. agpncando.com/clinical_education/index. html.

Psychoactive drug misuse

29

Adam R. Winstock

CHAPTER CONTENTS

is thought to be the central neurotransmitter in this process it is becoming clear that many others such as glutamate, 5HT and GABA have major but as yet unclear roles.

The reinforcing properties or the use/abuse liabilities of substances differ between drug classes but can also be impacted significantly by a number of other factors, namely the 'effect profile' (intensity of the effect, the speed of onset and duration of action), which is impacted upon by the dose, preparation, purity and route of administration. The effect profile and its relationship to abuse liability can be broadly expressed in an equation:

$$\text{Abuse liability} = \frac{\text{Intensity of effect}}{\text{Speed of onset} \times \text{duration of action}}$$

Generally, the quicker the onset (smoking and injecting), the shorter the high (crack) and the more intense the high (crack) the more reinforcing the substance and the more frequent the desire and/or need for administrations. Higher potency preparations of a substance are typically more reinforcing than less potent ones (e.g. cocaine powder versus coca leaves) because they are associated with higher plasma levels which in turn are often related to the more direct routes of administration that purified products permit. For example, cigarettes act as a highly reinforcing nicotine delivery system that requires smokers to light up hourly as plasma levels drop to the point where craving begins. An understanding of the interplay between route and duration of action helps explain why slower delivery systems such as patches are used to wean smokers off nicotine since longer-acting less intense effects are less reinforcing and easier to refrain from. A similar explanation in part helps us understand why long-acting orally active methadone is used in the management of opioid dependence.

The effect of drugs

The effect of a drug will depend upon the interplay of cognitive 'set' (mood state the person was in at the time of drug consumption), environmental 'setting' (social situation – including the mood of those one is with – in which the drug was taken) as well as the dose, type and purity of drug. As the dose of a drug increases, the role of the environment becomes less while the pharmacologically mediated ones of arousal or sedation become more marked.

Prevalence of substance abuse

Almost two-thirds of those aged 16–24 years have taken an illicit drug in 'the last year'. In the UK, cannabis is the mostly widely used drug with almost 3 million users reporting use in the last year. There has been an increase in *last year* use of Class A drugs among 16–59-year-olds between 1996 (2.7%) and 2008/2009 (3.7%), largely attributable to the rise in the use of cocaine (0.6–3%). It is also probable that there is an increasing population of those over 60 who use drugs but they are missed in general population studies and may be more likely to present through general medical and old age psychiatry services.

The 1996 OPCS survey of psychiatric morbidity in the UK population showed the prevalence of substance abuse to be 4.7% for alcohol dependence and 2.2% for drug dependence (Meltzer et al 1996). The American 1991 ECA study (Reiger et al 1990) reported even higher figures, with a lifetime prevalence of 13.5% alcohol abuse; 6.1% substance abuse disorder; 3.2% co-morbid substance abuse and other mental disorder; with male:female ratios of 2:1 for alcohol and 4:1 for substance use disorders.

Aetiology

Constitutional, environmental and childhood factors contribute the majority of risk for developing substance use disorders (Fig. 29.1). Often, there is an interplay of various risk factors, each compounding the other, giving rise to an 'interactive web of causation'. Risk factors such as: positive family histories; childhood abuse; disorganized neighbourhoods; poor academic attainment; limited opportunity and expectation for success; conduct disorder; attention deficit hyperactivity disorder (ADHD); depression or post-traumatic shock disorder (PTSD), often exist in a matrix devoid of protective factors, such as love, achievement, family and religion. Some of the most important aetiological factors are briefly covered below.

Individual factors

Genetics

Overall, the heritability of dependence (not use or abuse) is believed to be around 30–40%. It has been suggested that certain D2 polymorphisms coding for the dopamine receptor may underlie vulnerability to substance dependence through coding for personality traits (Blum et al 1995) such as a 'reward deficiency syndrome'. Similarly the DA D4 polymorphism, associated with the behavioural trait of thrill seeking and attention deficit disorder is considered by some to be an indirect risk factor for substance abuse. Genes also modify the subjective responses to drugs and may influence the risk of abuse by predisposing to psychiatric and personality disorders.

Personality

Despite 100 years of searching, the Holy Grail of the addictive personality remains elusive, probably because it does not exist. What has become recognized are a number of personality traits that may predispose to or otherwise associate with drug use. For example, both dissocial personality disorder and emotionally unstable 'impulsive' (borderline) personality disorder are associated with substance use, with early antisocial behaviour being one of the best predictors of later drug dependence. Both novelty seeking and low impulse control are also associated, with Cloniger (1994) suggesting that those who are high in novelty seeking and low in harm avoidance may be more prone to substance misuse. Experimentation with drugs is one of number of risk activities that many people engage in at some point in their lives. Whether or not initial use progresses to abuse and dependence will be the result of large number of other factors.

Psychological models

See section on Alcohol aetiology in Chapter 28.

Social

Social deprivation, dysfunctional neighbourhoods, childhood abuses, peer group selection and influence, familial drug use, cultural attitudes and drug availability all contribute to the social matrix that the individual's drug use is placed within. Demographic variables such as unemployment, gender, and age are obviously also important.

Dual diagnosis

Given the ubiquitous presence of drug misuse across social classes and races, the likelihood of psychiatric patients presenting with problems related to their use is commonplace. Consequently, the dual diagnosis patient (one with a severe mental illness and co-morbid problematic use of substances, not just dependence), is becoming the rule and not the exception in many inner cities and now represents perhaps the most needy, but most poorly-resourced group in the whole of psychiatry.

Two recent community studies reveal the high rates of co-existence of these disorders. A Camberwell study (Johnson 1997) reported about one-third of patients attached to a community mental health team had concurrent alcohol or substance misuse problems. A more recent four-city study of community mental health attendees suggested even higher figures with 44% reporting past year harmful use of alcohol and or problem drug use. Conversely, three-quarters of drug service and over 80% of alcohol service clients reported past year psychiatric disorder (Weaver et al 2003). Cannabis was the drug most frequently reported by problem drug users, although one-quarter also reported drinking at harmful levels, with 10% experiencing severe alcohol problems.

The co-morbidity of substance use and mental illness results in uniformly poor prognosis (Box 29.1). Adherence to treatment by people with psychiatric disorders is often poor. It is even worse among those who use substances. For example, Owen et al (1996) looked at compliance among 161 patients with schizophrenia and found that they were eight times more

Box 29.1

Associations of co-morbidity

- Increased rates of psychiatric admission – longer admissions, shorter remissions, higher rates of sectioning
- Increased rates of violence
- Increased rates of suicidal behaviour
- Increased rates of health service utilization
- Increased rates of non-compliance with treatment
- Increased rates of depot and high dose neuroleptic treatment
- Increased rates of homelessness, unemployment and imprisonment
- Poorer treatment access and efficacy
- Poorer treatment outcomes in both substance use and psychiatric treatment populations.

Box 29.2

How drugs exacerbate mental illness through their pharmacological effects

- Compound pre-existing 'cognitive set', e.g. anxiety, paranoia
- Direct pharmacological effects, e.g. positive symptoms with stimulants
- Antagonize medication effect centrally, e.g. cannabis on neuroleptic medication
- Metabolic interactions, e.g. cytochrome P450 induction/inhibition
- Impair already compromised information processing system reducing efficacy of psychological/cognitive therapies.

likely to be non-compliant with their medication than those who did not abuse substances and this was associated with worst symptoms at 6 months. Explanations for poorer compliance may include a poorer understanding of the nature of the illness and benefits of medication, more difficulty in engagement and retention in treatment contact outside the hospital setting, less family support and possibly higher rates of side-effects due to higher dose of medication. Higher doses may be needed because of drug-exacerbated positive symptoms, as well as direct antagonism of neuroleptics (e.g. cannabis). Compliance therapy based on motivational interviewing is useful in improving compliance and treatment outcome.

Possible explanations for the high rates of co-morbidity (other than a common environmental or genetic predisposition) include:

- Substance use may lead to psychological problems as a direct result of toxicity or indirectly as a consequence of the psychosocial consequences of drug use. Frequently, substance use will aggravate a pre-existing psychiatric condition (Box 29.2).
- Psychiatric illness may lead to self-medication with psychoactive substances in an attempt to relieve the distress of the illness or the side-effects of treatment they are prescribed, e.g. fatigue, mental sluggishness with neuroleptics.
- A shared common environment characterized by other factors such as socioeconomic disadvantage, emotional deprivation, social disorganization, childhood abuse, genetic loading and adult trauma.

Since high rates of co-morbidity initially found in clinical settings were replicated in the community, it is unlikely that the association is solely attributable to the over-representation of co-morbid cases in treatment settings.

Management

Current issues in service delivery to this group include polarization of specialities and the complexity and severity of the client group. In addition, specialist addiction services focus on alcohol and opiate dependence, while the most problematic and frequent substance use patterns for those in mental health are those of non-dependent use of cannabis, stimulants and alcohol. Harm reduction interventions should be a primary consideration, since this group are at higher than normal risk for blood-borne virus (BBV) transmission, and sexually transmitted diseases. Engagement with support focusing on the client's priorities such as housing and welfare then permit the opportunity for introducing other effective interventions such as cognitive behavioural therapy, motivational interviewing and compliance with appropriate pharmacotherapies. Those receiving supervised methadone or buprenorphine may usefully have their other psychotropic medication dispensed at the same time to enhance compliance. Unfortunately, they are a difficult group to engage and maintain contact with. This has prompted the development of small caseload, assertive outreach, dual diagnosis teams. There is little evidence so far to support any particular model for dual diagnosis care.

Taking a drug history

In order to provide the most optimal treatment, a complete assessment of drug use is required.

- **What drug/s:** what are they currently using (illegal, legal, prescribed, not prescribed, over-the-counter). The last three days' use is a good guide based on recent recall by the client.
- **How much:** quantity (weight, money spent, number of pills, etc.). The amount of a substance used frequently varies depending on the day of week, funds and other responsibilities. Ask minimum and maximum amounts used and consequences of binge use.
- **How often:** frequency (times per day, days in the last month), duration of consumption at current level and recent life events/stressors that may lead to a change in use.
- **How they are taken:** route of administration. Do not assume all drugs meant for oral consumption are swallowed. They may be injected.
- **The impact of their drug use:** explain to the client that you need to understand the impact their drug use has on their day-to-day activities. Asking about a typical day can highlight risky behaviours and reveal dependence criteria.
- **Ask at what time they wake up and why.** People may wake early because of depression or symptoms of withdrawal.
- **Ask them how they feel when they wake up.** Those dependent on drugs often report feeling 'sick' or unwell. If they report the latter, ask them to describe their symptoms of withdrawal. It may also be useful to ask those who do not wake because of withdrawal, how long after waking do they experience withdrawals and/or first use of a substance.
- **Ask where and when the first use takes place.** Do they leave enough drugs at bedtime to have something to *relieve withdrawal* in the morning or do they need to obtain drugs after waking? This may identify risky behaviours (e.g. sex work, criminal activity) or other priorities such as childcare or work commitments.
- **Ask them how their days start.** Do they shower? Do they have breakfast? (Lack of nutrition is common in this group.) Ask how they spend their day. Who do they see? Where do they go? This may identify high risk behaviours (e.g. sharing of injecting equipment), as well as evidence suggesting *prioritizing drug-seeking and drug-using behaviour over other activities and neglecting activities/people unrelated to use.* Ask whether their days were always spent like this or whether they used to get pleasure from other hobbies and interests. This may allow the client to reflect positively on non-drug-using periods. Ask if they have *difficulty controlling* their use, i.e. using more than they want to or for longer periods. Do they *crave* drugs?

- **Ask about their social networks.**
- **Ask about evening activities.** What do they enjoy? Do they find it easy to get off to sleep? Do they lie awake, do they sleep straight through? Many drug users sleep badly and may chase sleep with a cocktail of depressant drugs, which represents increased risk to the person.
- **Their drug use history.** The age of their first use, regular use, onset of *tolerance* and withdrawals, and where indicated the transition from smoking to injecting. Ask about adverse consequences of use upon health, relationships, work, etc. and identify *continued use despite problems*.
- **Past treatments:** e.g. counselling, AA, pharmacotherapies, detoxification, maintenance, in- vs outpatient. Duration and number of abstinent periods. Circumstances of relapse. Ask about *reinstatement of a dependent pattern of use* after relapse, people with a history of dependence are unable to control their use once they return to their substance and it is usually only a matter of days or a few weeks before they return to dependent uncontrolled use.
- **Complications of drug use:** psychological, social and physical.

Investigations

Substance misuse must always be considered in young people presenting with psychological problems. A full physical examination may reveal stigmata of substance use (e.g. recent injection sites, old tracks, venous scarring, 'puffy hand syndrome', abscesses) and evidence of malnutrition or undetected infection. Laboratory confirmation of self-reported use should be sought, most commonly with urinalysis, though false negatives can arise through dilution or contamination of samples. In most treatment settings self-report is fairly reliable. Urine tests and their results should not result in punitive consequences for the client (e.g. being discharged from the programme) but should be used in discussion about changes in treatment approach. Urine tests can tell you if a drug has been used recently but not how much, though sequential urine samples can detect reductions in cannabis levels with abstinence. The time windows for detection after last use of commonly used illicit substances are given in Table 29.1.

More recently, hair analysis has been used to retrospectively detect drug use, with most illicit drugs becoming incorporated into the hair follicle 7–10 days after ingestion. More recent use can be detected with oral fluid testing. This is becoming increasingly commonplace in treatment settings, the work place and at the road side. Oral fluid samples are obtained by placing a swab in the mouth and it is considered less invasive than collecting other biological samples. The observed concentrations of basic drugs such as the amphetamines, cocaine and some opioids

Table 29.1 Detection of drug use through urinalysis

Drug[a]	Detection window[b]
Cannabis	3 days to 6 weeks
Heroin	2–3 days
Methadone	7–9 days
LSD (photolabile–store away from light)	1 day
Stimulants	1–3 days

[a]Drug terminology and classification.
[b]Detection window – length of time urine remains positive after last use.

are similar or higher than those in plasma. Tetrahydrocannabinol (THC) is detectable but impacted significantly by very recent use and sequestration. There is wide intra- and interpersonal variation in detected levels (Drummer 2006). Other biological samples that may be used to detect substance use include blood, sweat, finger nails, buccal scrapings, breast milk and if one felt so inclined, even semen.

Viral screens

HIV and AIDS

Among injecting drug users, the risk of viral transmission is high and routine testing should be available with counselling. Infection rates show wide geographic variation reflecting differing injecting patterns. Rates of HIV have fallen since the mid-1980s, with recent studies suggesting rates of less than 1% among the UK injecting population (Crawford 1997). Much of this reduction in prevalence has been due to the widespread availability of 'needle exchange' services and provision of services focused towards 'harm minimization'. Rates in countries without such access are higher, e.g. in Eastern Europe and parts of South-East Asia. Although opiate users represent the largest group of injecting drug users, some evidence suggests that rates among those who inject stimulant drugs may be higher due to the higher daily rates of administration and socializing effects

of stimulant drugs. Other groups that are at high risk are prison populations, where restricted access to clean equipment means injecting is more likely to involve sharing of needles, syringes and related paraphernalia. Antiretroviral medications may interfere with the metabolism of methadone.

Hepatitis B and C

Rates of 70% for hepatitis C and 20–40% for hepatitis B infection are found among injecting drug users. The higher virulence and hardiness of hepatitis C explains the rates of infectivity and the need to advise users that risks of sharing extend beyond needles and syringes to include spoons, filters, tourniquets, water, etc. High levels of alcohol consumption, common in many methadone maintenance clients, worsens prognosis significantly as does co-infection with hepatitis B or HIV. Hepatitis C-positive injecting drug users should be made aware of their status, supported to adopt healthier lower risk behaviours and encouraged to seek treatment which can be curative in 50–80% depending on genotype. The UK is yet to introduce universal hepatitis B vaccination, despite WHO guidelines set out in 1997, instead relying on selective testing and vaccination in high risk groups. Clinicians should continue to offer opportunistic testing and vaccination to injecting drug users. Rapid vaccination schedules over 3 weeks and contingency management may increase the likelihood of vaccination schedule completion.

Drugs of abuse

These are covered individually below. See Tables 29.2 and 29.3 for an overview of drug classification and clinical signs suggestive of use.

Opiates: opium, heroin, methadone and buprenorphine

Opium is derived from the ripe seed capsule of the poppy, *Papaver somniferum*. The extract contains morphine and codeine, alkaloid opiate analgesics. Heroin (diamorphine) and

Table 29.2 Drug terminology, classification and cost (at time of writing)

Drug type	Example	Slang	Cost
CNS depressants	Heroin, benzodiazepines, alcohol, barbiturates, GHB	Smack, gear, brown, H, jellies, mazzies, barbs, GBH, liquid E	Heroin: £35–£70/g (£10 bag = 0.1 g)
CNS stimulants	Cocaine, amphetamine, ecstasy, methamphetamine	Blow, Charlie, whiz, E pills, ice pills, crystal	Cocaine: £40–£70/g Crack: £10 rock = 0.1–0.25 g E: £3–£10
Cannabis	Herbal marijuana, hashish resin, hash oil	Hash, weed, puff, spliff, skunk, black	Hash: £15 per 1/8 oz Skunk grass: £25 per 1/8 oz (3.5 g)
Hallucinogens	LSD, psilocybin, mescaline, DMT, ketamine, PCP	Tabs, trips, blotters, K	LSD: £2.50–£5/tab
Solvents, volatile substances	Toluene, butane, N20 nitrates, solvents, glue	Whippets, gas, tins	£3 for a lighter refill; £4.50 for small pot of glue

Table 29.5 Methadone and buprenorphine compared

	Methadone	Buprenorphine
Pharmacology	μ-receptor agonist	μ-receptor partial agonist
Practical pharmacokinetics	Bigger doses increase agonist effect	Bigger doses increase duration of action
Optimal maintenance doses	80–120 mg/day	12–16 mg/day
The stable dose for an individual	The right dose of methadone or buprenorphine is one that keeps a person free from withdrawal between doses, results in the abolition or significant reduction in craving for and use of illicit opiates without causing significant side-effects	
Route of administration	Oral	Sublingual
Induction rate	Start low (20–30 mg/day) increasingly gradually over weeks	Start 4–8 mg, increase rapidly over a few days
Induction risk	Overdose	Precipitated withdrawal
Overdose risk	High in non-tolerant persons	Ceiling on respiratory depression means much safer in overdose

Treatment options

Treatment options for opiate dependence can broadly be divided into maintenance treatment (substitution therapy), detoxification and aftercare (recovery). Methadone and buprenorphine are effective pharmacological interventions for the management of opioid dependence. These medications differ in both their pharmacological and risk profile (Table 29.5). A large body of research indicates that better treatment outcomes are achieved with longer treatment duration and doses of methadone >60–80 mg/day. Poor clinical outcomes are seen in patients precipitously discharged from treatment, including an increase in heroin use and mortality rates (Zanis & Woody 1998). As with other psychiatric disorders, medication-based treatments are most effective if given in conjunction with psychosocial interventions. Aside from opioid agonist medications and the treatment of co-morbid conditions, the major treatment modalities for heroin dependence are the psychological therapies, such as cognitive behavioural therapy, motivational interviewing, social skills training, contingency management, family therapy and self-help groups.

Methadone

Methadone is a synthetic orally effective, long-acting μ-receptor agonist developed by the Nazis in the 1940s as their access to opium became obstructed. It has been used as a treatment for opioid dependence since the 1960s and is the mostly widely used, evaluated and cost-effective treatment for opiate dependence. Methadone works by substituting for heroin at the μ-receptor and abolishing withdrawal. Through receptor occupancy and the induction of cross tolerance, higher doses (sometimes called 'blocking doses') also reduce the reinforcement (euphoria) obtained by the 'on top use of heroin', diminishing craving. Increasing the tolerance to other opiate drugs also protects against overdose.

Starting methadone treatment

Care is required during the induction of patients onto methadone. Doses as low as 30 mg can be fatal to the non-tolerant person. First doses should not usually exceed 30 mg/day and

ideally, patients should be monitored 2–4 h after the first dose. Methadone has a long half-life (24–48 h) and a steady state plasma level is thus not achieved until day 5–7. Because of rising plasma levels over the first 2–5 days of use (note there is also auto-induction of its metabolism), users are usually asked to attend a clinic or pharmacy daily for supervised consumption to make sure that they are not excessively sedated or showing other signs of toxicity (suggesting their dose exceeds their tolerance). The dose is increased gradually, with increments of 5–10 mg every 4–7 days occurring until withdrawal is abolished, craving reduced and tolerance to opiate significantly increased. There have been deaths recorded during unsafe and unmonitored induction onto methadone (Caplehorn & Drummer 1999), usually in opioid naïve persons or those using other depressant drugs such as alcohol and benzodiazepines. Confirmation of the patient's dependent status is therefore paramount, assessed by a careful and comprehensive assessment, observation, examination and where appropriate, objective confirmation by repeat urine drug screens and by direct observation of the patient while withdrawing and assessing the effect of an administered dose of methadone on site.

The response to ongoing use of heroin should usually be to increase the dose of prescribed opiate medication. A user should never be discharged from treatment for continuing to use illicit drugs or alcohol. The risk of overdose and other adverse outcomes will be higher than if they stay in treatment.

Starting buprenorphine (Subutex, Suboxone, Temgesic) treatment

Buprenorphine. Buprenorphine is a partial μ-receptor agonist. It has a ceiling effect on respiratory depression and is thus safer in overdose than methadone. It has a higher affinity for the μ-opioid receptor than pure agonists like heroin and methadone, but lower intrinsic activity. It has recently become an acceptable and effective alternative to methadone (Kosten 2003). Taken sublingually it has a bioavailability of 30–40%. It undergoes extensive first pass metabolism and thus oral bioavailability is poor. If it is taken within 6–12 h of heroin or 24–48 h of methadone, buprenorphine will displace the full agonist and precipitate withdrawal (*never give buprenorphine to a patient* *who has 'pinned pupils').* It is effective as a stabilization agent (where safe induction can be obtained within 2–3 days compared to 2–3 weeks for methadone). Typical maintenance doses are 8–16 mg/day with the maximum dose of buprenorphine to be given on any one day being 32 mg. Because of its high affinity and slow dissolution from the receptor, bigger doses of buprenorphine last longer (e.g. 32 mg may last 2–3 days) permitting less than daily dosing.

Like supervised methadone doses (which may be regurgitated or secreted in a bottle), buprenorphine can be diverted and injected. Supervised consumption is recommended for both methadone and buprenorphine, for at least the first 3 months of treatment. Careful observation initially at public clinics, then at community pharmacies is required to ensure that potentially abusable and lethal drugs are not diverted to the street drug market. However, stable patients should be given access to takeaway doses to enable them to work, study and reintegrate into a non-drug using environment.

Suboxone is buprenorphine combined with naloxone in a ratio of 4:1. Taken as directed sublingually, there is very poor bioavailability of naloxone compared with buprenorphine, thus the drug works similarly to buprenorphine. It is basically a less desirable injectable version of buprenorphine. However, when injected, the naloxone now is 100% bioavailable and depending on the current state of intoxication of the user, may precipitate withdrawal or at least be less reinforcing than buprenorphine alone. Whether such a combination preparation is significantly less abusable and divertable than the single product is as yet unclear. It has recently been introduced in the UK. There have been recent reports of both forms of buprenorphine being snorted and smoked.

Levo-alpha acetylmethadol (LAAM). This long-acting (48–72 h) μ-receptor agonist has been used in the treatment of heroin dependence since the 1960s. Although studies have demonstrated equivalence with other substitute therapies, it is not licensed for use in the UK because of concerns over the prolongation of the QT interval seen in some persons.

Other opiate pharmacotherapies: slow release oral morphine, injectable diamorphine and methadone and naltrexone

Slow release oral morphine and supervised injectable diamorphine and methadone are also used in some specialist settings. Although controversial in the UK, at the time of writing, positive results from randomized trial of supervised injectable diamorphine (RIOTT) suggest that such treatments might have a role in those who have failed to obtain benefit from oral opioid substitution treatments.

The long-acting orally active opiate receptor antagonist naltrexone can be used in the maintenance of abstinence of opiate dependents. Compliance with treatment is generally poor (and hence ineffective) unless supervised and part of wider treatment programmes. It is also associated with an increase in receptor sensitivity that means following the cessation of its use, people are particularly sensitive to the risk of overdose should they relapse. Recently, naltrexone implants and depot injections have been trialled and it may be that in certain populations, this way of enhancing compliance may be useful.

Long-term benefits of opiate substitution treatment (OST)

The National Treatment Outcome Research Study (NTORS) used a 5-year longitudinal, prospective cohort design to follow the outcomes of 650 persons admitted to opiate treatment services (community methadone and residential rehabilitation units) in 1995 (Gossop et al 1997). About one-quarter of those on methadone had become abstinent compared to 38% of those attending rehabilitation. Most of the improvement seems to have been achieved within a year, with levels sustained beyond this initial stage. Unfortunately, there was little positive impact on the use of crack cocaine or alcohol. Both substances, with their different mechanisms of actions, are probably perceived to be a more cost-effective intoxicant compared to heroin as the levels of opiate blockade increases. Results from the same group suggest that for every extra £1 spent on treatment, there is a return of more than £3 in cost savings associated with lower levels of victim costs of crime and reduced demands upon the criminal justice system. The benefits of opiate replacement therapy include:

- Reduced rates of injecting drugs
- Reduced rates of other illicit drug use
- Reduction in suicide/overdose
- Reduced rates of HIV and viral hepatitis
- Reduced rates of criminal activity
- Improvement in psychosocial and physical wellbeing.

Detoxification from heroin and coming off maintenance treatment

Detoxification is the first step to maintaining a period of abstinence. Many dependent users will seek detoxification at a time of crisis (see Ch. 28). Often the treatment episode is not completed. Users returning to the streets after detox or leaving midway though the process are at increased risk of overdose due to reduced tolerance therefore a decision to support detox should be carefully considered and generally not supported unless an aftercare plan is in place.

Opiate withdrawal is not life-threatening and can usually be managed safely in the community. Buprenorphine is the most effective agent for medically assisted detoxification and can safely be used in an outpatient setting where it is superior to symptomatic relief with μ2-agonists (although the two can also be combined). For those stopping heroin, a reducing dose over 5–10 days is usually adequate. Users should be rapidly stabilized on the dose where they experience no withdrawal symptoms (typically 8–16 mg/day) and then it is reduced over a week or so. The initial relief of withdrawal on buprenorphine may lead some users to consider a period of maintenance. This should be supported. Adjunctive medications such as simple analgesics, antiemetics and sedation can safely be used in combination with buprenorphine if required.

An alternative approach that avoids the use of an opioid is the use of the μ2-agonists, clonidine and lofexidine, that work at pre-synaptic adrenergic receptors, and suppress the central noradrenergic hyperactivity that is responsible for many of the symptoms of opiate withdrawal. The dose of μ2-agonists should be titrated against the symptoms and signs of withdrawal, while being careful to avoid hypotensive episodes (less common with lofexidine) and can be used both within outpatient and inpatient settings. They are often used in conjunction with other medications such as benzodiazepines for sleep, muscular cramps and agitation; and hyoscine for abdominal cramps; NSAIDs and paracetamol for pain and antiemetics, such as promethazine or metoclopramide.

For those wishing to come off maintenance, both methadone and buprenorphine doses may be gradually reduced over a few months. Unfortunately, while meta-analyses have identified advantages in the use of buprenorphine for heroin withdrawal, available research demonstrates no clear advantage in different approaches to withdrawal from long-term OST regarding medication approach (e.g. use of adrenergic agonists, methadone or buprenorphine tapering) or counselling interventions. Whether novel treatments, such as transfer to buprenorphine, treatment with very low naltrexone doses or long-acting naltrexone products may have a role is unclear. In the absence of a 'best treatment' to help people get off OST, providing stable patients with a menu of treatment options and supporting individual patient choice is the best therapeutic strategy, while accepting that supporting cessation of treatment for many patients, especially when they are unstable, may carry significant clinical risks.

Prescribing drugs to opiate addicts

In the UK, all doctors may prescribe methadone for the treatment of dependence and other opiates for analgesia and other clinical indications, but not dependence. Doctors should be wary of behaviours that are suggestive of possible 'abuse' of prescribed opiates. These include using the prescription up early, losing a prescription, asking for escalating doses and attending multiple prescribers. Although the attribution may be incorrect and there may be genuine reasons for the requests, it is the doctor's responsibility to ensure that the drugs are being used as directed.

Other treatment interventions

Psychological

There are numerous psychological approaches that are currently used to help those with substance-related problems reduce their use of drugs and the harm associated with them, including cognitive behavioural therapy (CBT), relapse prevention (RP) and psychotherapy (individual, family and group). The most influential approach in recent years has been the relapse prevention mode, which includes the identification of cues or triggers for craving (often people, places or paraphernalia or a certain mood state such as boredom or stress) and the learning of techniques (distraction, relaxation, imagery) to handle high-risk situations in which relapse is more likely. Motivational interviewing based on the work of Bill Miller in the USA has become increasingly popular. It aims to move the client along a 'cycle of change' (Miller & Rollnick 1991) (see Ch. 28). Involvement with Narcotics Anonymous and support groups such as Mainliners should be encouraged. Augmenting current approaches with contingency management is becoming increasingly common.

Physical

High levels of physical and psychiatric morbidity are compounded by poor nutrition, homelessness, financial hardship and poor access to primary care. Dentition is often particularly bad. Although methadone reduces salivary flow, poor nutrition, dental hygiene and the masking of dental pain probably contribute more significantly. Efforts at reducing injecting and related risk behaviours are a priority. Safer injecting techniques, sharps boxes, needles and syringe outlets and disposal bins should be combined with advice on safer sex, contraception and general healthcare. Models of shared care (between GP, specialist services, pharmacists and clients and specialized primary care health teams) have been successful in proactively engaging clients and service providers to effect the delivery of care to this multiply-disadvantaged high risk group. Special attention should be focused on provision of hepatitis testing and vaccination to all users.

Social and educational

High rates of early school drop-out and lower levels of employment skills hamper efforts at reintegration into the community as a non-drug user. All available potential supports should be considered, including family, friends, social services or voluntary sector supports, user advocate groups, religious communities and spiritual support groups such as Narcotics Anonymous. Providing credible accessible accurate health information as part of harm prevention initiatives foster a positive alliance with using communities and assist in promoting safer drug using practices with consequent benefit to the individual and society. Therapeutic communities and 'concept houses' based on a religious or abstinent theme offer longer-term care.

Pregnancy

The maternal use of opiates has consequences for both mother and child with increased rates of stillbirth, prematurity, low birth weight, IUGR and vertical HBV/HIV transmission risk. This group should be given priority access to coordinated treatment services with effective liaison between patient, family, antenatal, drug and social support services. In general, the aim of treatment should be to engage the mother and reduce risk-taking behaviours, e.g. injecting and stabilizing on methadone (buprenorphine is not yet licensed for use in pregnancy or while breast-feeding). Liaison with antenatal and primary care and social services through a multidisciplinary programme ensures the wellbeing of the mother and her environment. Pregnancy should be regarded as a window of opportunity in the drug user.

If considering detoxification, this should be done in the middle trimester. However, the risk of relapse and loss of engagement with services means that many specialists recommend that a woman remains on methadone. Although some women can manage a slow reduction through pregnancy, many may require an increase in dose in the last trimester. There is no relationship between the incidence or severity of neonatal withdrawal and the dose of methadone. Pregnant women should be advised to increase their dose if withdrawal is experienced. Both benzodiazepines and opiates are slowly metabolized by the newborn infant, so that peri-delivery administration may result in hypotonia and respiratory depression. Both opiates and benzodiazepine dependence in the mother may be associated with protracted withdrawal syndromes in the baby. The neonatal abstinence syndrome seen in babies born to opiate-using mothers is characterized by signs and symptoms in the gastrointestinal tract, respiratory system and autonomic nervous system, with failure to thrive and the risk of seizures. Withdrawal incidence and severity is poorly correlated with dose of methadone, but may be prolonged, requiring hospitalization. Management is with morphine and occasionally barbiturates.

Criminal justice system

Prisoners

The last decade has seen an increased focus on addressing drug use among those committing crime. Drug intervention programmes (DIP) involve identifying Class A drug-misusing offenders as they enter the criminal justice system and providing rapid access to treatments of both drug use and offending behaviours. About one in four prisoners are drug injectors and up to half of the prison population have a substance use disorder, most commonly alcohol and opiates. Access to illicit substances is not easily prevented by imprisonment, indeed some users may first 'pick up heroin' or increase their 'habit' while in prison. Prison may, however, be a chance for good drug treatment to be provided, especially if combined with good post-release programmes. Education and good primary healthcare are vital. The rate of fatal overdose is increased 50-fold in the week after release from prison among those with opioid dependence released without substitute pharmacotherapy.

HIV-positive

Reducing high-risk behaviours by those with HIV is important to limit the spread of the disease. Stabilization on opioid substitution treatment with abstinence from injecting, sharing and unprotected sex should be encouraged. Liaison with medical and psychiatric services is important.

Outcome

Opioid dependence is a chronic relapsing condition. People do well if they stay in treatment and if they are compliant. Longer treatment is associated with better outcomes. Abstinence rates following treatment completion vary widely, but between 60–85% are back using heroin within 6 months. Not surprisingly, users with multiple co-morbid diagnoses and severe dependence psychopathology have the poorest outcomes. Among the strongest correlates of mortality in this group are level of disability, heavy alcohol use, heavy criminal involvement and tobacco use. Longer treatment contacts tend to be associated with better outcomes (Simpson et al 1997). Annual mortality rates are between 1% and 2%, with between a third and a half accounted for by suicide and accidental overdose (an excess mortality ratio of 12). On average, heroin users die 15–20 years earlier than their non-drug using counterparts.

Stimulants: amphetamines, cocaine and MDMA ('ecstasy')

D-amphetamine and methamphetamine

Structurally similar to dopamine, amphetamines are synthetic *sympathomimetic drugs*. Stimulant amphetamines such as Dex-amphetamine and methyl amphetamine act through inhibition of central presynaptic reuptake of catecholamines (DA<NA) as well as indirect sympathomimetic effects secondary to disruption of vesicular storage of monoamines and inhibition of their breakdown by monoamine oxidases. Initially marketed as a treatment for nasal congestion, amphetamines became popular in the 1950s as appetite suppressants and continue to be used in the treatment of ADHD and narcolepsy.

Illicit amphetamine is typically a low purity (5%) combination of D- and L-amphetamine, typically taken orally, intranasally or intravenously. Methylamphetamine (methamphetamine, 'ice' 'crystal') is a more potent, often much purer (up to 80%) lipophilic, longer acting smokeable form of amphetamine that is common in South-East Asia, the USA and Australia. An intermediate product known as 'base' or 'paste' may be up to 40% purity. At present, methamphetamine remains uncommon in the UK, although reports of it within the gay dance scene have occurred. Prescribable stimulants such as methylphenidate (Ritalin) and diethylpropion (Tenuate) are also open to abuse. Other more recently available therapeutic stimulant drugs such as modafinil may also have the potential to be abused. At the time of writing, there are number of 'legal highs' available, with marked stimulant effects, including 4-methylmethcathinone (4MMC) related to the active constituent in khat.

Pattern of use

Users may be classified as recreational, functional or dependent. People who use amphetamine-type stimulants regularly in high doses, especially if they inject or smoke, develop tolerance rapidly and risk becoming dependent. However, unlike other drugs of dependence, daily use is less common, since it can lead to insomnia, anorexia and exhaustion. Paranoid psychotic symptoms including hostility, aggressiveness, suspicion and hallucinations may occur after heavy binges. Periods of intense use are ended in conjunction with depressant drugs (alcohol, heroin, benzodiazepines). The immediate period after use has been referred to as the crash or come down. It is characterized by hypersomnolence, hyperphagia, lethargy and low mood, and lasts 2–4 days.

Heavy users may inject several grams per day and can increase their number of injections to more than 20/day. Recreational users may use the drug sporadically, using considerably less. In such cases, amphetamines are taken orally or snorted, often in conjunction with other 'dance drugs' and alcohol. Amphetamines will tend to offset the sedating effects of alcohol in the same way as cocaine. Functional users include students and long-distance lorry drivers, who use the drug to enhance performance and stamina. Some may also use the drug to control weight but tolerance develops rapidly.

MDMA inhibition of the rate limiting enzyme (tyrosine hydroxylase in the case of MDMA).

Use leads to sympathomimetic effects, not unlike those seen with amphetamine and cocaine, including marked mydriasis, piloerection, hypertension, hyperthermia and increase in locomotor activity. Physical effects of MDMA include:

- Tachycardia, increased blood pressure and respiratory rate
- Hyperthermia, increased sweating, dehydration, sweaty palms, hot and cold flushes
- Dilated pupils, blurred vision
- Tremor, increased motor activity, agitation, dry mouth
- Teeth grinding, jaw tightening (bruxism)
- Anorexia, weight loss
- Insomnia and abnormal sleep architecture.

Metabolism

MDMA is primarily metabolized by demethylation by the enzyme CYP 2D6, of which two phenotypes predominate in the population, with 9% being 'poor metabolizers'. There is no evidence, as yet, to support the notion that this group may be at greater risk of fatalities associated with its use.

Patterns of use and sought after effects

MDMA is usually taken orally, either as a pill or powder. It may also be injected, snorted or used rectally ('E by bum'). In the UK, 1–4 tablets are often taken over a night usually in combination with other drugs such as alcohol, cocaine, GHB, ketamine or cannabis. Sought after affects include energy, euphoria, empathy and heightened sensory perception. Peak effect is 1–2 h after consumption with tolerance to empathogenic effects developing rapidly. Significant effects persist for a further 3–6 h, followed by a gradual 'come down'. Diminishing effects from subsequent doses are seen because of monoamine depletion and irreversible inhibition of the rate limiting enzyme tyrosine hydroxylase. The price of 'pills' has fallen to as little as £2–£5 in many places, making them an attractive and cost-effective alternative or additive to alcohol consumption

Unwanted effects

Adverse symptoms such as anxiety, panic and paranoia often develop, and a range of psychiatric disorders from psychosis to neuroses and affective disorders have been described following its use. Often, there is also nausea, reduced appetite and insomnia. Both auditory and visual hallucinations have been described as have delusions and suicidal feelings.

Neurotoxicity

There is reasonably strong evidence of dose-related selective 5HT neurotoxicity from both animal and human studies though the *in vivo* consequences in man continued to be debated. Histopathological studies suggest dose-related reduction in 5HT activity following chronic exposure, with abnormal axonal regrowth seen in rats. Key risk factors in animal models for increasing neurotoxicity are increased temperature, dehydration and dose (aggregation toxicity). The effect of MDMA on thermal regulation is dependent upon the ambient temperature, causing hypothermia in cooler conditions and hyperthermia in hotter ones. PET studies in humans suggest that there may be

structural damage to the serotonergic nerve terminal (McCann et al 1998). Some studies have suggested reduced serotonin transporter levels or ligand binding. The functional significance of these remote markers is unclear, and it is probable that whether an individual goes on to develop longer-term problematic psychological or behavioural problems following use of MDMA will depend upon the amount consumed, any genetic loading for psychopathology, their baseline balance and level of 5HT activity, and any neuroplasticity that may compensate for any neuronal dysfunction and other drug use. Theoretically, any vulnerability to mental disorders will be become more evident over the next decade as the generation who first popularized ecstasy reach middle age. Any loss that occurred from MDMA use may lead to early decompensation and functional loss.

Psychiatric and cognitive co-morbidity and MDMA

It has been difficult to assess the MDMA attributable fraction of depression and other psychopathology in the community. Ecstasy users typically consume a wide variety of substances and baseline levels of depression and other factors contributing to pre-morbid risk are not readily assessed by retrospective examination. Despite these factors, studies of ecstasy-using populations consistently report higher depression ratings on clinical scales than non-using controls. There appears to be a dose effect, with psychobiologic deficits more marked in heavy users. Women appear more sensitive to both acute short effects (mid-week blues and hallucinations at higher doses) but also possibly the longer-term neurotoxic ones (Maxwell 2003). Despite its prevalence over the years, the number of actual case reports of psychiatric conditions associated with the use of MDMA is small. Those reported include: depression, anxiety, panic, social phobia, bulimia, sleep disorders, paranoia, cognitive disorders, prolonged depersonalization/derealization, suicide, psychotic episodes, flashbacks and increased impulsivity (Guillot and Berman 2007). Factors that appear to increase susceptibility to psychiatric disorders with MDMA include female sex, dose, frequency and duration of use, polydrug use and constitutional vulnerability. There is no specificity to the disorders that have been reported with MDMA; indeed those reported are those common in the general population. The direction of causality of drug use and mental disorder is further confused by evidence that poor pre-morbid adjustment is itself associated with drug use.

Whether there are specific cognitive deficits specifically associated with MDMA continues to be a contentious issue with confounding drug use, especially cannabis, making it difficult to assess the degree of association (Morgan 2000). The most consistent deficits recorded in MDMA users are in immediate and delayed verbal recall (Hanson and Luciana 2004), although deficits in other areas such as verbal fluency, impulse control and processing speed have also been reported.

Dependence

Given the prevalence of MDMA use and the reported patterns of use, the possibility of a dependence syndrome similar to that seen with other stimulant drugs, remains. Since the dopaminergic system is also influenced by MDMA, it is likely that the ventral tegmental dopaminergic reward pathway underlies much of the reinforcement of MDMA. Users do report tolerance, loss of control and behavioural and lifestyle changes supportive of a dependence syndrome (Winstock et al 2001). However, no withdrawal has been reported and there is no specific pharmacological intervention in the management of its use. MAOIs and selective serotonin reuptake inhibitors (SSRIs) should be used with caution since concurrent consumption may place the person at risk of the 5HT syndrome, its reinforcing potential, and as such the possibility for the development of a dependence syndrome remains. A diagnosis of depression in current users should be deferred until a period of at least a few weeks abstinence has been obtained and their mental state reviewed.

Physical morbidity

There are 40–50 deaths recorded each year in the UK related to ecstasy consumption, most in conjunction with other substances. They account for less than 1% of all drug deaths recorded each year. Although most deaths are idiosyncratic and unrelated to dose, pathologies related to its stimulant activity are seen, including arrhythmias, cerebral hemorrhages, rhabdomyolysis, dehydration and malignant hyperthermia. Very rarely metabolic acidosis, seizures, SIAHD, acute kidney failure and acute liver failure have been reported. Context dependent risk can be reduced by maintaining good hydration, taking breaks from exertional activities such as dancing to cool down, avoiding alcohol and avoid mixing with other stimulant drugs.

γ-Hydroxybutyrate (GHB, GBH, liquid ecstasy)

GHB (Rodgers et al 2004) is an endogenous short-chain fatty acid found in the central nervous system (hippocampus, hypothalamus, cerebellum), kidney, heart, skeletal muscle and brown fat. It is probably derived from GABA (transamination to succinate aldehyde, reduced to GHB). A putative neurotransmitter, its role is unclear though specific binding sites have been identified in the hippocampus, which are linked to DA neurons. It was originally developed as an intravenous anaesthetic induction agent in 1964 but was not successful, causing unacceptably high levels of vomiting, and tonic–clonic jerks of hand and face at anaesthetic doses. Since the 1980s, it has been used as a supplement by body builders, as a sleep agent, a detox agent and most recently, as a dance drug. Usually used in the form of a liquid (also available as capsules, powder or crystals), it is colourless and odourless, with a slightly salty, acidic taste, often sold in little plastic 'sushi soy fishies'. Until a few years ago, the end-product and the key ingredients were widely available on the net. However, recent legislations have led to a reduction in its use but a corresponding rise in its procompounds GBL (γ-butyl-lactone) and 1,4 butanediol (soon to be banned).

Although probably derived from GABA, it has little effect on GABA-A or -B receptors at submillimolar concentrations. It does, however, readily cross the blood–brain barrier. Acutely it leads to a transient decrease followed by increase in dopamine levels (accompanied by increase in endogenous opioid release). Increases in Ach, GABA, 5HT are also seen. It exhibits some partial GABA-B activity at high levels (epileptogenic).

Taken orally, the drug has a rapid onset of action (<15 min) and a half-life of 27 min, being broken down to CO_2 and H_2O.

It exhibits peak effects after 60 min with the total duration of action being 2–4 h.

GBH and GBL have been popular on the dance music and gay club scenes for many years. At low doses they induce euphoria, stimulation and arousal. Effects are dose-related, however, and there is a steep dose–response curve with a narrow margin between untroubled and unconscious.

Clinically, GHB or GBL use should be suspected in particular groups such as clubbers and body builders who present with nystagmus, ataxia, nausea, vomiting, bradycardia and hypotension. Overdose risk is compounded by combined use with other depressants (especially alcohol), as well as wide fluctuation in purity, tolerance, context and other drugs consumed. The drug can also be associated with agitation, anxiety, aggressive behaviour, confusion, transient delirium and amnesia, especially on waking. Psychotic episodes have been reported when GHB is combined with stimulant drugs (massive increase in dopamine). Other problems include increased vomiting, aspiration, weakness, sedation, coma, amnesia and collapse. There has also been a single case report of Wernike–Korsakoff syndrome.

There has been recent concern that GHB is a common date rape drug. Theoretically it may be an efficient 'Micky Fin', since it leads to the onset of rapid coma and amnesia, but the evidence suggests that alcohol alone is by far the most common 'date rape' drug.

GHB and GBL dependence does occur. Users develop tolerance and may experience a rapid onset, severe waxing and waning, protracted alcohol withdrawal like syndrome, though with less autonomic arousal and risk of seizures but marked confusion, delirium and hallucinations. Management may require large doses of benzodiazepines over a waxing and waning 2-week period.

Hallucinogens: lysergic acid diethylamide (LSD), ketamine and psilocybin – mushrooms

Lysergic acid diethylamide (LSD)

Leaving his laboratory one day in 1943, the Swiss chemist Hoffman forgot to wash his hands, and accidentally discovered what a little bit of acid could do. Popular in the 1960s, LSD has now lost ground to other hallucinogens such as ketamine and is less commonly used than 20 years ago. The drug may be absorbed transdermally, but is usually taken orally after absorption onto a piece of blotting paper, a gelatine square (window panes) or on a sugar cube. Doses as low as 20–50 μg cause marked perceptual distortion with visual illusions and hallucinations, without any associated lowering of consciousness. Effects start after 30–90 min and may last ≥3–12 h. The half-life is 3 h.

Mechanism of action

LSD is an indoleamine hallucinogen and binds to $5HT_1$, $5HT_2$, $5HT_5$ and $5HT_7$ receptors. Hallucinogenic potency in man is closely related to $5HT_2$ binding affinity in animals. Further evidence for the major role of 5HT comes from recent human trials, demonstrating that the hallucinogenic effects of psilocybin can be attenuated by pre-treatment with the $5HT_2$ receptor antagonist ketanserin or the atypical antipsychotic risperidone, but not haloperidol, with hallucinogenic effects probably mediated by the agonist action at the $5HT_2$ receptor. However, LSD also has significant stimulant effects mediated through the release of dopamine. Tolerance occurs rapidly due to receptor desensitization, which is evident after 3 or 4 days consecutive use, explaining the absence of a dependence syndrome.

Clinical features

Marked perceptual changes, with an alteration in state of awareness and euphoria, are common. Visual (and less commonly auditory and other modality) hallucinations and distortions are frequently reported, as is the phenomenon of 'synaesthesia' with loss of the normal boundaries between sensory modalities (e.g. sounds are 'seen', colours are 'heard'). At higher doses, its sympathomimetic effects become evident, including hyperreflexia and hyperthermia. Sympathetic overactivity may also help explain adverse symptoms, such as anxiety and panic (the so-called 'bad trip'). As with other psychoactive drugs, use may precipitate a severe mental illness in some vulnerable individuals. Approximately 15% of users report 'flashbacks', a recurrence of experiences previously associated with LSD use, while the individual is drug free.

Treatment

The 'bad trip' usually responds to a supportive and reassuring environment (so-called 'talking down'), but if appropriate, benzodiazepines or low dose neuroleptics may be used.

Flashbacks may be associated with an underlying disorder such as anxiety and may be brought on by other drugs such as cannabis. Usually remitting with time, they may remain distressing for a minority. Overall, problems with LSD and other hallucinogens such as mushrooms are usually self-limiting, though persistent symptomatology may arise in those with a predisposition of psychosis.

Ketamine

Ketamine is a non-competitive antagonist at NMDA receptors. It is similar in action to PCP (but shorter acting), with binding to the cation channel of NMDA receptor being responsible for its analgesic/dissociative and purported neuroprotective effects. It also enhances monoamine transmission resulting in significant sympathomimetic properties. It also has analgesic opioid receptor mediated effects. The induction of an anaesthetic state and subsequent hallucinations are thought to be due to inhibition of central and peripheral cholinergic transmission.

Ketamine shows marked first pass metabolism and is fairly ineffective when taken orally. More commonly and efficiently, ketamine is snorted or injected. It exhibits dose-related psychedelic effects, which show a linear relationship at low doses. Effects are highly sensitive to age, dose, route, sex and setting and include:

- Rapid onset, short duration of action (1 hour), wide safety margin
- Dissociative anaesthesia 'somatosensory blockade' (analgesia without anaesthesia): analgesia
- Perceptual distortion/hallucinations/near death

- Out-of-body experience
- Sympathetic stimulation
- Emergence phenomena
- Cognitive impairment
- Thought disorder/synaesthesia
- Little effect on cough reflex
- Hypersalivation.

At low doses, sought-after experiences are primarily stimulant and elevation of mood. Psychedelic effects commence at higher doses. The Harvard academic Timothy Leary described it as 'the ultimate psychedelic journey'. Users describe entering the 'K hole' where they experience visits to God, aliens, their birth, past lives and the 'experiences of evolution' (Dillon et al 2003).

Detection by clinical examination relies on identifying mydriasis, tachycardia, elevated blood pressure, slurred speech, blunted affect, ataxia, delirium and nystagmus. Urine drug screens do not routinely detect it.

Adverse effects are short-lived (<5 h) and include: frightening hallucinations/out of body experiences; thought disorder; confusion; dissociation; chest pain; palpitations and tachycardia; nausea; stomach cramps; vomiting; difficulty with and burning on micturition; difficulty breathing; ataxia; temporary paralysis/inability to speak; blurred vision; no awareness of pain; derealization/depersonalization and amnesia. A psychotic picture that can briefly mimic schizophrenia can also be seen.

Management is by supportive monitoring (CVS) in a quiet, low-stimulation room with symptomatic treatment with benzodiazepines if needed. CVS excitation can sometimes be helped by using propranolol. Death is rare and usually only occurs when used in combination with alcohol and other respiratory depressants. Prolonged periods of immobility and unconsciousness may result in rhabdomyolysis. Chlorpromazine should be avoided (because of anticholinergic effects) and haloperidol is largely ineffective. One volunteer study found benefit from using lamotrigine.

Ketamine dependence has been described, with compulsive use a primary symptom. Although tolerance develops, there is no evidence for a withdrawal syndrome. Other risks associated with its use include accidents, trauma, risky sexual behaviour and cognitive impairment that appears to be persistent in heavy users.

'Magic mushrooms'

This is the street name for a variety of hallucinogenic fungi that contain the naturally occurring substituted tryptamines, psilocybin and psilocin. Taken orally (either raw or cooked), mushrooms produce a variable but dose-related psychedelic effect that comes on 30–60 min after consumption and lasts for 4–8 h. Hallucinogenic potency in man is closely related to $5HT_2$-binding affinity in animals. Although psilocybin causes mydriasis, unlike other psychedelics, its autonomic activity is modest. As with other hallucinogens such as LSD, rapid tolerance develops after repeated use over a few days.

A broad range of acute psychopathology may be seen with psilocybin, including panic, amnesia, acute toxic stuporous states and occasionally a short-lived psychotic syndrome, with changes in sensory perception and cognition, affective functioning and loosened associations. The pattern of thought and ego disturbance seen may resemble an acute schizophrenic episode. Apart from the acute risk of significant adverse psychological effects and precipitation and exacerbation of mental health problems, physical use is generally safe, with fewer than half a dozen fatalities reported. One of the greatest risks, however, is posed by the ingestion by mistake of a similar looking fungus. Psychiatrists should consider mushroom or other psychedelic intoxication in young people, and be prompted in their suspicion by a clinical examination revealing dilated pupils and behavioural disturbance, in the absence of significant sympathetic stimulation. A urine specimen should be taken and if possible, a sample of the consumed fungus obtained.

General sedatives: benzodiazepines and barbiturates

Benzodiazepines

Chlordiazepoxide was the first benzodiazepine to be made available, 2 years before diazepam, in 1962. At their peak, up to one in six of the adult population in many European countries had used a benzodiazepine in the preceding year, although since the mid-1980s this has fallen to approximately one in ten (Hallstrom 1993). National guidelines and education have led to changes in prescribing patterns over the last 20 years, with a fall in the prescription of benzodiazepines as hypnotics by a third, although levels of anxiolytic prescribing remain fairly level.

Mechanism of action

Acting on a specific receptor site on the GABA-A receptor, benzodiazepines enhance the response of the GABA-A receptor to GABA. This leads to hyperpolarization by increasing the frequency of opening of the chloride channel.

Metabolism

Bioavailability following oral administration is almost complete, with peak plasma concentrations being reached after 30–90 min. Being highly lipid-soluble and highly bound to albumin, drugs such a diazepam have a wide volume of distribution and diffuse rapidly across the blood–brain barrier and the placenta and appear in breast milk. They may also be given rectally, intravenously or intramuscularly, although this latter method may lead to unpredictable rates of absorption, as well as local tissue damage. Benzodiazepines undergo significant hepatic degradation with many compounds having active metabolites, whose half-lives exceed that of the parent compound (see Ch. 39).

Tolerance

Tolerance to the different effects of benzodiazepines occurs at different rates. Tolerance to the sedative and anticonvulsant effects begin after 2 or 3 days and are marked by 2–3 weeks. Tachyphylaxis has also been reported. Tolerance to their anxiolytic effects occurs much more slowly. The mechanisms underlying tolerance to benzodiazepines are not fully understood but may be mediated by changes in receptor sensitivity, altered expression of receptor subtypes or uncoupling of the links between the receptor and ligand.

Dependence

Those who become dependent upon benzodiazepines can be broadly divided into two groups. The first includes the iatrogenic user who, having had their use initiated by a doctor, shows no escalation of dose and at least initially, may derive benefits of improved psychosocial functioning. This group are typically older women, with a history of chronic psychiatric or physical illness. Gradual tapering off with psychological support and management of underlying co-morbid conditions can be an effective approach in this group.

The other group are polysubstance users, often those dependent on opioids. Although there may be an underlying anxiety disorder in some users, non-prescribed and uncontrolled use is usually unhelpful. Among those on methadone, the use of benzodiazepines is a risk factor for overdose and their provision to opioid dependent users should be avoided when possible. Use is characterized by increased doses, a desire for euphoria and consequent psychosocial problems. Addressing benzodiazepine use among polydrug users is challenging.

More commonly seen with short-acting, high-potency preparations, benzodiazepine dependence and withdrawal was first highlighted by Petursson and Lader in 1984 (Box 29.3). Longer periods of regular use are more likely to lead to dependence. Estimates suggest that very few people become dependent with periods of use of less than 3 months. Between 3 and 12 months of use, 10–20% will become dependant, rising to 20–45% after periods longer than a year. Some patients will be more prone to developing dependence than others. Risk factors for developing dependence on benzodiazepines include:

- High doses for long periods, shorter half-life drugs
- Previous history of substance dependence
- Those with chronic dysphoria, insomnia and vivid dreams
- Cognitive style: low self-esteem, tendency to catastrophize
- Those who have psychiatric causes for insomnia
- Passive dependent personalities
- Female sex.

The risk of developing dependence on benzodiazepines can be minimized by not prescribing them for periods longer than 14–28 days and discussing the issues of abuse and dependence early in treatment. Tolerance to the therapeutic effects of benzodiazepines such as sedation and anxiolysis develop within a few weeks.

Withdrawal

The decreased functioning of the GABA-BDZ complex (and its knock-on effects on other neurotransmitters) is probably responsible for most of the withdrawal syndrome. There do appear to be prolonged changes in GABA release following withdrawal and this may underlie protracted symptoms some patients experience. Typically, withdrawal commences 2–3 days after stopping, being maximum on days 7–10, usually abating by the end of the second and third weeks. The onset of withdrawal is more rapid with shorter acting preparations. Withdrawal symptoms may be confused with an unmasking of the original problem or with rebound anxiety. Differentiation should be based on the time sequence of its development and symptoms of sensory disturbance, such as hyperacusis,

cannabis users have higher levels of anxiety, the nature of the relationship is not clear.

Laboratory detection

In urine samples, inactive fat soluble metabolites of cannabis (THC-11-oic acid) are detectable for considerable periods of time after last consumption, ranging from 1 week for the casual user to 8+ weeks for the heavy chronic user, depending on the cut-off point for detection. Saliva, buccal scrapings, and clothes sprays are other methods employed to detect recent use of cannabis.

Dependence

Dependence on cannabis is the most common, but most under-recognized consequence of cannabis use, with around 1 in 10 regular users becoming dependent (Hall et al 1994). Effective treatments include CBT, MI, contingency management and RP. Concurrent tobacco smoking, which is prevalent in cannabis smokers, is a predictor of poor outcome, so NRT should be encouraged. Three-quarters of dependent users experience withdrawal discomfort on cessation, comprising insomnia, irritability, restlessness, loss of appetite, low mood, craving, sweating and vivid dreams. Peaking on day 2 or 3, most withdrawal symptoms have gone after 7–10 days. Management is largely symptomatic with short-term night sedation, caffeine avoidance, sleep hygiene and NRT being the most important aspects to address. There is no role for any specific pharmacotherapy to assist in the maintenance of abstinence from cannabis.

Volatile substances

The inhalation of volatile substances is commonly known as 'glue sniffing', 'chroming' or 'huffing'. Cheap, easily and widely available, volatile substance abuse (VSA) continues to be common among UK teenagers. The range of abused compounds and the variety of preparations is vast (Table 29.7). It is responsible for about 100 deaths each year with a modal age of 15 years.

Epidemiology

Studies suggest a prevalence of between 5% and 10% among secondary school children, with higher rates associated with poverty and deprivation. Although prevalence studies suggest equal sex distribution, deaths are far more likely in males, probably due to a different pattern of use. Most commonly a group

Table 29.7 Abused volatile substances

Type of product	Volatile constituent
Adhesives	Toluene
Aerosols	Propellant 11 and 12
Cleaning solvent products	Tetrachloroethylene
Fuel gases	n-butane, isobutane and propane
Inhalational anaesthetics	Halothane and nitrous oxide

activity, popular after school or during school holidays, only 2–5% will persist with solitary use.

Mechanism of action

These substances are diverse in chemical structure but all probably act through a similar mechanism of alteration of the lipid-rich neuroglial membrane. Metabolism mainly occurs in the liver and kidney. Animal studies confirm their reinforcing nature (e.g. rats will self-administer toluene) and although tolerance does develop fairly quickly, there is no evidence of a withdrawal syndrome.

Method of administration

Most commonly, the substance will be placed in a bag, where the fumes are allowed to gather, before inhalation. Other solvents (trichloroethane) may be absorbed onto material such as clothing and inhaled. Aerosols may be inhaled directly or through rebreathing with a bag.

Effects

The inhalation of these substances causes a rapid onset of emotional, perceptual and cognitive change lasting about 30 min, with hallucinations, a euphoric mood and an altered state of awareness. At higher doses, ataxia, nystagmus, frightening hallucinations and confusion may occur with the associated risks of accidental injury.

Complications

Adverse psychological reactions and accidents due to intoxication may occur. A study of 605 deaths from VSA (Esmail et al 1993) showed a male:female ratio of 5:1, with 70% of deaths in those under 18 occurring in the 14–16 age range. At the age of 15 years, 10% of all deaths and 20% of accident/violent related deaths are due to VSA. Death may result from arrhythmias, respiratory depression, inhalation of vomitus, laryngeal spasm with cardiac arrest secondary to vagal stimulation.

Chronic use

Chronic use has been associated with a cerebellar syndrome, while inhalation of lead-containing petrol has been linked with cognitive decline. Liver damage and peripheral neuropathies have also been reported.

Recognition

A high level of awareness and education among parents, teachers and children is needed in order to detect and avert future use in children. Markers of solvent abuse include:

- Apparent intoxication with giggling and confusion
- Smell of glue or perioral dermatitis
- Decline in academic performance or attendance
- Erratic, irritable behaviour
- Glue stains on clothing.

Stricter controls, limiting the variety and access to VSA by age-limits in combination with high-profile education of relevant parties are required to impact on a vulnerable group

Areca (betel) nut

Use of betel nut (areca nut) and its products is widespread, particularly in Indo-Chinese countries, being the fourth most widely used substance after tobacco, alcohol and caffeine, affecting approximately 20% of the world's population. There is some evidence of a dependence syndrome, although the greatest risk is oral submucous fibrosis and malignancy. Betel nut, with or without admixed tobacco, is widely used among UK Indo-Asian immigrants, particularly Gujarati speakers. The chemical composition of the nut is varied, containing a number of psychoactive alkaloids, with arecoline being the one present in the greatest quantity. Arecoline may act as a GABA-uptake inhibitor, as well as a sympathetic stimulant. Anecdotally, the nut and arecoline have significant medicinal properties ranging from an anti-helminthic and astringent to an aphrodisiac, digestive enhancement and psychomotor stimulant.

Legal highs

So-called 'legal highs' represent a diverse group of substances, from synthetic compounds (e.g. BZP, TFMPP and GBH) to traditional plant-based products, such as herbs (e.g. *Salvia divinorum*), seeds (e.g. Hawaiian Baby Woodrose) and fungi (e.g. 'magic mushrooms' and fly agaric). At the time of writing, the UK Government is considering passing legislation against several of these substances including GBL, piperazine derivatives (such as BZP) found in legal high party pills and a host of synthetic cannabinoid analogues that were found to be the active constituents of smoking blends marketed as incense. It is very likely that the next few years will see the appearance of more novel or rebranded compounds designed to provide intoxication within the confines of existing legislation. The psychiatrist should be aware that these substances have the potential to induce a wide range of psychopathological experiences related to their stimulant and psychedelic properties and that their use may not be reported on routine enquiry and may not be detected by urine drug screens. Some may have the potential to cause dependence.

References

Altman, J., Everitt, B.J., Glantier, S., et al., 1996. The biological, social and clinical basis of drug addiction: commentary and debate. Psychopharmacology 125, 285–345.

Andreasson, S., Allebeck, P., Engstrom, A., et al., 1987. Cannabis and schizophrenia: a longitudinal study of Swedish conscripts. Lancet 2, 1483–1486.

Atakan, Z., 2008. Cannabis use by people with severe mental illness – is it important? Advances in Psychiatric Treatment 14, 423–431.

Baker, A., Lee, N., 2003. A review of psychosocial interventions for amphetamine use. Drug Alcohol Rev. 22, 323–335.

Blum, K., Sheridan, P.J., Wood, R.C., et al., 1995. Dopamine D2 receptor gene variants: association and linkage studies in impulsive-addictive-compulsive behaviour. Pharmacogenetics 5, 121–141.

British Crime Survey, 2009. Home Office statistical bulletin1, Vol. Home Office, London.

Caplehorn, J.R., Drummer, O.H., 1999. Mortality associated with New South Wales methadone programs in 1994: lives lost and saved. Med. J. Aust. 170, 104–109.

Cloninger, C.R., 1994. Temperament and personality. Curr. Opin. Neurobiol. 4, 266–273.

Crawford, V., 1997. Injecting drug use. Curr. Opin. Psychiatry 10, 215–219.

Degenhart, L., Hall, W., Lynskey, M., 2003. Exploring the association between cannabis use and depression. Addiction 98, 1493–1503.

Dennis, M., Babor, T.F., Roebuck, M.C., et al., 2002. Changing the focus: the case for recognizing and treating cannabis use disorders. Addiction 97 (Suppl. 1), 4–15.

Dillon, P., Copeland, J., Janen, K., 2003. Patterns of use and harms associated with non-medical ketamine use. Drug. Alcohol Depend. 69, 23–28.

Drummer, O.H., 2006. Drug testing in oral fluid. Clin. Biochem. Rev. 27, 147–159.

Edwards, G., Gross, M., 1976. Alcohol dependence: provisional description of a clinical syndrome. Br. Med. J. 1, 1058.

Esmail, A., Meyer, L., Pettier, A., et al., 1993. Deaths from volatile substance abuse in those under 18 years: results from a national epidemiological study. Arch. Dis. Child 69, 356–360.

Fleming, P.M., Roberts, D., 1994. Is the prescription of amphetamine justified as a harm reduction measure? J. R. Soc. Health 114, 127–131.

Frischer, M., Bloor, M., Goldberg, D., et al., 1993. Mortality among injecting drug users: a critical reappraisal. J. Epidemiol. Community Health 47, 59–63.

Gossop, M., Marsden, J., Stewart, D., et al., 1997. The NTORS in the UK. Six month follow up outcomes. Psychol. Addict. Behav. 11, 324–337.

Goudie, A.J., Emmett-Oglesby, M.W. (Eds.), 1989. Psychoactive drugs: tolerance and sensitisation. Humana Press, New Jersey.

Guillot, C.R., Berman, M.E., 2007. MDMA (Ecstasy) use and psychiatric problems. Psychopharmacology 189, 575–576.

Hall, W., 2006. Is cannabis use psychotogenic? Lancet 367, 193–195.

Hall, W., Solowij, N., Lemon, J., 1994. The health and psychological consequences of cannabis use. National Drug Strategy Monograph Series No 25. Australia Government Publishing Service, Canberra.

Hallstrom, C., 1993. Benzodiazepine dependence. Oxford Medical, Oxford.

Hanson, K.L., Luciana, M., 2004. Neurocognitive function in users of MDMA: the importance of clinically significant patterns of use. Psychol. Med. 34, 229–246.

Hunter, G.M., Donoghue, M.C., Stimpson, G.V., 1995. Crack use and injection on the increase among injecting drug users in London. Addiction 90, 1397–1400.

Johnson, S., 1997. Dual diagnosis of severe mental illness and substance misuse: a case for specialist services? Br. J. Psychiatry 171, 205–208.

Kosten, T.R., 2003. Buprenorphine for opioid detoxification. Addict. Disord. Their Treat. 2, 107–112.

Lambert, M., Conus, P., Lubman, D.I., et al., 2005. The impact of substance use disorders on clinical outcome in 643 patients with first-episode psychosis. Acta Psychiatr. Scand. 112, 141–148.

Lingford-Hughes, A., Nutt, D., 2003. Neurobiology of addiction and implications for treatment. Br. J. Psychol. 182, 92–100.

Maxwell, J.C., 2003. The response to club drugs. Curr. Opin. Psychiatry 16, 279–289.

McCann, U.D., Szabo, Z., Scheffel, U., et al., 1998. Positron emission tomographic evidence of toxic effect of MDMA ('Ecstasy') on brain serotonin neurones in human beings. Lancet 352, 1433–1437.

Meltzer, H., Gill, B., Hinds, K., et al., 1996. OPCS surveys of psychiatric morbidity in Great Britain. HMSO, London.

Miller, W.R., Rollnick, S., 1991. Motivational interviewing: preparing people to change addictive behaviour. Guilford Press, New York.

Morgan, M., 2000. Ecstasy (MDMA): a review of its possible persistent psychological effects. Psychopharmacology (Berlin) 152, 230–248.

Owen, R.R., Fischer, E.P., Booth, B.M., et al., 1996. Medication non compliance and substance abuse among patients with schizophrenia. Psychiatr. Ser. 47, 853–858.

Pecknold, J.C., Swinson, R.P., Kuch, K., et al., 1988. Alprazolam in panic disorder and agoraphobia: discontinuation effects. Arch. Gen. Psychiatry 45, 429–436.

Petry, N.M., 2006. Contingency management treatments. Br. J. Psychiatry 189, 97–98.

Petursson, H., Lader, M., 1984. Dependence on tranquillizers. Oxford University Press, Oxford.

Power, K.G., Markova, I., Rowlands, A., et al., 1992. Intravenous drug use and HIV transmission amongst inmates in Scottish prisons. Br. J. Addict. 87, 35–45.

Powis, B., Strang, J., Griffiths, P., et al., 1999. Self reported overdose among injecting drug users in London: extent and nature of the problem. Addiction 94, 471–478.

Reiger, D.A., Farmer, M.E., Rae, D.S., et al., 1990. Co-morbidity of mental disorders with alcohol and other drug abuse: results from the Epidemiological Catchment Area (ECA) Study. J. Am. Med. Assoc. 264, 2511–2518.

Rodgers, J., Ashton, H., Gilvarry, E., et al., 2004. Liquid ecstasy on the dance floor. Br. J. Psychol. 184, 104–106.

Schuckit, M.A., 2006. The treatment of stimulant dependence. Addiction 89, 559–563.

Simpson, D., Joe, G., Brown, B., 1997. Treatment retention and follow up outcomes in the drug abuse treatment outcomes study (DATOS). Psychol. Addict. Behav. 11, 294–307.

Sugranyes, G., Flamarique, I., Parellada, E., et al., 2009. Cannabis use and age of diagnosis of schizophrenia. Eur. Psychiatry 24, 282–286.

Verdoux, H., Ginde, C., Sorbora, F., et al., 2003. Effects of cannabis and psychosis vulnerability in daily life: an experience sampling study. Psychol. Med. 33, 3–6.

Volkow, N.D., Fowler, J.S., Wang, G.J., 1999. Imaging studies on the role of dopamine in cocaine reinforcement and addiction in humans. J. Psychopharmacol. 13, 337–345.

Weaver, T., Madden, P., Charles, G., et al., 2003. Co-morbidity of substance misuse and mental illness in community mental and substance misuse services. Br. J. Psychol. 183, 304–313.

Winstock, A.R., Griffiths, P., Stewart, D., 2001. Drugs and the dance music scene: a survey of current drug use patterns among a sample of dance music enthusiasts in the UK. Drug Alcohol Depend. 64, 9–17.

Wolff, K., Farrell, M., Marsden, J., et al., 1999. A review of biological indicators of illicit drug use, practical considerations and clinical usefulness. Addiction 94, 1279–1298.

Yücel, M., Solowij, N., Respondek, C., et al., 2008. Regional brain abnormalities associated with long-term heavy cannabis use. Arch. Gen. Psychiatry 65, 694–701.

Zammit, S., Moore, T.H., Lingford-Hughes, A., et al., 2008. Effects of cannabis use on outcomes of psychotic disorders: systematic review. Br. J. Psychiatry 193, 357–363.

Zanis, D.A., Woody, G.E., 1998. One-year mortality rates following methadone treatment discharge. Drug Alcohol Depend. 52, 257–260.

The organization and development of mental health services

Michael Phelan

CHAPTER CONTENTS

Introduction

Much of the history of psychiatry relates to an ever-changing debate about how services should be organized and delivered to patients. The arguments and uncertainty continue today. There is some agreement about the guiding principles for service developments, but far less consensus on how these principles should be put into practice and the differing priorities. For many readers, this may appear to be a dull and esoteric topic, hardly relevant to a busy doctor. Yet little written elsewhere in this book can be put into practice, unless psychiatrists are working in effective and efficient services which are accessible to patients from all backgrounds. Psychiatrists need to know how services can be developed and organized so that they are in a position to take an influential and leading role in future progress.

In Box 30.1, some of the key principles of any mental health service are listed. In the asylum era, patients were frequently housed and treated many miles from their families and homes, in isolated and restricted environments. In contrast, it is now recognized that services should be provided as close as possible to where people live, and in the least restrictive environment. When possible services should be provided in people's homes, so that family support is not lost, and so that disruption to someone's life is kept to a minimum. The development of local mental health services must be dictated by the needs of the population, not by past service provision, which may have grown up in a haphazard way. Services should be focused on those in most need, rather than just on responding to demand. This requires a proactive response from staff. The needs of people with mental illness are often numerous and complex, frequently including social as well as health needs. No single professional group can hope to meet this diverse range of needs, and multidisciplinary teams are required. The providers of services must never lose sight of who they are trying to help, and they should be involved in a regular dialogue with service users, who should be actively involved at all levels of service planning and development. The demanding and vital role of carers is often under-recognized. They also need a voice in the development of services, as well as individual assessment and support. Service users need different types and intensities of help at different times, and must be easily able to access all elements of a service. Ethnic and other minority groups are especially vulnerable to mental illness and services should be able to respond to special needs, for instance by having easy access to interpreting services. Services should be constantly evaluated and able to change in response to the changing needs of the population, while providing the best evidence-based treatments. This evaluation should be focused on actual patient outcomes that are important to

The Care Programme Approach

In the UK, the Care Programme Approach (CPA) introduced the principles of case management into all routine mental health practice (Box 30.4). The aim of the CPA was to promote interprofessional communication and coordination of care among specialist mental health services, and thus reduce the likelihood of people with severe mental illness falling through the safety net of care. During the years after its introduction, failure to implement the CPA was frequently blamed on a lack of mental health resources. It was also hampered by staff having inadequate training and supervision and being reluctant to extend their specialist roles. However, perseverance has produced results and the CPA is now the bedrock of community services in the UK. Recent changes have helped to reduce the bureaucracy of the system (DoH 2008).

Needs assessment

Community services should be dictated by the needs of the people served. The CPA brought the concept of need into everyday mental health practice, by insisting that all service users had a regular assessment of their needs. A need can best be defined as 'what people benefit from', and can be distinguished from demand (what people ask for) and supply (what is provided). An assessment of need will be dependent on who is making the assessment. Need as assessed by a professional is termed 'normative need' and will often differ from the perceived needs of the patient. For instance, staff may well believe that a man needs to be in supported accommodation while he feels that he needs a flat of his own.

Individual needs assessment

Although there is agreement that the assessment of need of individuals should be conducted and be the basis of subsequent care, there is less agreement on exactly how needs should be

Box 30.4

The basic requirements of the CPA

1. **Needs assessment:** a systematic and comprehensive assessment of the social and health needs of any person who appears to require community services
2. **Care plan:** decided upon in conjunction with the service user and carers. It should list identified health and social needs, and planned interventions. Crisis and contingency plans must be included, as well as a risk assessment and risk management plan. Unmet needs should also be included (e.g. when someone refuses a service), and the plan should be flexible and adaptable to change as the service user's needs change. Care plans must take into consideration cultural needs
3. **Care coordinator:** a member of staff is assigned as the focal point of contact for the service user and his or her carers. The care coordinator is responsible for keeping in close contact with them, and for monitoring and coordinating care
4. **Reviews:** care plans are reviewed regularly, and changed when appropriate. Sometimes, this will require a multidisciplinary meeting, but reviews can take place with just the care coordinator and service user. Dates for future reviews must be agreed and recorded.

Box 30.5

Areas of potential need included in the CAN

Basic needs:
- Accommodation
- Food
- Occupation

Health needs:
- Physical health
- Psychotic and neurotic symptoms
- Drugs and alcohol
- Safety to self and others

Social needs:
- Company
- Intimate relationship
- Sexual expression

Functioning:
- Household skills
- Self-care and child care
- Basic education
- Budgeting

Service receipt:
- Information
- Telephone
- Transport
- Welfare benefits.

assessed. If a care plan is to be agreed with a patient, then clearly the initial assessment of need should incorporate the views of the patient (and possibly the carer) as well as the staff. Any assessment must cover a wide range of health, social and basic needs. Many identified needs will be universal, such as the need for food, occupation and money, whereas others will be more specific to a particular patient group (e.g. need for treatment of psychotic symptoms). The Camberwell Assessment of Need (CAN), is a rating scale original designed to quantify need in adults with severe mental illness (Phelan et al 1995) (Box 30.5), and subsequently adapted to cover other groups such as people with learning disabilities and mothers with mental illness. Such an approach has uses in routine clinical work as well as research and evaluation.

Population needs assessment

The ideal way to plan local services would be to assess the needs of all people identified as mentally ill in the area, aggregate the data, and base local service provision on this information. Unfortunately, such detailed information is rarely available. Service planners therefore use a range of proxy measures, which are known to give some approximation of the level of need in a population. These measures include sociodemographic information (e.g. proportion of people from an ethnic minority), previous service utilization, and estimates of the prevalence of specific mental disorders. Such assessments are used to decide on the distribution of mental health resources in different areas. It is hoped that the recent emphasis on needs assessment in healthcare will result in a more equitable distribution of resources, and the provision of more appropriate and targeted help to individuals.

Multidisciplinary working

A prominent characteristic of modern mental health practice is multidisciplinary team (MDT) working. This requires close working links across professions, and some loosening of traditional interprofessional links. For instance, a community psychiatric nurse (CPN) needs to identify him- or herself with a community team composed of different professions, rather than a CPN department. In multidisciplinary teams, there is a risk that staff will feel isolated and be concerned that their core professional skills are not recognized or valued. There is an inevitable tension between the need for team management and the necessity for staff to be supervised by someone from their own profession. Successful teams are those that possess a strong sense of team cohesion, and where individual members are clear about their roles.

Multidisciplinary working has led to the use of terms that are acceptable to different professionals, and reflect the multi-professional input, e.g. mental health services rather than psychiatric services, client or service user rather than patient.

Advocacy and service user involvement

A common problem for people in contact with mental health services is to get staff to understand what they want, and to obtain information about their condition, treatment and rights. This is especially important for those who are compulsorily detained, or who are newly diagnosed with a mental illness. Advocacy and the promotion of user empowerment has been initiated and supported by voluntary organizations such as MIND, Rethink and UKAN (United Kingdom Advocacy Network; see Ch. 12). These, and other organizations, vary in their membership and views, but together have been instrumental in giving patients and their carers a voice in how mental health services are organized, as well as providing support and information to patients and their families. When consulted about local service developments, common priorities among users include:

- The need for advocacy services
- Urgent support out of hours when needed
- Improved communication and information from professionals
- Side-effects of medication
- More psychological therapies
- Quality of care in residential and inpatient settings
- Reducing stigma.

The importance of service user involvement in the development of health services has been widely recognized by the UK government, and is demonstrated by the increasing prominence given to service user views and satisfaction in recent policy and legislation. They also have an important role to play in the teaching and training of psychiatrists and other mental health professionals.

Specific service elements

Community mental health teams

Over the last decade community mental health teams (CMHTs) have been the central point of most adult local mental health services. There are substantial variations in the size and format of CMHTs. Catchment areas can range from 20 000 to 70 000, and staff caseloads can vary from <20 to >40. The two main functions of a CMHT are to provide assessment and short-term treatment for less severe and time limited disorders, and provide on-going care for people with severe mental health illness, especially those who have complex needs and where there are significant risk factors. CMHT staff must work closely with colleagues in other parts of the service, such as the inpatient unit and assertive outreach team, and have effective links with a wide range of services in the community. For instance, a CMHT should have regular contact with the local police, housing department, welfare benefits advisor and local day-care providers. It is also essential that there are excellent links with local primary care teams; this can be encouraged by teams accepting referrals from specific GPs, rather than from a fixed geographical area.

By accepting a wide diversity of referrals and supporting individuals across the spectrum of mental health problems, they usually provide good continuity of care and clear accountability. However, this can all too easily lead to them becoming overwhelmed by the multiple expectations of patients and external agencies. Workload on staff can be excessive as they struggle to deliver evidence-based treatments (e.g. psychological therapies for people with schizophrenia) and do not have the opportunities to develop expertise in specific aspects of practice. Research has highlighted the high levels of stress among community mental health workers in multidisciplinary teams. Prosser et al (1996) found staff to have higher levels of depression and anxiety, and to be more 'emotionally exhausted' than hospital inpatient, day-care or outpatient staff. Job satisfaction among staff appears to be related to having team role clarity, and identification with the team.

Inpatient care

The number of psychiatric hospital beds in England and Wales has fallen by around 75% over the last 50 years, and similar reductions have occurred in most industrialized countries. There is considerable variation in the number of beds across the UK, with 3–4-fold differences in different areas. Even wider differences are seen across European countries. It is never possible to predict exactly how many beds are required, because of the multiple influences (levels of deprivation, alternative provision, local models of care), and although the need for hospital beds can never be entirely replaced by community services, it is not clear whether future reductions are advisable or possible.

The atmosphere and functions of inpatient units have changed markedly as the numbers of beds have fallen. Admissions are now much shorter, patients are more ill, and ward environments are more disturbing. With so much emphasis on the provision of effective community services and alternatives to admission, research and policy into inpatient units lagged behind, and there has been criticism and dissatisfaction about standards of care (DoH 2002a,b). Poor physical environments, reliance on bank staffing, lack of activities, over occupancy and poor multidisciplinary working are some of the difficulties (Brennan et al 2006). Having dedicated inpatient consultant psychiatrists appears to help lift standards, and specific admission wards may improve efficiency and reduce length of stay.

Crisis care

Caring for people in crisis is a core role for mental health services, but emergency services often receive the fiercest criticism from service users. The provision of crisis services poses some specific problems. There is the broad spectrum of problems that present to emergency mental health services, ranging from acute psychosocial crises through to possible organic confusional states. Services need to be provided on a 24-h basis, and this will usually require a degree of centralization, and subsequent difficulties in communication with sectorized daytime services. Staff working in emergency services have to cope with frequent intense encounters with distressed and at times aggressive and violent patients. The pressures on staff are compounded by the need to make rapid management decisions, based on limited information.

Crisis resolution teams

Numerous studies have compared the outcome of acutely ill people managed by a team providing intensive multidisciplinary home support, compared with hospital treatment (e.g. Hoult 1986; Muijen et al 1992). These studies varied in terms of the patients accepted, the characteristics of the local population and the intensity of care provided. However, they all reached broadly similar conclusions: many acutely ill patients can be managed effectively and safely outside hospital; such care does not result in significant differences in clinical or social outcome compared with hospital treatment but is usually more popular with patients; and the costs of community treatment are the same as, or less than, hospital care.

Crisis resolution teams (CRTs) are now incorporated routinely into many local mental health services throughout the UK. They offer a 24-h, 7-day-a-week rapid response service, which can provide an alternative to hospital admission for patients with acute and severe mental health problems. Staff focus on administering medication, providing practical help with the basics of daily living, and working closely with the client's normal support network, which may include family, friends and neighbours. Teams usually consist of around 15 staff members, and have between 20 and 30 clients on their caseload. Contact is intense, but time-limited. Clients may be visited several times a day if necessary, but contact will usually be limited to a few days, or at the most a few weeks. Johnson et al (2005) have demonstrated that in routine practice, such teams appear to be able to replicate the previous experimental work in keeping a significant proportion of patients out of hospital. If CRTs are not able to transfer clients rapidly to local community mental health teams, they quickly become swamped and ineffective.

Acute day hospital care

Day hospitals have traditionally been used to support and rehabilitate people with long-term illnesses, and are perceived as not having a significant role in crisis care. However, this view has been challenged, and research has indicated that many acutely ill people can be effectively and safely managed in a day hospital setting (Creed et al 1991). This is dependent on having adequate staff, however, including medical staff in a day hospital, and on patients having a supportive and secure home to return to at night.

Non-hospital residential care

Crisis respite care in a non-hospital setting is frequently asked for by service users, but rarely provided by statutory services. There are difficulties in providing a safe level of staffing in small residential units, and there can be opposition to opening such units in residential areas. In the UK, there does appear to have been a small and patchy increase in such provision during the last 10 years, but it remains an uncoordinated and under-evaluated element of service provision (Johnson et al 2009).

A&E departments

The first point of contact for many people with a mental health crisis is the accident and emergency (A&E) department of a general hospital. The attitudes of A&E staff towards psychiatric patients can be dismissive and hostile. Junior psychiatrists may have to conduct assessments in noisy and unsafe rooms that lack privacy. The appointment of specific mental health liaison nurses can help to improve communication with other agencies, and tackle negative attitudes among other staff.

Assertive outreach teams

Research suggests that some mentally ill people benefit from long-term community follow-up that is more intensive and assertive than that provided by community mental health teams, and in particular the amount of time that people spend in hospital can be reduced (Mueser et al 1998). Much of this research was conducted in the USA and Australia but nevertheless, such findings have led to the development of assertive outreach teams (AOTs) into mainstream mental health services in the UK. They provide care for people with a severe mental illness, who have a past history of heavy hospital use, difficulty in maintaining contact with standard services, and who have multiple and complex needs. AOTs will usually have a total caseload of around 90 clients, and individual staff will have caseloads of ≤15. Teams may operate 7 days a week, and often work extended hours. There is a strong emphasis on team working, with all staff having some knowledge of all the clients, and teams will persevere for months or even years to develop meaningful engagement with reluctant clients, with the aim of promoting recovery.

The REACT study conducted in London (Killaspy et al 2007) demonstrated that the AOT teams were more likely to remain in contact with clients but did not demonstrate any reductions in bed usage or other significant positive clinical outcomes. One possible reason for this difference, compared with the original research in the USA and Australia, is that the 'standard care' comparison groups in the original studies was of a lower standard than that now routinely provided.

Early intervention teams

There is a strong belief that early treatment in psychosis is crucial. The hope is that early treatment will help to improve long-term outcomes. Currently, there is often a significant period between the onset of symptoms and diagnosis and treatment (Birchwood et al 1997). Early intervention teams (EITs) provide a service for young people (usually 14–35 years) presenting with psychotic symptoms for the first time, and aim to reduce the duration of untreated psychosis (DUP). Such teams concentrate on administering the best possible pharmacological treatments and specialist psychological treatments, while focusing on the needs of the young person, such as their education and employment. As the incidence of schizophrenia and psychosis is low, EITs usually cover a population of up to 1 million, and expect to see around 150 new cases a year. There are some excellent examples of successful services, but it is not yet clear whether they will become a permanent established part of mainstream mental health services. Although these teams appear to produce better outcomes than routine care and to be cost-effective, there are mounting concerns that these gains are lost when care is transferred back to generic teams (Singh 2010).

Primary care

In 1973, The World Health Organization (WHO) stated that 'primary care physicians should form the cornerstone of community psychiatry' as they 'are best placed to provide long-term follow-up and be available for successive periods of illness'. In the UK, there is a unique and extensive network of primary care, which makes this declaration feasible. About 98% of the population are registered with a general practitioner (GP) and 60% consult at least once each year. Several studies have confirmed that 25–30% of patients attending primary care services have a significant psychiatric disorder, much of which may be 'hidden' or unrecognized by the GP (Goldberg & Blackwell 1970). Each GP will have on average around seven people with a severe and enduring mental illness on the list, and between 300 and 600 people with depression and anxiety. Although some patients with a severe mental illness have little or no contact with a GP, the majority have frequent contact and the GP has an opportunity to monitor their mental state and drug treatment, as well as their physical health. Approximately one-quarter of people with schizophrenia have no contact with specialist services and only see their GP.

Deinstitutionalization and short inpatient stays have had an inevitable impact on primary care workload. It is essential for specialist mental health services to work in close collaboration with primary care services, to ensure that the relatively small number of people with severe mental illness receive the necessary physical care, and that GPs are fully supported in caring for the far larger numbers of people with less severe disorders.

In the UK, there has been recent investment in improving access to psychological therapies (IAPT) within primary care. This is in recognition of the fact that minor mental health problems are common and that early appropriate interventions appear to be cost-effective by getting people back to work.

Day-care and occupation

As long-stay patients were discharged from asylums, day hospitals and sheltered workshops were the main providers of rehabilitation and day-care. Although providing a useful service, they were increasingly perceived as being another form of institution, and perpetuating segregation from the wider community. As a result, a wide range of different models of day-care and vocational programmes have developed, but in the UK, provision remains patchy, and for many service users, the options are still limited. There needs to be strong user involvement in any occupational programme to ensure that it is meeting the needs of those that it serves. Most importantly, real jobs for real pay should be available for as many as possible, through vocational support and supported employment schemes.

Housing

No chapter on the organization of mental health services would be complete without at least a mention of the importance of housing. If vulnerable mentally ill people are to survive out of hospital, it is essential that they are provided with adequate and secure accommodation and the appropriate level of support. No amount of nursing or other input will compensate for poor housing. The range of accommodation required in any area to cater for different patients will include 24-h staffed hostels, daytime staffed hostels, group homes with staff visiting and supported flats. Community mental health teams need to develop cooperative links with local housing workers, who are often the first to notice that a tenant is not well when they stop paying rent or fail to look after their property.

There are high rates of mental illness among the homeless, and providing psychiatric services to them requires expertise and hard work. To be successful, services must first address the priorities of the homeless person, such as food and shelter, as well as trying to treat specific psychiatric disorders. Specialist multidisciplinary teams need to balance offering a flexible non-coercive approach, with a therapeutic focus and emphasis on the patient's right to receive treatment (see Ch. 7).

Conclusions

Mental health services are in a constant state of flux. An era of long-term coercive asylum-based care came to a gradual end 50 years ago as services began to focus on acute and 'normalized' care. This then led to an era of 'community care' with more attention given to long-term monitoring and support to the most needy patients. In recent years, the predominance of generic

Any links are also influenced by crime rates, prevalence of psychiatric disorders and application of the criminal justice system as well as how health and social policies are applied to mentally disordered offenders.

It can be helpful to look at the different kinds of offences that are committed before trying to link these with any particular mental disorder.

Crimes committed by mentally disordered offenders are essentially the same as those committed by the general population. They include:

- Violent offences – from minor assault to homicide
- Sexual offences – from indecent assault to rape
- Property offences – acquisitive and destructive offences.

Violent crimes

Violent crimes include the following:

- Wounding:
  - with intent to cause grievous bodily harm (section 18, Offences Against the Person Act 1861)
  - with no intent to cause grievous bodily harm (section 20 of the same act).
- Assault:
  - occasioning actual bodily harm (section 47 of the same Act)
  - common assault.

As with homicide, such offences can be associated with any form of mental disorder in the offender.

The contemporary terminology of 'child abuse and neglect' encompasses non-accidental injury, child neglect, non-organic failure to thrive and sexual and emotional abuse. Abuse varies from the most minor of assaults to the most life-endangering. Cordess (1995) provided a helpful illustration of the classification of child abuse and neglect, and child abduction.

Homicide is the general term for the killing of one human being by another. Legally, homicide is classified into lawful and unlawful homicide. Lawful homicide includes justifiable killings (e.g. on behalf of a state) and excusable homicide (e.g. an accident or reasonable mistake, self-defence). Unlawful homicide was previously defined in common law as 'the unlawful killing of any reasonable creature or being and under the Queen's peace, the death following within a year and a day of the deed'. The Law Reform (Year and a Day Rule) Act 1996 abolished the 'year and a day' rule. Now, a prosecution where a death occurs more than 3 years after an injury can be instituted with the consent of the Attorney General.

Homicide includes murder, manslaughter, killing of infants, which includes child destruction (a killing of a child before birth), infanticide and death by dangerous driving.

There are many motivations for why homicides are committed, including political, during the course of a crime, and 'normal' emotional, such as shame, jealousy, anger or revenge. Alcohol and substance misuse are significant disinhibiting factors for perpetrators of homicide. A small proportion of homicides are committed by offenders with a psychiatric disorder.

Sexual offences

The Sexual Offences Act 2003 defines in detail a wide range of categories of sexual offences against both adults and children:

1. Rape
2. Assault by penetration
3. Sexual assault
4. Causing sexual activity without consent
5. Causing a person to engage in sexual activity without consent
6. Rape and other offences against children under 13
7. Child sex offences
8. Abuse of position of trust
9. Familial child sex offences
10. Offences against persons with a mental disorder impeding choice
11. Inducements, etc. to persons with a mental disorder
12. Care workers for persons with a mental disorder
13. Indecent photographs of children
14. Abuse of children through prostitution and pornography
15. Exploitation of prostitution
16. Trafficking
17. Preparatory offences (e.g. administering a substance with intent)
18. Sex with an adult relative
19. Other offences (exposure; voyeurism; intercourse with an animal; sexual penetration of a corpse; sexual activity in a public lavatory).

In UK law, a child under 13 years in age is not able to consent to a sexual act. A person aged 18 or over commits a sexual offence if he intentionally touches another person, the touching is sexual, and either the child is under 16 and the adult does not reasonably believe that the child is 16 or over, or the child is under 13.

There are various theories of sexual offending against children: Finkelhor's four preconditions model (1984), Wolf's multi-factor model (1985) and Ward and Siegert's pathway model (2002). (There is a chapter on the assessment and management of sexual offenders offering psychodynamic perspectives in 'The New Oxford Textbook of Psychiatry', see Hale et al 2000).

Violent sexual assault against adults includes:

- Rape (rape is seen predominantly as an act of violence expressed in sexual terms)
- Buggery (this is anal intercourse with males or females, and anal or vaginal intercourse with animals, i.e. bestiality)
- Indecent exposure (exhibitionism) (indecent exposure is an offence whereas exhibitionism is a paraphilia).

Ward and Beech (2006) provide an extensive review of the current theoretical understanding of adult sexual offending.

Property offences

Acquisitive property offences are:

- Theft and handling stolen goods, including shoplifting
- Taking and driving away (motor vehicles)

- Robbery
- Blackmail
- Burglary
- Fraud and forgery.

Psychiatric illness is only rarely obviously associated with the above. Shoplifting is predominantly carried out by 10- to 18-year-olds and those dependent on illicit drugs, but a small percentage of such offending is associated with an affective disorder in middle-aged women in particular. Personality and developmental difficulties of adolescence are associated with the taking and driving away of motor vehicles.

There is no specific psychiatric condition associated with burglary, but substance misuse and/or dependency is a common feature in such offenders. Burglaries of domestic dwellings sometimes result in opportunistic acts resulting in crime not apparently planned, for example, in the sexual assault of a victim who happens to be at home during a burglary. In the assessment of such a case, one would have to take into consideration the nature of the psychopathology of the offender, whose disturbed internal world contained the ingredients for this opportunity to arise. In convicted prisoners, a history of burglary has been found to be a factor in the prediction of reconviction for general, sexual, and violent reconvictions.

Destructive (also described as expressive) offences are:

- Criminal damage
- Arson (fire-setting).

Criminal damage is commonly part of a wider antisocial behaviour.

Lewis and Yarnell (1951) and Prins et al (1985) have provided useful classifications of arson. There is no specific mental disorder associated with arson (fire-setting). Historically, the regular requests for psychiatric assessments of arsonists is most likely due to the public's concern about the dangerousness of the behaviour and the view that arsonists must surely be mentally disturbed. The majority of apprehended (most are not) fire-setters, however, are referred to the psychiatric services for assessment, although no particular psychiatric diagnosis is associated with fire-setting. However, a recent Swedish case-controlled study (Anwar et al 2009) concluded that individuals with schizophrenia and other psychoses have a significantly increased risk of an arson conviction.

There are some interesting psychoanalytic speculations about the relationship between fire-setting and early disturbed sexual development, and attempts are being made to address this association more scientifically. Most arsonists are managed within the criminal justice system although some do find their way to secure psychiatric hospitals. In terms of future dangerousness, studies show that about 30% repeat an arson offence but many will commit other types of offences.

Over recent years, forensic psychiatry has also expanded its interest into specific types of offending such as stalking, the 'fixated', 'violent true believers' (individuals committed to an ideology or belief system, which advances homicide and suicide as a legitimate means to further a particular goal), white collar crimes, domestic violence, perversions and child internet pornography.

Specific mental disorders and offending

The relationship between mental disorder and violence is undeniably complex. In the public eye, there has long been an association between the two and the archetypal image of a 'killer schizo' has no doubt been further perpetuated by the development of the entertainment and mass media industries in the modern age. Although, in the past, clinicians were often eager to stress the absence of any association between mental disorder and violence, there is a body of evidence demonstrating a clear statistical link (Hodgins 1992; Mullen 1997; Wallace et al. 1998; Harris & Lurigio 2007). An estimate of the frequency of association between the various kinds of mental disorder and offending is of value in helping to determine the nature and extent of facilities required for appropriate treatment.

Organic disorders

Lishman (1968) found that among head-injured people, post-traumatic antisocial behaviour was rare and almost exclusively confined to those with injuries of the frontal lobe. Subsequent studies have reconfirmed the importance of the frontal lobe or frontotemporal damage but also emphasized that pre-morbid personality traits may be as important as the location and extent of the injury in determining subsequent behavioural disturbances. In 1996, a report from the Vietnam Head Injury Study found that patients with frontal ventromedial lesions consistently demonstrated Aggression/Violence Scale scores significantly higher than controls and patients with lesions in other brain areas. It was concluded that ventromedial frontal lobe lesions increase the risk of aggressive and violent behaviour (Grafman et al 1996). A meta-analysis of studies between 1966 and 2008 found that traumatic brain injury modestly increased the risk of violence (Fazel et al. 2009). A survey of sentenced prisoners in England and Wales (Gunn et al 1991), evaluating a wide offender constituency, including non-violent offenders, found that approximately 1% of them suffered from organic brain disorder.

Schizophrenia

Over recent decades, there has been a growing body of evidence to suggest a putative link between schizophrenia and violence. Clinicians have, at times, been somewhat taciturn in accepting this, however, perhaps because overall rates of violent crime remain, in reality, relatively low in the UK. Serious violence perpetrated by people with schizophrenia is, therefore, a rarity. There have also been a number of prominent studies which have found little or no association between schizophrenia and violence in the absence of co-morbid substance abuse. The influential cross-sectional study by Steadman et al, as part of the McArthur Risk Assessment Study (1998) estimated the prevalence of violence by discharged patients in the community, by diagnosis. The study concluded that discharged patients diagnosed as having schizophrenia were more likely to be violent disorders. It is important to note that there is a close link between having a diagnosis of a personality disorder and suffering from neurotic symptoms whether or not these would amount to a separate diagnosis of neurotic disorder. It can be helpful to examine these neurotic conflicts and the symbolic meanings of particular offences for a given individual through offering psychodynamic psychotherapy.

Epilepsy

The belief in an association between epilepsy and violence has persisted for centuries, peaking in the nineteenth century when Cesare Lombroso, an Italian Criminologist, put forward his theory of a common neurological origin of criminality, genius, and epilepsy. Chiswick (1993) stated that serious violence as an ictal phenomenon is exceedingly rare but, despite this, people with epilepsy were shown to be over-represented in the prisoner population compared with the general population (Gunn 1977), although this study has not been repeated. There is no evidence of a relationship between epilepsy and crimes of violence (Gunn & Taylor 1993). Indeed, a recent meta-analysis of studies between 1966 and 2008 found an inverse relationship between a diagnosis of epilepsy and violence (Fazel et al 2009). It is possible that some degree of brain damage could be responsible for both the epilepsy and antisocial behaviour. Whitman et al (1980) concluded that the important socio-economic correlate of epilepsy accounts for the association and some intrinsic link between epilepsy and violence. Similarly, violence in temporal lobe epilepsy is not simply an ictal phenomenon (Herzberg & Fenwick 1998).

The mentally disordered offender and the criminal justice system

Pre-trial stage issues

Patients can be referred for various reasons before a trial. A court may either remand a defendant into custody and request a psychiatric report from there or bail him and ask for a psychiatric report to be prepared as either an in-patient or an outpatient. There are provisions in Part 3 of the 1983 MHA as amended (sections 35 and 36) that empower the court to remand a defendant to hospital for assessment or treatment. Requests for psychiatric assessment and reports can be from the court, the Crown Prosecution Service, the defence solicitor or the probation service. Generally, reports are requested as a routine for those persons charged with murder. A prison inreach team will make a referral to the local forensic psychiatric service if there are concerns about an inmate's mental health and request that he is transferred urgently for treatment under section 48 of the Mental Health Act 1983 as amended.

A defendant's solicitor will instruct a forensic psychiatrist for a psychiatric report if there are any concerns regarding the defendant's fitness to plead, either arising from mental disorder or learning disability, if a psychiatric defence is potentially available to him/her, or if there are possibly mitigating factors arising from the defendant's mental disorder that could reduce his culpability for the alleged offence (see trial stage issues).

The age of criminal responsibility in England and Wales is now 10 years, whereas it was previously a requirement to prove whether criminal responsibility was possible between the ages of 10 and 14 years. This strict delineation can be seen as a retrograde step, possibly taken following certain high profile cases of children between the ages of 10 and 14 years carrying out serious violent offences including homicide (Bulger case 1993) in order to satisfy society's need for retribution.

Court diversion

Court diversion schemes were introduced in England and Wales in 1989, underpinned by the philosophy that the mentally ill should be treated rather than punished. There is an important role at the interface between the criminal justice system and mental health assigned to diversion, which is loosely defined as a means of ensuring that people with mental health problems who enter the criminal justice system are identified and directed towards appropriate mental health care, particularly as an alternative to imprisonment. Furthermore, prison healthcare wings are not designated as hospitals within the meaning of the National Health Services Act 1977, and treatment cannot be given in prison under the Mental Health Act 1983 as amended.

The court diversion scheme is a means of identifying defendants with mental illness and/or learning disability early on in their journey through the criminal justice system and for putting appropriate interventions in place when their mental health needs are properly identified. Court-based schemes perform three main functions: the screening and assessment of detainees; a negotiation for community-based treatment as an alternative to further involvement in the criminal justice system; referral to local community mental health services.

Trial stage issues

Fitness to plead

The definition of unfitness to plead is based in common law in England and Wales and was first formulated in 1836. The issue of fitness to plead can be raised before a trial starts and the subsequent findings are made by a judge, in the absence of a jury. To be fit to plead, a defendant should be able to:

- Understand the charge(s) and its implications
- Enter a plea of guilty or not guilty
- Challenge jurors
- Instruct counsel
- Follow the evidence in court.

Unfitness can be raised by the defence, prosecution or judge. If found unfit to plead, there is a trial of facts. If the defendant is found not to have committed the offence, he/she is released by the court. If hospital treatment is required following this and the person will not accept it voluntarily, admission would then be under civil section. If the defendant is found to have committed the offence, the judge now has discretion as to disposal.

Following the introduction of The Domestic Violence, Crime and Victims Act 2004, three options for disposal are now available:

- **Hospital Order:** this is equivalent to a Hospital Order under section 37, with or without a Restriction Order under section 41 of the amended 1983 Mental Health Act.
- **Supervision Order:** this is equivalent to a probation order with a condition of psychiatric treatment. (section 9(3), Criminal Justice Act 1991).
- **Absolute Discharge:** this is the disposal where the offence is a minor one and there are no indications for treatment and supervision in the community.

Legal defences

An accused may be found not guilty by reason of insanity under the McNaughten Rules if it can be demonstrated, at the time of committing the act, the party accused was 'labouring under such a defect of reason, from a disease of mind, as not to know the nature and quality of the act he was doing or, if he did know it, that he did not know he was doing what was wrong'. Medicolegal issues centre on the definition of 'disease of mind', which is not a medical concept and has been held to include any disease which affects normal mental functioning. A wide range of illnesses including epilepsy, cerebral arteriosclerosis, diabetes and even sleepwalking are covered by this definition, many of which would not medically or indeed colloquially, be considered insanity. The disease of the mind, once established, must be shown to have caused a defect of reason which resulted in the accused either not understanding the physical nature and quality of what he is doing or not knowing that what he is doing is legally wrong. Delusional beliefs regarding the moral nature of a defendant's actions are therefore not relevant to the defence.

Diminished responsibility

Diminished responsibility is a defence available only for the charge of murder. If successful, it reduces a murder conviction and subsequent mandatory life sentence to a conviction of manslaughter. Diminished responsibility has its roots in the common law of Scotland and was introduced into English law by the Homicide Act 1957 (section 2.1), which states that:

'Where a person kills or is a party to the killing of another, he shall not be convicted of murder if he was suffering from such abnormality of mind (whether arising from a condition of arrested or retarded development of mind, or any inherent cause or induced by disease or injury) as substantially impaired his mental responsibility for his acts and omissions in doing or being a party to a killing'.

An abnormality of mind is defined as a state of mind which a reasonable man would consider abnormal. This wide definition allows the defence to cover many conditions which would not meet the criteria for the insanity defence. Although the abnormality must cause a substantial impairment of mental responsibility, the impairment need not be total. The defendant may therefore know what he is doing and be aware that it is wrong but he must find it substantially more difficult than a normal person to control his actions. The burden of proof is on the defendant, on the balance of probabilities. It is accepted in about 80% of pleas for diminished responsibility.

Automatisms

Medical and legal concepts of automatism differ considerably. Progressive judgements on automatism have changed legal interpretation over the years, though the use of this defence remains rare. Automatism itself has defied a clear medical definition. Fenwick (1990) stated that an automatism is an involuntary behaviour over which an individual has no control. The behaviour itself is usually inappropriate to the circumstances, and may be out of character. It may be complex, coordinated and, apparently, purposeful and directed, though lacking in judgement. Afterwards, the individual may have no recollection, or only partial and confused memory, for his actions. In organic automatisms, there must be some disturbance of brain function, sufficient to give rise to the above features. In psychogenic automatisms, the behaviour is complex, coordinated, and appropriate to some aspects of the patient's psychopathology. The sensorium is usually clear, but there will be severe or complete amnesia for the episode (see Ch. 27).

In legal terms, the defence of automatism applies to a situation where the defendant has a total lack of voluntary control over his actions. Automatism was defined by Lord Denning 'an act which is done by the muscles without any control by the mind, such as a spasm, a reflex action or a convulsion; or an act done by a person who is not conscious of what he is doing, such as an act done while suffering a concussion or sleepwalking'. In the appeal hearing of the same case in 1983, the Lord Chancellor, Viscount Kilmiur, further defined automatism as 'the state of the person, though capable of action, is not conscious of what he is doing. It means unconsciousness, involuntary action and it is a defence because the mind does not go with what is being done'.

The legal concept of automatism is effectively divided into two types: insane automatism and non-insane or true automatism. In cases of non-insane automatism, the lack of control must be due to an external factor, for example a head injury, the effect of an anaesthetic or insulin-induced hypoglycaemia. Alternatively, if the lack of control is caused by an internal factor, such as epilepsy, diabetes or a cerebral tumour, it would be considered an insane automatism (in effect legal insanity) as the cause constitutes a disease of the mind in legal terms.

Intoxication

Under certain circumstances, one may expect an intoxicated individual who commits a crime not to have the necessary *mens rae* (guilty mind) at the time of the act. This should, strictly speaking, result in the individual being acquitted. In order to prevent defendants avoiding conviction on the basis of intoxication, the law has evolved in terms of policy rather than legal logic. Crimes are distinguished between those of basic intent, where the *mens rae* necessary is no more than the intentional or reckless commission of the act (such as rape, various offences of assault and manslaughter) and those of specific intent (such as murder, theft and any attempted crime). Voluntary intoxication is not a defence to a crime of basic intent but there are situations where it may be put forward as a mitigating factor, such as in crimes of specific intent.

Multi-agency public protection arrangements (MAPPA)

Multi-agency public protection arrangements (MAPPA) were established by the Criminal Justice and Court Services Act (2000). The arrangements require police and probation to work together to manage the risk posed by dangerous offenders in the community. The MAPPA Guidance was revised in 2009 to achieve greater consistency of practice across different areas of the country. The plan was for the Prison Service to become part of the responsible authority with the police and the National Probation Service. Furthermore, there would be a statutory duty to cooperate by those agencies that, although not part of the Criminal Justice System, work with sex offenders. These agencies include local health authorities and NHS trusts, housing authorities and registered social landlords, social services departments, social security and employment service departments, youth offending teams, local education authorities and electronic-monitoring providers. There are four key features within MAPPA:

1. **Identifying Offender to be Supervised under MAPPA**

   This is generally determined by offence and sentence but is also assessed by perceived risk. There are three formal categories of offender:

   ○ Category One: registered sex offenders. There were around 32 000 category one offenders identified in 2008/2009.

   ○ Category Two: violent offenders or other sex offenders. There were approximately 11 500 within this category in 2008/2009.

   ○ Category Three: other offenders. This category comprised of around 900 individuals in 2008/2009.

2. **Sharing of Information about Offenders**

   MAPPA aims to promote information sharing between all relevant agencies with a view to establishing more effective supervision and better public protection. In practical terms this can, on occasion, raise issues of confidentiality.

3. **Assessing Risk Posed by Offenders Supervised under MAPPA**

4. **Managing Risk Posed by Offenders Supervised under MAPPA.**

Offenders are managed within one of three levels, depending on the degree of supervision they require. *Level One* offenders are assessed as presenting low or medium risk of serious harm to others and are managed under normal agency management. Just under 75% of MAPPA offenders were managed at this level in 2008/2009. *Level Two* offenders are assessed as posing a high or very high risk of harm and are designated as requiring local inter-agency risk management. They accounted for approximately 22% of MAPPA cases in 2008/2009. *Level Three* offenders are those who pose the highest risk of causing serious harm and whose management is so problematic that multi-agency cooperation and oversight at a senior level is required, with the authority to commit what

is termed, exceptional resources. In 2008/2009, 2% of MAPPA cases fell into this category.

Prison psychiatry

Psychiatric healthcare in prisons has been a cause for concern over the centuries, particularly the availability and quality of the care. The primary aim of prison is custody of its inmates; institutional practices are therefore of the utmost importance, and this places medical care in general in a less important role.

Gunn et al (1991) surveyed a prison population based on a 5% sample of men serving sentences. They looked at 406 young offenders and 1478 adult men, 404 and 1365, respectively who agreed to be interviewed. A total of 37% of the men had psychiatric disorders diagnosed, of whom 0.8% had organic disorders, 2% psychosis, 6% neurosis, 10% personality disorder and 23% substance misuse. Some 35% were judged to require transfer to hospital for psychiatric treatment; 5% required treatment in a therapeutic community setting and a further 10% required further psychiatric assessment or treatment within the prison. By extrapolation, the sentenced prison population includes over 700 men suffering from psychoses and around 1100 who would warrant transfer to hospital for psychiatric treatment.

The ONS survey of psychiatric morbidity among prisoners in England and Wales (Singleton et al 1998) was commissioned by the Department of Health in 1997 to provide up-to-date baseline information about the prevalence of psychiatric problems among male and female, remand and sentenced prisoners in order to inform policy decisions about services. Among those who had a clinical interview, the prevalence of any personality disorder was 78% for males on remand, 64% for males sentenced and 50% for female prisoners. Antisocial personality disorder had the highest prevalence of any category of personality disorder.

The prevalence rates for any functional psychosis in the past year (2009) based on the clinical interview data were 7% for males sentenced, 10% for males on remand and 14% for female prisoners. Schizophrenic or delusional disorders were more common than affective disorders. These rates are far higher than found in the earlier survey of the general household population in which a rate of 4/1000 (0.4%) was found. Elevated rates of neurotic symptoms, PTSD symptoms, suicidality, history of hazardous drink and substance misuse were also identified.

In 1996, Her Majesty's Chief Inspectorate of Prisons for England and Wales identified serious problems in prison healthcare delivery, which was then provided by prison medical and nursing services employed directly by the Home Office. Problems included poor quality of care and impoverished links with the NHS. It was decided that the NHS should deliver prison healthcare and in 1997, the Prison Service Health Advisory Committee formally stated that prisoners are entitled to access the same range and quality of health services as the general public. From 2001, mental health 'inreach' teams were brought into prisons. These were intended to function in a similar fashion to community mental health teams. Inreach teams are multidisciplinary, managed by NHS Trusts and commissioned by local Primary Care Trusts.

Risk assessment and risk management

Risk assessment and risk management has become an essential and prominent part of almost all mental health practice. Western society over the last few decades have become increasingly intolerant of risk, with an increasing 'culture of blame' and a desire for the eradication of risk of untoward events. It is of course impossible to practise psychiatry without some uncertainty, although mental health professionals have a duty to provide the best treatment to and management of any given patient they have assessed.

One key event in California in the late 1960s has influenced how psychiatry and psychotherapy is practiced. The *Tarasoff* decisions arose when the parents of Tatiana Tarasoff (a student at the University of California), who had been killed in 1968 by fellow student Prosenjit Poddar, sued Poddar's treating mental health professionals and their employer, the University of California. While Tatiana was away on holiday, Poddar had told his psychologist that he was thinking about killing a particular young woman. The psychologist guessed who the woman was and informed the university campus police. Although the police checked up on Poddar, they did not detain him. Poddar stopped seeing his psychologist, and fatally stabbed Tatiana after she returned to California.

In its first decision on this matter, in 1974, the California Supreme Court ruled that the psychologist's response had been insufficient. The Court ruled that the psychologist should also have warned Tatiana about the danger Poddar posed to her. After a re-hearing was requested, the California Supreme Court issued a second ruling that described the clinician's duties even more broadly: 'once a therapist does in fact determine, or under applicable professional standards reasonably should have determined, that a patient poses a serious danger of violence to others, he bears a duty to exercise reasonable care to protect the foreseeable victim of that danger'. In other words, whereas the general public have a moral (but not a legal) duty to inform a potential victim of the danger someone may pose to them, mental health professionals have a legally enshrined duty to disclose a specific and credible threat.

Risk-thinking, in terms of both risk assessment and risk management evolved significantly since the 1970s, when in 1974 The American Psychiatric Association issued the following pronouncement: 'We are not able to predict who will be violent'. Unstructured clinical risk assessment has evolved to 2nd generation actuarial tools and progressed to the current use of 3rd generation 'Structured Clinical Guides'. Much of the research and the development of risk assessment tools has originated from North America. In forensic mental health settings and in the criminal justice system, being able to predict the likelihood that an individual poses a risk of committing a serious act of physical or sexual violence has significant consequences. For example, psychiatric evidence given at a sentence hearing could be used to determine whether or not a defendant is dangerous could impact on the length or nature of a custodial sentence and when making pre-release decisions. Risk assessment will also determine whether a mentally disordered offender would require admission to a secure psychiatric hospital, the level of security and determine pre-discharge decisions and the level of community psychiatric supervision and monitoring.

It is important to point out the difference in language used by forensic mental health practitioners and the criminal justice system. The terms 'dangerous' and 'risky' should not be seen as interchangeable. Dangerousness is a legal concept, and, since the Criminal Justice Act 2003 came into force, it remains an issue forensic psychiatrists are asked to address when instructed to assist the court in making sentencing decisions.

'Dangerousness' is a rather vague term with numerous different meanings. It has been seen to imply a relatively enduring and stable characteristic of a person and not take into account specific dynamic factors or environmental triggers that may increase the likelihood of a particular individual deciding to commit a violent act. It can also be a label that is easy to attach to someone but far harder to remove.

The shift of emphasis away from 'dangerousness' and towards a broader concept of risk assessment was summarized by Steadman (1993):

* A move from a legal concept of dangerousness to a 'decision-making concept' of risk
* That prediction should be considered as being on a continuum rather than a 'yes/no' dichotomy
* That there should be a shift away from the notion that there can be single prediction of risk, to a recognition that there is a continuing process of risk assessment that must be incorporated into the day-to-day management of mentally disordered people.

Early research on the ability of mental health professionals to assess dangerousness in people with mental disorder produced less than encouraging results. Monahan's comprehensive review in 1981 of the existing studies (first generation) at the time concluded:

> 'The 'best' clinical research currently in existence indicates that psychiatrists and psychologists are accurate in no more than one out of three predictions of violent behaviour over a several-year period among institutionalized populations that have both committed violence in the past (and thus have a high base rate for it) and who were diagnosed as mentally ill'.

Subsequent studies (second generation) suggested that mental health professionals had at least a modest ability to predict violence and that their predictions were significantly more accurate than chance. The most common type of incorrect predictions were false positives, i.e. incorrectly predicting an individual would go on to commit a violent act.

Mossman's review (1994) of risk prediction studies over the past two decades concluded:

1. Clinicians were able to distinguish violent from non-violent patients with a 'modest, better-than-chance level of accuracy'.
2. Predictive ability in second generation studies appeared to be better than in the first generation studies.
3. The accuracy of short-term predictions was not significantly different than the accuracy of long-term predictions.
4. Past behaviour was a robust predictor of future behaviour.

proceedings, including evidence required to determine fitness to plead or for the purpose of sentencing.

Part 33.2 of the Act describes an expert's duty to the court:

1. An expert must help the court to achieve the overriding objective by giving objective, unbiased opinion on matters within his expertise.

2. This duty overrides any obligation to the person from whom he receives instructions or by whom he is paid.

3. This duty includes an obligation to inform all parties and the court if the expert's opinion changes from that contained in a report served as evidence or given in a statement under Part 24.

Part 33.3 states an expert's report must:

1. Contain details of the expert's qualifications, relevant experience and accreditation

2. Contain details of any literature or other information that the expert has relied on in making the report

3. Contain a statement setting out the substance of all facts given to the expert that are material to the opinions expressed in the report or upon which those opinions are based

4. Make clear which of the facts stated in the report are within the expert's own knowledge

5. State who carried out any examination, measurement, test or experiment which the expert has used for the report and –
   a. Give the qualifications, relevant experience, and accreditation of that person
   b. Say whether or not the examination, measurement, test or experiment was carried out under the expert's supervision
   c. Summarize the findings on which the expert relies

6. Where there is a range of opinion on the matters dealt with in the report –
   a. Summarize the range of opinion, and
   b. Give reasons for his own opinion

7. If the expert is not able to give his opinion without qualification, state the qualification

8. Contain a summary of the conclusions reached

9. Contain a statement that the expert understands his duty to the court, and has complied and will continue to comply with that duty

10. Contain the same declaration of truth as a witness statement.

Planning the written report

1. Ensure the interview is carefully recorded, including the history and the mental state examination of the subject of the report. Handwritten notes should be structured, legible and comprehensive.

2. The expert should be prepared to reveal everything in the report. However, if it is either advisable or necessary to exclude any material, explicit reference should be made so that the parties or the Court can decide whether or not they should see it, although it may not be revealed in open court.

3. State the name and date of birth of the person assessed.

4. Provide an introductory paragraph indicating who instructed you, the basis for the instruction, the defendant's current situation (e.g. on bail, in prison) and any relevant Mental Health Act they may be detained under.

5. If the defendant has been charged, then state what charge(s) he/she faces with and how he/she is pleading.

6. Refer to the dates and places of interviews held and all other information made available to you.

7. Summarize the prosecution's account of the (alleged) offence from information available such as witness statements. Any aspects of the person's mental state at the time should be documented. Summarize the police interview(s) transcript(s) and indicate if there is anything unusual in the transcript suggestive of an abnormal mental state.

8. Ask the interviewee for an account of the (alleged) offence. If he/she has yet to enter a plea or has entered a not guilty plea, frame the question in terms of what the allegations consist of.

9. Proceed with a background history, including a picture of the family dynamics if this is possible from the material available. This can be followed by the personal history, including birth and early childhood development, schooling, delinquency in adolescence, academic qualifications, employment record, drugs and alcohol history, forensic history, medical history, psychosexual history and psychiatric history.

10. The defendant's mental state at the time of both the (alleged) offence and the assessment should now be described.

11. In the conclusions section, begin with a very brief resumé of the background and personal history.

12. Give your opinion of any diagnosis/es with clear evidence to support your opinion and whether the interviewee is detainable under the Mental Health Act.

13. Give your opinion on the person's mental state at the time when the (alleged) offence was committed. Give an opinion on whether intoxication with alcohol, illicit drugs, psychological factors or active symptoms of mental disorder affected the person's behaviour at that time.

14. It can be helpful to a court to include a psychodynamic formulation which contains current psychopathology, aetiological factors and any maintaining factors. The purpose of this would be to try to offer a picture of the offender's internal world to the court as a way of increasing everybody's understanding of the offence in relation to that particular individual, and thereby improve the chances that the person will receive the most appropriate disposal.

15. An opinion on suitability for treatment should be given if possible. If treatment is recommended, then it ought to be specified.

16. The recommendations must be within the remit of the court and should be available. It is sensible to make any recommendations respectfully to the court and to mention any concerns you might have should those recommendations not be followed. A comment on prognosis is appreciated but not always possible.

17. State your name and qualifications at the end and your current status within your profession. Date the report.

Appearing in court

Before attending court to give oral evidence, read your report again to be familiar with its contents. It can be helpful to read any literature which can support your opinion and recommendations. If a long time has lapsed since the preparation of the report, you may need to consider a further interview with the person and provide an addendum to your report prior to the hearing.

It is helpful to make yourself familiar with court procedures as this can help overcome feelings of anxiety induced by what may be perceived as a strange, threatening or even hostile atmosphere. Note which court you are appearing in, e.g. Magistrates' Court, Crown Court, High Court or Central Criminal Court.

It is best to respect dress code and time. Generally, courts are very appreciative of professionals giving their time to assist.

The following notes apply to all courts:

- Announce your arrival to the clerk.
- Bow to the bench when you enter.
- You will be shown where to sit.

- Be prepared for how you will want to be sworn in, as you will be asked.
- When you say the oath, use this as an opportunity to gauge your voice projection.
- Check how to address the bench (e.g. the judge will be addressed as 'Your Honour' in Crown Court, or 'My Lord' or 'My Lady' in High Court).
- In the witness box, bring only your report and any notes you have prepared that you have checked can be disclosed, as this may be requested.
- Answer questions succinctly and do not attempt to answer questions beyond your remit, especially when you are feeling pressed to do so.
- When asked a question by a barrister or Queen's counsel, turn towards the bench when replying. He/she is the person you are answering to.
- Remember that you are an impartial witness there to assist the court.
- When you leave the court, bow again.

It may be helpful to discuss your experience in court with colleagues afterwards, especially if you have had a difficult cross-examination.

Further reading

Bluglass, R., Bowden, P. (Eds.), 1990. Principles and practice of forensic psychiatry. Churchill Livingstone, London.

Chiswick, D., Cope, R. (Eds.), 1995. Seminars in practical forensic psychiatry. Royal College of Psychiatrists, London.

Cordess, C., Cox, M. (Eds.), 1998. Forensic psychotherapy: crime, psychodynamics and the offender patient. Jessica Kingsley, London.

Doctor, R. (Ed.), 2003. Dangerous patients: a psychodynamic approach to risk assessment and management. Karnac, London.

References

Anwar, S., Langstrom, N., Grann, M., et al., 2009. Is arson the crime most strongly associated with psychosis?—A national case-control study of arson risk in schizophrenia and other psychoses. Schizophr. Bull. 0, sbp098v1–sbp098 [Epub ahead of print].

Appelbaum, P.S., Robbins, P.C., Monahan, J., 2000. Violence and delusions: data from the MacArthur Violence Risk Assessment Study. Am. J. Psychiatry 157, 566–572.

Blair, J., Mitchell, D., Blair, K., 2005. The psychopath: emotion and the brain. Blackwell, Oxford.

Chiswick, D., 1993. Forensic psychiatry. In: Kendell, R.E., Zealley, A.K. (Eds.), Companion to psychiatry studies. Churchill Livingstone, London.

Cleckley, H., 1941. The mask of sanity. Mosby, St Louis MO.

Cordess, C., 1995. Crime and mental disorder: 1. criminal behaviour. In: Chiswick, D., Cope, R. (Eds.), Practical forensic psychiatry. Seminars in practical forensic psychiatry. Redwood Press, Wiltshire.

Day, K., 1994. Male mentally handicapped sex offenders. Br. J. Psychiatry 165, 630–639.

Department of Constitutional Affairs, 2006. Criminal Procedure Rules. Part 33. Expert evidence. The Stationery Office, London.

Dien, K., Woodbury-Smith, M., 2010. Asperger syndrome and criminal behaviour. Advances in Psychiatric Treatment 16, 37–43.

Fazel, S., Danesh, J., 2002. Serious mental disorder in 23,000 prisoners: a systematic review of 62 surveys. Lancet 359, 545–550.

Fazel, S., Philipson, J., Gardiner, L., Merrit, R., Grann, M., 2009. Neurological disorders and violence: a systematic review and meta-analysis with a focus on epilepsy and traumatic brain injury. J. Neurol. 256, 1432–1459.

Fenwick, P., 1990. Automatism. In: Bluglass, R., Bowden, P. (Eds.), Principles and practice of forensic psychiatry. Churchill Livingstone, London.

Finkelhor, D., 1984. Child sexual abuse: new theory and research. Free Press, New York.

Freidman, S., Howitz, S., Resnick, P., 2005. Child murder by mothers: a critical analysis of the

current state of knowledge and a research agenda. Am. J. Psychiatry 162, 1578–1587.

Grafman, J., Schwab, K., Warden, D., et al., 1996. Frontal lobe injuries, violence, and aggression: a report of the Vietnam Head Injury Study. Neurology 46, 1231–1238.

Gunn, J., 1977. Epileptics in prison. Academic Press, London.

Gunn, J., Taylor, P.J. (Eds.), 1993. Forensic psychiatry clinical, legal and ethical issues. Butterworth-Heinemann, Oxford.

Gunn, J., Maden, A., Swinton, M., et al., 1991. Treatment needs of prisoners with psychiatric disorders. Br. Med. J. 303, 338–340.

Hale, R., Dhar, R., 2008. Flying a kite – observations on dual (and triple) diagnosis. Crim. Behav. Ment. Health 18, 145–152.

Hale, R., Minne, C., Zachary, A., 2000. Assessment and management of sexual offenders. In: Lopez-Ibor, , Andreasen, (Eds.), The new Oxford textbook of psychiatry. OUP, Oxford, pp. 2061–2066.

Hare, R.D., 1991. The Hare psychopathy checklist. Multi-Health Systems, New York.

5%, respectively in those over 75 years with dementia. Alzheimer disease is more common in men and vascular dementia is more common in women.

The prevalence of dementia in nursing and residential home populations is 35–50% for mild/moderate dementia and around 30% for severe dementia. The prevalence of dementia among acutely ill and continuing care geriatric inpatients is 35–61% and up to 90%, respectively.

Depression

The reported prevalence of depression in the elderly ranges from 11% to 16%. There is evidence that prevalence of depression increases with age in women (Copeland et al 1987). The prevalence of depression in residential and nursing home populations is about 35%. The prevalence of depression in acutely ill and continuing care geriatric inpatients of up to 50% and 38%, respectively has been reported.

Neurosis

The Liverpool study reported a prevalence of 2.4% for all neuroses (Copeland et al 1987). The Guy's/Age Concern survey reported prevalence of 3.7% for generalized anxiety and 10% for phobias (7.8% agoraphobias, 1.3% social phobias and 2.1% specific phobias) (Lindesay et al 1989). However, many of these individuals also had co-morbid depression and thus, the prevalence of pure neurosis is likely to be lower. Personality disorder has not been systematically studied in the elderly.

Schizophrenia and late paraphrenia

In the Liverpool study, the prevalence of these disorders was 0.1% (Copeland et al 1987).

Dementia

Definition

The ICD-10 defines dementia as follows: dementia is a syndrome due to disease of the brain, usually of chronic or progressive nature, in which there is impairment of multiple higher cortical functions, including memory, thinking, orientation, calculation, learning capacity, language and judgement. Consciousness is not clouded. The cognitive impairments are commonly accompanied, and occasionally preceded, by deterioration in emotional control, social behaviour or motivation. This syndrome occurs in Alzheimer disease, in cerebrovascular disease, and in other conditions primarily or secondarily affecting the brain.

Thus, dementia implies global intellectual deterioration. Moreover, functional impairment is a necessary prerequisite for the diagnosis of dementia (see Ch. 27 and Box 32.1).

Box 32.1

Diagnostic guidelines for ICD-10 diagnosis of dementia in Alzheimer disease

The following features are essential for a definite diagnosis:
- Presence of dementia as described above
- Insidious onset with slow deterioration. While the onset usually seems difficult to pin-point in time, realization by others that the defects exist may come suddenly. An apparent plateau may occur in progression
- Absence of clinical evidence, or findings from special investigations to suggest that the mental state may be due to other systemic or brain disease which can induce a dementia (e.g. hypothyroidism, hypercalcemia, vitamin B_{12} deficiency, niacin deficiency, neurosyphilis, normal pressure hydrocephalus, or subdural)
- Absence of a sudden, apoplectic onset, or of neurological signs of focal damage such as hemiparesis, sensory loss, visual field defects, and incoordination occurring early in the illness (although these phenomena may be superimposed later).

Non-cognitive features

In addition to cognitive impairment, dementia encompasses several non-cognitive domains, including disorders of behaviour, personality, mood, thought content and perception and functional disability. These are nowadays referred to as behavioural and psychological signs and symptoms of dementia (BPSD).

Behaviour disturbances including agitation, aggression, wandering, pacing, restlessness, sleeplessness and sexual disinhibition are not uncommon and occur in over 50% of patients during the course of dementia (Burns et al 1990a). Personality changes, including emergence of new personality features or an exaggeration of pre-morbid personality traits, are common in dementia (Jacomb & Jorm 1996). Personality in this context includes the ability to express and experience emotions, however inappropriate.

The prevalence of depressive symptoms and depressive illness in Alzheimer disease are 0–87% (median 41%) and 0–86% (median 19%), respectively (Wragg & Jeste 1989). The prevalence of depressive symptoms and syndrome is generally greater in vascular dementia than Alzheimer disease.

Auditory, visual and olfactory hallucinations have been described (Burns et al 1990b). A former classification of delusions (simple persecutory, complex persecutory, grandiose and those associated with specific neurological deficits) has been modified into delusions of theft, delusions of suspicion and systematized delusions (Burns et al 1990c). Four types of misidentification syndromes have been described (Burns et al 1990b): people in the house, misidentification of mirror image, misidentification of television and misidentification of people. The prevalence of delusions, hallucinations and misidentification syndromes in Alzheimer and vascular dementia varies: 20–50%, 17–36% and 11–34%, respectively (Burns et al 1990b,c).

Alzheimer disease

Definition

The essential features for an ICD-10 diagnosis of dementia of Alzheimer type are listed in Box 32.1. ICD-10 further classifies this dementia into four sub-groups: dementia in Alzheimer disease with: (i) early onset, (ii) late-onset, (iii) atypical or mixed and (iv) unspecified. The DSM-IV definition of Alzheimer disease is similar.

Pathology

Pathological changes include widening of sulci, narrowing of gyri and ventricular enlargement consistent with brain atrophy. Histological changes include senile plaques, neurofibrillary tangles, granulovacuolar degeneration and amyloid deposition in blood vessel walls in cortical and subcortical grey matter. Amyloid has been identified as the main ingredient of senile plaques. The severity of cognitive impairment and neurotransmitter changes are associated with the number of senile plaques (see Ch. 27).

Aetiology

First-degree relatives of Alzheimer disease sufferers have a three-fold higher risk of developing the disorder, although most cases are sporadic. Three specific pathogenic loci and several risk-associated loci have been identified using linkage studies of family pedigrees. Autosomal dominant pattern of inheritance is observed in some families with early-onset disease. Patients with Down syndrome, with trisomy 21 and variants, have a higher risk of developing Alzheimer disease. Mutations in the amyloid precursor protein (APP) gene located on chromosome 21 have been identified as a cause of early-onset Alzheimer disease. APP is a transmembrane glycoprotein and its derivative, β-amyloid peptide, is found in amyloid plaques. APP gene mutations can cause the three secretase enzymes involved in the cellular processing of APP to produce more β-amyloid. Mutations on presenilin-1 gene, located on chromosome 14, account for some early-onset familial Alzheimer disease. A homologous gene, presenilin-2, on chromosome 1 has a similar effect. The precise function of the presenilin genes is unclear, but they may be involved in the transport and processing of APP within the nerve cell (see Ch. 3).

Apolipoprotein is found both in plaques and tangles. Moreover, Alzheimer disease is associated with apolipoprotein E genes (ApoE) located on chromosome 19 (Saunders et al 1993). ApoE exists in three forms in the following order of frequency: ε3, ε4 and ε2. The various permutations individuals can have are ε3ε3, ε3ε2, ε3ε4, ε4ε4, ε4ε2 and ε2ε2. Having one ε4 allele increases the risk of having Alzheimer disease four-fold and having two ε4 alleles increases the risk 16-fold. Presence of ε4 alleles can reduce the age of onset. However, about 40% of Alzheimer disease patients do not possess an ε4 allele, so its presence is not necessary or sufficient for the development of Alzheimer disease. Other risk modifying genes of possible importance include $α_1$-antichymotrypsin gene and possible candidate genes on chromosome 12 (see Ch. 3).

Other risk factors include age, infections, autoimmune conditions, head injury, hypertension and hypotension, aluminium, previous history of depression, advanced maternal age at birth and thyroid disease. Diagnosis of rheumatoid arthritis, long term prescription of non-steroidal anti-inflammatory drugs, steroids and oestrogens are reported to be protective against the development of Alzheimer disease.

Vascular dementia

Definition

The ICD diagnosis of vascular dementia assumes the general definition of dementia described earlier. ICD-10 vascular dementia is divided into several categories including acute onset, multi-infarct, subcortical vascular dementia, mixed cortical and subcortical dementia, other vascular dementia and unspecified. The DSM-IV criteria are similar. The probability of the diagnosis is increased by abrupt onset (possible index vascular event), stepwise decline (possible recurrent vascular events), presence of associated arteriosclerosis, focal neurological signs and symptoms, patchy cognitive deficits, relative preservation of personality, nocturnal confusion, hypertension and evidence of cardiovascular disease.

Pathology

In vascular dementia there may be gross or localized brain changes with atrophy and ventricular dilatation. There may be evidence of ischaemia and infarction in brain tissue, and arteriosclerosis in the major blood vessels. There are no characteristic neurochemical changes (see Ch. 27).

Aetiology

Risk factors for the development of vascular dementia include male sex, increasing age, oriental culture, hypertension, heart disease, strokes, diabetes, cigarette smoking and hyperlipidaemia.

Dementia with Lewy bodies

This dementia, also called cortical Lewy body disease and Lewy body dementia, is characterized by Lewy bodies in the cerebral cortex and the substantia nigra (see Ch. 27). It is also associated with reduction in acetylcholine transferase in the neocortex and reduced dopamine in the caudate nucleus. Variable prevalence of 6–15%, depending on sample types, has been reported.

Clinical features include fluctuating cognition with pronounced variations in attention and alertness, recurring visual hallucinations, which are typically well formed and detailed, spontaneous motor features of parkinsonism and neuroleptic sensitivity (Consensus Guidelines for the Clinical Diagnosis of Dementia with Lewy Bodies, DLB 1996). Repeated falls, transient disturbance of consciousness, systematized delusions and hallucinations in other modalities also occur. Mortality is increased in patients treated with neuroleptics. Severity of cognitive impairment is associated with the density of cortical Lewy bodies.

Other dementias

A number of other dementias occur in old age, including those due to alcohol, fronto-temporal dementias, normal pressure hydrocephalus, neurosyphilis, and those due to vitamin deficiencies (see Ch. 27).

The management of dementias

The government has made dementia a national priority and recently published the National Dementia Strategy for England (DoH 2009). It aims to ensure that significant improvements are made to dementia services across three key areas: improved awareness, earlier diagnosis and intervention, and a higher quality of care. The strategy lists 17 key objectives which are outlined in Box 32.2.

Diagnosis

A detailed history from the patient and informants, mental and physical state examination, and special investigations are required for accurate diagnosis. The history should also address any sensory impairment and loss of function. A detailed cognitive assessment will allow accurate identification of the precise cognitive deficits and their functional consequences. This can be further supplemented by formal neuropsychometric assessment by a clinical psychologist, particularly when there are doubts about diagnosis. Physical examination will allow identification of the aetiology of dementia and any associated

delirium, the severity of self-neglect due to dementia and sensory impairment. This should facilitate distinction between dementia, delirium superimposed on dementia, delirium alone and other mental illness. Table 32.1 illustrates some of the distinguishing features between delirium and dementia (see Ch. 27).

In general, the findings of the history and examination will guide as to which special investigations are needed (listed in Box 32.3) in order to further identify reversible causes of dementias and super-added delirium and identify the severity of self-neglect. MRI and CT scans may allow identification of other structural pathologies like tumours and help in the differential diagnosis of dementias. They can help identify ischaemic

Table 32.1 Distinction between dementia and delirium

	Dementia	Delirium
Onset	Insidious	Acute
Decline	Relatively slow	Rapid
Level of consciousness	Alert	Clouding of consciousness
Sensory	No hypersensitivity	Hypersensitivity (e.g. perceptions hyperacusis)
Visual hallucinations	Less common	More common
Stability of mental	Fairly stable state	Fluctuating

Box 32.2

National Dementia Strategy: Key objectives

1. Raise awareness of dementia and encourage people to seek help
2. Good quality early diagnosis, support and treatment for people with dementia and their carers, explained in a sensitive way
3. Good quality information for people with dementia and their carers
4. Easy access to care, support and advice after diagnosis
5. Develop structured peer support and learning networks
6. Improve community personal support services for people living at home
7. Implement the new deal for carers
8. Improve the quality of care for people with dementia in general hospitals
9. Improve intermediate care for people with dementia
10. Consider how housing support, housing-related services, technology and telecare can help support people with dementia and their carers
11. Improve the quality of care for people with dementia in care homes
12. Improve end of life care for people with dementia
13. An informed and effective workforce for people with dementia
14. A joint commissioning strategy for dementia
15. Improve assessment and regulation of health and care services and of how systems are working
16. Provide a clear picture of research about the causes and possible future treatments of dementia
17. Effective national and regional support for local services to help them develop and carry out the Strategy.

Box 32.3

Special investigations in mental illness in the elderly
Commonly indicated

- FBC
- ESR
- U&Es
- Calcium
- TFT
- LFT
- Glucose
- B_{12}
- Folate
- Lipid profile
- Syphilis serology
- MSU
- Chest X-ray
- CT brain
- ECG

Sometimes indicated

- EEG
- Lumbar puncture
- MRI scan.

changes and areas of infarction in vascular dementia and characteristic radiological features of normal pressure hydrocephalus. Functional MRI scanning, positive emission tomography (PET) and SPEC scanning are not normally used in routine clinical practice, but may be needed.

General treatment

A simple explanation of the diagnosis, management plan and possible sequelae should be given to the patient and the professional or family carer. Box 32.4 illustrates some of the specific issues that should be addressed during such explanations. Professional carers and relatives often require considerable support to understand and cope with the behaviour disturbance. Both groups of carers may also require opportunities to ventilate their feelings. Relatives may be able to join support groups such as the Alzheimer Disease Society in the UK, which provide information and peer group support.

Almost all drugs can cause delirium and many exacerbate the cognitive impairment of dementia. Thus, indications for their continued use should be reviewed. Any potentially reversible or partially reversible causes of dementia, hypothyroidism or neurosyphilis for example, should be treated. Common causes of delirium and behaviour disturbance such as pain, constipation, urinary tract infection and chest infection should be rigorously sought and treated, and advice from specialist geriatric medicine services should be sought when appropriate. Optical, ophthalmology or audiology opinion should be sought when sensory impairment is identified because their correction may improve cognitive deficits.

Early identification and intervention may avoid a full-blown crisis. Both professional and non-professional carers could be advised to use some simple calming strategies. Disturbed patients should be approached from the front, gently and calmly. Communication should be clear and unambiguous. Judicious use of touch and non-threatening postures may also be of value (see Ch. 34).

Box 32.4

Specific areas of information shared with carers

- Diagnosis of dementia and its implications
- Behaviour problems in dementia
- Possible causes of the behaviour problem
- How the problems are going to be managed
- Results of any special investigations
- Role of medication, if any
- Need for day-care
- Need for respite-care
- Need, if appropriate, for admission into hospital
- Need to refer to psychogeriatric services
- What resources may be available to carers
- Need for placement into a residential facility
- Management of financial resources (power of attorney or Court of Protection), health and social welfare
- Ability to drive a car.

Pharmacological treatments

Acetylcholine deficit is common in Alzheimer disease. Drugs designed to inactivate the acetylcholinesterase enzyme, which breaks down acetylcholine in the synaptic cleft, have been advocated to improve cognition. Three drugs in this group, donepezil (Gauthier et al 2002), galantamine (Tariot et al 2000) and rivastigmine (Rosler et al 1998) are available in the UK and have modest efficacy for improving cognitive impairment in mild to moderately severe Alzheimer disease (see Ch. 39). There is increasing evidence that these drugs also improve behaviour and psychotic symptoms of dementia (BPSD) and function. Furthermore, rivastigmine has been shown to improve cognitive impairment and BPSD including apathy, anxiety, delusions and hallucinations in dementia with Lewy bodies (McKeith et al 2000).

In the UK, the amended National Institute of Clinical Excellence (NICE) guidelines (see: www.nice.org.uk) recommend that only those with a diagnosis of moderate Alzheimer disease and a Mini Mental State Examination score of 10–20 should be prescribed these drugs, usually in secondary care. Where MMSE is not an appropriate tool to be used (e.g. in presence of learning disability, or other disabilities, communication/linguistic difficulties), other appropriate methods should be used. Another drug called memantine, which works by reducing overstimulation of the N-methyl-D-aspartate (NMDA) receptor by glutamate (memantine is NMDA antagonist) improves cognition and also produces global improvement (Reisberg et al 2003). However, even though it is licensed, it is not recommended for clinical use in UK.

The efficacy of other psychotropic drugs in the treatment of BPSD is unclear and probably modest. Research in this area is open to criticism because of poor methodology and it has been argued that psychotropics simply sedate the patient rather than modify target behaviour (Shah & Thomas 2006). The Committee on Safety of Medicines has advised against using risperidone and olanzapine in dementia because they both increase the risk of strokes and for olanzapine mortality is also increased. Because of altered pharmacokinetics and pharmacodynamics in the elderly, small doses should be used with careful observations for side-effects.

Short-acting benzodiazepines or clomethiazole may be helpful in the management of acute disturbance in patients with dementia. However, tolerance, dependence and other side-effects mandate that they should be used briefly and avoided if at all possible. Carbamazepine and sodium valproate may have efficacy in the treatment of aggressive behaviour.

Antidepressants have proven efficacy for the treatment of depression in dementia. Ideally one of the newer antidepressants from the selective serotonin uptake inhibitor (SSRI) group or other newer antidepressants should be used because they have fewer anticholinergic side-effects. The SSRI citalopram has been shown to decrease agitation in double-blind studies and other drugs acting on the serotonin system have anecdotally been reported to reduce aggressive behaviour in dementia.

Depression

Clinical features

The clinical features of depression in the elderly are essentially similar to those in younger individuals. Agitation, retardation, hypochondriasis, cognitive impairment and delusions of physical ill-health, persecution, poverty, self-blame, worthlessness and guilt are common; nihilistic delusions may occasionally occur. Hallucinations are unusual, but when they occur they are usually second person auditory hallucinations with a derogatory content (and are mood congruent). Cognitive impairment in depression may be mistaken for dementia, a phenomenon referred to as depressive pseudodementia. This can be discriminated from dementia by the clarity of onset, relatively rapid onset, its duration and speed of cognitive decline, the manner in which the patient answers the questions, presence or absence of higher cortical deficits and/or other depressive symptoms (Table 32.2).

Aetiology

The aetiology of depression can be divided into predisposing factors, precipitating factors and perpetuating factors. Predisposing factors can be classified into genetic factors, physical health, personality and social support. Up to 30% of late-onset depressions have a family history. Physical illness and its treatment may predispose to depression in up to 50% of medically ill elderly inpatients. Occult malignancies may present with depression and drugs like corticosteroids can produce depressive side-effects. Late-onset depression may be associated with anxiety-prone, avoidant and dependent personality. The association between depression and the presence of a confidante or an intimate relationship are unclear, with some studies supporting and others refuting such a relationship.

Precipitating factors include independent adverse life events, which are important in precipitating depression and are frequent in the preceding year. Bereavement is an important life event associated with depression in the elderly. However, not everyone with depression has experienced adverse life events and not everyone experiencing such events becomes depressed. Thus, other factors must operate. Personality traits, including an inability to form close relationships, a tendency to be helpless and hopeless, an inability to tolerate change and loss of control, and feelings of loneliness, despair and dependence on others may be vulnerability factors predisposing to depression. Both precipitating and predisposing factors may also act as perpetuating factors.

Management

An accurate diagnosis is essential in the treatment of depression and this can be achieved by satisfactory history from the patient and a collateral source, mental state examination and a thorough physical examination. This process will also allow exclusion of differential diagnoses. Box 32.2 summarizes the most significant differences between dementia and depressive pseudodementia. Physical examination and selected special investigations from the list in Box 32.3 will allow identification of self-neglect (e.g. dehydration or anaemia) and other physical illnesses (e.g. hypothyroidism or hypercalcaemia mimicking depression).

Treatment plans should be tailored to individual patients with regard to the severity of the depression and its aetiology. Treatment should be directed at predisposing factors, precipitating factors and perpetuating factors on the social, psychological and biological axis. NICE (see: www.nice.org. uk) recommends the stepped care model aiming to match patient needs to the most appropriate services. Where possible, rectification or adjustment of correctable factors should be effected. Treatment should be divided into three phases: acute, aimed at remission of the index episode; continuation, aimed at preventing relapse of the index episode after treatment; and maintenance, aimed at prevention of new episodes. First-line pharmacological treatment should be with newer antidepressants (selective serotonin reuptake inhibitors and related drugs, selective noradrenaline (norepinephrine) reuptake inhibitors and reversible monoamine oxidase inhibitors), which are as potent as older antidepressants but have fewer side-effects (see Ch. 39). In the elderly, due to altered pharmacokinetics and sensitivity, it is wise to start at small doses and increase doses slowly with close monitoring for side-effects. Efficacy may begin at 3 weeks but may not be observed for up to 10 weeks in some patients. After recovery antidepressant medication should continue for a longer period than in younger patients. The multicentre study from the Old Age Depression Research Interest Group (1993) suggests a minimum maintenance period of 2 years, although a study did not show efficacy for sertraline in relapse prevention over a 2-year follow-up period (Wilson et al 2003).

Should an antidepressant appear ineffective, the adequacy of dosage, compliance and treatment duration, improvement of perpetuating factors and the accuracy of the diagnosis should be examined before changing medication. If all these factors are satisfactory, consideration should be given to changing the antidepressant to one from another chemical group. There are no hard and fast rules with regard to which

Table 32.2 Significant clinical differences between depressive pseudodementia and dementia

	Pseudodementia	Dementia
Onset	Acute	Insidious
Course	Rapid	Insidious
Duration	Relatively brief	Permanent
Main complaint	Impaired memory	No complaints
Cognitive questioning	Cannot respond or does not know answer	Incorrect response
Higher cortical functioning	Intact	Impaired
Mood congruent delusions	Common	Uncommon

treatment to adopt after first-line antidepressants fail. It will be dictated by previous response, patient and carer preference and psychiatrist's preference. Choices include a different SSRI, mirtazapine, moclobemide, reboxetine or lofepramine. Venlafaxine can be given for more severe depression, taking into account the special considerations as outlined by NICE.

ECT is well tolerated in the elderly (Benbow 1994). However, the recent NICE (www.nice.org.uk) guidelines recommend that ECT should only be used to achieve rapid and short-term improvement of severe symptoms, after an adequate trial of other treatments has proven ineffective or when the condition is thought to be potentially life threatening, in individuals with severe depression (catatonia, a prolonged, or a severe episode of mania). It controversially suggests caution in the use of ECT in the elderly. Depressive delusions, psychomotor retardation, agitation and other biological symptoms predict a good response (Benbow 1994). If exacerbation of confusion is an issue, unilateral ECT may be considered.

Most depressed elderly patients benefit from supportive psychotherapy and some may need more formal counselling. Cognitive–behavioural therapy and group psychotherapy are effective, while reminiscence therapy, problem-solving therapy, family therapy and more in-depth interpersonal psychotherapy may be of benefit but have not been systematically evaluated. Psychotherapeutic techniques must take account of factors associated with old age including memory, sensory deficits and articulation difficulties.

Over a 12-month follow-up period, between 35% and 68% of treated depressed patients remain well, between 14% and 29% remain continuously depressed, and between 12% and 19% relapsed (Baldwin & Jolley 1986). Over a 3-year follow-up period between 22% and 31% achieved lasting recovery, between 28% and 38% had a further episode with recovery, between 23% and 32% achieved partial recovery, and between 7% and 17% remained continuously ill (Baldwin & Jolley 1986). Mortality is also increased among depressed elderly patients.

Mania

The prevalence of mania decreases with increasing age, but among patients with bipolar illness, mania may not infrequently present for the first time in old age. Up to 50% of 1st-degree relatives of such patients have affective disorders and such a family history is associated with early onset of illness. Two subtypes of mania have been described in elderly patients:

- Affective disorder with depression in middle age and manic episodes late in life
- Secondary mania in which the first affective episode is associated with coarse neurological disorder in an individual with low genetic loading.

The clinical presentation of mania in old age is similar to that seen in younger patients.

The pharmacological treatment of mania is essentially similar to that in younger patients, but should allow for the age-related altered pharmacokinetics and prolonged half-life of various drugs. Neuroleptics are of value in acute mania. Lithium and anticonvulsants, like carbamazepine and sodium valproate, can be of value in acute mania, but are also used for prophylaxis.

Late paraphrenia

In ICD-10 and DSM-IV late paraphrenia is subsumed under paranoid schizophrenia or persistent delusional disorder. Patients with late paraphrenia present for the first time in old age with persecutory delusions, auditory and/or visual hallucinations and Schneiderian first rank symptoms. Delusions of reference, hypochondriasis and grandeur, misidentification syndromes and hallucinations in other modalities may also occur. Affective symptoms are concurrently present in up to 60% of cases. Late paraphrenia patients do not show an obvious marked cognitive decline, but their performance on some cognitive test batteries is worse than normal ageing.

Late paraphrenia is commoner in women. They have sensory deficits including auditory and visual impairment. Personality features of suspiciousness, sensitivity, quarrelsomeness and unsociability are also associated with this disorder.

There are no controlled trials of neuroleptic usage in late paraphrenia, but anecdotally neuroleptics are accepted as the treatment of choice. Correction of sensory deficits may also help. All this should be coupled with social, psychological and occupational support.

Squalor syndrome

This syndrome is characterized by extreme self-neglect, domestic squalor, social withdrawal, apathy, tendency to hoard rubbish and lack of shame (Snowdon et al 2007). The annual incidence has been estimated as 0.5/1000 population over the age of 60 years. Sex ratio is unclear with conflicting reports. The vast majority of these individuals live alone and many are known to the community authorities, but they tend to decline offers of help. Financial hardship may be absent, many own properties and they come from all social classes. Physical illness and biochemical and haematological abnormalities commonly occur in these individuals. Deafness and visual impairment are common accompaniments.

Normal mental state is observed in up to 50% of cases. The remainder have the following diagnosis in order of decreasing frequency: dementia, paraphrenia or chronic schizophrenia, alcoholism and manic-depressive illness. Their subjectively measured personality characteristics are domineering, quarrelsome and independent.

Management should be along the lines of principles described for individual disorders earlier and consistent with general principles of management in old age psychiatry described below. Use of various legislations, including the Mental Health Act in the UK, in this syndrome has been described (Shah 1995).

development of a single assessment process across different disciplines and agencies, and agreed protocols between primary and secondary care for the assessment and management of dementia and depression.

Patients may require follow-up for further assessment, treatment, rehabilitation, monitoring of side-effects, monitoring of mental state, support for patient or carers and advocacy (Shah & Ames 1994). This may be at home, in the outpatient clinic or at a day-hospital.

Outpatient clinics

Outpatient and specialist memory clinics can complement home visits with detailed neuropsychometry, and blood and radiological investigations (Shah & Ames 1994). Such clinics are being increasingly located in the general hospital because it allows access to a wide range of facilities. Memory clinics offer elective, detailed assessment of patients with dementia and related disorders, but due to the lengthy assessments such clinics are able to evaluate a relatively small number of patients. However, through Standard 7 of the NSF, the development of memory clinics is encouraged.

Day hospitals

Day hospitals are an important component of old age psychiatry services. They allow assessment, treatment, rehabilitation, long-term support, development of a social network and support for carers (Shah & Ames 1994). The UK Royal College of Psychiatrists recommend 90 day places for a population of 30 000 over 65-year-olds. Day hospitals cater both for functionally and organically ill patients, either in separate units or on separate days, and flexible day hospitals which are open at the weekend and during the evening are slowly emerging, with obvious advantages. In rural areas travelling day hospitals have been developed.

Inpatient care

There are three types of hospital admissions: assessment and/ or treatment, respite and continuing care. The UK Royal College of Psychiatrists recommends 45 acute beds and 90 continuing care beds for a population of 30 000 over the age of 65 years.

Factors that may contribute to an inpatient admission include severity of the illness, severity of the sequelae of the illness, insufficient social and community support at home, need for more detailed and intensive assessment, and implementation of certain treatments like ECT. Respite admissions can be in standalone units, acute admissions wards or continuing care wards. They are usually intended to give carers a break. Some patients may require long-term (continuing care) admissions. In the UK, continuing care admissions are regulated by locally agreed criteria (between different agencies) following a department of health directive.

Role of the general practitioner

General practitioners play a vital role in the satisfactory functioning of psychogeriatric services. They see a significant amount of psychiatric morbidity and have good ability to recognize both depression and dementia, but adopt less good treatment strategies. The latter could be facilitated by the psychogeriatric service providing support and back-up with liaison clinics in general practice involving psychiatrists, community psychiatric nurses and social workers. Standard 7 of the NSF promotes close working between primary care and specialist old age psychiatry services through a range of models such as above and through development of agreed protocols for assessment and management of dementia and depression.

Liaison service

Psychiatry of old age services should provide a liaison service to departments of geriatric medicine and general hospitals, residential and nursing homes, social service and voluntary agency day facilities, voluntary organizations and other local government facilities. The liaison service should aim to share knowledge about psychiatry of old age with others and improve the ability of non-specialist professionals to detect and manage mental illness. This can be done on a case by case basis (consultation model) and by contributions to their meetings and open forum seminars (liaison model) or by both models.

Depressed medically ill elderly inpatients experience severe psychological distress, have more severe physical illnesses, have physical illnesses that are difficult to treat, are poorly compliant with treatment, have longer hospital admissions and have a higher mortality. Moreover, depression is poorly recognized and treated among geriatric inpatients and more than 80% of depressed elderly patients have no documented plans for the management of their depression following discharge. Furthermore, less than half of all elderly medically ill in-patients with depression are referred to psychiatrists and antidepressants are used infrequently and at inadequate doses.

The prevalence of mental illness in residential facilities including sheltered homes, hostels, residential homes, special accommodation homes and nursing homes is considerable. Residential facility staff and nursing home staff have limited psychiatric training, so psychiatric morbidity is often unrecognized in such facilities or, when recognized, poorly treated. There is considerable need for liaison service development in this area.

Mental health legislation and elderly patients

The application of mental health legislation to elderly patients is essentially the same as its application to younger patients in most jurisdictions. Thus, in England and Wales, for example, the various sections of the amended Mental Health Act 2007 apply equally to elderly and young patients. The Mental Capacity Act 2005 (MCA 2005) (Department of Constitutional Affairs 2005) allows for treatment of incapacitated patients if this in their best interests. For incapacitated patients who cannot be detained in hospital under the Mental Health Act, the Mental Health Act 2007 has introduced Deprivation of Liberty Safeguards into the MCA 2005 (DoH 2007). It allows detention of patients in hospitals and care homes, but gives no formal powers of treatment.

References

Baldwin, R.C., Jolley, D., 1986. The prognosis of depression in old age. Br. J. Psychiatry 149, 574–583.

Benbow, S.M., 1994. Electro-convulsive therapy in later life. In: Chiu, E., Ames, D. (Eds.), Functional psychiatric disorders of the elderly. Cambridge University Press, Cambridge, pp. 440–460.

Burns, A., Jacoby, R., Levy, R., 1990a. Psychiatric phenomena in Alzheimer disease IV: disorders of behaviour. Br. J. Psychiatry 157, 86–94.

Burns, A., Jacoby, R., Levy, R., 1990b. Psychiatric phenomena in Alzheimer disease. II Disorders of perception. Br. J. Psychiatry 157, 76–81.

Burns, A., Jacoby, R., Levy, R., 1990c. Psychiatric phenomena in Alzheimer disease. I: Disorders of thought content. Br. J. Psychiatry 15, 72–76.

Consensus Guidelines for the Clinical and Pathological Diagnosis of Dementia of Lewy Body Type (DLB), 1996. Report of the Consortium on DLB International Workshop held in Newcastle, UK 1996 for diagnosis. Neurology 47, 1124–1134.

Copeland, J.R.M., Dewey, M.E., Woods, N., et al., 1987. Range of mental illness among the elderly in the community. Prevalence in Liverpool using the GMS AGECAT package. Br. J. Psychiatry 150, 815–823.

Department of Constitutional Affairs, 2005. The Mental Capacity Act 2005. Online. Available: www.opsi.gov.uk/acts/acts2005/20050009.htm.

DoH, 2001. National Service Framework for Older People. Department of Health, London.

DoH, 2007. Mental Health Act 2007. Online. Available: www.england-legislation.hmso.gov.uk/acts2008/pdf/ukpga_20070012_en.pdf.

DoH, 2009. Living Well With Dementia: A National Dementia strategy. www.dh.gov.uk/en/Publicationsandstatistics/Publications/PublicationsPolicyAndGuidance/DH_094058.

Gauthier, S., Feldman, H., Hecker, J., et al., 2002. Functional, cognitive and behavioural effects of donepezil in patients with moderate Alzheimer disease. Curr. Med. Res. Opin. 18, 347–354.

Harwood, D., Hawton, K., Hope, T., et al., 2001. Psychiatric disorder and personality factors associated with suicide in older people: a descriptive and case-control study. Int. J. Geriatr. Psychiatry 16, 155–165.

Jacomb, P., Jorm, A., 1996. Personality change in dementia of Alzheimer type. Int. J. Geriatr. Psychiatry 11, 201–207.

Lindesay, J., Briggs, K., Murphy, E., 1989. The Guy's/Age Concern survey. Prevalence rates of cognitive impairment, depression and anxiety in an urban community. Br. J. Psychiatry 154, 2317–2329.

McKeith, I., Del Ser, T., Spano, P., et al., 2000. Efficacy of rivastigmine in dementia with Lewy bodies: a randomised, double-blind, placebo-controlled international study. Lancet 356, 2031–2036.

Old Age Depression Research Interest Group, 1993. How long should the elderly take antidepressants? A double blind placebo controlled study of continuation/prophylaxis therapy with dothiepin. Br. J. Psychiatry 162, 175–182.

Reisberg, B., Doody, R., Stoffler, A., et al., 2003. Memantine in moderate-to-severe Alzheimer disease. N. Engl. J. Med. 348, 1333–1341.

Rosler, M., Retz, W., Retz-Junginger, P., et al., 1998. Effects of two-year treatment with cholinesterase inhibitor rivastigmine on behavioural symptoms in Alzheimer disease. Behav. Neurol. 11, 211–216.

Saunders, A.M., Strittmater, W.J., Schmechel, D., et al., 1993. Association of apolipoprotein E allele E4 with late-onset familial and sporadic Alzheimer disease. Neurology 43, 1467–1472.

Shah, A.K., 1995. The use of legislation in cases of squalor. Med. Sci. Law 35, 43–44.

Shah, A.K., Ames, D., 1994. Planning and developing psychogeriatric services. Int. Rev. Psychiatry 6, 15–27.

Shah, A.K., De, T., 1998. Suicide in the elderly. Int. J. Psychiatry Clin. Pract. 2, 3–17.

Shah, A.K., Thomas, C., 2006. Pharmacological interventions in behavioural and psychological symptoms of dementia. In: Ritchie, C., Ames, D., Masters, C., et al. (Eds.), Treatment strategies in dementia. Clinical Publishing, London, pp. 203–226.

Skegg, K., Cox, B., 1991. Suicide in New Zealand 1957–1986: the influence of age, period and birth-cohort. Aust. N.Z. J. Psychiatry 25, 181–190.

Snowdon, J., Halliday, G., Shah, A.K., 2007. Severe domestic squalor: a review. Int. Psychogeriatr. 19, 37–51.

Tariot, P.N., Solomon, P.R., Morris, J.C., et al., 2000. A 5-month, randomised, placebo-controlled trial of galanthamine in AD. The Galanthamine USA-10 Study Group. Neurology 54, 2269–2276.

Wilson, K.C.M., Mottram, P.G., Ashworth, L., et al., 2003. Older community residents with depression: long-term treatment with sertraline. Br. J. Psychiatry 182, 492–497.

Wragg, R.E., Jeste, D., 1989. Overview of depression and psychosis in Alzheimer disease. Am. J. Psychiatry 146, 577–587.

PART 3

Diagnosis, investigation and treatment

Clinical examination of psychiatric patients

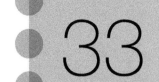

Pádraig Wright   Julian Stern   Michael Phelan

CHAPTER CONTENTS

Introduction

The psychiatric interview is undertaken primarily in order to establish a diagnosis. It includes history-taking and the clinical examination of the mental state. However, the psychiatric interview is much more than a diagnostic process. It also helps to establish rapport between patient and doctor and to educate and motivate the patient.

Interviewing patients also serves an important therapeutic purpose. This is the goal for patients during psychotherapeutic consultations, but it also applies to all other patients for whom the opportunity to discuss problems with a sympathetic listener is often helpful. The many functions of the psychiatric interview are described in Box 33.1.

The diagnostic process in psychiatry differs from that in other medical disciplines in that:

- It relies almost exclusively on history-taking and clinical examination
- The account obtained from the patient must be corroborated by information from the patient's partner, children or other relatives, or from the family doctor, social worker or teacher, as appropriate.

Interviewing such third parties should only be undertaken with the patient's fully informed consent. However, such corroborative interviews should be the rule rather than the exception because psychiatric patients may, consciously or unwittingly, conceal important information. Verbal accounts from patients and third parties should be supplemented by written records from family doctors, hospitals or schools when appropriate. This is especially the case for events that occurred many years ago or for which the patient has only a second-hand account from parents or others.

Psychiatric interviews should be conducted in macroscopic settings that facilitate the patient's privacy and comfort and ensure the doctor's safety. These goals are relatively easy to achieve in psychiatric outpatient clinics but present challenges when patients are interviewed in their home (privacy and safety) or in general medical hospital departments (comfort, privacy and safety), and may be impossible to achieve in some settings, for example police stations or prisons.

The microscopic setting of the interview also warrants attention. Patients feel more at ease if seated at the same level as, and to one side of, rather than opposite, the doctor. One tried and trusted arrangement (Fig. 33.1) is for the doctor to sit at a fixed desk with the patient seated in a heavy or fixed chair to the

Box 33.1

The functions of the psychiatric interview

- **History-taking:** undertaken in order to elicit the patient's account of problems and establish a differential diagnosis
- **Mental state examination:** undertaken in order to establish the presence or absence of specific psychiatric symptoms and thus confirm a diagnosis on which treatment may be based
- **Establishing rapport**
- **Education and motivation of the patient:** undertaken in order to advise the patient about their illness or its treatment, about prognosis, and indeed about the processes of psychiatric evaluation and treatment
- **Treatment:** may be the primary goal of the interview as in a formal psychotherapeutic interaction, or it may be an additional function as in the standard clinical interview.

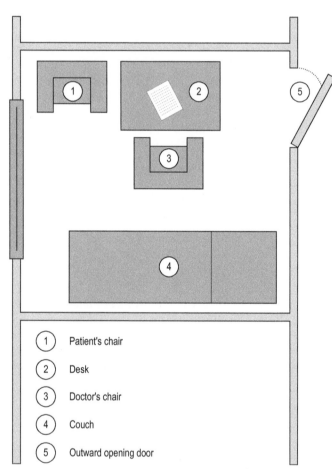

① Patient's chair

② Desk

③ Doctor's chair

④ Couch

⑤ Outward opening door

Figure 33.1 • The layout of a room suitable for history-taking and clinical examination of psychiatric patients.

doctor's left. The door should be to the doctor's right and should open outwards. This arrangement facilitates writing (for a right-handed doctor), eye contact between patient and doctor and safety (the desk and patient's chair are virtually immobile, the door can be reached and opened quickly and, given that it opens outwards, cannot be barricaded from within the room). Safety is enhanced by ensuring that there are no potential weapons such as lamps, electrical cables or coat hangers in the interview room, and by telling a receptionist, nurse or other colleague that the interview is taking place.

The taking of a psychiatric history, assessment of a patient's personality and performance of a mental state examination will now be described. Psychodynamic aspects of clinical examination and difficulties that may be encountered when interviewing psychiatric patients will also be discussed.

Taking a psychiatric history

Prior to the interview, care should be taken to ensure that patients and those accompanying them know the interviewing doctor's name and the location of coffee shops, toilets, etc. The interview should commence with introductions, a brief explanation of the purpose of the interview, and an estimate of the time available or required. Explain the need to take notes and reassure the patient about confidentiality. If the interview is medicolegal in nature, the doctor should explain who has requested and who may see any resulting report.

Establishing the reason for referral and the presenting complaint

Note-taking should commence with a brief record of the reason the patient was referred (e.g. depression not responding to antidepressant treatment), the referring source (e.g. general practitioner) and the expected outcome of the referral (e.g. confirmation of diagnosis or initiation of other treatment).

History-taking proper should commence with the collection of demographic details. This is both necessary and, being emotionally neutral information as distinct from emotionally laden information, helps to establish rapport. Some patients may remain ill at ease at the end of this stage of the interview and it may be appropriate to continue eliciting relatively neutral information by proceeding with personal history and family history details, only returning to the presenting complaint and history of the presenting complaint later in the interview. Otherwise, it is best to proceed as outlined in Box 33.2 and invite the patient to describe his/her problems. This is undertaken in order to establish the presenting complaint and to get a brief overview of the difficulties the patient is currently experiencing. A few words or a short phrase may be sufficient to describe the presenting complaint and it is usual to record the patient's own words. Thus, it is preferable to write, e.g. 'I feel utterly miserable – there is absolutely no hope for me', rather than the word 'depression'.

Establishing the history of the presenting complaint

The duration of the patient's difficulties should next be established by asking, 'When did you last feel perfectly well?' or 'When were you first troubled by these problems?' Having established the nature and duration of the patient's problems, their history (potential precipitants, mode of onset of symptoms, severity of symptoms and treatment received to date) should next be established.

Box 33.2

A scheme for eliciting and recording clinical information

The reason for referral

- Brief demographic details
- The reason the patient was referred (depression not responding to treatment)
- The referring source (general practitioner, community nurse)
- The expected outcome of the referral (confirmation of diagnosis, admission)

The presenting complaint

- The presenting complaint (e.g. 'I feel miserable. Completely without hope')

The history of the presenting complaint

- The duration of the presenting complaint
- Potential precipitants
- The mode of onset of symptoms
- The severity of symptoms and their impact on the patient's life

Establishing the family history

- Age, marital status, occupation, physical and mental health, and/or cause of death of 1st-degree relatives
- The personality of each 1st-degree relative and the relationship each has with the patient
- Family history of psychiatric illness (especially alcohol and drugs, psychiatric hospitalizations, and suicide)
- Psychiatric illness in members of the extended family
- Possible impact of events such as births, marriages and deaths upon the patient

Establishing the personal history

- Gestation and birth, early development and ages at which milestones were attained
- Childhood relationships with parents and siblings
- Ages of starting and finishing school
- Relationships with peers and teachers
- Academic and sporting achievements
- Employments (listed chronologically), reasons for changes in employment
- Age at menarche and details of sexual relationships, sexual experiences, contraception and terminations of pregnancies
- Age at marriage, duration of relationship before marriage, spouse's age, health and occupation, and sex and age of any children
- The quality of the relationship between patient and spouse, and patient and offspring
- Significant illness and surgical procedures
- Psychiatric illnesses (durations of each, treatment received, doctor and/or hospital)
- Previous episodes of unrecognized psychiatric illness
- Current social situation (accommodation arrangements, income, make-up of household, domestic or financial difficulties)

Establishing the forensic history

- Arrests, cautions, convictions, imprisonment or other punishment
- Crimes admitted to but not detected.

Potential precipitants should be identified when possible and may include psychosocial stresses (unemployment, domestic strife, poverty), physical illness (influenza, cancer) or its treatment, or non-adherence to maintenance therapy with antidepressants, antipsychotics or mood stabilizing drugs. An attempt should be made to differentiate between independent precipitants and those which may have arisen because of the patient's deteriorating mental health. Loss of employment because of poor performance consequent upon mental illness is but one example of the latter.

The mode of onset of symptoms is important in establishing a diagnosis and in determining a prognosis. Thus, symptoms of sudden onset often suggest an identifiable and potentially treatable cause (head injury, psychosocial stress or illicit drugs) and a better outcome, whereas insidiously developing symptoms are more often associated with disorders with ill-defined aetiologies, symptomatic or no treatment and poor outcomes. The severity of the patient's illness and the disability it causes must be evaluated by questions about changes in appetite, weight, sleep pattern and sexual behaviour, and by enquiries about how symptoms impact on the patient's personal, domestic, occupational and social functioning. Finally, the nature, duration and effect of any treatment received to date should be noted.

Establishing the family history

The age, martial status, occupation, physical and mental health, and cause of death of each of the patient's 1st-degree relatives (parents, siblings and offspring) should next be recorded. In addition, an attempt should be made to evaluate the personality of each 1st-degree relative, living or deceased, and to assess the relationship each has or had with the patient. A family history of psychiatric illness is often difficult to obtain because of stigma (see Ch. 12), because some mental illnesses are accepted as the norm within the family, or because alcohol or substance abuse is not regarded as mental illness. Specific questions must therefore be asked about alcohol and drugs, psychiatric hospitalizations and suicide. In addition to information about first-degree relatives, information about psychiatric illness in members of the extended family should be sought. Finally, the possible impact of events such as births, marriages and deaths upon the patient and upon the atmosphere in the patient's home, both during childhood and currently, should be considered. The most important family history data may usefully be recorded in a genogram (see Fig. 33.2 for an example).

Establishing the personal history

A record of the patient's personal development, sexual development and relationships, past medical and psychiatric history, and current social circumstances is next obtained. Information is first collected about the patient's gestation and birth, early development and the ages at which milestones (sitting upright, standing upright, walking, talking and bladder and bowel control) were attained. The patient's childhood relationships with parents and siblings should also be evaluated, and the ages of starting and finishing school, relationships with peers and teachers, and academic and sporting achievements should be noted. Following

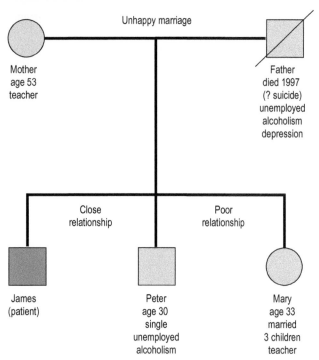

Figure 33.2 • The use of a genogram for recording history information.

this, employments should be listed chronologically and the reasons for changes in employment noted. It is especially important to note if new jobs represent advancement or decline in terms of responsibility and remuneration, because the latter may reflect progressive impairment consequent upon mental illness.

Following this, age at menarche and details of sexual relationships, sexual experiences, contraception and terminations of pregnancy are obtained as appropriate. Age at marriage, duration of relationship before marriage, spouse's age, health and occupation, and the sex and age of any children should also be recorded. The quality of the relationship between patient and spouse, and patient and offspring, should also be enquired into.

Details of all significant illness and surgical procedures are next recorded, followed by details of any psychiatric illnesses, including the durations of each, the treatment received, and the doctor and/or hospital attended. It is important to note that while patients may have no formal past psychiatric history, they may nonetheless have had previous episodes of psychiatric illness, recognized or unrecognized – such episodes must be enquired about.

The patient's current social situation refers to accommodation arrangements, income (from employment or from social welfare payments), make-up of household, and any domestic or financial difficulties. The suitability of accommodation and the patient's income and financial status are especially important as problems in these areas may impact upon psychiatric illness.

Establishing the forensic history

Forensic details may be elicited by asking the patient if they have ever been in trouble with the police (arrests, cautions, convictions, imprisonment or other punishment). Delinquency or

crimes admitted to but not detected should also be noted and alcohol and/or substance abuse may also be enquired about at this time. It may be appropriate to corroborate the forensic history by reviewing police or court records in the case of some patients.

Assessing a patient's personality

It is extremely difficult to evaluate a patient's pre-morbid personality during a psychiatric consultation and any opinion formed must be constantly reviewed in light of further contact with the patient and additional information from informants. Questions such as, 'If I had met you before you became ill, would I notice many differences between you then and you now?', 'How would your best friend (or spouse or work colleague) describe you?' or 'How would you deal with a serious financial difficulty (unemployment, illness in your family)?' may allow some access to the patient's personality. Further information may be gained by enquiring about the patient's relationships (many or few friends, deep or superficial friendships), character (confident or self-deprecating, impulsive or cautious, independent or dependent, shy or gregarious) and usual mood (cheerful or despondent, optimistic or pessimistic, stable or emotional). Personal habits (tobacco, alcohol and substance use/abuse, when first used/abused and current quantity used/abused per day, and expenditure on this) and attitudes (religious and moral, and also attitudes to psychiatry and psychiatric treatment) should also be enquired into. Finally, an individual's preferred leisure activities may reflect a preference for company or solitude, or intellectual, physical, competitive or creative pursuits. A brief enquiry into the patient's plans for the future may also be informative, although it is important to note that such plans may be heavily influenced by current symptoms, especially depression.

Performing a mental state examination

The doctor will have become aware of many symptoms (and of the patient's cognitive ability) during the process of history-taking, but in performing a mental state examination, only those symptoms the patient is experiencing or exhibiting at the time of the examination should be recorded. History-taking will almost certainly indicate a probable diagnosis but it is nevertheless important to confirm this and to rule out other diagnoses by a systematic mental state examination, which carefully considers the patient's appearance, posture and movement, behaviour, speech, mood and affect, thought, perception, cognition and insight (Box 33.3). The many clinical features that may be detected during the mental state examination are described in detail in Chapter 6 and are only referred to briefly, and in order to ensure continuity, below.

Appearance

Personal care may be impaired (schizophrenia, depression, dementia or alcohol or substance abuse), bizarre clothing or accessories may be worn (mania, depression, schizophrenia, dementia, anorexia nervosa, or organic psychiatric disorder),

Box 33.3

A scheme for eliciting and recording the mental state examination

Appearance
- Personal care and clothing
- Stigmata suggestive of drug abuse
- Facial appearance

Posture and movement
- Posture
- Movements
- Tension, hypervigilance, excessive sweating
- Mannerisms, stereotypies, echopraxia, flexibilitas cerea, negativism or excitement
- Parkinsonism, akathisia, tardive dyskinesia, tics
- Responding to auditory hallucinations

Behaviour
- Irritability, distractibility and apathy
- Overfamiliarity, importunateness, sexual inappropriateness
- Social withdrawal, no eye contact, little conversation
- Perplexity
- Aggression and violence

Speech
- Quantity of speech
- Rate of speech
- Volume of speech
- Neologisms, thought disorders, punning, clang associations, flight of ideas, poverty of the content of speech
- Perseveration, dysphasia or dysarthria

Mood and affect
- Depression (enquire about suicide)
- Elation
- Anxiety
- Depersonalization or derealization
- Affect (appropriateness of mood, rate of change of mood)

Thought
- Rate of thinking
- Form of thought
- Content of thought (delusions, over-valued ideas and obsessional thoughts)

Perception
- Illusions
- Hallucinations

Cognition
- Orientation in time, place and person
- Serial sevens, months of the year or days of the week backwards
- Repeat and later recall the names of three unrelated objects (short-term memory)
- Recount recent political or sporting news items (recent memory)
- Dates of distant events, birth dates of close relatives (remote memory)
- Mini-mental state examination if appropriate

Insight
- Illness
- Nature of illness
- Appropriate treatment.

or stigmata suggestive of intravenous drug abuse or solvent abuse may be apparent.

Patients with dyspraxia may wear clothing backwards, may not wear underclothing, or may fasten buttons incorrectly. Facial appearance may reflect underlying mood, parkinsonism caused by antipsychotic medication, or organic disorder (thyroid disease, Parkinson disease or supranuclear palsy), while tearfulness and crying are features of many psychiatric disorders, most noticeably depression.

Posture and movement

Patients may exhibit a slumped posture with slowed movements if depressed, while manic patients are usually overactive. Anxious patients may appear tense and hypervigilant and may sweat excessively. Patients with schizophrenia may exhibit mannerisms, stereotypes, echopraxia, flexibilitas cerea, negativism or excitement, and parkinsonism, akathisia and tardive dyskinesia associated with antipsychotic treatment may also be evident. Schizophrenic patients may also be observed attending to or responding to auditory hallucinations. Patients with social phobia will appear extremely anxious in the presence of other people and the rituals undertaken by patients with obsessive–compulsive disorder may be evident. Tics may occur in isolation, in patients with anxiety disorders (especially obsessive–compulsive disorder) and in Gilles de la Tourette syndrome.

Behaviour

In addition to the abnormalities of posture and movement described above, patients with psychiatric illness frequently exhibit abnormal general and social behaviour. This may be observed during the patient's interaction with relatives, other patients and hospital personnel, as well as during the formal psychiatric interview. Abnormalities of general behaviour include irritability (mania, agitated depression, alcohol withdrawal), distractibility (depression, mania, dementia) and apathy (depression, dementia).

Social behaviour is often severely compromised by psychiatric illness. Manic patients are overfamiliar and importunate, attempt to engage those around them in conversation and may behave in a sexually inappropriate manner. Patients with schizophrenia or depression are often socially withdrawn, may not make eye contact, and do not easily engage in conversation, while demented patients may appear perplexed and may ignore social conventions. Aggression and violence are relatively uncommon but may be especially associated with mania, personality disorder, schizophrenia and alcohol or drug abuse.

Speech

The patient's speech is observed throughout the psychiatric interview and verbatim examples of speech should be recorded in order to illustrate the symptoms described below and in order to note the content of conversation which may reflect underlying psychopathology. Speech may be abnormal in quantity, rate, volume and/or tone.

a time limit – whether he/she reacts to the announcement in a particular way (moaning, complaining, grateful or seemingly disinterested), and whether they make use of the time constructively or spend the session on seemingly trivial issues and then complain when the session ends that they have not been given the opportunity to talk about the real problem. This latter might occur in a patient with a paranoid and passive–dependent personality.

Information gathering, in the formal sense described in the first part of this chapter, is important. However, there is much additional non-verbal and non-explicit information to be gleaned from the patient. Use is made of the stethoscope, the sphygmomanometer and of laboratory apparatus that measures arterial blood gas concentrations in cardiology. In psychiatry, the best instruments – metaphorical stethoscopes – are the psychiatrist's own emotions.

Transference, counter-transference, projective identification and acting out

The concepts of transference, counter-transference, projective identification and acting out are of crucial importance and are described in more detail in Chapter 37.

What are the expectations which both doctor and patient bring to the interview? They are partially socially determined, to do with the traditional power relationships and status of the doctor, hospital and patient (Mechanic 1968). But they are also personal, depending on the patient's earliest experiences with parents and carers, subsequent experiences with other figures of authority (teachers, grandparents, carers), and experiences with medical professionals. Thus the patient's (often unconscious) attitude, demeanour, and behaviour towards the doctor may reflect all sorts of past experiences and internalizations.

Similarly, the doctor brings his or her own set of attitudes, memories, and internal figures. One cannot expect to have the same underlying attitude towards an elderly woman who reminds one of a dearly loved grandmother as towards a young, arrogant man who reminds one, only too clearly, of an obnoxious younger sibling who might have displaced one from one's mother's breast when one was a mere toddler.

So each encounter involves the patient's transferences and the counter-transference of the practitioner. A traditional method for dealing with counter-transference in medicine in general, and in psychiatry in particular, is to pretend that it does not exist by employing a formulaic mode of history-taking and case management. However, Winnicott (1957), in his seminal paper 'Hate in the counter-transference', described the psychiatrist caring for a psychotic or difficult patient as similar to a mother caring for a demanding baby: 'However much he loves his patients he cannot avoid hating them and fearing them, and the better he knows this the less will hate and fear be the motives determining what he does to his patients'.

Counter-transference, hate and malignant alienation

If counter-transference hatred is not recognized, the hateful feelings will be repressed and/or projected elsewhere. Watts and Morgan (1994) have described the defences used to avoid

knowledge of counter-transference hate as including repression, reaction formation, projection and distortion/denial (see defence mechanisms in Ch. 37):

- Repression may seem safe as far as the psychiatrist is concerned, but the hatred may be conveyed by non-verbal messages such as inattentiveness, yawning, or watching the clock.
- With reaction formation (attempting to turn hate into its opposite, love), the psychiatrist becomes oversolicitous and may meddle, overprescribe or hospitalize the patient excessively.
- Projecting counter-transference hate, by thinking, e.g. 'I do not wish to harm that patient, it is he who wants to kill himself', can lead the psychiatrist towards a nihilistic view of the patient as a 'hopeless case', to which the response may be either to do nothing or make a zealous attempt to control the patient.
- Distortion/denial implies that the psychiatrist selectively attends to clinical facts which support his views of the patient, and repudiates or devalues the patient's own experiences.

Watts and Morgan go on to describe a scenario of 'malignant alienation'. In this situation, patients, often with severe personality disorders, suicidal depression, longstanding violent tendencies, or those described as 'withdrawn psychotic' patients, have longstanding difficulties in communicating their needs effectively. They evoke counter-transference hate and this hatred is acted out by carers, rather than understood and made conscious. The 'difficult patient' is alienated and may finally be placed at high risk of suicide.

The concept of projective identification is of great importance (see Ch. 37). Steiner (1976) gives an example of a competent and experienced psychiatrist treating an anorexic woman. She came into the consulting room 20 min late for her appointment, sullen, aggressive and critical of the psychiatrist. He started off sympathetically, but found himself feeling increasingly inadequate. Eventually he commented, 'You do seem to find everything I say useless'. Later on he told her he was going to be leaving her in a couple of months and this evoked a furious outburst from her, with the patient accusing him of letting her down, and in particular of unreliability. The psychiatrist felt overwhelmed with guilt, and although he knew that in fact it was the patient who had been chronically unreliable over the period he had treated her, he was unable to recognize that her fury had to do with the fact that he had actually been helpful to her and how helpless she felt at the prospect of him abandoning her.

Through projective identification, this patient induced in her psychiatrist a state of mind in which he felt inadequate and unable to deal with her as he should. This was precisely the state of mind of the patient. Making him feel useless and helpless, and yet (later on) feeling that he could contain these feelings for her without being overwhelmed as she was, seemed to provide an important sense of relief for her. Thus projective identification, by producing such a state of mind in the doctor, can be seen as a primitive form of communication, 'through which a patient hopes that the doctor or therapist can experience something of what it is like to be in the patient's state of mind' (Steiner 1976).

The task of the psychiatrist is thus to respond to the patient's behaviour with firmness, understanding and empathy, to contain the projections, and not be provoked into inappropriate actions by them, and this requires external and internal stability.

External and internal stability

External stability can be facilitated by the provision of a stable setting – the same room, the avoidance of unnecessary interruptions during a consultation, informing the patient in advance of the duration of the session and so on. Psychiatrists in training may be obliged to be constantly available via pagers, but interruption of a session by pagers or telephones is antithetical to a good therapeutic alliance. It repeatedly indicates to the patient that time with the psychiatrist is not regarded by the psychiatrist as protected or precious in any way. The telephone on the desk, the pager in the pocket and even the writing of notes may serve as a defensive armour (akin to a white coat and stethoscope) that prevents intimacy. If the phone is always about to ring, the pager about to go off, the door about to be knocked on, how deeply involved can the patient and the psychiatrist become?

Thus, consultations should take place in a setting that is safe and not prone to unnecessary interruption. The psychiatrist should review the patient's notes before the session so that the first minutes of the session are not occupied with the psychiatrist reading letters of referral or previous notes, while the patient waits. If possible, the psychiatrist should avoid writing notes during the session and should focus fully on the patient's verbal and non-verbal communications, and on the psychiatrist's own affective responses towards the patient.

Support for this work is vital, and detailed, regular external supervision from a senior colleague (usually the consultant) is essential during the training phases of a psychiatrist's career. Thereafter, regular supervision remains desirable. Indeed, such supervision is a hallmark of the ideal practice of psychotherapy. Regrettably, most consultant psychiatrists receive no formal ongoing supervision of their work.

The work of a psychiatrist is often very different to that of a psychotherapist, but there are many areas of overlap and cross-fertilization. Thus, the recommendations of the Royal College of Psychiatrists (1998) that each trainee psychiatrist in the UK have direct, supervised experience of treating patients using a number of psychotherapeutic modes, are significant. The concepts of transference, counter-transference, projective identification and acting out will only become meaningful when experienced in this way, and only then can they be harnessed throughout the rest of one's work in other fields within psychiatry. Other forms of support include staff support groups (optimally facilitated by an outside facilitator) and case discussion workshops during which 'difficult cases' may be considered. Personal psychotherapy or analysis will help one understand oneself, one's motivations, anxieties, blind-spots and prejudices, and will make one aware of one's own counter-transference and thus minimize the risk of inappropriate acting out with patients, colleagues and others.

Difficulties that may be encountered when interviewing psychiatric patients

Psychiatrists need to elicit a great deal of information in a short time and ensure that patients are as comfortable as possible while doing so. They often fail to do this, and research has identified a number of common reasons. First, all doctors frequently fail to clarify exactly what a patient means, and will often accept the patient's jargon (e.g. 'My nerves are driving me mad, doc'). A second common mistake is that of failing to respond to non-verbal cues. If a patient appears to be on the point of crying, for example, the doctor can usefully comment on the fact that the patient appears upset, rather than ignore it or move to another topic. A further common mistake that doctors may make is that of providing premature reassurance during interviews. By prematurely reassuring patients, a doctor effectively prevents them from fully explaining their concerns, and is more likely to cause upset than to reassure.

Psychiatrists need to be aware that there are many different ways to ask questions. At the beginning of an interview, it is appropriate to use open-ended questions (e.g. 'Tell me about your problems' or, 'What is your sleep like?') that are then followed-up with closed questions to clarify certain points (e.g. 'Did you first feel depressed or first feel anxious?' or 'Do you have difficulty in falling asleep?'). Leading questions that imply an answer (e.g. 'You don't sleep very well, do you?') are generally best avoided, as are questions with multiple themes (e.g. 'What are your sleep, appetite and energy like?'). Facilitating techniques should be used to encourage disclosure. These include silences that allow the patient time to think about a reply, brief empathic statements such as, 'That must have been extremely upsetting for you', the use of non-verbal cues such as nodding, and the maintenance of appropriate eye contact while the patient is speaking. It is very useful to present the patient with a brief summary of your understanding of their account of their problems, both in order to ensure an accurate record has been obtained and to impress upon patients that they have been listened to and their difficulties understood.

Certain types of patients and interview situations present particular difficulties to the psychiatrist. These are now discussed individually.

The stuporose patient

Stupor may be caused by schizophrenia (catatonic stupor), affective disorder (depressive or, very rarely, manic stupor) or hysteria (dissociative stupor), or by posterior diencephalic/upper mesencephalic lesions. Stuporose patients are mute, motionless and unresponsive to stimulation, but are otherwise completely conscious, aware and alert. They must be evaluated by observation of their behaviour, by physical examination and by interviewing an informant. Catatonic stupor is suggested by negativism, waxy flexibility and other schizophrenic movement disorders (see Ch. 19), depressive stupor by tearfulness and a sad expression, and dissociative stupor by closed eyes and resistance to passive eye-opening. Evidence of diencephalic/mesencephalic lesions includes abnormally reacting, unequal pupils. Both stuporose patients and patients who exhibit mutism may sometimes communicate by reading and writing.

The elderly patient

The assessment of elderly patients differs from that of other patients in that sensory impairment may present difficulties and cognition and physical health must be thoroughly evaluated. Impaired hearing and vision may be overcome by conducting the interview in a quiet, well-lit room, by speaking slowly and clearly (not loudly) and by using written material and functioning hearing aids. It is often invaluable to have the help of a relative or friend who can communicate readily with the patient.

The mentally handicapped patient

Short, clear questions should be used when interviewing mentally handicapped individuals and any account obtained should be supplemented with an account from an informant. Particular attention must be paid to changes in behaviour and to biological features of psychiatric illness. Thus a mentally handicapped patient may be unable to complain of feeling depressed but may exhibit increased irritability, loss of appetite and weight, sleep disturbance and tearfulness. A definitive assessment and diagnosis may be impossible in the case of some severely mentally handicapped individuals, and it may be necessary to undertake a trial of treatment with, for example, antidepressants if depression is suspected.

The agitated patient

Interviewing agitated patients is difficult and may be dangerous (see Ch. 36). The doctor may have to confine questions to those that are immediately important, only completing the evaluation when the patient has improved following treatment. Agitated patients respond best to a quiet calm manner of questioning, and are most appropriately interviewed in open areas where they do not feel restrained. Help must always be readily available in the event that the patient becomes violent.

Interviewing patients via an interpreter

The ability to conduct an interview via an interpreter is an essential skill for any psychiatrist. Although it may often be necessary to utilize the interpreting skills of the patient's friends or relatives, a trained interpreter should always be used if available. This ensures privacy for the patient and precludes the risk of relatives allowing their own views of the situation to modify their translation. When working with an interpreter, three chairs should be arranged in a triangle and the doctor should speak directly to the patient, addressing them in the second person. The doctor can help the patient feel at ease and feel understood by paying attention while the patient answers and by responding to the patient's non-verbal cues. Summarizing and asking the patient to repeat important points will help ensure that the patient understands all questions and that the doctor has obtained an accurate account. Similar principles apply when interviewing a deaf person via a sign interpreter. However, it is best if the signing interpreter sits slightly behind and to one side of the doctor, and it is important that good lighting is provided, in order that signing can be seen clearly and interpreted accurately.

Emergency consultations

Emergency consultations often take place in less than ideal settings (e.g. in patients' homes, in police stations or with several other individuals present) and sufficient time for a through assessment is rarely available. Nonetheless, the doctor should attempt to obtain an outline personal history and a clear account of the presenting complaint, its duration, and the mode of onset and severity of symptoms. This should suggest a probable diagnosis and the mental state examination should then concentrate on the symptoms associated with this diagnosis. Alcohol and drugs should be enquired about and a brief targeted physical examination undertaken if appropriate. A corroborating history from a relative or friend may be especially helpful during emergency consultations. In exceptional circumstances, this may be obtained without the patient's consent (see Ch. 36).

References

Folstein, M.F., Folstein, S.E., McHugh, P.R., 1975. 'Mini mental state' –a practical method for grading the cognitive state of patients for the clinician. J. Psychiatr. Res. 12, 189–198.

Mechanic, D., 1968. Medical sociology. Free Press, New York.

Royal College of Psychiatrists, 1998. Higher specialist training handbook, eighth ed. Royal College of Psychiatrists, London.

Steiner, J., 1976. Some aspects of the interviewing technique and their relationship to the transference. Br. J. Med. Psychol. 49, 65–72.

Watts, D., Morgan, G., 1994. Malignant alienation: dangers for patients who are difficult to like. Br. J. Psychiatry 164, 11–15.

Winnicott, D.W., 1957. The child, the family and the outside world. Penguin, London, pp. 49–78.

Diagnosis and classification in psychiatry

34

David J. Castle   Assen V. Jablensky

CHAPTER CONTENTS

Introduction

Classification in psychiatry has a long history, a story eloquently told by Berrios (1999: 145), who makes the point that most reviews of classification systems in psychiatry have been 'written in terms of a "received view"', and that 'this contains two assumptions, that: (1) the activity of classifying is inherent to the human mind; and (2) psychiatric "phenomena" are stable natural objects'. He articulates instead a 'conceptual history', assuming that all psychiatric classification systems are 'cultural products', and concludes, inter alia, that classifications are only valuable if they 'can release new information about the object classified'.

The history of the evolution of our major modern psychiatric diagnostic and classification systems, namely the American Psychiatric Association's 'Diagnostic and Statistical Manual' (DSM) and the World Health Organization's 'International Classification of Diseases' (ICD) is rather more dry, and how much these systems really 'release new information' is debatable. But diagnostic criteria and classification systems in psychiatry are useful for a number of other reasons, as outlined by Jablensky (1999):

1. The enhancement of diagnostic agreement among clinicians, allowing improved reporting

2. Improving reliability of diagnosis in research, such that comparisons can be made across studies

3. Provision of an international reference system that ensures less 'idiosyncrasy' in teaching

4. A 'demystification and transparency' in reporting and communication about psychiatric disorders and enhancing communication with non-professionals.

Also, as Kendell and Jablensky (2003) articulate, even if we do not accept many putative diagnostic entities in psychiatry as valid (i.e. as 'real'), it does not mean that they do not have utility. Indeed, Kendell and Jablensky (2003: 4) conclude that, 'Although most diagnostic concepts have not been shown to be valid [in the sense of having demonstrable natural boundaries], many possess high utility by virtue of the information about outcome, treatment response, and aetiology that they convey. They are therefore invaluable working concepts for clinicians.'

Thus, this chapter provides a broad overview of diagnosis and classification in psychiatry. Some detail is given on our two predominant world systems, DSM and ICD, before a consideration of more generic issues, such as how one determines whether a particular set of symptoms constitute a 'disorder'; and how one goes about deciding whether disparate putative disorders relate to each other. We then consider alternative approaches to psychiatric classification, and close with a glimpse of what future psychiatric classifications might look like.

Types of classification systems in psychiatry

Broadly, psychiatry has embraced classification systems that fall into three main types, namely:

1. **Symptom based:** this approach is commonly used in psychiatry. There is a long tradition to this approach, notably formulated comprehensively by Kraepelin, whose multi-edition 'Textbook' became the basis of modern psychiatric classification systems. Kraepelin (1893) not only took account of cross-sectional psychopathology, but also

the manifestation of positive psychotic symptoms to occur in the setting of substance use, in individuals who have a vulnerability to psychosis (see Verdoux 2004). Also, the affective disorder exclusion criterion belies the fact that many people with schizophrenia also exhibit depressive symptoms at some stage of their illness course (Siris 1991) and the lack of any consistent delineation of so-called 'schizoaffective' disorder.

One of the other problems associated with attempting to define a core entity that really 'is' schizophrenia, is that sets of criteria tend to be rather arbitrary and this may have profound implications for research as they force a circularity into the consideration of these putative disorders. For example, defining schizophrenia as a disorder with at least 6 months illness duration, as in DSM-IV (APA 1994), necessarily biases samples towards a poor outcome group; Research Diagnostic Criteria (RDC; Spitzer et al 1978) have an only 2-week illness stipulation, with the inclusion of more patients with a relatively benign outcome. DSM-III (APA 1980) arbitrarily imposed an age-at-onset cut-off for schizophrenia at 45 years, biasing samples towards younger ages, and Feighner criteria (1972) give loadings for a family history of schizophrenia, a long illness duration, and an early onset. The effect of such restrictions is evident in the male:female ratios for the different sets of diagnostic criteria. Thus, in a register-based first episode sample (Castle et al 1993), more lenient RDC produced a male:female ratio of 1.2:1; for DSMIIIR (APA 1987) the ratio was 1.3:1; and for DSMIII (APA 1980), 2.2:1. The stringent criteria of Feighner et al (1972) excluded many more females than males, with a resultant gender ratio of 2.5:1.

The problem of co-morbidity

Another problem with many psychiatric classification systems is the implicit attempt to pigeon-hole individuals and apply diagnostic labels to them. Regrettably, this denies the fact that many people have more than one psychiatric disorder. Indeed, having one psychiatric disorder increases the risk of having another one. For example, in the National Comorbidity Survey in the USA (Kessler 1995), if a respondent had one psychiatric disorder, they had a 56% chance of having another one as well. For example, it appears that people with schizophrenia have a particular predilection to depression, and certain anxiety disorders, notably obsessive–compulsive disorder (see Castle et al 2008); whether the latter association indicates similar pathogenetic factors, remains a point of conjecture (see Gross-Isseroff et al 2003).

Psychiatrists tend to be taught, and to think, in a very hierarchical way, such that certain diagnoses 'trump' others (Foulds 1976). This can result in patients not being assessed or treated adequately in terms of the extent of their psychopathology. For example, it is well recognized that 'negative' symptoms of schizophrenia can be secondary to, for example, depression, and the implicit belief by the clinician that such symptoms as social withdrawal and apathy are part and parcel of the schizophrenia process may leave depression undiagnosed and untreated.

There is also the problem that as we cleave more and more putatively discrete disorders from the core, the core

becomes the rag-bag 'deficit' diagnosis. This is evidenced by the anxiety disorders, where panic disorder, the phobic disorders, and obsessive–compulsive disorder have been reified, leaving 'generalized anxiety disorder' as something of a default diagnosis (Tyrer 1984). The problem with this is that it may be seen as a general diagnostic dustbin, with a residue of a number of disorders that happen not to 'fit' within the current nosology.

The problem of the Axes

Both ICD-10 and all editions of the DSM since 1980 encompass the notion that psychiatric disorders can be conceptualized on a number of different Axes. The multiaxial approach was foreshadowed by Rutter and colleagues (1969) in their classification of childhood psychiatric disorders, where developmental stage and intellectual functioning are classified on Axes separate from the primary clinical diagnosis. DSM-III took the bold step of classifying personality disorders on a separate Axis (Axis II); this was not the case in ICD-10. While the DSM approach to personality disorders has been praised in that it raised the profile of the personality disorders and enhanced the consideration of personality pathology, the downsides have been considerable. Perhaps most concerning is the implicit belief that disorders on Axis II are 'untreatable'. Indeed, when the Axis II disorder 'depressive personality disorder' was found to respond to antidepressants, it was elevated to Axis I (as 'dysthymia') (Akiskal et al 1977); a similar tale can be told of cyclothymic personality disorder and cyclothymia (Akiskal 1983).

The obverse problem arises for schizotypal personality disorder, which can increasingly be considered a *forme fruste* of schizophrenia (see Battaglia & Torgersen 1996), in that it aggregates in families of probands with schizophrenia, shows similar eye tracking abnormalities as people with schizophrenia, and responds to antipsychotic medication.

Another problem is that of the labelling, usually pejorative, of people with 'personality disorders' (Lewis & Appleby 1988). What is too often the case is that the behaviours of such individuals are considered a manifestation of their Axis II pathology, whereas they are just as vulnerable (if not more so) to a number of Axis I disorders. Thus, people with so-called borderline personality disorder share many psychosocial risk factors with people with post-traumatic stress disorder (e.g. early sexual abuse) and depression (lack of supporting relationships, unemployment).

In fact, the whole personality disorder issue has been an ongoing headache for those engaged in classification systems. Westen and colleagues (2006) found that clinicians tended not to find DSM-IV Axis II diagnoses very useful in clinical practice, and more readily endorsed a 'prototype' approach. But Rottman et al (2009) reported that clinicians did not readily endorse the dimensional 'five factor model' for personality disorders, retreating instead behind the relative certainty of DSM-IV. Axis II is perhaps one of the major areas of controversy in the planning towards DSM-V (e.g. Skodol & Bender 2009).

How to determine whether a putative diagnostic entity belongs with others

A further consideration is how to determine whether one disease entity should be grouped with others. An example of such groupings of disorders is the so-called obsessive–compulsive (OC) spectrum of disorders, in which disorders are grouped because they share certain symptoms. In its broad conceptualization, the OC spectrum encompasses (see Hollander 1993):

1. Disorders associated with *bodily preoccupation*, including body dysmorphic disorder (BDD), anorexia nervosa, and hypochondriasis
2. *Neurological disorders*, including Tourette syndrome and autism
3. *Impulse control disorders*, including pathological gambling, kleptomania and trichotillomania.

Decisions about inclusion in the OC spectrum have been based on similarities with OCD in a variety of domains, such as symptoms, demographic features, course of illness, co-morbidity, treatment response, joint familial loading and presumed aetiology (reviewed by Castle & Phillips 2006). The symptom domain (i.e. the presence of obsessions and/or repetitive behaviours) is the usual initial reason for considering a given disorder to be a potential spectrum candidate. However, it is clear that disorders should not be grouped together and considered related to one another on the basis of shared symptomatology alone. Indeed, the brain has a fairly limited repertoire in terms of the symptoms it produces. The fact that positive psychotic symptoms, for example, occur in schizophrenia, temporal lobe epilepsy, cannabis intoxication, borderline personality disorder, and Huntington disease does not imply that these disorders should be grouped together or considered related disorders (see Castle & Phillips 2006).

A powerful potential 'grouping' variable for psychiatric disorders is shared aetiological factors. In terms of the OC spectrum, our knowledge of aetiology is limited, and the extent of 'sharing' of such parameters among putative members of the spectrum is uneven. For example, BDD shows some familial aggregation with OCD, but other psychiatric disorders such as depression show much higher rates of aggregation in families of people with BDD. In a controlled family study, Bienvenue et al (2000) found increased rates of BDD alone or BDD with hypochondriasis in relatives of probands with OCD, but hypochondriasis alone and impulse control disorders did not show any excess. In a separate study, somatization disorder, but not OCD, aggregated in family members of probands with hypochondriasis (Noyes et al 1997). Thus, overall family studies of the OCD spectrum give only mixed support for aetiological links amongst some putative members.

Longitudinal course is also very variable amongst members of the putative OC spectrum. Thus, BDD tends to onset in the teens and is fairly stable throughout life, if untreated (this is very similar to social anxiety disorder, not a member of the 'spectrum'), while the onset-age and longitudinal course of trichotillomania, for example, is far more unpredictable. Demographic parameters also differ between members of the spectrum. Whilst OCD shows a roughly equal gender representation (males have a mean onset earlier than females), as does BDD (but no clear difference between the genders in onset-age), anorexia nervosa is essentially a disorder of girls.

Treatment response has been put forward as one of the most compelling justifications for grouping disorders in the OC spectrum. Again, the degree of support is variable across conditions. Thus, while OCD and BDD tend to respond the serotonergic antidepressants (SRIs) and cognitive behaviour therapy (CBT), trichotillomania does not (Van Minnen et al 2003). And in any event, other disorders also appear to respond selectively to SRIs, notably premenstrual dysphoric disorder (PMDD; see Grady-Weliky 2003). A further twist is that some people with OCD do not respond to SRIs, suggesting to some observers that subtypes of OCD might have different biological underpinnings. For example, the findings that OCD in conjunction with tics tends to require the use of a dopamine-D2 receptor blocker suggests dopaminergic involvement in what might be a relatively distinct subtype (see Lochner & Stein 2003).

Thus, the attempt to group a number of psychiatric disorders under the OC umbrella, while heuristically of potential utility, is defensible to a reasonable degree for only some members of the proposed spectrum, while the claim for other of the disorders is far more tenuous. Furthermore, if one were to accept for membership of the OC spectrum all of the potential candidate disorders, one would encompass a large slice of the entire DSM, raising further questions about the usefulness of such an exercise.

Classifying behaviours

Another matter worthy of consideration is those psychiatric classification systems that have attempted to classify certain behaviours, rather than disorders as such. A good example is Pilowsky's (1978) classification of 'abnormal illness behaviours'. This is a brave attempt to make some meaning out of how people manifest illness behaviours, and the 'motivations' behind the behaviours. This approach implicitly encompasses the sociological notions of 'illness behaviour' ('the ways in which given symptoms may be differentially perceived, evaluated and acted (or not acted) upon by different kinds of person' (Mechanic & Volkert 1960) and 'sick role') a 'partially and conditionally legitimated state whereby the ill individual is granted certain societal privileges, but is expected to desire wellness, and act in a way compatible with professional advice, in getting better' (Parsons 1964).

Thus, Pilowsky (1978) considers 'abnormal illness behaviour' as those forms of illness behaviour that is 'either deemed ill suited to the most effective and parsimonious way of maximizing health, or judged to deviate markedly from the usual range of particular organismic states, or both'. To incorporate all manifestations of abnormal illness behaviour, Pilowsky's (1978) classification encompasses both 'somatically focused' as well 'psychologically focused' behaviours, which may be either 'illness affirming' or 'illness denying'. There is a further subdivision, such that the motivation may be predominantly conscious or predominantly unconscious (see Box 34.1 for a full exposition).

This scheme has an admirable comprehensiveness to it, but is compromised by the fact that individuals may adopt a number of different 'illness behaviours', either in parallel or in different

Box 34.1

Pilowsky's classification of abnormal illness behaviour (Pilowsky 1978)

Somatically focused abnormal illness behaviour

I Illness affirming:

A. Motivation predominantly conscious:
1. Malingering
2. Munchausen syndrome

B. Motivation predominantly unconscious:
1. Neurotic:
   * Conversion reaction
   * Hypochondriacal reaction
2. Psychotic:
   * Hypochondriacal delusions associated with:
     a. Psychotic depression
     b. Schizophrenia
     c. Monosymptomatic hypochondriacal psychosis

II Illness denying:

A. Motivation predominantly conscious:
1. Illness denial in order to obtain insurance cover, employment
2. Denial to avoid feared therapies

B. Motivation predominantly conscious:
1. Neurotic:
   * 'Flight into health', e.g. non-compliance with therapy after myocardial infarct
   * Counterphobic behaviour, e.g. risk-taking associated with haemophilia
2. Psychotic:
   * Psychotic denial of somatic symptoms, e.g. as part of a hypomanic reaction
3. Neuropsychiatric:
   * Anosognosia, e.g. denial of hemiparesis.

Psychologically focused abnormal illness behaviour

III Illness affirming:

A. Motivation predominantly conscious:
1. 'Pseudopatients' (simulation for research purposes)
2. Compensation seeking
3. Ganser syndrome ('hysterical pseudodementia')

B. Motivation predominantly unconscious:
1. Neurotic:
   * 'Psychic hypochondriasis'
   * Dissociative reactions
   * Psychogenic amnesia
2. Psychotic:
   * Delusions of memory loss

IV Illness denying:

A. Motivation predominantly conscious:
1. Denial of psychotic symptoms to avoid stigma, hospitalization or gain discharge from care
2. Denial of psychotic illness to avoid perceived discrimination by, e.g. employers

B. Motivation predominantly unconscious:
1. Neurotic:
   * Refusal to 'psychological' diagnosis or treatment in the presence of neurotic illness, personality disorder of dependency syndromes
2. Psychotic:
   * Denial of illness ('lack of insight') in psychotic depression, mania, schizophrenia
3. Neuropsychiatric:
   * Confabulatory reactions in, e.g. Korsakoff psychosis.

---

settings at different times. An example is so-called 'accident neurosis', which Miller (1961) famously and polemically dismissed as essentially malingering, but which increasingly is recognized a complex set of reactions to an accident, compounded to various degrees by legal processes and the potential for monetary 'reward'. Mayou (1996) has warned against the potential reification of post-traumatic stress disorder in this context, as a legally 'legitimized' disorder, the criteria for which the individual must meet in order to obtain legal redress and compensation.

Are dimensional approaches better?

Dimensional approaches to psychiatric classification have mostly been championed by psychologists rather than psychiatrists. Perhaps the best known is Eysenck's (1970) dimensional approach to personality. Thus, people are considered in terms of their behaviours and attitudes, to 'rate' along three dimensions, namely 'introversion-extroversion', 'neuroticism' and 'psychoticism'. While useful enough in considering the personal make-up of individuals, and being to some extent predictive of psychiatric disorders *per se*, the approach does not help very much in deciding diagnosis or treatment. Thus, while dimensional approaches overall might be a closer reflection of 'truth', their utility in terms of whether

they actually enhance our ability to treat people effectively and reliably is questionable. It is of interest that current considerations of how classification will look in DSM-V are strongly influenced by a dimensional approach, perhaps a reflection of the criticisms of categorical systems (e.g. Oosthuizen et al 2008; Regier et al 2009). But whether clinicians will be able to utilize dimensions in clinical practice remains to be seen (e.g. Rottman et al 2009); perhaps some combination of dimensional and categorical approaches will be seen as a compromise model, as have been put forward for psychosis (Demjaha et al 2009).

Alternative approaches to psychiatric classification

There is little doubt that DSM-IV and ICD-10 are major achievements in that they bring in clarity, explicit rules and reference points in the field of clinical investigation which has been beset with problems of low reliability and with scepticism about the value of diagnosis to the extent of perceiving it as an obstacle to the management of patients. However, it would be unfortunate if the acceptance of the present diagnostic systems stifles further discussion of their limitations, shortcomings and potential for misuse. Also, the need must be recognized for renewed research leading to alternative or complementary solutions for the classification problems in psychiatry.

One recent trend is in restoring to psychiatric research the syndromes and symptoms as basic units of observation by adopting a primarily syndromological approach to the clinical study of psychiatric conditions. The proposed rationale for this is that with the use of present-day research technologies it is more likely that significant associations between dynamic cerebral processes and psychopathology will eventually be found at the level of symptoms and syndromes rather than at the level of disorders as defined in the current diagnostic systems. Systematic studies of this kind have been proposed, and van Praag (1993) coined the term 'functional psychopathology' for this reorientation of psychiatric research, in the expectation that 'functional psychopathology would be to psychiatry what physiology is to medicine'.

Similarly, the study of selected neurophysiological, cognitive, and neurochemical markers, assessed as dimensions across the conventional diagnostic groups and in the general population, may reveal unexpected patterns of association with clinically significant symptoms, behaviour, or personality traits that might result in refined definitions of clinical entities and in better validated phenotypes for genetic research.

A third trend is the application of new statistical models to the analysis of the validity of existing systems and the generation of novel and, sometimes, radically different approaches to classification. One such approach focuses on the concept of prototype (Cantor et al 1980) as an alternative to the classical category as the basic unit of classification. The difference here is that while a category must be defined in terms of necessary and sufficient characteristics, a prototype only requires a correlation with its defining features. The difficulty of fitting psychopathology and behaviour into tightly defined disease categories, which explains some of the shortcomings of the current diagnostic systems, is eliminated in a prototype-based classification by fiat, if we decide to forgo the objective that a psychiatric classification should mirror all the features of a biological classification. An extension of the prototype approach, using mathematical set theory and a generalized form of latent class analysis as a computational method, proceeds on the assumption that the concept of a discrete, 'crisp' disease entity may not be applicable to psychiatric disorders which could be better represented by 'fuzzy' sets, allowing for considerable variation and heterogeneity. Some early results of the application of this model to large psychiatric data sets on psychoses (Manton et al 1994) suggest that it may be possible to develop a classification based on a series of empirically derived 'ideal' or 'pure' types of disorders; that individuals may show quantifiable degrees of membership in more than one such 'pure' type; and that the classification has clinical relevance, including a high prognostic validity.

Future prospects: clinical or biological classification in psychiatry?

A point of view which is sometimes expressed – mainly by researchers with a biological orientation – is that clinical neuroscience will eventually replace psychopathology in the diagnosis of mental disorders, and that the phenomenological study of subjective experience of people with psychiatric illnesses will be relegated to the domain of applied anthropology. For example, increases in knowledge about the biological causes and processes in schizophrenia would gradually lead to a model of clinical practice which regards psychopathology as an epiphenomenon that is of secondary importance for the diagnosis and treatment. This belated transformation of clinical psychiatry would simply reproduce developments in other medical disciplines where biochemical, electronic and imaging tools have replaced ancient, finely honed clinical skills like the ability to elicit by palpation over 50 characteristics of the arterial pulse wave. Once the genes causing, or predisposing to, psychiatric disorders are mapped and cloned, diagnostic applications may become feasible in at least some disorders, as recent advances in familial Alzheimer disease suggest. In time, such developments would result in a completely redesigned classification of mental disorders, based on genetic aetiology. The categories of such a classification and their hierarchical ordering may recombine the present clinical diagnostic entities in many unexpected ways. Such a classification, the argument goes, would for the first time approximate a 'natural' classification in psychiatry.

This, indeed, is already happening in general medicine where molecular biology and genetics are transforming dramatically medical classifications. New organizing principles are producing new classes of disorders, such as mitochondrial diseases (Johns 1995). Large chapters of neurology are being re-written to reflect novel taxonomic groupings like diseases due to nucleotide triplet repeat expansion (Rosenberg 1996). The potential of molecular genetic diagnosis in various medical disorders is increasing by leaps and bounds and it looks unlikely that it would bypass psychiatric disorders (Farmer & Owen 1996).

Although the majority of psychiatric disorders now appear to be much more complex from a genetic point of view than has been hitherto assumed, there can be little doubt that molecular genetics and neuroscience will eventually have a major impact on our understanding of the aetiology and pathogenesis of psychiatric disorders. This is also likely to include a better understanding of the role of environmental and behavioural factors and of gene-environment interactions at different stages of individual development. However, the exact nature and extent of the impact of such advances on the diagnostic process in psychiatry and on the classification of psychiatric disorders is extremely difficult to predict. The outcome will ultimately depend not so much on the knowledge base of psychiatry *per se*, as on the social, cultural and economic forces that shape the societal perception of mental illness and thereby determine the nature of the clinical practice of psychiatry.

One possible outcome is, of course, what Eisenberg (1986) called 'mindless psychiatry' – a psychiatric practice guided by biological models of mental disorders, in which the subjective experience of psychopathology is an epiphenomenon. It corresponds exactly to what Karl Jaspers called 'the somatic prejudice' – one of the six fallacies that Jaspers identified in psychiatry, namely the belief 'that all psychological interest in schizophrenia will vanish when once the morbid somatic process that underlies it is discovered' (Jaspers 1963).

Another possible outcome is that clinical psychiatry will retain psychopathology at the core of its identity as a medical discipline uniquely dealing with the abnormal representations of reality in everyday consciousness. And, since classification is not only an abstract system representing the natural order of things, but also a tool of communication servicing practical needs, it must retain a relationship to the subjective world and to behaviour. Therefore, the speculation is that in the future psychiatry will evolve towards a dual classification – one grounded entirely within the realm of biological and medical classifications, with molecular genetic and neuroscience concepts as organizing principles, and another, dimensional or prototype-based which would be unapologetically naturalistic

in its design and isomorphic to the reality of clinical phenomenology. To prevent or redress the cognitive impoverishment of the discipline that might result from an uncritical adoption of a classification system as its *one* language, it behoves clinicians, researchers and teachers to reflect on the two realities and two cultures that meet on the common ground in psychiatry and ensure its vitality and relevance.

What is inevitable is that further iterations of ICD and DSM will eventuate, and to what extent they embrace the concepts outlined above, will be to some extent an ongoing balancing of utility and validity (see Kendell & Jablensky 2003). And to what extent ICD and DSM will be able to be 'harmonized' remains to be seen (First 2009).

References

Akiskal, H.G., 1983. Dysthymic disorder: psychopathology of proposed depressive subtypes. Am. J. Psychiatry 140, 11–20.

Akiskal, H.G., Djenderedjian, A.H., Rosenthal, R.H., et al., 1977. Cyclothymic disorder: validating criteria for inclusion in the bipolar affective group. Am. J. Psychiatry 134, 1227–1233.

APA, 1980. Diagnostic and Statistical Manual of Mental Disorders, third ed. American Psychiatric Association, Washington DC.

APA, 1987. Diagnostic and Statistical Manual of Mental Disorders, third ed., revised. American Psychiatric Association, Washington DC.

APA, 1994. Diagnostic and Statistical Manual of Mental Disorders, fourth ed. American Psychiatric Association, Washington DC.

APA, 2000. Diagnostic and Statistical Manual of Mental Disorders, fourth ed., text revision (DSM-IV TR). American Psychiatric Association, Washington DC.

Battaglia, M., Torgersen, S., 1996. Schizotypal disorder: at the crossroads of genetics and nosology. Acta Psychiatr. Scand. 94, 303–310.

Berrios, G.E., 1999. Classifications in psychiatry: a conceptual history. Aust. N.Z. J. Psychiatry 33, 145–160.

Bienvenue, O.J., Samuels, J.F., Riddle, M.A., et al., 2000. The relationship of obsessive-compulsive disorder to possible spectrum mechanisms: results from a family study. Biol. Psychiatry 48, 287–293.

Cantor, N., Smith, E.E., French, R.S., et al., 1980. Psychiatric diagnosis as prototype classification. J. Abnorm. Psychol. 89, 181–193.

Castle, D.J., Ames, F.R., 1996. Cannabis and the brain. Aust. N.Z. J. Psychiatry 30, 179–183.

Castle, D.J., Phillips, K.A., 2006. The OCD spectrum of disorders: a defensible construct? Aust. N.Z. J. Psychiatry 40, 114–120.

Castle, D.J., Wessely, S., Murray, R.M., 1993. Sex and schizophrenia: effects of diagnostic stringency, and associations with premorbid variables. Br. J. Psychiatry 162, 658–664.

Castle, D.J., Knoesen, N., Wykes, T., 2008. Depression and anxiety in schizophrenia. In: Castle, D.J., Copolov, D., Wykes, T. et al.,

(Eds.), Pharmacological and psychosocial treatments in schizophrenia. second ed. Informa Healthcare, London, pp. 61–80.

Demjaha, A., Morgan, K., Morgan, C., et al., 2009. Combining dimensional and categorical representation of psychosis: the way forward for DSM-V and ICD-11? Psychol. Med. 39, 1943–1956.

Eisenberg, L., 1986. Mindlessness and brainlessness in psychiatry. Br. J. Psychiatry 148, 497–508.

Eysenck, H.J., 1970. A dimensional system of psycho-diagnosis. In: Mahrer, A.R. (Ed.), New approaches to personality classification. Columbia University Press, New York, pp. 169–207.

Farmer, A., Owen, M.J., 1996. Genomics: the next psychiatric revolution? Br. J. Psychiatry 169, 135–138.

Feighner, J.P., Robins, E., Guze, S.B., et al., 1972. Diagnostic criteria for use in psychiatric research. Arch. Gen. Psychiatry 26, 57–63.

First, M.B., 2009. Harmonisation of ICD-11 and DSM-V: opportunities and challenges. Br. J. Psychiatry 195, 382–390.

Foulds, G.A., 1976. Hierarchical nature of personal illness. Academic Press, London.

Glass, I.B., 1989. Alcoholic hallucinosis: a psychiatric enigma. Br. J. Addict. 84, 29–41.

Grady-Weliky, T.A., 2003. Premenstrual dysphoric disorder. N. Engl. J. Med. 348, 433–438.

Gross-Isseroff, R., Hermesh, H., Zohar, J., et al., 2003. Neuroimaging communality between schizophrenia and obsessive-compulsive disorder: a putative basis for schizo-obsessive disorder? World J. Biol. Psychiatry 4, 129–134.

Hollander, E., 1993. Obsessive-compulsive spectrum disorders: an overview. Psychiatric Annals 23, 355–358.

Huntington Disease Collaborative Group, 1993. A novel gene containing a trinucleotide repeat that is expanded and unstable in Huntington's disease chromosomes. Cell 72, 971–983.

Jablensky, A., 1999. The nature of psychiatric classification: issues beyond ICD-10 and

DSM-IV. Aust. N.Z. J. Psychiatry 33, 137–144.

Jaspers, K., 1963. General psychopathology (J. Hoenig, M.W. Hamilton, Trans.). University Press Manchester, Manchester.

Johns, D.R., 1995. Mitochondrial DNA and disease. N. Engl. J. Med. 333, 638–644.

Kendell, R.E., Brockington, I.F., 1980. The identification of disease entities and the relationship between schizophrenic and affective psychoses. Br. J. Psychiatry 137, 324–331.

Kendell, R.E., Gourlay, J., 1970. The clinical distinction between the affective psychoses and schizophrenia. Br. J. Psychiatry 117, 261–266.

Kendell, R., Jablensky, A., 2003. Distinguishing between validity and utility of psychiatric diagnoses. Am. J. Psychiatry 160, 4–12.

Kessler, R.C., 1995. The epidemiology of psychiatric comorbidity. In: Tsuang, M., Tohen, M., Zahner, G. (Eds.), Textbook of psychiatric epidemiology. Wiley, New York, pp. 179–198.

Kraepelin, E., 1893. Psychiatrie, fourth ed. Barth, Leipsig.

Lewis, G., Appleby, L., 1988. Personality disorder: the patients psychiatrists dislike. Br. J. Psychiatry 153, 44–49.

Lochner, C., Stein, D.J., 2003. Heterogeneity of obsessive-compulsive disorder: a literature review. Harv. Rev. Psychiatry 11, 113–132.

Manton, K.G., Korten, A., Woodbury, M.A., et al., 1994. Symptom profiles of psychiatric disorders based on graded disease classes: an illustration using data from the WHO International Pilot Study of Schizophrenia. Psychol. Med. 24, 133–144.

Masters, C.L., Beyreuther, K., 1994. Alzheimer's disease: a clearer definition of the genetic components. Med. J. Aust. 160, 243–244.

Mayou, R., 1996. Accident neurosis revisited. Br. J. Psychiatry 165, 399–403.

McCarley, R.W., Wible, C.G., Frumin, M., et al., 1999. MRI anatomy of schizophrenia. Biol. Psychiatry 45, 1099–1119.

Mechanic, D., Volkert, E.H., 1960. Illness behaviour and medical diagnosis. J. Health Hum. Behav. 1, 51–58.

Miller, H., 1961. Accident neurosis. Br. Med. J. 919–998.

Murray, R.M., O'Callaghan, E., Castle, D.J., et al., 1992. A neurodevelopmental approach to the classification of schizophrenia. Schizophr. Bull. 18, 319–332.

Noyes Jr., R., Holt, C.S., Happel, R.L., et al., 1997. A family study of hypochondriasis. J. Nerv. Ment. Dis. 185, 223–232.

Oosthuizen, P., Emsley, R., Niehaus, D., et al., 2008. The multidimensional assessment of psychopathology in mood and psychotic disorders. A proposal for Axis II in DSM-V/ICD-11. Afr. J. Psychiatry 11, 260–263.

Parsons, T., 1964. Social structure and personality. Collier-Macmillan, London.

Pilowsky, I., 1978. A general classification of abnormal illness behaviours. Br. J. Med. Psychol. 51, 131–137.

Prince, M., Cullen, M., Mann, A., 1994. Risk factors for Alzheimer's disease and dementia: a case-control study based on the MRC elderly hypertension trial. Neurology 44, 97–104.

Regier, D.A., Narrow, W.E., Kuhl, E.A., et al., 2009. The conceptual development of DSM-V. Am. J. Psychiatry 166, 645–650.

Robins, L., Guze, S.B., 1970. Establishment of diagnostic validity in psychiatric illness: its application to schizophrenia. Am. J. Psychiatry 126, 983–987.

Rosenberg, R.N., 1996. DNA-triplet repeats and neurologic disease. N. Engl. J. Med. 335, 1222–1224.

Rottman, B.M., W-k, Ahn, Sanislow, C.A., et al., 2009. Can clinicians recognize DSM-IV personality disorders from five-factor model descriptions of patient cases? Am. J. Psychiatry 166, 427–433.

Rutter, M., Lebovici, L., Eisenberg, L., et al., 1969. A tri-axial classification of mental disorders in childhood. J. Child Psychol. Psychiatry 10, 41–61.

Schneider, K., 1959. Clinical psychopathology (M. W. Hamilton, Trans.). Grune & Stratton, London.

Siris, S.G., 1991. Diagnosis of secondary depression in schizophrenia: implications for DSM-IV. Schizophr. Bull. 17, 75–98.

Skodol, A.E., Bender, D.S., 2009. The future of personality disorders in DSM-V? Am. J. Psychiatry 166, 388–391.

Spitzer, R.L., Endicott, J., Robins, E., 1978. Research Diagnostic Criteria (RDC): rationale and reliability. Arch. Gen. Psychiatry 35, 773–782.

Szasz, T., 1976. Schizophrenia: the sacred symbol of psychiatry. Br. J. Psychiatry 129, 308–316.

Toone, B.K., 1991. The psychoses of epilepsy. J. R. Soc. Med. 84, 457–459.

Tyrer, P., 1984. Classification of anxiety. Br. J. Psychiatry 144, 78–83.

Van Minnen, A., Hoogduin, K.A., Keijsers, G.P., et al., 2003. Treatment of trichotillomania with behavioural therapy or fluoxetine: a randomised, waiting-list controlled study. Arch. Gen. Psychiatry 60, 517–522.

van Praag, H.M., 1993. Make-believes in psychiatry or the perils of progress. Brunner Mazel, New York.

Verdoux, H., 2004. Cannabis and psychosis proneness. In: Castle, D.J., Murray, R.M. (Eds.), Marijuana and madness. Cambridge University Press, Cambridge, pp. 75–88.

Westen, D., Shedler, J., Bradley, R., 2006. A prototype approach to personality disorder diagnosis. Am. J. Psychiatry 163, 846–856.

WHO, 1992. The ICD-10 Classification of mental and behavioural disorders: clinical descriptions and diagnostic guidelines. World Health Organization, Geneva.

Wing, J., Nixon, J., 1975. Discriminating symptoms in schizophrenia. Arch. Gen. Psychiatry 32, 853–859.

Electroencephalography and neuroimaging

35

Pádraig Wright   Thordur Sigmundsson   James V. Lucey

CHAPTER CONTENTS

Introduction

Psychiatrists often bemoan the absence of biological markers for the diseases they study and treat, and critics of psychiatry frequently cite this absence as evidence that psychiatric illness does not exist. Electroencephalography has been used to investigate psychiatric illness for more than half a century but it has contributed little to our understanding of such illness.

However, the use of increasingly sophisticated structural and functional neuroimaging, and indeed electrophysiological, techniques offers hope that we will soon more fully understand the neurophysiological correlates of psychiatric illness. Current and potential future applications to psychiatry of electroencephalography and of structural and functional neuroimaging will be discussed in this chapter.

Electroencephalography in psychiatry

The normal electroencephalogram

An electroencephalogram (EEG) is a recording of the electrical potential of the brain made at the scalp surface. The EEG α rhythm was first recorded with an Einthoven string galvanometer by Austrian psychiatrist Hans Berger in 1929, and until recently, the EEG was the only non-invasive means of assessing brain function (Berger 1931).

An EEG is a recording of the electrical potential produced by inhibitory and excitatory post-synaptic electrical discharges from neuronal dendrites at the cortical surface. Such neurons constitute less than 5% of all neurons in the brain. The voltage recorded on an EEG is only 10% of that recorded on an electrocardiograph because the electrical resistance of the skull is high. An individual's EEG is largely genetically determined and several investigations have reported that EEGs recorded from monozygotic twins were almost identical (Dummermuth 1968). The EEG records changes in the electrical potential of the brain, which are detected as variations in voltage (10–100 microvolts, μV) and frequency (0.5–40 Hz).

When recording an EEG, electrodes (usually 21) are placed on the scalp in a standard (or international) 10/20 arrangement, in which the electrodes are placed at points either 10% or 20% of the total distance along an imaginary line between two anatomical landmarks, e.g. the nasion and inion. Negative potentials cause an upward deflection on the EEG record, and either bipolar (between two electrodes) or common (between any single electrode and a fixed electrically neutral site such as the nose or ear lobe) reference potentials may be recorded. The arrangement of recording electrodes in use at a given time is referred to as a montage.

EEG recordings may be made with the patient either lying still or ambulatory, and nasopharyngeal (inserted via the nares) or sphenoidal (inserted inferior to the zygomatic arch) electrodes may be used to allow recordings from the inferior temporal lobe, especially prior to temporal lobe surgery. Depth electrodes are occasionally placed in the brain via burr holes, and electrocorticography may be undertaken by placing electrodes directly on the brain intraoperatively. More recent technological advances allow continuous portable EEG recording for ≥ 24 h, simultaneous videotape display and recording of a subject's behaviour and EEG and thus their potential correlation, and the rapid computerized analysis of digitized EEG data. This latter facilitates brain mapping, in which EEG voltages or amplitudes are plotted on a map representing the brain and for which extensive comparative data from both healthy and psychiatric subjects are available (Fenwick 1992).

Normal EEG frequencies

The normal EEG frequencies are as follows:

- δ rhythm = 0.1–3.9 Hz
- θ rhythm = 4.0–7.9 Hz
- α rhythm = 8.0–13.0 Hz
- β rhythm = 13.0–40.0 Hz

The α rhythm (30–50 μV) is the normal rhythm seen in a subject who is awake with his eyes closed. It is maximal over the occipital and, to a lesser extent, the parietal regions, and is often less evident over the dominant hemisphere. The β rhythm is present over the remaining frontocentral areas of the scalp. If the subject opens his eyes or undertakes mental activity, the α rhythm blocks or attenuates and is replaced by β rhythm all over the scalp. The β-waves from different sites are out of phase and are said to be desynchronized. The δ and θ frequencies occur during sleep but are not present during wakefulness in adults, while τ- and μ-waves occur over the occipital and motor cortices respectively, and are caused by minimal ocular (scanning) and limb movements. A hypnotized subject exhibits the same EEG as one who is awake and alert, and minor abnormalities are common in EEGs recorded from healthy individuals.

Age and the EEG

Although EEG activity is evident from at least the 2nd trimester of gestation (Eeg-Olofsson 1970), the EEG of a normal neonate reveals relatively little rhythmic electrical activity. Desynchronized δ- and θ-waves are evident in recordings from alert older infants. With increasing age, these are replaced by α rhythm from frontal, through temporal and parietal, and thence to occipital regions. In general, the EEG is dominated by δ rhythm until about the age of 2 years, by θ until about the age of 5 years, and by α activity thereafter until the adult EEG emerges.

The adult pattern of dominant α rhythm described above becomes evident in late adolescence and is referred to as the mature EEG. Frontal θ and posterior temporal δ-waves may persist in some young adults (referred to as a maturational EEG)

and there is some evidence that these rhythms are associated with personality disorder when they are present in later adulthood (referred to as an immature EEG).

From the seventh decade of life onwards, α-waves are of lower voltage and frequency, and low-frequency rhythms such as δ-waves may reappear. These changes are more evident in men than in women and may be accompanied by clinically insignificant temporal slow-wave foci (Obrist & Busse 1965).

Activation of the EEG

Suspected EEG abnormalities may not be evident during a standard recording. These may be revealed if the brain is stressed or otherwise activated in some way. The techniques used to unmask abnormalities hidden in the resting EEG record include:

- Hyperventilation, which induces cortical hypocapnia, cerebral vasoconstriction and hypoxia, and may allow epileptic foci to become evident
- Photic stimulation, in which a strobe light flashing at 8–15 Hz is used to capture the occipital α frequency, that is the α frequency adjusts to match that of the strobe light (photic driving). This may allow epileptic foci to be seen and may even induce epileptic seizures, as may a flickering television screen
- Barbiturates and neuroleptics, which may both be used to unmask epileptic foci.

The EEG and sleep

Sleep is similar to coma, in that it consists of inactivity and loss of awareness and responsivity. In contrast to the comatose individual, however, the sleeping individual either awakens spontaneously or can be roused. The EEG has been used extensively in the investigation of both the physiology of sleep and sleep disorders. Indeed physiological sleep is divided into five stages purely on the basis of changes observed in EEG recordings taken from sleeping subjects.

During sleep, the rhythm recorded on an EEG changes from the β rhythm of wakefulness, through occipital α rhythm when the eyes are closed, to the sleep EEG. Stages I (transitional sleep), II, III and IV of the sleep EEG are referred to as non-rapid eye movement (non-REM) or orthodox sleep, during which parasympathetic tone is increased, while Stage V is referred to as rapid eye movement (REM) or desynchronized sleep, during which sympathetic tone is increased. Stages III and IV are characterized by slow waves and are therefore sometimes referred to as slow wave sleep (SWS), or as synchronized sleep. The principal EEG features of sleep stages I to IV are summarized in Box 35.1.

Stage V or REM sleep is also called paradoxical sleep because, while deep unconsciousness and marked atonia occur, paradoxically the EEG resembles that recorded during Stage I (transitional) sleep, or when a subject is awake with his eyes closed. Thus low voltage, variable frequency waves and occasional α rhythm are recorded. The eyes exhibit rapid conjugate movements and physiological arousal is evident as tachycardia, tachypnoea, systolic hypertension, increased oxygen consumption, dilated pupils, penile tumescence or vaginal lubrication, increased cerebral perfusion and occasional myoclonic jerks.

Box 35.1

EEG features of sleep

Stage I

- The α rhythm gradually disappears
- Low-voltage desynchronized slow waves (δ and θ) appear
- High-voltage sharp waves occur at the vertex

Stage II

- Low voltages and δ and slower frequencies dominate the recording
- Sleep spindles occur (sinusoidal 12–14 Hz of 0.5 s)
- K complexes occur (high-amplitude sharp positive/negative deflections)

Stage III

- High-voltage slow waves all over the scalp
- δ-waves account for <50% of rhythm
- Sleep spindles and K complexes diminish

Stage IV

- High-voltage slow (δ) waves dominate the EEG
- δ-waves account for >50% of rhythm
- Sleep spindles and K complexes are absent.

Dreaming is reported (and is vividly recalled) by 60–80% of individuals awakened from REM sleep, as compared to about 20% of subjects awakened from non-REM sleep. REM accounts for over 50% of sleep in childhood, for 25% in adulthood and for 10% of sleep in old age. REM changes on an EEG recorded during the daytime suggest either sleep deprivation, withdrawal from alcohol or from drugs that suppress REM (barbiturates, benzodiazepines), or narcolepsy.

The cycle from Stage I to V takes about 1.5 h and is repeated four or five times per night (Fig. 35.1). Thus, sleep during the early part of the night is largely SWS; sleep during the later part of the night is largely REM sleep, and overall most time is spent in Stage II sleep. The normal sleep/wake cycle is of 25 hours' duration (not 24 h) and if deprived of sleep (or selectively of REM sleep) extra REM sleep, called REM-rebound, occurs when normal sleep is again possible. However, the function of sleep in general, and of REM sleep in particular, is unknown. Both total sleep deprivation and selective REM deprivation have real but relatively modest effects on formal tests of cognitive function, which can largely be compensated for by increased effort, at least in the short term. This cognitive deficit has been quantified as equivalent to that caused by a blood alcohol level of 0.05% (Falleti et al 2003). However, performance on formal tests of cognitive function are not good indicators of occupational or other performance and there is growing evidence that sleep deprivation significantly impairs the working ability of, e.g., doctors (Samkoff & Jacques 1991). It is important to note that sleep requirements vary greatly both between individuals and within individuals at different times and that 5 or 6 hours' sleep is sufficient for many people. In particular, sleep requirements diminish with age.

The circadian rhythm of secretion that hormones such as cortisol, prolactin, growth hormone and insulin exhibit is well known and some hormones exhibit a similar secretory pattern (which may be superimposed on the circadian pattern) during the sleep cycle. Thus, growth hormone levels are maximal during SWS, prolactin levels peak during early Stage I and later Stage IV sleep, and testosterone levels increase continuously during sleep. There is also increasing evidence that seasonal and circadian patterns of hormone levels and behaviour may be controlled by rhythmic secretion of melatonin from the pineal gland. Melatonin levels are low during REM sleep and may be controlled by a putative biological clock in the suprachiasmatic nucleus of the hypothalamus, which responds to light falling on the retina. Melatonin is effective in alleviating jet lag (during which the normal diurnal variation in body temperature and in cortisol and catecholamine secretion is disrupted) but there is no evidence that phototherapy for seasonal affective disorder acts by increasing melatonin levels.

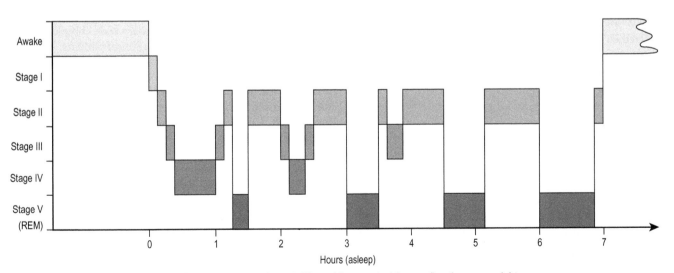

Figure 35.1 • The cycle from sleep Stage I–V takes about 1.5 h and is repeated four or five times per night.

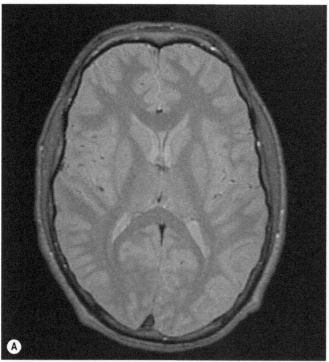
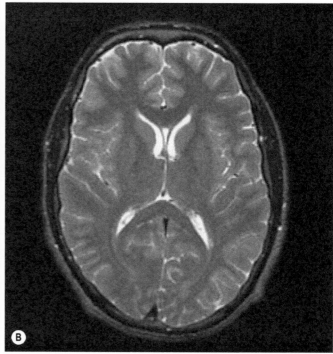

Figure 35.3 ● (A) and (B) are proton density and T2-weighted axial MRI images respectively taken from the same anatomical location in the head of a patient at the level of the basal ganglia. (Images courtesy of Neuroimaging Department, Maudsley Hospital, London.)

Box 35.4

Clinical indications for structural brain scans

- Dementia
- Delirium
- Catatonia
- Movement disorder
- Acute change in personality
- First onset of psychosis
- History of head trauma
- History of seizures
- Eating disorder
- Electroencephalographic abnormalities
- Focal neurological abnormalities
- First onset of psychiatric symptoms after age 50 years
- Atypical symptoms or course of illness.

---

cross-sections on CT scans. MRI subsequently provided the opportunity to examine both smaller structures poorly visible on CT (temporal lobe, cerebellum) and images of the brain in different planes. MRI also provided excellent separation between white and grey matter, which allowed segmentation of the brain into three components – white and grey matter, and cerebrospinal fluid (CSF). It is usual to refer to specific brain regions being investigated with CT or MRI as regions of interest (ROI), the volumes of ROIs being compared between groups either manually (by tracing them on a computer monitor and multiplying the area by the slice thickness to get the volume for each slice, the cumulative volume of ROIs on all slices providing an estimate of the volume of the structures being examined) or automatically (by using computer programs capable of segmenting the brain into grey and white matter and CSF and of calculating the volume of each component separately). More recently, it has become possible to analyse structural imaging data using methods first developed for analysing functional neuroimaging data (the recording of images with a template image in stereotactic space and the analysis of differences in grey or white matter intensities on a voxel (volume element) by voxel basis). In addition to the search for brain abnormalities specific to individual neuropsychiatric disorders, structural neuroimaging has also been used to monitor disease progress in patients with degenerative brain disorders (Fox et al 1996), examine the effects of pharmacological treatments such as increased basal ganglia volume in patients treated with antipsychotic drugs (Chakos et al 1995), and to co-register structural and functional neuroimaging data, e.g. PET with MRI.

Functional neuroimaging in psychiatry

Four functional neuroimaging techniques have established themselves in psychiatric research and their clinical applications are becoming increasingly important. Single photon emission tomography (SPET) and positron emission tomography (PET) depend on the administration of radioactive isotopes and the subsequent detection of γ-photons and positrons respectively. Functional MRI (fMRI) and MR spectroscopy (MRS) utilize MRI technology as described above.

Positron emission tomography (PET)

PET is the benchmark technique for functional imaging of metabolic processes such as regional cerebral blood flow (rCBF) or regional cerebral metabolism of glucose (rCMG). It involves the combination of two technologies, tracer kinetic assay (TKA) and CT. TKA involves the use of a radiolabelled, biologically active compound (the radionuclide tracer) and a mathematical model of its kinetics as it participates in a biological process. The PET scanner measures the tissue concentration of the tracer and produces a three-dimensional image of the anatomical distribution of the biological process being investigated.

The radionuclide tracers used during PET imaging are natural substrates or their analogues, combined with radioactive forms of natural elements (labels) such as ^{11}C, ^{13}N, ^{15}O and ^{18}F. These radiolabels emit radiation in the form of positrons that pass through the body and are detected externally, but that do not alter the biological process being investigated. Positrons are positively charged electrons that are emitted from the nucleus of some radioisotopes because they have an excess of protons and a positive charge, and are thus unstable. An emitted positron collides with electrons until it comes to rest and then combines with an electron to become a positronium. Since the positron is an anti-electron, the positron and electron annihilate each other and their masses are converted into electromagnetic energy. The mass of the electron and positron are equal, and equivalent to 511 kiloelectronvolts (keV) of energy. In a collision referred to as a true coincidence, the annihilation produces two 511 keV photons 180° apart. The scanner detects this energy. This is annihilation coincidence detection (ACD). Only true coincidences produce valid spatial information, so scanner designs try to maximize true coincidences and minimize scatter coincidences that produce 'noise'.

PET imaging (Fig. 35.4) requires a charged particle accelerator or cyclotron to produce positron-emitting isotopes and over 500 such isotopes have been produced by labelling with ^{15}O, ^{13}N, ^{11}C or ^{18}F. Compounds used with PET include H_2O^{15} for rCBF measurement and ^{18}F deoxyglucose (DG) for rCMG. PET imaging benefits from a low radiation exposure time:imaging time ratio, because PET radionuclides have short half-lives (^{15}O = 2 min, ^{18}F = 110 min). Dosimetry (here, used to ascertain the relationship between the radiation dose administered to the subject and the quality of the image detected) is determined by effects on organs throughout the body and not only by effects on the organ under investigation. In ^{18}F-DG PET imaging, 77% of the radiation dose is accounted for by photons of emitted ionization, and only 23% by annihilation of positrons.

The CT technique in PET uses rigorous mathematical algorithms to produce tomographic images of projections from an object. PET scintillation detectors produce light when struck by radiation and image resolution depends on both detector resolution and the radiation cut-off frequency used. The signal to noise ratio is high and the tomographic planes are usually perpendicular to the long axis of the body. Early tomographic systems used ROI (regions of interest) analysis relying on manual placement of templates upon reconstructed images (see above). These were prone to inter-rater and intra-rater variability because anatomical localization was relatively unreliable. Modern

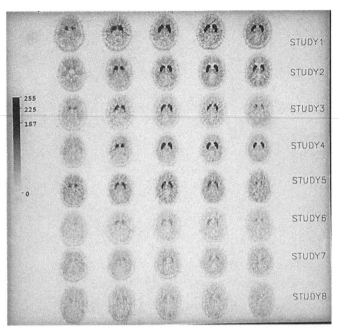

Figure 35.4 • PET images of ^{11}C raclopride, a dopamine D_2 receptor ligand. The images are darkest in the striatum where the highest levels of ^{11}C raclopride occurs. Subject study 4 had placebo, and subject studies 1–3 and 5–8 had increasing doses of ziprasidone (2, 5, 10, 15, 20, 40 and 60 mg). The images show decreasing binding of ^{11}C raclopride due to ziprasidone's increasing occupancy of the dopamine D_2 receptor. (Image courtesy of Dr C. Bench, MRC Cyclotron Unit, Hammersmith Hospital, London.)

PET imaging depends on computerized and automated systems for PET data analysis such as the Statistical Parametric Mapping or SPM system. Moreover, simultaneous anatomical localization of PET data using MRI – a process known as MRI co-registration – is increasingly available.

Single photon emission tomography (SPET)

SPET refers to a computerized emission tomographic system that depends on isotopes that emit single photons (as distinct from positrons in PET). Single photons are detected singly rather than in coincident pairs (as in PET). Collimation – the trapping of emitted photons and their direction towards the detector – is required because single photons are scattered randomly, and this means that most photons are absorbed by collimators and thus go undetected. Thus only a fraction of emitted photons are counted by SPET detector systems and SPET resolution is achieved at the expense of SPET sensitivity. The sensitivity of SPET is the degree to which the system responds to an incoming signal measured as counts per second (CPS) per slice (megaBequerel per litre or MBq/L). The most frequently used detector systems in clinical practice are rotating γ cameras.

Once acquired, SPET data are organized as slices, and reconstructed separately from projections spaced over a 360° arc of rotation about the subject. The SPET detector system behind the collimator is made of sodium iodide crystals with photomultiplier tubes (PMTs) and SPET detector systems may have one

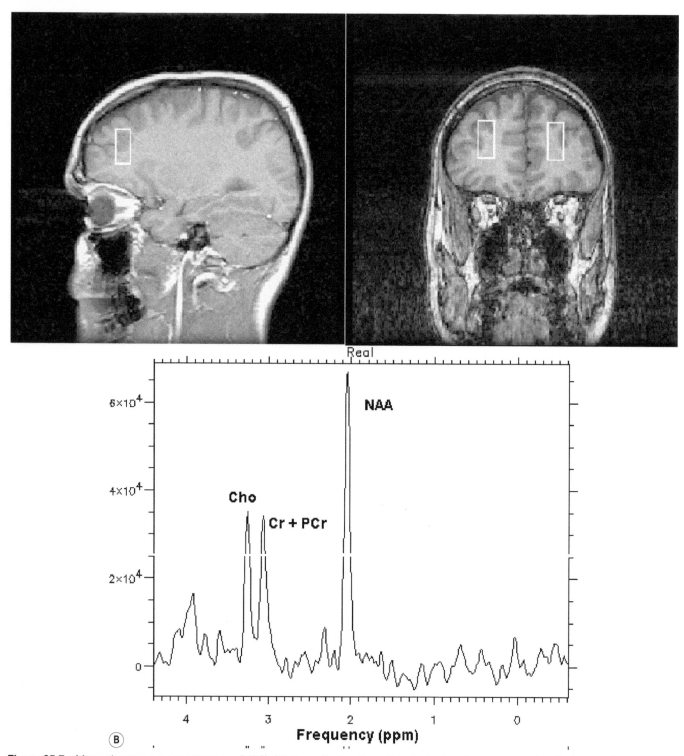

Figure 35.7 • Magnetic resonance spectroscopy (MRS). (A) shows the location within the brain using coronal and sagittal magnetic resonance images of spectroscopic voxels from which a processed proton MRS spectrum may be derived. (B) displays a typical processed proton MRS spectrum from the frontal lobe in a healthy volunteer. The major metabolite peaks, N-acetyl aspartate (NAA) – an amino acid found only in neurons and therefore used as a neuronal marker, choline (Cho) and creatine and phosphocreatine (Cr1PCr), are indicated. (Images courtesy of Neuroimaging Department, Maudsley Hospital, London.)

(Lim et al 1998). In addition to protium (^{1}H), other isotopes that possess nuclear spin include fluorine (^{19}F), sodium (^{23}Na), phosphorus (^{31}P) and lithium (^{7}Li). This allows MRS detection in the brain of molecules that incorporate these isotopes, and phosphorus and proton MRS have been used extensively to investigate brain energy metabolism. Furthermore, the preliminary use of MRS in the evaluation of psychopharmacological compounds has already been reported (Maier 1995). It therefore appears likely that MRS, like fMRI, will soon have a place in clinical psychiatric practice (Malhi et al 2002).

References

Berger, H., 1931. Uber das electroenkephalogramm des Menschen III. Arch. Psychiatr. Nervenkr. 94, 16–22.

Blackwood, D.H.R., Muir, W.J., 1990. Cognitive brain potentials and their application. Br. J. Psychiatry 157 (Suppl. 9), 96–101.

Chakos, M.H., Lieberman, J.A., Alvir, J., 1995. Caudate nucleii volumes in schizophrenic patients treated with typical antipsychotics and clozapine. Lancet 345, 456–457.

Dummermuth, G., 1968. Variance spectra of EEGs in twins. In: Kellaway, P., Peterssen, I. (Eds.), Clinical electroencephalography of children. Grune and Stratton, New York.

Eeg-Olofsson, O., 1970. The development of the EEG in normal children and adolescents from the age of 1 through 21 years. Acta Paediatr. Scand. 208 (Suppl), 1+.

Falleti, M.G., Maruff, P., Collie, A., et al., 2003. Qualitative similarities in cognitive impairment associated with 24 h of sustained wakefulness and a blood alcohol concentration of 0.05%. J. Sleep Res. 12, 265–274.

Fenwick, P.B.C., 1992. Use of the EEG in psychiatry. In: Weller, M., Eysenck, M. (Eds.), The scientific basis of psychiatry. WB Saunders, London.

Fox, N.C., Freeborough, P.A., Rossor, M.N., 1996. Visualisation and quantification of rates of atrophy in Alzheimer's disease. Lancet 348, 94–97.

Jakobi, W., Winkler, H., 1927. Encephalographische studien auf chronisch schizophrenen. Arch. Psychiatr. Nervenkr. 81, 299–332.

Johnstone, E.C., Crow, T.J., Frith, C.D., et al., 1976. Cerebral ventricular size and cognitive impairment in chronic schizophrenia. Lancet ii, 924–986.

Larkin, E.P., 1985. The X-ray department and psychiatry. Br. J. Psychiatry 146, 62–65.

Lim, K.O., Adalsteinsson, E., Spielman, D., et al., 1998. Proton magnetic resonance spectroscopic imaging with spiral-based k-space trajectories. Arch. Gen. Psychiatry 55, 346–352.

Maier, M., 1995. In vivo magnetic resonance spectroscopy: applications in clinical psychiatry. Br. J. Psychiatry 167, 299–306.

Malhi, G.S., Valenzuela, M., Wen, W., et al., 2002. Magnetic resonance spectroscopy and its applications in psychiatry. Aust. N.Z. J. Psychiatry 36, 31–43.

Muller, T.J., Kalus, P., Strik, W.K., 2001. The neurophysiological meaning of auditory P300 in subtypes of schizophrenia. World J. Biol. Psychiatry 2, 9–17.

Obrist, W.D., Busse, E.W., 1965. Wilson, W.P. (Ed.), Applications of electroencephalography in psychiatry. Duke University Press, Durham NC.

Samkoff, J.S., Jacques, C.H., 1991. A review of studies concerning effects of sleep deprivation and fatigue on residents' performance. Acad. Med. 66, 687–693.

Emergency psychiatry

Peter Fitzgerald   John M. Cooney

CHAPTER CONTENTS

Introduction

Emergency psychiatry encompasses that clinical practice which is directed towards the treatment of distressed patients with acute psychiatric disorders. Such treatment may involve reassurance, direction to other medical or non-medical resources, the prescribing of medication or admission to hospital. Whatever intervention is indicated, a psychiatric emergency demands that it be provided immediately. Thus, the role of the psychiatrist or mental health professional is primarily to make a decision on the further management of the patient. It follows therefore, that adequate information about the patient's presenting problem, and assessment of the individual and their circumstances in an objective manner, is critical. At all times, consideration must be given to the safety of patients, professional colleagues and third parties.

Emergency psychiatry has considerable overlap with general psychiatry but it warrants consideration as a specialist topic for several reasons. The trend towards deinstitutionalization means that vulnerable patients are exposed to rigours of daily life that are demanding and may be overwhelming. Psychiatric patients are more conspicuous in the community and in the media through the reporting of episodes of violence and this leads to subsequent public disquiet. This makes patients more likely to attend an emergency service either at their own request or at that of a third party. Debate continues as to the true prevalence of violent incidents committed by psychiatric patients and as to whether community care has resulted in their increase. There is no debate that one consequence of community care for psychiatrists and their colleagues is that risk has assumed primacy when dealing with patients. This is nowhere more evident than in emergency psychiatry – safe, coherent and rapid decision-making is paramount.

Clinicians working in an emergency situation must deal primarily with symptoms rather than with diagnoses. The environment in which emergency psychiatry is practised is often less controlled than a ward setting or a community base and patients or their relatives or friends may be unable or unwilling to provide collateral information. The clinical approach is therefore necessarily pragmatic and directed towards finding the best-fit solution within the constraints of the patient's symptoms and available services, effectively implementing this solution, and most importantly, documenting the process and decision. This calls for considerable common sense and judgement on the part of the clinician, as well as knowledge of psychiatry and of the applicable ethical and medicolegal environment.

This chapter will consider the general clinical approach to patients in the emergency context. Special consideration will be given to clinical presentations that are common, that cross

Aggression and violence in the emergency setting

Most aggression and violence in society is not due to mental illness. However, epidemiological studies have shown that people with mental disorders are more likely to be violent than community controls and that this increased risk is largely mediated by the presence of either co-morbid personality disorders, substance misuse or active psychotic symptoms (Swanson et al 1990; Steadman et al 1998).

When violence occurs, the issues of importance for the emergency psychiatrist are safety, recognition of the causative factors and initiation of measures to reduce the possibility of recurrence. Thus the psychiatrist must be able to:

- Recognize signs of incipient violence and prevent it from occurring
- Manage violent incidents
- Prevent recurrence of violence.

The literature describing inpatient violence has been reviewed previously, initially by the Royal College of Psychiatrists in its clinical practice guidelines on the management of imminent violence (Royal College of Psychiatrists 1998) and subsequently by the National Institute for Clinical Excellence in its guidelines on the short-term management of violent (disturbed) behaviour (NICE 2005).

Threatened violence

The general principles outlined in the assessment process above should always be applied. When a request for an emergency consultation is made there will usually be some indication of the potential for violence. The details of this must be pursued before the patient is assessed. This is critical because while non-psychiatrists can physically restrain the patient only a psychiatrist can apply the knowledge base required to examine for psychopathology and subsequently determine and implement an appropriate course of action. The emergency psychiatrist should therefore gather the available information and resist the urge to 'do something'. Safety requires adequate consideration of the site of the interview and the personnel who should be present, care should be taken with clothing, and potential weapons such as jewellery or scarves, etc. should be avoided.

Clues to incipient violence will come from observation of the patient's appearance and behaviours – glaring, muscular tension, restlessness, and movements that are more rapid or deliberate are all warning signs, while speech that is louder, more strident and more profane reflects a patient's arousal and irritability.

The patient's anger should be managed with a measured and reasonable response employing de-escalation techniques prior to any other interventions. When these fail to calm a person, it should be remembered that further physical interventions are used if appropriate only as a support to, and never as a replacement for, on-going verbal de-escalation efforts.

De-escalation techniques

De-escalation (or 'defusing') involves the use of techniques aimed at calming disruptive behaviour and thus preventing the development of violence. Stevenson and Otto (1998) define it is as an interactive process in which a patient is redirected towards a calmer inner personal space. While there are several different theoretical approaches to de-escalation, all share the same principal components, which are assessment of the circumstances, a style of communication designed to facilitate cooperation and a problem-solving strategy (Dix 2001). In assessing the aggressive incident, it is helpful to attempt to understand it as an interactive process involving external and internal cues leading to over-arousal, evoking an emotional response and a behavioural result.

In managing a person threatening violence, the clinician should follow the below approach:

- First, manage the environment, e.g. removing other patients from the area, creating a safe space and enlisting the help of colleagues as appropriate
- Attempt to establish a rapport and emphasize cooperation. Address the patient with respect, using their title (Mr, Mrs, etc.) and make a clear introduction
- Ensure that one's own non-verbal communication remains non-threatening, calm and confident throughout the interaction without being dismissive or overbearing. Adopt a neutral posture with hands kept in the midline and allow a greater personal space than normal. Standing at a slight angle rather than face to face and avoiding prolonged direct eye contact will also aid in presenting in a non-provocative manner
- Ask open questions and enquire about the reason for the person's anger in an empathic and non-judgemental manner. Focus on the emotional content of their response
- Offer and negotiate realistic options and avoid threats or confrontation. Try to focus on elements of the person's problem that can be agreed upon and resolved. It is important to avoid making the person lose face and to promote a sense of autonomy if possible, for example by offering medication if appropriate or by acknowledging the person's capacity to harm others but offering the alternative solution of dialogue. One should present oneself as someone who can solve the problem, as a listener and not a restricter. However, it must be professionally and dispassionately conveyed that violence is unacceptable.

Where de-escalation techniques have failed to calm a patient, or when the situation is acutely dangerous, it may be necessary to make use of additional interventions such as physical restraint, rapid tranquillization and seclusion to manage the incident (as outlined below). The choice of intervention(s) should be guided primarily by the clinical needs of, and risks to, the disturbed patient in addition to the protection of staff and others.

The intervention selected must amount to a proportionate and reasonable response to the risk posed as each of these interventions has rare but potentially fatal complications.

Actual violence

It is usually not possible to complete a thorough history from an acutely agitated patient and it is often necessary to accept some degree of diagnostic uncertainty in the early stages of management. Nevertheless, when violence occurs, the emergency psychiatrist must consider three principal differential diagnoses, which will guide management:

1. Violence of organic origin:
   - Drugs (iatrogenic and of abuse) and alcohol
   - Brain trauma, tumours, infections, infarctions, inflammation, demyelination, degeneration and epilepsy. Systemic disorders including metabolic disturbances such as porphyrias, hypoglycaemia, electrolyte imbalances, uraemia, hepatic encephalopathy, and hypoxia. Endocrine dysfunction as in Cushing and Addison diseases, thyroid disease (hyper- and hypo-), vitamin deficiency, infections and poisoning
2. Violence of psychotic origin:
   - Affective disorder and schizophrenia
3. Violence of non-organic, non-psychotic (behavioural disturbance) origin:
   - Where there is no acute or gross abnormality of brain or mind but when there may be abnormality of emotional development or maturation.

The management of violence will depend on which category the disturbed behaviour falls into. The general measures available to manage violence include:

- Psychological:
  - Establish a relationship
  - Provide alternatives to violence, such as taking medication or discussion
- Social:
  - Practical problem-solving about precipitants, e.g. advising about access to benefits
- Physical:
  - Restraint
  - Seclusion
  - Medication (rapid tranquillization).

More specific measures for managing violence depend upon which of the three causes is involved.

Violence of organic origin

Safety and containment of violence have primacy, following which the underlying cause should be sought and treated. Verbal diffusion may be appropriate initially and frequent orientation of the patient is often helpful. Psychotropic agents should be used sparingly and titrated carefully against changes in mental state examinations. An intensive level of nursing care and observation should always be provided.

Violence of psychotic origin

Safety and containment of violence have primacy. Consideration should be given to an organic cause in a patient known to suffer with a chronic psychotic disorder in the presence of new or uncharacteristic behaviour. Verbal diffusion should be attempted as a first option. If necessary, psychotropic agents should be administered initially for their psychomotor effects and should be titrated against arousal and agitation. Patients should subsequently be maintained on antipsychotic medication necessary to resolve psychotic symptoms. An intensive level of nursing care is necessary.

Violence of non-organic, non-psychotic (behavioural disturbance) origin

Safety and containment of the patient are the first priorities. An organic or psychotic origin should be excluded in the course of the assessment. It is important to establish the basis for the incident in an empathetic and non-judgemental manner. Verbal diffusion may be possible, for example by outlining options including medication (taking care that this was not the goal of the outburst in the first place). It may be useful to apportion responsibility for the disturbance as this clarifies the situation and is educational for perpetrator, psychiatrist and colleagues.

Physical restraint

Physical restraint should be used with consideration for the self-respect, dignity and privacy of the patient (Royal College of Psychiatrists 1998).

The aim of physical restraint is to safely immobilize the individual and thus prevent harm from occurring either to themselves or to others. It is a temporary measure, and should be employed only until other interventions can be administered as appropriate (e.g. rapid tranquillization) and its prolonged use should be avoided. It is vital that all staff restraining patients be properly trained in order to minimize risk of injury both to themselves and to the patient: fatalities have been known to occur secondary to asphyxia or over-arousal in context of underlying heart disease or drug effects (O'Halloran & Frank 2000; Norfolk, Suffolk and Cambridgeshire Strategic Health Authority 2003). Attempts to restrain a patient should not be undertaken when alone or in the absence of adequate numbers of personnel who have received training in restraint techniques. Ideally, this implies at least five people – one per limb and one to control/protect the patient's head. It is preferable that one trained person be team leader and coordinate the response, and for the interviewing doctor to withdraw and allow the emergency team to act.

Seclusion

Seclusion is the formal placing of a patient in a specially designated room for the short-term management of disturbed/violent behaviour.

Indications for seclusion include:

- To prevent imminent harm to others, namely staff and other patients, if other means are inappropriate or ineffective
- To prevent imminent harm to the patient if other means are inappropriate or ineffective
- To decrease the stimulation the patient receives
- At the patient's request.

The emergency psychiatrist must be aware of the standards of good practice when seclusion is used, such as those produced by the Royal College of Psychiatrists (1998), and the NICE guidelines (2005), which are as follows:

- Particular care is needed in heavily medicated, physically unwell or intoxicated patients
- An observation schedule must be specified
- A doctor must be present within the first few minutes of seclusion
- A nurse must be in sight or sound throughout (present if the patient is sedated)
- There must be a nursing review every 15 min and a medical review every 4 h
- The patient must not be deprived of clothing and must be able to call for assistance
- A full record of the seclusion incident must be made according to a specified format.

Seclusion must never be used as part of a treatment plan or as a punishment and it is not a substitute to having adequate staffing of highly trained personnel on the unit. Clear protocols for the observation and physical monitoring of secluded patients are vital to its effective, safe practice.

It is noteworthy that patients have expressed a preference for medication, rather than prolonged restraint or seclusion, in situations where they have behaved violently (Royal College of Psychiatrists 1998). This report confirms previous work by Harris et al (1989), in which the following hierarchy of preferred treatments was conceived by patients and nursing staff:

- Manual restraint and oral medication
- Removal of clothing and intramuscular medication
- Seclusion and restraint with constant observation.

Pharmacotherapy (rapid tranquillization)

Rapid tranquillization is the term used to describe the acute treatment of aggression or violence by pharmacological means with the aim of urgently but safely sedating a patient in order to reduce both suffering and the risk of harm. A state of calm rather than deep sedation or sleep is considered to be the desirable endpoint and the patient should ideally be able to respond to the spoken word throughout the period of tranquillization.

The trend in recent years has been for the use of lower doses of neuroleptics because of their cardiotoxicity in patients who may be dehydrated, nutritionally depleted, intoxicated or otherwise physically compromised. Benzodiazepines are used increasingly in parallel with antipsychotics in emergencies. In general, oral administration of medication is preferable, although clearly not always practicable. The emerging evidence base for parenteral administration of atypical antipsychotics is useful in focusing attention on this sometimes difficult to manage and difficult to study population (Brier et al 2002; Wright et al 2001). It should be borne in mind that the efficacy of newer agents has been established in patients who have been able to give consent and by definition, are not the most severely disturbed. Clinical practice will help the further evaluation of these agents in this more severely ill population. There is little

difference in terms of time to onset of action between orally and intramuscularly administered medication (Dubin 1985). Faced with a violent patient, these differences may seem relevant, however, and of course patients who refuse orally administered medication may require parenteral treatment.

The most important pharmacological recommendations made by NICE in their 2005 guidelines on the short-term management of disturbed/violent behaviour in inpatient psychiatric settings and emergency departments are as follows:

- Oral administration of medication is preferred to parenteral administration from the perspective of patient's dignity
- When parenteral administration of medication is required, intramuscular administration is preferred to intravenous administration from the perspective of patients' safety
- The intramuscular drugs recommended for rapid tranquillization are haloperidol, lorazepam and olanzapine
- When the behavioural disturbance occurs in a non-psychotic context, it is preferable to initially use lorazepam alone
- When the behavioural disturbance occurs in the context of psychosis, an oral antipsychotic in combination with oral lorazepam should be considered in the first instance. Where parenteral therapy is indicated, then the combination of an intramuscular antipsychotic (haloperidol) and an intramuscular benzodiazepine (lorazepam) is recommended
- While i.m. olanzapine may also be considered in the context of behavioural disturbance associated with psychosis, intramuscular lorazepam should not be given within 1 hour of i.m. olanzapine, and oral lorazepam should be used with caution
- If haloperidol (or another typical antipsychotic drug) is administered intramuscularly, an anticholinergic drug should be immediately available in order to reduce the risk of acute dystonia and other extrapyramidal side-effects
- Diazepam (intramuscularly) and chlorpromazine (oral or i.m.) are not recommended for use in rapid tranquillization.

There are specific risks associated with the medications that are used in rapid tranquillization. In relation to antipsychotics the main concerns relate to extrapyramidal effects and cardiac effects (drug induced arrhythmias and sudden cardiac death). Respiratory depression is the chief risk for benzodiazepines.

The three drugs recommended by NICE for intramuscular use during rapid tranquillization will now be described.

Haloperidol

This is probably the most widely used drug at present. It is a high-potency agent with low cholinergic, adrenergic, serotonergic and histaminergic binding, but it frequently causes extrapyramidal symptoms which can generally be rapidly reversed by giving antiparkinsonian medication such as procyclidine and may be prevented with prophylactic anticholinergics if susceptibility is known. It is important to note that sudden death has occurred in the context of rapid tranquillization with haloperidol, probably due to exacerbation of the already prolonged QTc associated with acute behavioural disturbance (McAllister-Williams & Ferrier 2002). The i.v. route is not recommended as, while i.v. haloperidol produces a slightly more rapid onset of action, mean aggression scores fall only slightly more rapidly than following i.m. administration, and i.v. administration is associated with a higher risk of adverse effects. The usual initial dose is 5–10 mg (half this for the elderly), which may be repeated within 1 hour, as necessary. Although the maximal licensed daily intramuscular dose is 18 mg, on occasion it may be necessary to exceed this. In such circumstances, vigilance towards monitoring the patient's physical condition, including vital signs, is important and an ECG tracing should be obtained as soon as is practical.

Lorazepam

This short-acting (half-life 10–18 h) benzodiazepine has inactive glucuronide metabolites and is well absorbed following intramuscular administration (in contrast to diazepam whose absorption is impaired by the acidic environment of active muscles). Effects are evident within 1 hour and persist for up to 6 hours. Acute dosage is 2–4 mg, which may be repeated after 2 hours.

Benzodiazepines are the treatment of choice in those sensitive to antipsychotics (e.g. with a history of neuroleptic malignant syndrome) or in those with specific physical health concerns (e.g. significant cardiac disease). With all benzodiazepines there is a risk of respiratory depression, and their effects can be reversed by the antagonist flumazenil. There is also a risk of paradoxical behavioural disinhibition in some who receive benzodiazepines, such that these drugs may be inappropriate in some cases (Fava 1997).

Olanzapine

Reduction in agitation and disturbed behaviour is evident within 15 min (T_{max} is 30–40 min) and increases to a maximum at 2 hours (Wright et al 2001) following 10 mg of olanzapine administered intramuscularly.

Extrapyramidal effects are much less likely in comparison with haloperidol and the intramuscular preparation appears to have a low risk of prolonged QT interval. Other potential side-effects include dizziness or collapse due to vasovagal bradycardia/syncope and thus caution is required when combined with other drugs that can induce bradycardia or are depressants of the respiratory or central nervous systems (Macpherson et al 2005). It is recommended that intramuscular olanzapine and parenteral benzodiazepine should not be given simultaneously, with at least 1 h separating their use.

Self-harm and attempted suicide in the emergency setting

Although one should realize that the majority of episodes of self-harm never reach the health service, those which do represent 4–5% of all attendances at emergency departments, thus making it one of the top five causes of acute medical and surgical admission in the UK (Gunnell et al 1996). Each year, up to 170 000 people in the UK attend an emergency department having self-harmed. Between 0.5% and 1% of these people

will die by suicide during the subsequent year, rising to 4–5% over longer-term follow-up, while up to 25% will engage in a repetition of self-harm at some point (Hawton et al 2003; Owens et al 2002).

When a patient who has self-harmed attends the emergency department, it is important that a psychosocial assessment not be routinely delayed until after medical treatment is complete, unless obviously the patient is incapable of being assessed. Delays in the provision of medical treatment and psychosocial assessment may often be perceived by patients who self-harm as punitive and can lead to increased distress or absconding. Therefore, if a person who has self-harmed has to wait for treatment, he or she should be offered an environment that is safe and minimizes distress, such as a separate quiet room with adequate supervision to ensure safety.

Assessment of needs

All people who have self-harmed should be offered an assessment of needs, which should be comprehensive and adhere to the biopsychosocial model of care. Important components include evaluation of the motivational factors specific to the act of self-harm, current suicidal intent and hopelessness, as well as a full mental health and social needs assessment (Box 36.1). A formulation can then be formed which will combine vulnerability factors (both long term and short term) and precipitating factors to describe as fully as possible the antecedents of the episode of self-harm.

Patients vary enormously in the amount of information that they will disclose about their motivation, the circumstances of the act and other important details. This may be because they are psychomotor retarded by depression and feel worthless and unable to trust anyone, or because they are embarrassed, or angry at not succeeding or at not being taken seriously. There are many reasons for reticence and it is essential for the evaluating psychiatrist to gain sufficient information despite this. Generalizations about patients are dangerous (the clinical adage that the more readily patients disclose their suicidality, the less likely they are to be suicidal is almost certainly incorrect) and counter-transference can distort clinical judgement, leading to over-identification and inappropriate reassurance that all will

Box 36.1

The main components of assessment of need after self-harm

1. Psychiatric history and mental state examination, including any history of previous self-harm and alcohol or drug use
2. Recent life events and current difficulties
3. Social situation (including current living arrangements, work and debt)
4. Personal relationships (including recent breakdown of a significant relationship)
5. Recent life events and current difficulties
6. Enduring psychological characteristics that are known to be associated with self-harm
7. Motivation for the act.

be well. The opposite reaction may also occur and it is not uncommon for psychiatrists and colleagues to feel hostility towards patients they perceive as manipulating them. Such feelings can distort the information-gathering process and must be recognized and used as clues to the objective clinical state of the patient.

Assessment of risk

Risk assessment is vital and mandatory for all people who present with self-harm; this assessment should include identification of the main clinical and demographic features known to be associated with risk of further self-harm and/or suicide, and identification of the key psychological characteristics associated with risk, in particular depression, hopelessness and continuing suicidal intent.

The assessment of suicide risk may be informed by epidemiological data but must be firmly based on assessment of the individual patient, including evaluation of both risk factors and protective factors. The risk of suicide is not static and an attempt to gain a longitudinal view of its course from both patient and collateral sources is very useful. It is noteworthy that risk factors for non-fatal repetition of self-harm are different from the risk factors most commonly reported for completed suicide, but there is clearly some overlap (Box 36.2).

Intent is best estimated by considering sequentially the patient's preparation (planning, and so-called terminal events such as writing a note or letter, or making a will), the circumstances of the attempt (alone, precautions taken against discovery, belief that planned act was lethal), and the aftermath (not

---

Box 36.2

Risk factors for self-harm and suicide

A: Risk factors for non-fatal repetition of self-harm

- A history of self-harm prior to the current episode
- Psychiatric history (especially inpatient treatment)
- Current unemployment
- Lower social class
- Alcohol or drug-related problems
- Criminal record
- Antisocial personality
- Uncooperativeness with general hospital treatment
- Hopelessness
- High suicidal intent.

B: Risk factors for suicide

- Older age
- Male
- Previous attempts
- Psychiatric history (especially inpatient treatment)
- Unemployment
- Poor physical health
- Living alone
- Medical severity of the act – especially near-fatal self-harm
- Hopelessness
- Continuing high suicidal intent.

---

seeking help, stated wish to die, regret of failure). A first attempt that occurred impulsively, with rescue inevitable and using a method of low lethal potential may suggest an attempt by the patient to effect change, a degree of ambivalence, and a lower risk of completion.

Mental illness is a major risk factor for suicide and 90% of those completing suicide have a mental disorder. On the other hand, the majority of psychiatric patients do not kill themselves despite the high prevalence of suicidal ideation. This is not a cause for complacency but an attempt to put mental illness and suicide in perspective.

Of those with mental illness completing suicide, approximately 45% suffer with an affective disorder. In relation to depression, the single most important risk factor in the mental state is hopelessness, while patients with psychotic depression have a five-fold increase in risk relative to patients with major depression without psychotic features. Co-morbid alcohol or drug abuse or dependence significantly escalates the risk. The lifetime suicide risk for patients with an affective disorder is generally quoted as 15%, although recent reappraisal of data with sophisticated statistics yields a lower estimate of 6% (Inskip et al 1998). From a clinical perspective, however, the presence of affective disorder significantly increases the risk of suicide for an individual patient, particularly in the period immediately following diagnosis.

The lifetime risk of suicide for patients with schizophrenia is 10% and is greatest soon after the diagnosis and during any post-psychotic depressive phase, particularly if associated with demoralization and hopelessness. The post-discharge period also represents a time of great risk, requiring particular vigilance.

Alcohol dependence is associated with a lifetime risk of 15% for completed suicide and this risk does not diminish with the passage of time from diagnosis, while about 3–8% of patients with borderline personality disorder kill themselves (McGlashan & Heinssen 1988; Stone et al 1987). These latter are at risk because of the instability of interpersonal relations, self-image and affect, and the impulsivity that characterize the disorder. Thus, while chronic self-harm may be a way of coping with life for such patients, it is important to recognize co-morbid disorders, such as depression and clearly evaluate such patients in a systematic manner when they present following self-harm (Kernberg 1984).

About 1% of patients presenting with deliberate self-harm will go on to complete suicide during the following year (the majority during the following 6 months) (Hawton & Fagg 1988). The rate of psychiatric disorder among this latter group is approximately 20% and thus, the majority of patients presenting with deliberate self-harm do not suffer from a mental illness but have other problems that led them to act in this manner. Identification of the pertinent issues and definition of these problems is required as is explanation so that alternatives may be considered by the patient. Thus, it is vital to establish the level of domestic and social support available to the patient and to gauge their own personal resources as indicated by their capacity to form relationships, maintain employment, deal with adversity and have insight into, and some control over, their emotional state. This approach will facilitate the generation of a problem list (which may include a psychiatric diagnosis) and the clarification of risks and possible alternatives.

Management of the patient will depend on this process and upon the personal, domestic, social and statutory supports available.

As with any other treatment, the overarching aims are to reduce harm and improve survival while minimizing the harm that may result from the treatment. The key aims and objectives in the treatment of self-harm, as outlined by the National Institute of Clinical Excellence (NICE 2004) guidelines, should include:

- Rapid assessment of physical and psychological need (triage)
- Effective engagement of the patient (and carers where appropriate)
- Effective measures to minimize pain and discomfort
- Timely initiation of treatment, irrespective of the cause of self-harm
- Harm reduction (from injury and treatment; short term and longer term)
- Rapid and supportive psychosocial assessment (including risk assessment and co-morbidity)
- Prompt referral for further psychological, social and psychiatric assessment and treatment when necessary
- Prompt and effective psychological and psychiatric treatment when necessary
- An integrated and planned approach to the problems of people who self-harm, involving primary and secondary care, mental and physical healthcare personnel and services, and appropriate voluntary organizations.

In many hospitals, more than half of attenders are discharged from the emergency department without specialist assessment. Patients who leave hospital direct from an emergency department without a psychosocial assessment are obviously less likely to have been offered follow-up (Kapur et al 1998) and furthermore, there is evidence that those who do receive a psychosocial assessment may be less likely to repeat an act of self-harm (Hickey et al 2001; Kapur et al 2002).

Referral for further assessment and treatment should be based upon the combined assessment of needs and risk. Temporary admission, which may need to be overnight, should be considered following an act of self-harm, especially for people who are very distressed or for those who may be returning to an unsafe or potentially harmful environment. Reassessment should be undertaken the following day or at the earliest opportunity thereafter.

All acts of self-harm in people older than 65 years of age should be regarded as evidence of suicidal intent until proven otherwise with serious consideration given to admission for further mental health risk and needs assessment. This is because the number of elderly people who go on to complete suicide is much higher than in younger adults that present with self-harm.

Conclusions

Emergency psychiatry cuts across all areas of psychiatric specialization and expertise. What distinguishes it as a speciality is the requirement to make a rapid and effective decision to resolve some need that has provoked presentation by the patient. To do this, the clinician simultaneously operates in two related but distinct clinical dimensions. The first dimension is represented by the need to assess the patient in a logical and methodical manner while all the time attending to safety. This process of assessment and attention to safety requires objectivity at a time and in a situation where there may be immense pressure to act immediately to resolve the problem. This is where the second dimension – the expertise and experience of the psychiatrist – can provide the comprehensive approach that is necessary for the safe and effective resolution of emergencies.

References

Brier, A., Meehan, K., Birkett, M., et al., 2002. A double-blind, placebo-controlled dose response comparison of intramuscular olanzapine and haloperidol in the treatment of acute agitation in schizophrenia. Arch. Gen. Psychiatry 59, 441–448.

Dix, R., 2001. De-escalation techniques. In: Beer, D., Pereira, S., Paton, C. (Eds.), Psychiatric intensive care. Greenwich Medical Media, London.

Dubin, W.R., 1985. Rapid tranquillization, the efficacy of oral concentrate. J. Clin. Psychiatry 46, 475–478.

Fava, M., 1997. Psychopharmacologic treatment of pathologic aggression. Psychiatr. Clin. North Am. 20, 427–451.

Gunnell, D.J., Brooks, J., Peters, T.J., 1996. Epidemiology and patterns of hospital use after parasuicide in the south west of England. J. Epidemiol. Community Health 50, 24–29.

Harris, G.T., Rice, M.E., Preseon, D.L., 1989. Staff and patients' perceptions of the least restrictive alternatives for the short-term

control of disturbed behaviour. J. Psychiatry Law 17, 239–263.

Hawton, K., Fagg, J., 1988. Suicide and other causes of death following attempted suicide. Br. J. Psychiatry 159, 359–366.

Hawton, K., Zahl, D., Weatherall, R., 2003. Suicide following deliberate self-harm: long-term follow-up of patients who presented to a general hospital. Br. J. Psychiatry 182, 537–542.

Hickey, L., Hawton, K., Fagg, J., et al., 2001. Deliberate self-harm patients who leave the accident and emergency department without a psychiatric assessment: a neglected population at risk of suicide. J. Psychosom. Res. 50, 87–93.

Inskip, H.M., Harris, E.C., Barraclough, B., 1998. Lifetime risk of suicide for affective disorder, alcoholism and schizophrenia. Br. J. Psychiatry 172, 35–37.

Kapur, N., House, A., Creed, F., et al., 1998. Management of deliberate self-poisoning in adults in four teaching hospitals: descriptive study. Br. Med. J. 316, 831–832.

Kapur, N., House, A., Dodgson, K., et al., 2002. Does the general hospital management of deliberate self-poisoning make a difference to outcome? A cohort study. Br. Med. J. 325, 866–867.

Kernberg, O.F., 1984. Severe personality disorders: psychotherapeutic strategies. Yale University Press, New Haven CT.

Macpherson, R., Dix, R., Morgan, S., 2005. A growing evidence base for management guidelines. Revisiting guidelines for the management of acutely disturbed psychiatric patients. Advances in Psychiatric Treatment 11, 404–415.

McAllister-Williams, R.H., Ferrier, I.N., 2002. Rapid tranquillisation: time for a reappraisal of options for parenteral therapy. Br. J. Psychiatry 180, 485–489.

McGlashan, T.H., Heinssen, R.K., 1988. Hospital discharge status and long-term outcome for patients with schizophrenia, schizoaffective disorders, borderline personality disorder and unipolar affective disorder. Arch. Gen. Psychiatry 45, 363–368.

NICE, 2004. Self harm. The short-term physical and psychological management and secondary prevention of self-harm in primary and secondary care (Clinical Guideline 16). National Institute for Clinical Excellence, London.

NICE, 2005. The short-term management of disturbed/violent behaviour in in-patient psychiatric settings and emergency departments (Clinical Guideline 25). National Institute for Clinical Excellence, London.

Norfolk, S., Cambridgeshire Strategic Health Authority, 2003. Independent inquiry into the death of David Bennett. NSCSHA, Cambridge.

O'Halloran, R.L., Frank, J.G., 2000. Asphyxial death during prone restraint revisited. A report of 21 cases. Am. J. Forensic Med. Pathol. 21, 39–52.

Owens, D., Horrocks, J., House, A., 2002. Fatal and non-fatal repetition of self-harm. Systematic review. Br. J. Psychiatry 181, 193–199.

Royal College of Psychiatrists, 1998. Management of imminent violence. Clinical practice guidelines to support mental health services (Occasional Paper OP41). Royal College of Psychiatrists, London.

Steadman, H.J., Mulvey, E.P., Monahan, J., et al., 1998. Violence by people discharged from acute psychiatric inpatient facilities and by others in the same neighborhoods. Arch. Gen. Psychiatry 55, 393–401.

Stevenson, S., Otto, M.P., 1998. Finding ways to reduce violence in psychiatric hospitals. J. Healthc. Qual. 20, 28–32.

Stone, M.H., Stone, D.K., Hurt, S.W., 1987. Natural history of borderline patients treated by intensive hospitalization. Psychiatr. Clin. North Am. 10, 185–207.

Swanson, J., Holzer, C.E., Ganju, V.K., et al., 1990. Violence and psychiatric disorders in the community: evidence from the Epidemiologic Catchment Area surveys. Hosp. Community Psychiatry 41, 761–770.

Wright, P., Birkett, M., David, S.R., et al., 2001. Double-blind, placebo-controlled comparison of intramuscular olanzapine and intramuscular haloperidol in the treatment of acute agitation in schizophrenia. Am. J. Psychiatry 158, 1149–1151.

Psychotherapy – individual, family and group

37

Julian Stern

CHAPTER CONTENTS

Introduction

This chapter reviews those psychotherapies derived from or related to the psychodynamic model, i.e. individual, group and family therapies. (Cognitive and behavioural models are described in Chapter 38.)

Psychotherapy is 'essentially a conversation which involves listening to and talking with those in trouble, with the aim of helping them understand and resolve their predicament' (Bateman et al 2000).

It is a broad term used to describe many modes of treatment ranging from psychodynamic therapies to more focused (e.g. cognitive–behavioural) therapies, and may involve individual patients, families, couples or groups of otherwise unconnected patients. Therapists may work alone or in couples, supervised 'live' (as in some models of family therapy) or retrospectively.

The psychotherapeutic model also informs much of the work performed in other psychiatric settings, and psychotherapists are often called upon to perform functions within psychiatry (and more broadly, medicine) other than the treatment of patients, for example consultations to staff groups or the offering of an opinion on a complicated patient on a ward. Thus, Gabbard (2000: 4) describes a model of psychodynamic psychiatry that is 'an approach to diagnosis and treatment characterized by a way of thinking about both patient and clinician that includes unconscious conflict, deficits and distortions of intrapsychic structures and internal object relations, and that integrates these elements with contemporary findings from the neurosciences'.

Jerome Frank's 'common features'

Jerome Frank (1961) identified a number of features that are common to all of the psychotherapies. These include:

- An intense emotionally-charged relationship with a person or group
- A rationale or myth explaining the distress and methods for dealing with it
- The provision of new information about the future, the source of the problem and possible alternatives that hold a hope of relief
- Nonspecific methods of boosting self-esteem
- Provision of success experiences
- Facilitation of emotional arousal
- The therapy takes place in a locale designated as a place of healing.

While all these factors might describe some of what occurs in psychotherapy, it is difficult to give a real 'flavour' of what goes on within a therapeutic relationship, until one takes on a patient for psychotherapy under supervision, (or undergoes one's own therapy). Then the full complexity, intrigue and interest of the relationship, of the patient's life, of terms such as 'transference' or 'counter-transference', come alive. Psychotherapy can then begin to make sense, both as an explanatory model and as a method of treatment. It is in recognition of this, that the Royal College of Psychiatrists (2009) has made the psychotherapeutic treatment of patients – using at least two different modalities – a mandatory part of the training of each junior psychiatrist in the UK. '[Trainees should] with appropriate supervision, commence and monitor therapeutic treatment in patients, based on a good understanding of the mechanism of their actions... [They should be able to] demonstrate the capacity to deliver basic psychological treatments in at least 2 modalities of therapy in both longer and shorter durations' ('Intended learning outcome 5', Royal College of Psychiatrists 2009: 23).

Psychodynamic/psychoanalytic psychotherapy

This mode of therapy, often just termed 'psychotherapy', derives from the work of Sigmund Freud. 'The technique of psychodynamic therapy is a focus on the provision of conscious understanding, primarily through the use of interpretation of the patient's verbalizations and behaviour during the (psychotherapy) session' (Roth & Fonagy 1996: 5).

'The best way of understanding psychoanalysis is still by tracing its origin and development', wrote Freud in 1923, and it remains enlightening and enjoyable to read Freud's original works.

Box 37.1 presents an extremely condensed summary of Sigmund Freud's life (see Gay 1995) and writings.

Freud's models of the mind

Freud's theories of the mind progressed through three main phases (Bateman & Holmes (1995): the 'affect trauma' model; the topographical model; and the structural model.

The earliest model is the *affect trauma model*, where Freud was influenced by casualties of the Franco-Prussian war (where such casualties included cases of hysterical paralysis). The idea was of an accumulation of 'dammed up' effects inside the patient which, if released, would threaten psychic equilibrium, and potentially lead to symptoms.

A treatment gradually developed, initially involving hypnosis and subsequently the 'ventilation' of these affects and memories, leading to an emotional 'catharsis' via the fundamental rule of 'free association', with particular reference to repressed childhood memories of physical or sexual trauma. 'Free association' is a key technique in psychoanalysis, in which the patient is invited to talk about anything that comes into his/her mind as completely as possible, no matter how trivial or 'irrational' it may seem (see Akhtar 2009 & Rycroft 1972, for useful definitions of many of the terms used here).

Despite having been impressed by Charcot's work with hysterics in Paris, and Janet's descriptions of the successful use of hypnosis in the treatment of hysterics, Freud subsequently abandoned hypnosis. The reasons are multiple: first, Freud found it difficult to hypnotize some patients, and was also concerned about the possible role of suggestion in such treatments. Furthermore, in the case of Anna O., whom his colleague Breuer had treated (Freud & Breuer 1895), the importance of (sometimes erotic) transference had become manifest.

Freud's biographer, Ernest Jones (1961: 148), described the erotic transference that Anna O. developed towards Breuer:

'(Breuer) decided to bring the treatment to an end... and bade her (Anna O.) goodbye. But that evening he was fetched back to find her in a greatly excited state, apparently as ill as ever. The patient, who according to him had appeared to be an asexual being and had never made any allusions to such a forbidden topic throughout the treatment, was now in the throes of an hysterical childbirth, the logical termination of a phantom pregnancy that had been invisibly developing in response to Breuer's ministrations. Though profoundly shocked, he managed to calm her down by hypnotising her, and then fled the house in a cold sweat.'

Box 37.1

Sigmund Freud (1856–1939)

- 1856 – is born in Freiburg (Moravia)
- 1860 – family moves to Vienna
- 1873 – Freud enters medical school in Vienna
- As a medical student, he made original contributions to neurohistology
- As a neurologist, he made original contributions in the fields of aphasia and cerebral palsy
- 1885 – visits Charcot in Paris
- 1886 – returns to Vienna and marries Martha Bernays
- 1895 – publishes, with Breuer, *Studies on Hysteria*
- 1896 – publishes *Heredity and the aetiology of neuroses* in French. The word 'psychoanalysis' appears for the first time
- For the next four decades, he was extremely prolific, and his works are collected in the 24-volume 'Standard Edition'
- Among his most famous cases were:
  - Anna O. (with Breuer): *Studies on Hysteria* (Freud & Breuer 1895)
  - Dora: *Fragment of an analysis of a case of hysteria* (1905a)
  - Little Hans, a boy with a phobia of horses, whose father Freud saw: *Analysis of a phobia in a five year old boy* (1909a)
  - Rat Man: *Notes upon a case of obsessional neurosis* (1909b)
  - Schreber, a case of paranoia whom Freud wrote about but never saw as a patient: *Psychoanalytic notes on an autobiographical account of a case of paranoia (Dementia paranoides)* (1911a)
  - Wolf Man: *From the history of an infantile neurosis* (1919)
- 1923 – first operation on his jaw and palate for what was incorrectly diagnosed as leukoplakia, but was cancer. He eventually undergoes more than 20 operations
- 4 June 1938 – after the Nazis march into Austria, and Anna Freud is questioned by the Gestapo (in March 1938), Freud and his family leave Vienna for Paris and then arrive in London 2 days later
- September 1938 – the Freuds move to 20 Maresfield Gardens in Hampstead, London, Freud's last home and now the home of the Freud museum
- 23 September 1939 – Freud dies.

Breuer, terrified by Anna O.'s symptoms and infatuation with him, fled Vienna together with his wife, and never returned to work in the developing field of psychoanalysis.

Unlike Breuer, Freud was able to recognize the importance of transference (see below), and over the next decade (1897–1908) abandoned hypnosis in favour of free association.

The second model, i.e. the *topographical model*, implies a spatial model, in which different psychological functions are located in different places. The division of the mind into the unconscious, preconscious and conscious systems (Freud 1900) ushered in the second phase of Freud's work, still containing echoes of cerebral localization.

A fundamental idea derived from this phase is the contrast between the two principles of mental functioning, i.e. primary process and secondary process. *Primary process* thinking occurs in dreaming, fantasy and infantile life; here the distinctions between opposites need not apply, nor do the differences between past, present and future. *Secondary process* thinking is rational and follows the principles of logic, time and space.

Freud differentiated between *unconscious and preconscious* phenomena. Unconscious phenomena are not available to the conscious mind, and have been actively repressed because of their unthinkable nature – a memory, feeling or thought that conflicts with our view of ourselves and of what is acceptable, and which would cause too much guilt, anxiety or psychic pain if it were acknowledged. These are to be distinguished from phenomena that are unconscious in a descriptive sense, but which are easily brought to mind, and therefore are neither subject to repression nor operating under the sway of primary process thinking, i.e. the system 'preconscious'. The preconscious in the topographical model has a role both as a reservoir of accessible thoughts and memories, and as a censor capable of modifying instinctual wishes of the system unconscious, to render them acceptable to the conscious system.

In his book *The Interpretation of Dreams* (1900), Freud called dreams, 'The royal road to the unconscious'. Other routes to the unconscious include the unravelling of 'parapraxes' (so-called Freudian slips), and interpretation in analysis, especially transference interpretations (see below).

Structural theory was described in 1923 by Freud, and remains firmly embedded in instinct theory. It does not replace the above models, although in this model, there is more emphasis on three structural components of the personality, i.e. the id, super-ego and ego.

The 'id' operates under the sway of the pleasure principle, and is the part of the personality concerned with basic inborn drives, and sexual and aggressive impulses. The id is the 'dark, inaccessible part of our personality; what little we know of it we have learnt from our study of dream-work and the construction of neurotic symptoms, and most of that is of a negative character, and can be described only as a contrast to the ego... we call it a chaos, a cauldron full of seething excitations' (Freud 1933: 105–106). It is filled with energy reaching it from the instincts but it has no organization, and strives to satisfy instinctual needs subject to the observance of the pleasure principle – the achievement of pleasure and the avoidance of unpleasure or tension.

Undoing is also referred to as 'magical undoing' or 'doing and undoing'. Undoing allows the person to reverse hostile wishes which he believes he has already perpetrated in the 'doing'. This is seen most frequently in patients with obsessional symptoms.

In obsessional neurosis the technique... is first met with in the 'diphasic' symptoms, in which one action is cancelled out by the second, so it is as though neither action had taken place, whereas in reality, both have (S. Freud 1926).

The attempt to undo has a magical quality, aiming to reverse time, to attack the reality of the original hostile wish or thought, and recreate the past as though such intentions had never existed in the first place.

Splitting

This term refers to a splitting or division of an object into good and bad, 'idealized' and 'denigrated'. The child, according to Kleinian theory, will keep the mother split into two separate persons – the good, nurturant provider (idealized) and the mother who is unavailable, depriving, frustrating (denigrated). This 'split' characterizes the 'paranoid-schizoid' position (see below) and is gradually diminished with the acquisition of the 'depressive position', where there is a recognition of good and bad in the same person, and the development of 'ambivalence'.

A male patient may tell his female psychiatrist that she is the only person who has ever understood him; she is destined for great things, and has remarkable empathy (idealization). After she disappoints him by being unavailable one day, he describes her as useless, incompetent and irrelevant (denigration). Splitting can also occur within a team, for example the same patient may describe some team members as hopeless and others as excellent. Splitting is seen as a primitive defence mechanism.

Acting out

'Acting out' is the direct expression of an unconscious impulse in order to avoid the awareness of the accompanying affect. This concept was initially described by Freud, in his paper 'Remembering, Repeating, and Working Through' (1914), in which he describes how we all have a tendency towards unconsciously repeating relationships with important figures (primarily our parents). This links closely with the concept of transference. Freud wrote about a 'repetition compulsion' and a tendency towards 'acting out' in the transference, i.e. acting towards one's therapist as if he/she were one's father, mother, etc. One of the aims of psychoanalysis or psychotherapy is to allow the patient to see his/her tendency towards such acting out, and to 'work through' this compulsion rather than repeatedly 'acting it out'.

Subsequent writers have distinguished between acting out within a psychotherapy session and outside a session, and some have suggested that the term 'acting out' should be reserved for events outside the session and 'acting in' for events inside the session. There is further confusion in that 'acting out' is a term now adopted within general psychiatry, usually with pejorative connotations, towards a patient who is 'misbehaving'. In addition, psychotherapists are now aware of the concept of 'acting out in the counter-transference', e.g. a tendency to behave sadistically with a patient who might, by a process of projective identification (see above), project his/her disowned violence onto the therapist or psychiatrist. The therapist or psychiatrist then 'identifies' with this, and instead of being able to make sense of what is going on, an enactment occurs with the patient.

Intellectualization

This refers to thinking and speaking in jargon, rather than feeling.

Sublimation

Sublimation is seen as a healthy defence mechanism – the indirect expression of instincts without adverse consequences, e.g. great works of art, or hostility channelled into sport.

Psychosexual stages

Central to much of Freud's work was an explicit focus on sexuality and sexual fantasies. His stages of sexual development are summarized in Table 37.2.

Freud viewed adult sexuality as the outcome of a libidinal drive present from birth, and progressing through a number of 'pre-genital' phases, with pleasure bring derived from particular erotogenic zones associated with particular stages. Thus, initially he proposed an 'oral' phase (before the age of 1), where the infant derives satisfaction via the mouth, from sucking for example the nipple, or thumb ('auto-erotic'). This satisfaction appears to be independent of any nutritional/hunger needs in the infant.

Second, he described the 'anal' phase (ages 1–3), where immense gratification and pride is derived from gaining control over defecation, or the retention of faeces. This is followed

Table 37.2 Freud's stages of sexual development

Age	Stage	Features
0–1 year	Oral	Gratification by oral means from the breast in particular
1–3 years	Anal	Gratification via control over defecation, a sense of self develops
3–5 years	Phallic	Further elaboration of oedipal configuration and fantasies, with castration complex fears
5–12	Latent	The infantile stage of sexuality ends with the repression of the Oedipus complex, ideas from previous stages are repressed and denied expression
12–20	Puberty	Sexual drives are reawoken under the influence of hormonal changes

by the 'phallic' phase, when the child develops more awareness and curiosity of his/her genitalia, with concomitant curiosity and anxiety about sexual differences. Freud also described the Oedipus complex and subsequent castration anxiety (see below) as pertaining to this phase. Following the phallic phase is 'latency' (ages 6–12), a period of relative quiescence of sexual interest, perhaps even prudishness, with the child's interests turning towards the outside world, and to intellectual pursuits at school. Latency ends with puberty, when hormonal changes re-ignite the sexual drive and the 'genital' phase starts.

The 'Oedipus complex'

For Freud, the 'Oedipus complex' was the nuclear complex from its discovery in 1897 to the end of his life. Derived from the Greek tragedy in which Oedipus unknowingly kills his father and has an incestuous relationship with his mother, the Oedipus complex is central to much of Freud's theorizing on psychosexual development, and has its female equivalent in the 'Electra complex'.

Modern analytic authors, especially those following Klein (see below), describe the 'Oedipus situation', which includes not only the sexual relation between the parents (the primal scene), but also focuses on the disappointment, sense of unfairness and wish for revenge evoked, when the young child is forced to confront the fact that his or her (assumed) exclusive two-person relationship with the mother is actually not so exclusive, that there is a third person involved (father), and that in many circumstances (in particular, those pertaining to adult sexuality) it is the child who is excluded by the mother–father dyad. 'Castration anxiety' is another term of Freud's, referring to the young boy's fear of castration as punishment for his oedipal longings towards his mother.

Freud has been accused of writing from a masculine-biased ('phallocentric' and 'patriarchal') point of view, especially pertaining to female sexuality and of ignoring many important socioeconomic and cultural dimensions. These critiques are beyond the scope of this chapter, but do have their impact on the contemporary theory and practice of psychoanalysis and psychoanalytic psychotherapy.

Dreams

Freud considered *The Interpretation of Dreams* (1900) as his finest and most personal work, laying the foundations for the entire edifice of psychoanalysis. Insight such as this, he wrote, 'falls to one's lot but once in a lifetime'. By analysing his own dreams, he came to the conclusion that 'a dream is the fulfillment of a wish'. Freed from the constraints of reality, under the sway of the pleasure principle, and in response to the day residue, i.e. recent events or preoccupations, the dreamer's deepest feelings and impulses are activated. The wishes, often of an infantile sexual nature are cleverly disguised by 'dream work', and the latent (underlying) content is disguised, censored, condensed, and displaced, emerging as the manifest content. Freud described four fundamental rules of dream work: condensation, displacement, conditions of representability and secondary revision.

In *condensation*, different elements are fused or combined into a single overdetermined image, which then requires unpacking. This is the means by which thoughts that are mutually contradictory make no attempt to do away with one another, but persist side by side.

Displacement resembles the work of a magician, the censor's attention being distracted by a shift of emphasis away from the area of maximal conflict or interest. Displacement allows an apparently insignificant idea or object to become invested with great intensity, which originally belonged elsewhere. This displacement takes place because consciousness finds the original object of these intense feelings (e.g. hatred or sexual longing towards a parent) unacceptable. The thoughts therefore undergo repression and appear in a disguised and displaced form.

A further aspect of dream work is what Freud describes as 'conditions of representability', whereby dreams represent words in figurative form, in images. Freud saw this as the most interesting form of dream-work. An example (Perelberg 2000) is the representation of an important person by someone who is 'high up', at the top of a tower in a dream.

All dreams are subject to '*secondary revision*', an attempt by the dreamer to organize, revise and establish connections in the dream to make its account intelligible.

Freud's distinction between the latent and manifest content of dreams is important. The work that transforms latent thoughts into manifest dream content is called 'dream work', while the work in the opposite direction is the work of interpretation. The process of interpretation allows access to the wish expressed in the dream.

Freud's works

Among Freud's most important works are the case histories in Box 37.1, and also:

- *Studies on Hysteria* (with Breuer) (Freud & Breuer 1895)
- *The Interpretation of Dreams* (Freud 1900)
- *Three Essays on the Theory of Sexuality* (Freud 1905b)
- *Totem and Taboo* (Freud 1913)
- *Remembering, Repeating and Working Through* (Freud 1914)
- *Mourning and Melancholia* (Freud 1917)
- *Beyond the Pleasure Principle* (Freud 1920)
- *Group Psychology and the Analysis of the Ego* (Freud 1921)
- *The Ego and the Id* (Freud 1923)
- *New Introductory Lectures on Psychoanalysis* (Freud 1933)
- *Moses and Monotheism* (Freud 1939).

Developments following Freud

All forms of dynamic psychotherapy stem from the work of Freud and psychoanalysis. C.G. Jung and Alfred Adler broke away before the First World War to form, respectively, the schools of analytic psychology (Jung) and individual psychology (Adler).

While the neo-Freudians (Adler, Horney, Stack-Sullivan, Fromm) shifted the emphasis from biological to social processes, Jung developed his own school of analytical psychology which moved away from man's biological roots to a study of the manifestation of his psychological nature in myths, dreams and culture.

Alfred Adler (1870–1937)

Adler split from Freud in 1910, and is an important member of the group of neo-Freudians. Adler emphasized social factors in development, and gave more importance to aggressive strivings and the drive to power. Acutely aware of sibling rivalry, he argued that neurosis originated in attempts to deal with feelings of inferiority, sometimes based on relative physical handicaps (organ inferiority), and this gave rise to a compensatory drive to power.

Similarly, he saw masculine protest in women as a reaction to their inferior position in society. He postulated an aggressive drive before Freud himself did, and although not mainstream, many of his ideas have been incorporated, e.g. inferiority complex, and the recognition that striving for power may reveal itself by its apparent opposite, i.e. retreat into manipulative weakness. He played a part in founding social and preventive psychiatry, and in the development of day hospitals, therapeutic clubs and group therapies.

Carl Gustav Jung (1885–1961)

Along with Adler, Jung was one of the first important figures to split away from Freud. He founded the school of analytic psychology. Jung started his psychiatric career working with psychotic patients in a hospital ('Burghölzli', a wooded hill in the district of Riesbach of southeastern Zürich). and was struck by the universal symbols ('Archetypes') in their delusions and hallucinations. A basic organizing assumption running through his work is that the mind consists of far more than can be gained by experience, and this additional part is termed the 'collective unconscious'.

Thus, there are three levels of the psyche – the conscious/unconscious (including the psyche), the 'personal unconscious' and the 'collective unconscious' (racial and universal features). He thus moved in an opposite direction from Adler and the neo-Freudians.

The persona is the outer crust of the personality, which is the opposite of the personal unconscious on a variety of dimensions, e.g. thinking vs feeling, sensuousness versus intuition, extrovert vs introvert (related to the direction of flow of mental energy).

For Jung, there was a deeper, transpersonal unconscious, something that reflects the history of the human species and indeed the cosmic order, and that arises prior to an individual's experience. Within this collective unconscious are the so-called archetypes, which may roughly be defined as universal nuclear mythic themes (The Hero, The Great Mother, etc.). The manifestations of the archetypes appear in a profusion of symbols that appear in dreams, disturbed states of mind and certain cultural products, e.g. he claimed to have objective evidence of archetypes in the form of spontaneous production of symbolism that could not have been known to the subject by ordinary means, e.g. a schizophrenic patient has a vision of the sun as a wheel, which matches a similar vision reported in an ancient and forgotten text.

Archetypes can be defined as generalized symbols and images within the collective unconscious, and include:

- Animus – the unconscious masculine side of the woman's female persona
- Anima – the unconscious female side of the man's persona
- Complex – a group of interconnected ideas that arouse associated feelings and effect behaviour.

Object relations theorists (Fairbairn, Guntrip, Balint, Winnicott)

The early psychoanalytic view of sexuality as a pleasure-seeking drive, present from birth, appeared for some theorists to be too centred on the individual and his gratifications. Object relations theorists have suggested that the primary motivational drive in man is to seek a relationship with others. Rather than the individual deriving satisfaction through different means at different stages, starting with the oral phase, he seeks relationships with others, starting with the mother. In psychoanalysis, the term 'object' refers to that (usually a person) which is used to gratify a need. The original 'object' in Freud's theories was a maternal breast. A 'bad object' is an object whom the subject fears or hates, who is experienced as malevolent. An 'internal object' is derived from an external object by the process of introjection, and is located in internal reality. Object relations theory is thus the psychoanalytic theory in which the subject's need to relate to objects occupies the central position, in contrast to instinct theory, which centres on the individual's need to reduce instinctual tension.

Object relations theory was underpinned by experimental work, including the work of Harlow, whose work on infant primates illustrates the drive for attachment to 'objects', and Bowlby, whose work on maternal deprivation and the effects of separation of mother from infant is described below.

Object relations theory has been one of the dominant schools in British psychoanalytic thinking, with key early figures including Ronald Fairbairn in Scotland, Harry Guntrip in Leeds, Michael Balint and Donald Winnicott (see below); it plays a major or dominant role in the three traditions within the British Psychoanalytical Society.

The three traditions or groupings that have emerged within the British Psychoanalytical Society are:

- Contemporary Freudians – Anna Freud, Joseph Sandler
- Middle/Independent group – Donald Winnicott, Michael Balint, Christopher Bollas
- Kleinians – Melanie Klein, Wilfred Bion, Donald Meltzer, Herbert Rosenfeld, Hanna Segal.

Donald Winnicott (1896–1971)

Winnicott trained initially as a paediatrician. He coined the following terms:

- Primary maternal preoccupation
- Good enough mother
- False self
- Transitional objects.

Winnicott noticed that a change in the mental state of the mother towards the end of pregnancy seemed to attune her particularly towards the needs of her new baby. He argued that, initially, the mother's attention to the baby's needs protects the infant from impingements that disturb his 'going-on-being', which is a prerequisite for integration. Any impingement, be it external or internal in origin, produces catastrophic disintegration.

In the first months, he argued, 'there is no such thing as a baby', i.e. there is only a mother–baby dyad. Slowly, by a process of gradual disillusionment, separation occurs. Initially the baby makes use of 'transitional objects', i.e. blankets, pieces of mother's clothing, etc. A 'transitional object' is treated by the subject as being halfway between himself and another person, typically a doll or piece of mother's clothing, which does not have to be treated with the consideration appropriate to that person. Such objects help children to make the transition from infantile narcissism to object-love, and from dependence to self-reliance.

The baby develops an ability to play, and an ability to 'be alone in the presence of the mother'. Play is an important concept in Winnicottian theory, and the ability to play is seen as similar to the ability to make use of therapy.

In his later writings he made use of the concepts 'true self' and 'false self'. Winnicott believed that the drive-driven child conjured up in his mind an object suited to his needs, especially when excited. If at this precise moment the 'good enough mother', i.e. a mother attuned to his needs, presents him with just such a suitable object, a moment of illusion is created in the baby, who feels (omnipotently) that he has 'made' the object himself. The repetition of these 'hallucinatory' wishes and their realization by the mother leads the infant to believe he has created his own world. This omnipotence is healthy, leading to the development of a creative and healthy self. Only once this 'true self' has been established, can omnipotence be abrogated and the reality of pain and loss be faced. A child who grows up with a mother who is unable to facilitate this and the subsequent gradual 'disillusionment', will develop a compliant 'false self' that conceals frustrated instinctual drives.

An extremely influential paper by Winnicott, 'Hate in the countertransference', was written in 1947. In it he describes various ways in which mothers may hate their children, and the parallels with hatred in the counter-transference for psychotherapists and health professionals more generally (see 'Transference' and 'Counter-transference' below).

John Bowlby and attachment theory

John Bowlby (1907–1990) was an eminent British researcher and psychoanalyst who is associated with the concepts of 'attachment' and 'separation'. The main features of 'attachment theory' have been summarized as follows (Holmes 1993):

- Lorenz's work with birds and Harlow's work with monkeys suggest that the mother–infant relationship is not necessarily mediated by feeding. Bowlby postulated a 'primary attachment relationship' developing in the human infant at around 7 months, the main evolutionary function of which was to protect the subject from predation.
- This attachment relationship is characterized by 'proximity seeking', activated in young children by separation from an attachment figure, and in later life by threat, illness and fatigue.
- Attachment results in the 'secure base phenomenon'. When an individual is securely attached, he or she can engage in 'exploratory behaviour'.
- Separation leads to 'separation protest', in which efforts are made, often angry or violent, towards reunion. Permanent separation, i.e. loss, impairs the capacity of the individual to feel secure and to explore his/her environment.
- The individual carries inside him/her an 'internal working model' of the world, in which are represented the whereabouts and likely interactive patterns between self and his/her attachment figures.
- The 'attachment dynamic' is not confined to infancy and childhood, but continues throughout life. Development is a movement from immature to mature dependence, or 'emotional autonomy'.

Although Bowlby found himself somewhat marginalized within UK psychoanalytic circles (Holmes 1993), his work remains important for both its clinical and research implications.

Mary Ainsworth, who worked with Bowlby at the Tavistock Clinic, subsequently developed the Strange Situation Test (SST) (Ainsworth et al 1978), a reliable instrument for rating the attachment and security of a 1-year-old infant to his/her parent, usually the mother. Three typical reactions to separation, reuniting with the mother and response to a stranger in the room were first described:

- The secure child – protests when mother disappears, but is easily pacified on her return and returns to exploratory play
- The insecure–avoidant child – does not protest much on separation, and on the mother's return hovers warily nearby, unable to play freely
- The insecure–ambivalent child – does protest, but cannot be pacified by the returning adult, pushing away toys and/or burying his/her head in the mother's lap.

Subsequently, a fourth category has been recognized:

- The insecure–disorganized child – freezes on separation and seems unable to sustain any organized pattern of behaviour.

Longitudinal studies have followed the progress of infants rated on the SST, and a striking finding is the stability of the attachment patterns over time.

Subsequently, Main (1990) has developed the Adult Attachment Interview (AAI), for studying attachment phenomena in adults. Adults are interviewed in a semi-structured interview, in which they are asked to describe early memories, feelings and thoughts about their own parents. The interview is supposed to 'surprise the unconscious', and reveal feelings about current and past attachments and separations, and to tap into emotional responses to loss and difficulty. The interviews are

Lacan did not stick rigidly to the 50-min hour (see below), and his writings are complex.

In Lacan's view, the oedipal child enters into the world of 'signs', which convey to him the meanings of self, gender and the body, just as he is similarly confronted by language and grammar that he must assimilate in order to become part of the linguistic community.

Lacan described three developmental stages:

* A primordial period of unconscious infantile 'desire'
* A world of the 'imaginary' emerging from the 'mirror stage' in which the child first confronts his image and narcissistically (therefore incorrectly) assumes this to be his true self
* Finally, the 'symbolic order' arising through the contact with language, the 'no(m) du pere', a linguistic expression of Freud's picture of the father's combined role as the necessary separator of child and mother, ego ideal and potential castrator.

At around the age of 2 years, the child begins to acquire self-awareness and language. A crisis of development occurs then, as the primitive pre-oedipal unity of mother and child is shattered by the advent of the 'no(m) du pere' – the name of the father and also the 'no' of the father, 'the prohibition placed like the archangel's sword at the gates of paradise by the jealous father' (Bateman & Holmes 1995).

The practice of psychotherapy and psychoanalysis

Psychotherapy is practised in a quiet, private room, with the therapist and patient either facing each other (sometimes at an angle) or with the patient lying on a couch, with the therapist sitting behind the patient's head. Sessions usually last 50 min (the so-called 'therapeutic hour') and direct questioning, reassurance and polite chatter are usually avoided. Sessions are at the same time every week, and may be as frequent as five times a week, or as infrequent as once a week, with the frequency fixed at the beginning of treatment (though subject to revision during the course of treatment). Treatment lasts many months, and often many years.

The boundaries and rules are strict, and therefore any 'boundary violation' or 'acting out', e.g. the patient arriving late, or storming out of the session, can be interpreted by the therapist at that time or at a later date. The deeper unconscious meanings of the patient's communications are of prime importance, and are brought to the surface through the process of interpretation rather than didactic teaching or coaching.

Psychoanalysis as a treatment

Psychoanalysis involves daily (four to five times per week) sessions (of 50 min), with the patient lying on a couch, and the analyst sitting behind the patient. The duration of treatment can be for many years, and psychoanalysis is thus both time- and resource-consuming. The practice of psychoanalysis is thus almost exclusively restricted in the UK, to the private sector,

although many patients are treated at training institutions for a reduced fee.

Psychoanalytic psychotherapy training and treatment clinics in the Freudian/Kleinian tradition, as well as Jungian analytic training organizations, are currently represented by an umbrella body, the BPC (British Psychoanalytic Council, see: www.psychoanalytic-council.org). Some of the less intensive psychotherapy training organizations and clinics are grouped under the auspices of the UKCP (United Kingdom Council for Psychotherapy, see: www.psychotherapy.org.uk), with counselling organizations brought together by the BACP (see: www.psychotherapy.org.uk).

The theoretical underpinnings of many of the briefer treatments (so-called brief dynamic therapy; see below) derive from psychoanalysis, and many practitioners, whether analysts, therapists or other mental health professionals, have undergone their own analytic therapy.

Shedler (2010) describes seven features which reliably distinguish psychoanalytic psychotherapy from other therapies, i.e.:

1. Focus on affect and expression of emotion
2. Exploration of attempts to avoid distressing thoughts and feelings
3. Identification of recurring themes and patterns
4. Discussion of past experience (developmental focus)
5. Focus on interpersonal relations
6. Focus on the therapy relationship
7. Exploration of fantasy life.

Key concepts

Transference and counter-transference

Freud first made use of the term 'transference' in 1895, and initially regarded it as an obstacle to treatment. The patient is 'frightened at finding that she is transferring onto the figure of the physician the distressing ideas that arise from the content of the analysis'. Freud saw this as a 'false connection' between a person who was the object of earlier– often sexual or erotic – wishes, and the doctor.

By 1909, he was beginning to see that this could be an agent for therapeutic change. Positive and negative transference was described, and transference interpretations became central to the practice of psychoanalysis, especially Kleinian analysis.

However, not all interpretations are transference interpretations, and there is debate in analytic circles as to whether everything should be interpreted with reference to transference or not.

A definition of transference by Greenson (quoted in Bateman et al 2000: 52) is as follows:

'Transference is the experiencing of feelings, drives, attitudes, fantasies and defences toward a person in the present, which do not befit the person but are a repetition of reactions originating in regard to significant persons of early childhood, unconsciously displaced onto figures in the present. The two outstanding characteristics of a transference reaction are: it is a repetition, and it is inappropriate.'

Transference occurs in many situations, including other doctor–patient relationships. One might treat a consultant, or a headmaster, or a priest in an inappropriate way, e.g. with anxiety, cheekiness, temerity, etc., unconsciously transferring one's basic attitude to one's father or another early authority figure onto the figure in the present.

Psychotherapy requires that a therapeutic or working alliance be set up between the adult part of the therapist and the adult part of the patient, in order that one can investigate the relationship between the child part of the patient and the therapist.

'Counter-transference' refers to the therapist's attitudes towards the patient. It was also initially regarded as a hindrance by Freud, and was one of the reasons why psychoanalysts and psychoanalytic psychotherapists are expected to undergo their own personal analyses. Any strong emotions the therapist felt towards the patient were initially seen to have originated from the therapist's own past, his/her own conflicts or unresolved problems, and thus inappropriately transferred onto the patient.

However, the concept was expanded to include not only the therapist's own personal 'baggage', but also particular affects and emotions which the patient evokes in his/her therapist, which had more to do with the patient than the therapist. Thus, a patient who is very 'passive–dependent' might project all of his/her unacknowledged hostility onto the therapist who then feels like getting rid of the patient. (The concepts of projection and projective identification as defence mechanisms are particularly relevant here.)

In an important paper Winnicott (1949) (see above) described 'Hate in the countertransference'. He described patients' capacity to evoke feelings of hatred in their helpers, which are in some way appropriate. He relates this to the various ways in which a mother may, on occasions, hate her own infants.

Like transference, counter-transference is ubiquitous, and it is essential that psychiatrists and mental health professionals learn to recognize it, and not act out their counter-transference wishes, for instance by prematurely discharging an irritating patient. A constant monitoring of one's own affective state is necessary, and at all times it is important to try to ascertain whether a strong emotion – sadness, a rescue fantasy, boredom, sadism, etc. is primarily emanating from the practitioner (fatigue due to a late night), or from the patient (sudden boredom, which may indicate the patient avoiding something, or the patient being subtly hostile to you).

Interpretations

Greenson (1967) has described three types of verbal communication contributing to therapeutic understanding, and all are used to a lesser or greater extent in therapy/analysis:

- Clarification
- Confrontation
- Interpretation.

Clarification involves rephrasing and questioning. Confrontation draws attention to what the patient is doing, often repeatedly and sometimes unawares, e.g. arriving late, forgetting to pay the bill, etc. Interpretation offers new formulations of unconscious meaning and motivation.

There are various types of interpretations, including:

- **Dream interpretations:** here the analyst discovers the latent (underlying) content of the dream by analysing its manifest content

- **Transference interpretations:** often held to be the most powerful, i.e. interpreting the patient's behaviour/attitude in the consulting room towards the analyst, e.g. 'you feel I am pushing you away when I go on my holiday, just as you felt pushed out when your younger brother was born and you were sent off to boarding school'
- **Correct interpretations:** those that both adequately explain the material being interpreted, and are formulated in such a way and communicated at such a time as to make sense to the patient.
- **Premature interpretations:** 'true' interpretations, but presented to the patient at a time when he/she is not yet ready to 'receive' or make sense of them.

Thus, just because a patient agrees with an interpretation, it does not follow that it is correct – the patient may just be very compliant. Conversely, if a patient disagrees with or dismisses an interpretation, it may be 'correct', but the patient may habitually reject the unpleasant truth about him/herself.

Therapeutic alliance

The term 'therapeutic alliance' refers to the ordinary, adult-to-adult relationship that the patient and therapist need to have in order to cooperate over their joint task. It involves the patient's willingness to abide by some of the basic rules (such as attendance, timekeeping, payment (in private sector psychotherapy)), and to be able to keep more primitive hostile impulses at bay (e.g. impulses towards acting out in a violent manner). In psychotherapy, the therapist thus sets up a therapeutic alliance between the adult part of the patient and the adult part of the analyst, in order to explore the way in which this relationship is distorted and coloured by the child part of the patient.

Psychotherapy can thus only be conducted satisfactorily if there is enough adult capacity or 'ego strength' in the patient to recognize, tolerate and sustain the paradox that, although he may have intense feelings towards the therapist 'as if' the latter were a parental figure, in reality this is not the case (see below).

Cawley's levels of psychotherapy

Cawley (1977) described 'Levels of psychotherapy', ranging from level 1 (informal, between friends) to level 2 (formal therapy, primarily supportive and non-interpretative) to level 3 (formal therapy dynamic/ analytic, interpretative) (Table 37.3).

While almost any person with difficulties may benefit from level 1 psychotherapy (supportive), a number of questions arise when considering patients for dynamic/analytic psychotherapy (level 3).

Selection of patients for dynamic psychotherapy

Bateman et al (2000: 190) list four selection criteria when considering who should be offered formal psychodynamic psychotherapy (level 3):

Table 37.3 Cawley's levels of psychotherapy

Level	Activity/process
1. Outer (support and counselling)	1. Unburdening of problems to a sympathetic listener 2. Ventilation of feelings within a supportive relationship 3. Discussion of current problems with helper
2. Intermediate	4. Clarification of problems, their nature and origins 5. Confrontation of the defences 6. Interpretation of the transference and unconscious motives
3. Deeper (exploration and analysis)	7. Repetition, remembering and reconstruction of the past 8. Regression to less adult and more primitive levels 9. Resolution of conflicts by 'working through' them

- That the person's difficulties are understandable in psychological terms
- That there is sufficient motivation for insight and change
- That the patient has the requisite ego strength
- That the person has the capacity to form and maintain relationships.

During the initial assessment interview, it should be possible to make a tentative psychodynamic formulation, which will take into account both the patient's past and his/her current difficulties. The patient's preparedness to think about problems is a parallel requirement. The patient's response to a trial interpretation can help in assessing this.

How does the patient respond to the therapist? Does he/she use excessive denial and/or projection as habitual defence mechanisms, disavowing all responsibility for all his/her difficulties, only blaming others. Does he/she 'really' want to change, or just moan at the therapist, using the therapist as a metaphorical dustbin?

What about 'ego strength'? The patient must be able to evaluate his/her experiences and integrate the competing demands of the motivational drives (id), conscience (super-ego) and external reality, while coping with the tensions they create. He/she needs to cope with emotions evoked without decompensating, acting too destructively, or becoming overwhelmed with anxiety. He/she also must keep in touch with the adult part of the self, i.e. maintain the working alliance with the therapist at the same time as getting into contact with the disturbed, needy, messy child within.

One therefore needs to know, whether the patient will cope with the end of each session, and with the therapist's absences? Hence there are a number of contraindications to psychodynamic psychotherapy (see below).

Gabbard (2000), provides an alternative set of criteria. He suggests that the presence of the following 11 features indicates an expressive exploratory emphasis in psychotherapy:

- Strong motivation to understand
- Significant suffering
- Ability to regress in the service of the ego
- Tolerance of frustration
- Capacity for insight (psychological mindedness)
- Intact reality testing
- Meaningful object relations
- Good impulse control
- Ability to sustain work
- Capacity to think in terms of metaphor and analogy
- Reflective responses to trial interpretations.

Contraindications to psychoanalytic psychotherapy include:

- A patient who is actively *suicidal* (unless also being cared for by a psychiatric team)
- Repeated suicide attempts
- A history of gross deliberate self-harm and/or violence towards others
- A current drug or alcohol *addiction* (Edwards & Dare 1996)
- Serious *psychosomatic* conditions (with very concrete thinking and no wish to view the illness in another light). In general, patients with a fixed and long-standing tendency towards somatization are not regarded as good candidates for psychodynamic therapy. They are seen to deal with psychic conflict by somatizing. Somatization is seen as a defence against coming into contact with very primitive, disturbing fears, fantasies and memories. Some analytic authors argue that somatization is a defence against psychosis. However, Guthrie et al (1991) have published a study indicating the value of psychodynamic psychotherapy for patients suffering from irritable bowel disorder with (see also Guthrie 1996). In general, the prognosis with such patients depends on the fixity and chronicity of the 'psychic solution' (see Sharpe et al 1996 for a trial of CBT for the management of patients with ME)
- Patients suffering from a *psychotic* illness such as schizophrenia. In such patients, the impaired ego boundaries generally make psychodynamic psychotherapy unviable. Unable to distinguish fantasy from reality, such patients are unable to distinguish between their own thoughts and those of others, and a psychotic transference may occur. Furthermore, engaging in therapy requires an 'as if' quality from the patient. For example: an elderly male therapist is not really your father, it is 'as if' he were your father. This 'as if' quality is lacking in the patient suffering from an acute psychotic episode. There are some patients with psychotic illnesses, especially bipolar affective disorder, who can benefit from dynamic therapy while in remission (preferably in a unit attached to a psychiatric hospital). And some dedicated and experienced psychotherapists have worked

effectively with patients suffering from an acute psychotic illness (Lucas 2009)

- No evidence of the capacity to *form and sustain relationships* (relative contraindication). The capacity to form and sustain relationships is important as a prognostic indicator, and this may sound cruel: the very people who find this difficult may be deemed 'not suitable' for therapy using this criterion. Nonetheless, if the patient has never sustained a close relationship, it is likely that he/she will flee from therapy, either finding it useless or finding the therapist's absences too difficult to bear. This is not an absolute contraindication, and many schizoid patients are seen in therapy.

Variants and developments of psychodynamic psychotherapy

Brief dynamic psychotherapy

Brief dynamic psychotherapy (BDP) is defined as a 'time-limited form of psychoanalytically-based therapy, usually lasting 6–40 sessions, characterized by a high level of therapist activity, and the attempt to work with a psychodynamic 'focus' which links presenting problem, past conflict or trauma and the relationship with the therapist' (Holmes 1994).

Indications for BDP usually include motivation for change, a circumscribed problem, evidence of at least one good relationship in the past, and the capacity for 'psychological mindedness' (see below). Malan (1963) listed contraindications for BDP, including:

- Chronic addiction
- Serious suicide attempts
- Chronically incapacitating phobic or obsessional symptoms
- Evidence of grossly destructive or self-destructive acting out.

The patient needs to have the 'ego strength' to cope with the psychological turmoil following an emotionally charged session, without drowning his/her sorrows in alcohol or drugs. He/she also must be able to resist hitting a partner/spouse/therapist/shopkeeper following such a session, and must also resist self-harm.

The defence mechanisms in many patients with severe phobias and chronic obsessive–compulsive disorder may respond poorly to dynamic therapy and are often treated, in the first instance at least, by focused therapies (cognitive–behavioural), even though psychodynamic therapists may contribute to an understanding of their aetiology).

The patient, once accepted for BDP, will be informed of the number of sessions, the length of the sessions, whether homework is required (e.g. in cognitive analytic therapy), arrangements for holidays, and a post-therapy follow-up.

A focus is found, which brings together the patient's presenting problem, a past difficulty (often relating to a past loss or trauma), and the current transferential relationship to the therapist. Various authors describe different models and metaphors; for instance, Malan uses two triangles – the triangle of person and the triangle of defence. The triangle of person links the relationship with the significant other with the therapist and the parental figure; the triangle of defence links a hidden impulse for forgotten feeling, a defence, and the resulting anxiety.

Other key names in the field of BDP include Malan, Davanloo, Michael and Enid Balint, Luborsky and Mann.

One of the key features in brief or focused therapy is the active therapist; another feature is the focus right from the start on the termination, which will inevitably re-evoke feelings of loss, so central to many patients' problems. Thus, a patient's habitual response to loss (e.g. turning a blind eye and denying or viciously attacking oneself) will be mobilized in the therapy.

In brief dynamic therapy, constant supervision for the therapist is necessary, and personal therapy for the therapist highly desirable.

Cognitive analytic therapy (CAT)

This therapy was devised by Anthony Ryle at St Thomas' Hospital, London, specifically for use in the UK National Health Service. It is a time-limited therapy, lasting 16 or sometimes 24 sessions. Ryle himself was influenced by the Russian cognitive scientist Vygotsky (Ryle et al 1992).

In the therapy there are three Rs, i.e. *reformulation* (the reshaping of the history and description of the present), therapy then being occupied with the patient being helped to *recognize* the recurrences of these unrevised patterns, so they can become open to *revision*.

The patient is given reading material from 'the psychotherapy file', which describes a number of patterns of unrevisable, maladaptive procedures termed traps, dilemmas and snags. The patient then identifies which ones apply to him/her:

- Traps: negative assumptions generate acts which produce consequences which reinforce the assumptions
- Dilemmas: the person acts as though available action or possible roles were limited to polarized alternatives (false dichotomies), usually unaware that this is the case
- Snags: appropriate roles or goals are abandoned either because the individual makes an assumption that others would oppose them, or because they are perceived as forbidden or dangerous.

At the fourth session, the therapist provides a summary of his or her understanding of the history and its meaning, and describes how the strategies, used historically as a way of surviving, may now be maladaptive.

A diagram (sequential diagrammatic representation, SDR) may be used, and the patient will keep this. The patient feels understood and 'held' and becomes less defensive. Dreams, memories and feelings become accessible. Sessions thereafter are usually unstructured although homework is given. At the end, a goodbye letter is given to the patient, and patients are also asked to write their own evaluation.

> 'The emphasis of this therapy is upon the formation and use of accurate descriptions and the aim is that patients may learn to recognize automatic procedures in time to consider alternatives.'
>
> (Ryle et al 1992: 402)

Foundations of family therapy

Family therapy has broadened the focus of treatment from the individual to the family and social context, contending that individuals live not in isolation but within a social context, and are best understood by examining their relationships to others and the environment in which they interact. The notion of holism underlines the central concept. The whole is made up of more than a group of individuals, as it also includes the relationships between its members. A central concept, therefore, is of circular causality. Circularity implies that every member in a system influences the others and is influenced by them. When such an assumption is applied to a family in therapy, blame for the problem is not attributed to individuals, and problems are viewed with respect to relationships between people, or other systems, and may be an inevitable result of change across time.

The family is seen as a dynamic system that co-evolves with its environment. The family experiences continual fluctuation as it moves through its own family lifecycle and time. Carter and McGoldrick (1984) have presented a framework which details the six stages of the family lifecycle and the changes required from the family in order for it to proceed developmentally.

The symptom is believed to have occurred when the family has not appropriately adjusted to disruptions or transition points in the family lifecycle. Such transition points may include changes in the composition of the family (e.g. births, deaths or divorces), particular developments by individual members (e.g. change in residence, school or workplace) and unexpected changes (e.g. illness or retrenchment). Such changes may require negotiation of new rules or family structures. It is believed that the family is self-regulating and thus will attempt to maintain stability or homeostasis. In response to fluctuations brought about by changes in the developmental lifecycle, or stresses from outside the family system, change in one family member may be counterbalanced by complementary changes in another member, in a process known as negative feedback.

Positive feedback has the opposite effect. A small deviation within the system may be exaggerated or amplified by other members. This process may explain how some problems develop and become out of control and how the same unhelpful solution is repeated.

A universal goal of family therapists is to remove the symptom and alleviate family distress, while other aims involve clarifying communication, solving problems and promoting individual autonomy. In most family therapies, there is the tendency to de-emphasize insight and promote action, and to concentrate on the present rather than the past (in contrast to individual psychodynamic psychotherapy). The therapist's role is as a change agent and is thus generally active and directive. The three main family therapy schools (structural, systemic, strategic) share these foundations. However, they differ in their levels of focus, methodology, and techniques.

In particular, systemic therapy (like psychodynamic psychotherapy) influences psychiatric practice way beyond the confines of particular patients being treated in specific psychotherapy settings. The systemic approach is well integrated, especially in the field of child and adolescent psychiatry, less so within general adult psychiatry (Asen 2002).

Group psychotherapy and analysis

Group psychotherapy and group analysis are popular and well-established modes of psychotherapy, practised, like individual and family therapy, both in the private and public sectors. Many of the founding figures in group therapy and analysis were also trained in individual psychoanalysis (e.g. Wilfred Bion). However, the theory and practice of group analysis is now a distinct discipline influenced not only by psychoanalysis but also by sociology, social psychology and organizational theory (Roberts 1995).

At least three models of group analytic practice can be discerned:

* *Analysis in the group* – where an individual may be treated within a group context
* *Analysis of the group* – where the leader/'conductor'/ therapist interprets the transference of the group to him/ herself
* *Analysis through and of the group* – especially associated with the work of Foulkes and the institute of group analysis.

Wolf and Schwarz are associated with analysis in the group, similar to individual therapy in a group setting. Bion and Ezriel are associated with analysis of the group. Henry Ezriel proposed that in every meeting of a group it is possible to identify a common group tension. His method was for the 'conductor' (therapist) to identify three types of object relationship emerging from the common group tension:

* The 'required' relationship – a socially acceptable, safe, defensive mode of functioning, e.g. 'I will miss the group during the summer break'
* The 'avoided' relationship – which might include feelings of murderous rage about the therapist's long indulgent summer break
* The 'calamitous' relationship – which is the feared outcome of the avoided relationship being consciously acknowledged, e.g. murderous wishes could destroy therapist and group, incestuous wishes would lead to dire punishment.

Foulkes is associated with analysis through the group, i.e. the awareness of transpersonal phenomena and multiple levels of group functioning, including:

* Level of current adult relationships
* Level of individual transference
* Level of shared feelings and fantasies (the level of archetypal universal images, similar to Jung's archetypes of the collective unconscious).

Yalom (1985) published *The Theory and Practice of Group Psychotherapy* having worked both in the USA and at the Tavistock Clinic in London. He describes a number of therapeutic factors specific to groups:

* Universality
* Altruism
* Corrective recapitulation of the family group, i.e. what went wrong in the early family group can be repeated and recognized in the group, where in a more open and experiential atmosphere less maladaptive ways can be worked out

- Imitative behaviour
- Interpersonal learning
- Cohesiveness
- Existential factors, which include the recognition of responsibility in the face of our basic aloneness and mortality
- Catharsis
- Insight
- Development of socializing techniques
- Guidance
- Instillation of hope.

Pairing and subgrouping can be destructive, as can inappropriate idealization of the therapist. In general, the maintenance of boundaries, including starting and finishing on time and preparation of the room, is part of the therapist's function.

While not all patients in the mental health setting will formally be involved in group therapy, all patients and staff are wittingly and unwittingly caught up in group processes. Hobbs (in Holmes 1991) usefully describes a number of group processes within psychiatry. It is in order to better understand these processes that some wards or psychiatric teams make use of an outside facilitator in a staff support group, or a case discussion seminar. Even within these groups, there are further group dynamics of which to be aware (see Stern 1996).

Therapeutic communities

The term 'therapeutic community' (TC) is generally used in the UK to describe small, cohesive communities where patients (sometimes referred to as 'residents') have a significant involvement in decision-making and the practicalities of running the unit. Key principles include collective responsibility, citizenship and empowerment, and TCs are structured in a way that deliberately encourages personal responsibility and discourages unhelpful dependency on professionals.

Patients are seen as bringing strengths and creative energy into the therapeutic setting, and the peer group is seen as all-important in the establishment of a strong therapeutic alliance. The belief in flattening of hierarchies and delegated decision-making may be seen by outsiders as facilitating something anarchic, but in reality there is a deep awareness of the need for strong leadership and a safe therapeutic frame (Campling 2001).

The power of groups was demonstrated in the UK in the Second World War by the Northfield experiments, named after the Northfield Hospital in Birmingham. Here, an army psychiatric unit was run along group lines, and some prominent figures, including Bion, Foulkes and Main, were involved. Bion went on to write about groups and became a prominent Kleinian theoretician (see above). Foulkes is one of the founding fathers of group analysis, and Main described the therapeutic community, an institution where 'the setting itself is designed to restore morale and promote the psychological treatment of mental and emotional disturbance'. Main went on to create the influential example of the Cassel Hospital in Surrey.

Maxwell Jones founded the Belmont in the 1950s, later called the Henderson Hospital, in Sutton, Surrey. Here, the community was the main focus, and careful procedures for admission, discipline and discharge were established over many years. The hospital treated patients with severe personality disorders, with a regime characterized by what the anthropologist Rapoport (1960) termed 'permissiveness, reality-confrontation, democracy and communalism'.

Permissiveness encourages the expression and enactment of disturbed feelings and relationships, so that they can be examined by patients and staff alike. Differences between patients and staff are minimized, and decisions are made with residents having a majority vote (and often being harsher than staff members themselves). Permissiveness is usually limited to the verbal expression of feelings, and would be strongly confronted if it led to other members of the TC being emotionally hurt or damaged, or feeling marginalized or excluded. Racist comments, for example, would not go unchallenged in modern TCs (Campling 2001).

A further important observation form Rapport's study was the repeated cycle of *oscillations*: times of healthy functioning, when residents were well able to manage responsibility and a level of therapeutic permissiveness; and other times when high levels of disturbed behaviour have meant that staff had to take a more active role. A further observation was the conflict between those whose main objective was preparing residents for the outside world, and those whose main objective was helping residents to better understand their inner worlds – a tension between 'rehabilitation' and 'psychotherapy' that still persists in many modern TCs. The Henderson was in many ways the prototypical therapeutic community.

Clark (1977) has described three important terms:

- *Therapeutic community or therapeutic community proper* refers to the specific type of therapeutic milieu set up by Maxwell Jones and followers, e.g. Henderson, 'a small face-to-face residential community using social analysis as its main tool'
- *Therapeutic milieu* is a social setting designed to produce a beneficial effect on those being helped in it, e.g. a sheltered workshop, hospital ward, hostel
- *Social therapy* is the least specific term, employing the idea that the milieu or social environment can be used as a mode of treatment.

TCs have a long history of involvement in research. Much of this has been from a social science perspective and qualitative in nature. Some of it is of importance to other areas of psychiatry, for example methodological approaches to develop, describe and measure the therapeutic milieu, of which the Ward Atmosphere Scale developed by Moos is the best example. Over the past decade, researchers based at both the Henderson and the Cassel hospitals have produced methodologically sound research demonstrating the cost-effectiveness of their treatments (Norton 1996).

TCs are seen to have a valuable role to play within the future of mental health services. Within the NHS in the UK, they have established a niche for those suffering from severe emotionally unstable personality disorder, a group of high risk patients who become heavy users of services if they do not receive the intensive long term psychosocial therapy they require.

The application of TC ideas, like ideas from psychodynamic, systemic and group therapy, has had an important impact on the general practice of psychiatry.

Research in psychotherapy

This is a vast topic, outside the realms of this chapter. The interested reader is referred to the recently published paper by Shedler (2010) (see below) and the publication by Roth and Fonagy (1996), in which they systematically and critically review the literature on:

* Which psychotherapeutic interventions are of demonstrable benefit to particular patient groups
* Research evidence that would help funders of healthcare decide on the appropriate mix of therapies for their population
* The extent to which one can draw on evidence of demonstrated efficacy in controlled research conditions and clinical effectiveness in services as delivered.

Three examples of methodologically sound research in psychotherapy are the work of Guthrie, Creed and colleagues in Manchester working with patients from a gastroenterology clinic; the work by Julian Leff and colleagues in London, researching systemic couple therapy for depression, and Barbara Milrod's studies (in New York, USA) of psychotherapy for panic disorder.

In their earlier study, Guthrie and colleagues (1991) studied the effects of psychodynamic interpersonal therapy on patients with irritable bowel syndrome (IBS). The treatment group received seven sessions of exploratory psychotherapy, while the control group received a similar number of sessions of supportive listening. At the end of the study a significantly greater improvement was found in the treatment group, rated by a gastroenterologist who was blind to the treatment groups. The study includes a placebo attention control and clearly showed that the improvement resulting from the psychotherapy was the result of the specific effect of the therapy, rather than as a result of spending time with an empathic and supportive therapist. In addition, only the most difficult patients, i.e. those with chronic, unresponsive symptoms, were included in the study.

A subsequent study by the same group (Creed et al 2003) has looked at the cost-effectiveness of psychodynamic interpersonal therapy and paroxetine in patients with severe IBS. The results showed that both treatments were superior to treatment as usual in improving the physical aspects of health related quality of life measures, but there was no difference in the psychological component. During the follow-up year, the psychotherapy but not paroxetine was associated with a significant reduction in healthcare costs compared with treatment as usual. (A recent study by Drossman and colleagues (2003) highlights the efficacy of cognitive–behavioural therapy (CBT), and to a lesser extent desipramine, in a similar population.)

In the study by Leff et al (2000), the relative efficacy and cost of couple therapy, antidepressant therapy and CBT were compared, for the treatment and maintenance of people with depression living with a critical partner or spouse. Patients in a long-term heterosexual relationship who met defined criteria for depression were randomly allocated to the three treatments mentioned above. (The CBT drop-out rate was so high that this treatment option was soon deleted from the trial.) The results

were striking: over half (56%) of those allocated to drug treatment dropped out of the treatment compared with 15% of those offered couple therapy. Subjects' depression improved in both groups, but couple therapy showed a significant advantage according to the Beck depression inventory, both at the end of treatment and after a second year off treatment. Overall, there was no difference in the total costs (adding the costs of psycho- or pharmacotherapy to the costs of other services used). The authors conclude 'For this group, couple therapy is much more acceptable than antidepressant drugs and is at least as efficacious, if not more so, both in the treatment and maintenance phases' (Leff et al 2000: 95).

Milrod et al (2007) conducted the first efficacy randomized controlled clinical trial of panic-focused psychodynamic psychotherapy. This was a manualized psychoanalytical psychotherapy for patients with DSM-IV panic disorder. Participants were recruited over 5 years in the New York City metropolitan area, all being adults with primary DSM-IV panic disorder. All subjects received assigned treatment, panic-focused psychodynamic psychotherapy or applied relaxation training in twice-weekly sessions for 12 weeks. The Panic Disorder Severity Scale, rated by blinded independent evaluators, was the primary outcome measure. The researchers found that subjects in panic-focused psychodynamic psychotherapy had significantly greater reduction in severity of panic symptoms. Furthermore, those receiving panic-focused psychodynamic psychotherapy were significantly more likely to respond at treatment termination (73% vs 39%), using the Multicenter Panic Disorder Study response criteria. The secondary outcome, change in psychosocial functioning, mirrored these results.

Three recently published reviews highlight the increasingly robust research base for short- and long-term psychoanalytic psychotherapy. Shedler (2010: 98) convincingly argues that 'empirical evidence supports the efficacy of psychodynamic therapy'. He shows that not only are effect sizes for psychodynamic therapy as large as those reported for other therapies, but that the therapeutic gains and maintained and indeed tend to improve after the therapy ends, in contradistinction to some other therapies. Furthermore, he writes 'nonpsychodynamic therapies may be effective in part because the more skilled practitioners utilize techniques that have long been central to psychodynamic theory and practice. The perception that psychodynamic approaches lack empirical support does not accord with available scientific evidence and may reflect selective dissemination of research findings.'

Lewis et al (2008: 445) review the field of Short Term Psychodynamic Psychotherapy (STPP) and find that there is an 'increasing body of evidence suggesting that STPP can be an effective psychological treatment for patients suffering from mental health problems', while Leichsenring and Rabung (2008) conclude in their meta-analysis that 'there is evidence that LTPP (long term psychodynamic psychotherapy) is an effective treatment for complex mental disorders'.

These studies (as well as the work of Bateman & Fonagy 2008, described above; and Dare et al 1990, on the treatment of anorexia nervosa, described above) and meta-analyses are methodologically very different from the traditional intensive, highly personal case study/research work carried out over months or years in psychoanalytic or psychotherapy practice. The tradition within most psychodynamic work remains that of detailed case histories, originating with Freud's own cases. Both are valuable sources of information about patients and psychological processes. Single case studies have a number of attractive features – they can be carried out in routine clinical practice, they do not necessarily require the facilities associated with more complex research, and can sometimes be completed fairly quickly. However, precisely because they are single case studies, the results cannot necessarily be generalized. The task of psychotherapy research in the future is to proceed with both modes of enquiry, and permit as much cross-fertilization between the two modes of research and practice as possible.

The role of psychotherapy and the psychotherapist within psychiatry – overt and covert functions

Within psychiatric practice in Britain, and perhaps throughout the world, psychotherapy occupies a unique role. Not only is it a mode of treatment for some patients, it is also an explanatory model; not only is the psychotherapist called upon to fulfil numerous overt functions within the institution, there are also all sorts of other functions which a psychotherapist may be called upon or expected to fulfil, some more appropriate than others.

The role of a psychotherapist within a medical hospital is equally interesting and complicated, see Stern (1999, 2010).

Overt roles of the psychotherapist

The 'overt roles' are the explicit functions for which the organization employs the practitioner. They are what might be described in a job description, and include:

- Assessment of patients referred for psychotherapy
- Treatment of such patients if appropriate – individual, groups, family, cognitive behavioural therapy, etc.
- Consultations to various teams in the hospital – for instance, a forensic or community mental health team
- Supervision of junior staff who are treating patients
- Formal teaching for junior psychiatrists, and medical students, including those preparing for examinations
- The running of staff support groups for junior doctors and/or other teams on wards/community
- Attending the weekly 'grand round'
- Research and audit
- *Ad hoc* consultations.

Over and above the many varied overt roles mentioned above, much more is provided.

Covert roles of the psychotherapist

First, through intensive contact with supervisees, much psychological support is provided for psychotherapists as they struggle to cope with what it takes to work with mental disturbance. The model is of long-term focused care on an individual, and tries to make sense of symptoms and behaviour that would otherwise be described as unintelligible.

There is also the presence in the hospital of someone who, while functioning (hopefully) effectively and creatively, also states implicitly or explicitly that he/she has had or is having his/her own psychotherapeutic or analytic treatment. This generally facilitates others to ask for it themselves, so that the psychotherapist is often called upon by colleagues to help find a suitable therapist for themselves or their family members.

An allied role is to provide 'meaning' to the work publicly. Constantly at weekly academic meetings or 'grand rounds', fascinating cases are presented – of pathologically jealous men, of depressed mothers, of lonely migrants who have lost everything and evoke sadness in their carers; but within some minutes of these presentations beginning, these people are transformed into cases of 'treatment-resistant depression', 'psychosis', 'post-traumatic stress disorder (PTSD)', and the actual patient seems to be lost to the discussion. It is not only the patients who are transformed – sensitive, creative psychiatrists compete with each other with regards to diagnosis, special investigations, reading the latest scan, and discussing the latest research. The patient and what he or she is, or means, or wishes, or fears, is lost.

This is where the psychotherapist may try and come in, with notions of the unconscious, or family dynamics, of conflict or of counter-transference, to try help make sense of what is going on internally, and between the patient and carer, and perhaps why some of the drugs are not being taken or are not 'doing the job properly'. On occasions, this is reassuring and helpful to the group and to the patient in the long run. On other occasions, especially when the level of anxiety in the room is too high, these comments are brushed aside, and the discussion continues, seemingly untouched.

A third covert function is to provide a place where 'impossible' patients can be disposed of. A number of patient groups come to mind:

1. So-called 'borderline' women: often self-destructive, sometimes causing splits within the team, these patients 'refuse' to improve on antidepressants and make the young psychiatry trainee (or not so young consultant) distinctly uneasy
2. Slightly older patients, again predominantly women, who somatize, re-enacting their sadomasochistic object relations through contact with the medical profession, as well as their social network, and once again frustrate psychiatrists by 'refusing' to get better
3. Men who are not quite violent or perverse enough to be referred to forensic services, but who are difficult to engage and treat in the context of a community mental health team (CMHT), and who once again tend not to improve on antidepressant therapy.

These patients are the ambivalently charged 'gifts' from psychiatric colleagues to the psychotherapy team. Many intelligent psychiatrists want to get rid of or dispose of these 'special' patients, and refer them to the psychotherapy department, even if they are unmotivated or unlikely to be suitable for psychological therapy.

Box 38.1

Definitions

- *Behaviour therapy* is a treatment approach originally derived from learning theory, which seeks to solve problems and relieve symptoms by changing behaviour and the environmental contingencies which control behaviour.
- *Behaviour modification* is an approach to change behaviour in clinical and non-clinical settings based on operant conditioning.
- *Cognitive therapy* is a treatment approach derived from cognitive theories which seeks to solve problems and relieve symptoms by changing thoughts and beliefs.
- *Cognitive behaviour therapy* (*behavioural–cognitive therapy*) refers to the pragmatic combination of concepts and techniques from these therapies in clinical practice.

a fear of the rat which generalized to other stimuli such as cotton wool and even gentlemen with white beards. Watson's pupils developed a method for deconditioning anxiety in children, which was probably the first example of behaviour therapy. Two types of conditioning exist: classical and operant (see also Ch. 5).

Classical conditioning

Watson was strongly influenced by the work of the Russian physiologist Pavlov. Pavlov's work on conditioning salivation in dogs is well known. In a typical Pavlovian experiment, a physiological response such as salivating to the sight of food is studied. The food is termed the *unconditional* stimulus (UCS) and salivation is termed the *unconditional response* or *reflex* (UCR). Presentation of the food is repeatedly paired with a *conditional stimulus* (CS), for instance a bell. When the bell is then rung without the food, the dog salivates. This salivation to the bell is the *conditional response* or *reflex*.

Pavlov found that the strength of conditioning is increased by a number of factors:

1. If the unconditional stimulus (food) follows the conditional one (bell)
2. If there is a short delay between the unconditional stimulus and the conditional stimulus
3. The intensity of UCS and CS: bigger pieces of food or a louder bell.

Behaviour therapists have been particularly interested in the application of classical conditioning theory to anxiety. Phobias in particular can be seen as forms of conditioned fear responses to given stimuli. This model has been applied to simple phobias, agoraphobia, social phobia and obsessive compulsive disorder. (As an explanation of the development of most phobias, the conditioned fear model is inadequate, e.g. only 23% of animal phobias are associated with a prior traumatic experience with the animal; McNally & Steketee 1985). This has led to the idea that we may be *prepared* to acquire certain fears on evolutionary grounds (Seligman 1971). The classical conditioning model has been very influential in the development of exposure therapy, because of the evidence from animal studies of how fears can be deconditioned. Joseph Wolpe was the first person to apply these principles in a significant way to psychiatric patients.

His method was based on the premise that one physiological state (relaxation) was incompatible with another (anxiety), a concept termed reciprocal inhibition. Thus, if a phobic patient could relax in the presence of a phobic stimulus, the anxiety response could be deconditioned. His *systematic desensitization* is a technique in which phobic patients are taught deep muscle relaxation, and then imagine feared stimuli in an increasing hierarchy of anxiety (Wolpe 1958). Exposure therapy for anxiety disorders depends on the process of *habituation*. This process, which is still incompletely understood, is one in which repeated exposure to a stimulus leads to a decrement in orienting responses and arousal within an exposure session.

Operant conditioning

Classical conditioning describes how an organism responds to its environment. Operant conditioning (Skinner) is more concerned with the way that behaviour acts or operates on the environment to produce consequences. Behaviour which gets the environment to react in a rewarding manner is more likely to be repeated. A *reinforcer* is any environmental response which increases the frequency of a behaviour. For animals this is often food, but for human beings more subtle things like money or social acceptance may be reinforcing. Animals and humans will be able to detect situations where they are more likely to receive a reward. These situations then *cue* a behavioural response which elicits reinforcement. For instance, if a mother gives a child a sweet to keep it quiet in a supermarket when it starts to shout, it will soon learn to have a tantrum every time it is taken there. The supermarket acts as a cue, the tantrum is the behavioural response and the sweet the reinforcement.

Modern developments of conditioning theories

Conditioning theories have progressed a long way since the days of Pavlov and Skinner. It has been established that this form of learning does not depend on the organism being a mere passive responder to the environment or just acting in a random way. Modern theories of conditioning emphasize how the process involves the acquisition of knowledge about the relationship between an action and the occurrence of a reinforcer, rather than a simple stimulus-response reflex (Adams & Dickinson 1981). If an animal is trained to perform an action to obtain food, and then the food is separately paired with an aversive stimulus, the simple conditioning model would predict that there would be no change in the trained behaviour: the behaviour would be reflexly conditioned, and so the animal would not predict that the result of the behaviour would be aversive. Of course, the animal is much less likely to perform the behaviour. The organism is therefore making predictions about the consequences of behaviour. These new ideas have some similarities with cognitive theories of learning and there is a rapprochement between the two approaches (Rapee 1991). More recently, a new group of cognitive behavioural therapies have emerged which unashamedly apply radical behavioural (Skinnerian) theories in a much more sophisticated clinical context. These include dialectical behaviour therapy (Linehan 1993, Linehan et al 2007) and acceptance and commitment therapy (Hayes et al 1999, 2004).

Characteristics of behaviour therapy

In contrast to psychoanalytic approaches to therapy, behavioural therapy is far more structured and directive. The emphasis is on here and now problems that can generate goals that are specific, measurable, and attainable. This allows desired outcomes to be defined and assessed. A patient with agoraphobia might set a goal of being able to travel by herself 10 stops on a tube train at rush hour. It is easy to decide if a goal as operationally defined as this has been met by the end of therapy. Therapists routinely measure outcomes with each patient and change therapy techniques on the basis of research evidence. The therapeutic relationship is collaborative, but the therapist is in control. Usually, the rationale for treatment is discussed with the patient and the patient set clear tasks within and between sessions. Because of this clear focus behaviour therapists are usually able to set criteria for the sort of patients they can treat. If a patient cannot identify clear problems and goals, or if a patient is not willing to accept and comply with the treatment plan they will not be taken on for therapy.

Exposure therapy

Exposure is a simple and easily learned treatment for anxiety disorders which has been shown to be effective in numerous clinical trials. Despite the attraction of more sophisticated cognitive models, 60–80% of patients with anxiety are likely to respond to straightforward behaviour therapy. Therapy for phobias (simple phobia, agoraphobia, social phobia) lasts for 8–15 sessions. Sessions involving therapist aided exposure may last 2 h, but other sessions, where homework is reviewed and new homework set, may only need 30 min. As with many cognitive and behavioural techniques, active participation of the patient is necessary for the therapy to be effective. Since this involves confronting the situation which the patient is avoiding, whether it be social gatherings, tube trains or dirt, the therapist needs to be skilled in persuading the patient to comply. The first step in therapy therefore involves the explanation of the rationale of exposure. Patients are taught about the nature and function of anxiety and told that symptoms, although unpleasant, are not dangerous. They are told that with exposure the anxiety symptoms will reduce within the session (*habituation*), and that with each successive session the initial anxiety response will become less. While a single very prolonged exposure session (*flooding*) may be sufficient to eliminate some phobias, most patients prefer to approach the problem in a more gradual way (*graded exposure*). The patient and therapist then construct a hierarchy of feared situations, and the patient is encouraged to enter these feared situations in a graded way. The hierarchy is constructed so that there is a gradual increase in the feared characteristics of the stimuli at each stage. Initial sessions may require therapist aided exposure, but most patients can then go on to carry out homework assignments on their own (Marks 1987). Modelling has also been employed as an aid to exposure (Bandura 1971): if a patient is too frightened to approach a feared stimulus themselves the therapist can model a coping response, e.g. by approaching and handling a spider. Many patients can carry out self-exposure effectively with only minimal

---

Box 38.2

Characteristics of effective exposure

1. Real life, rather than imagination (Emmelkamp & Wessels 1975)
2. Prolonged rather than brief (Stern & Marks 1973)
3. Makes use of regular self-exposure tasks (McDonald et al 1978).

---

intervention from the therapist (see Box 38.2), and Marks et al (2004) demonstrated that computer-aided self-exposure was more effective than a relaxation placebo and just as effective as therapist-led exposure.

Case example

Jim was a 50-year-old manager of a betting shop who had been seriously assaulted during a robbery. On his way back from depositing the day's takings he was attacked by two men who thought he still had the money. His front teeth had been knocked out and he suffered severe bruising. At the time, he feared for his life. A year later, when he was referred by his GP, he had still not been able to return to work. He had symptoms of post-traumatic stress disorder, including high levels of anxiety, hypervigilance, nightmares and avoidance of travelling alone in parts of the East End of London where he lived. Jim understood that he was overreacting to many situations, but still found himself irrationally afraid of any young men. He was able to draw up a hierarchy of feared situations and set about exposing himself to these systematically. Progress was not always smooth. Early on in the therapy, a local man with mental health problems threatened him with a gun in the street! He understandably needed encouragement to continue with the programme. With perseverance, he was able to spend longer periods helping out in the shop, and was very pleased to find that he could strike up mutually agreeable conversations without seeing the customers as potential attackers. At the end of 12 sessions of therapy, he was at the top of the hierarchy except for being able to carry and cash large sums of money. He decided that it was not a reasonable expectation of his firm that he should do this alone and he eventually left his job.

In obsessive–compulsive disorder, exposure is combined with *response prevention*. In this disorder, obsessional fears are usually neutralized by rituals, such as checking, handwashing, etc. The therapist helps the patient construct a hierarchy of stimuli which trigger intrusive thoughts, and then supports the patient in exposure to these cues without engaging in the neutralizing behaviour. For instance, a patient with a fear of contamination by dog faeces might scrub their hands many times a day, and avoid walking in places where they have seen dog faeces. Exposure could begin with the patient touching dusty surfaces and resisting the urge to wash their hands. As he or she progresses up the hierarchy, he or she could move on to touching carpets, shoes, etc. It would also be important to overcome avoidance by deliberately walking in the park or down a street where the patient had seen dogs defaecating. At home they might have elaborate rituals to prevent supposed contamination from getting into the house, e.g. taking off shoes with gloves and leaving them in a 'dirty' area of the house and having a shower. The behavioural programme would expect

The cognitive model of anxiety

In anxiety, the self is seen as *vulnerable*, the world *dangerous*, and the future *uncertain*. Schemas associated with vulnerability are seen to be of evolutionary usefulness in energizing the organism and preparing for fight or flight from danger (Beck et al 1985; Beck & Clark 1997). The problem in anxiety disorders is that these danger schemas are activated inappropriately in non-threatening situations. Once anxiety is present the cognitive apparatus selectively attends to threat (e.g. a grandparent suddenly becomes aware of all the dangers in a children's playground), overestimates the chance of disaster (the grandparent becomes convinced that their grandchild will inevitably fall off the climbing frame) and underestimates the opportunities for rescue or coping (the grandparent frets about what she will do if the child falls and fears she won't be able to cope). Once this selective attention is operating danger signals in the internal or external environment become predominant and this reinforces the anxiety. Again, avoidance and various safety behaviours are seen as maintaining factors in anxiety disorders. As in depression, there are underlying assumptions (this time about the world being a dangerous place, about the individual being vulnerable, etc.) which may be dormant until triggered by a life event.

Cognitive models of specific anxiety disorders

Cognitive therapists have taken this basic model of anxiety and modified it for panic (Clark 1996), generalized anxiety disorder (Wells 1997, 2000), hypochondriasis (Warwick & Salkovskis 1989) and social phobia (Clark & Wells 1995) and post-traumatic stress disorder (Ehlers & Clark 2000).

Much of this work has been carried out at Oxford, where the approach has been to identify the particular beliefs and behaviours that maintain the disorders. These models (Table 38.1) have in common a description of:

1. Bias in information processing
2. Selective attention
3. Maladaptive behaviours – avoidance and safety behaviours.

In panic disorder, there is a catastrophic misinterpretation of bodily sensations. The patient selectively attends to bodily sensations of autonomic nervous system activity and mistakes them for signs of impending disaster. The misinterpretations are specific to the sensation: breathlessness – suffocation, chest pain – heart attack, etc. Agoraphobic symptoms may arise out of avoidance of situations where panics have occurred. More subtle avoidance is seen when the person acts to prevent the feared catastrophe taking place, by avoiding exercise if they fear a heart attack. This prevents them from testing the negative belief and helps to maintain the disorder. In hypochondriasis, a similar process takes place, but the misinterpretations are not of impending disaster. The person with health anxiety will see bodily symptoms as signs of disease which might be life-threatening but which are not imminently life-threatening. Safety behaviours include reassurance seeking from family and medical professionals and obsessional checking for signs of disease. In panic and health anxiety the focus of attention is usually on bodily symptoms, but in generalized anxiety disorder it is worry which is the cause of distress. According to Wells (2000), any negative events can set off worry (e.g. unpleasant news, intrusive thoughts). Worry is then chosen as a coping strategy (often because of beliefs that it helps problem solving or prevents bad things happening), but once this happens negative beliefs about worry (e.g. that worry can cause stress or that the person will lose control of their thinking) set in and a vicious cycle is set up, perpetuating the anxiety. Clark (1996) has carried out a number of compelling experiments specifically designed to test his model of panic. The current empirical status of the model is reviewed in Clark and Beck (2010).

A similar approach has been taken by Salkovskis (1985) to obsessive compulsive disorder. Here, the source of the problem is not the intrusive thoughts themselves but the interpretation the person makes of them. Intrusive thoughts are actually quite common in the general population, occurring in 80% of individuals, and the content of normal and abnormal obsessions is similar (Rachman & de Silva 1978; Salkovskis & Harrison 1984), but in OCD these thoughts are seen as threatening. They usually imply that the person has some responsibility for their content of their thoughts. A man who had intrusive thoughts of jumping in front of a tube train, or swerving in the face of oncoming traffic, saw these as indications that he might be schizophrenic, and that he might actually lose control and do what he feared. Another patient experienced intrusive thoughts of friends and family being attacked. He believed that this meant that he was an evil person, otherwise why would he have these images? This overdeveloped sense of responsibility for intrusions leads the obsessional patient to try to suppress them. But these attempts at thought control paradoxically make the intrusions stronger and more frequent. Rituals are seen as strategies for neutralizing intrusive thoughts. So, the person who feared his

Table 38.1 Cognitive models of anxiety disorders

	Panic disorder	Hypochondriasis	Generalized anxiety disorder	Social phobia
Bias in information processing	Catastrophic misinterpretation	Non-catastrophic misinterpretation	Misinterpretation of any situation as threatening	Misinterpretation of social threat
Selective attention	Bodily sensations of autonomic nervous system activity	Any bodily sensations	Worrying thoughts	Image of self as a social object
Safety behaviours	Avoidance of exercise, controlling breathing	Reassurance seeking, checking for symptoms	Thought control, avoidance	Avoiding eye contact, monitoring of speech

images of violence meant he was bad would say to himself 'I'm not bad' and would make gestures with his arms to ward off the images. Someone with intrusive thoughts that he might forget to turn off the gas and so be responsible for the death of everyone in his house will obsessionally check the taps are turned off many times before he can leave the house.

Vulnerability to emotional disorder

So far, we have looked at the way in which cognitive theory explains different emotional disorders. In Beck's model, vulnerability to a disorder comes from the existence of underlying dysfunctional assumptions or schemas. We all need to have assumptions about the world in order to make sense of the 'blooming, buzzing confusion' of reality. Schemas help us to select and organize experience and predict what is going to happen next. If we have a stable, supportive family upbringing, we develop positive schemas. We see ourselves as basically worthwhile and competent. We see others as potentially supportive and well inclined. We see the world as generally a positive place. If on the other hand we have aversive experiences in childhood, we may see ourselves as worthless or incompetent, others as critical or abusive, and the world as dangerous or hostile. We all have some positive and some negative core beliefs. Often the negative beliefs remain dormant if we have positive life experiences in childhood and adulthood. Sometimes we avoid them by developing conditional assumptions about the world. These 'if–then' beliefs predicate self-worth on the world being a certain way. They are global, absolute and rigid, and predispose to emotional problems. Examples of dysfunctional assumptions predisposing to depression would be:

- I must always be nice to people.
- It is terrible to be rejected.
- I can only be happy if I have a successful life.
- If I make a mistake, it means I am a failure.
- If I do not have someone to love me, I must be worthless.

Critical incidents may lead to the activation of these beliefs and the core beliefs associated with them. Not all negative life events will lead to depression. The key is the personal meaning of the event, and whether or not it fits with a person's underlying assumption. Thus someone with a belief that he can only be happy if he is loved may cope with the loss of a job but not the loss of a relationship. Research has shown that a major negative life event is not always necessary to trigger depression. In fact, as people experience repeated depressive episodes the severity of precipitating events becomes milder, the so-called 'kindling' effect (Monroe & Harkness 2005). It appears that low mood activates the underlying assumptions of people who have had a previous depressive episode (Segal et al 1999) and this predicts future relapse. It also seems that 'cognitive reactivity' – fluctuations in attitudes to self in response to daily events – predicts the onset of a depressive episode (Scher et al 2005). In the light of these findings Beck has modified his cognitive theory of depression. He proposed (Beck 1996) that the cognitive, affective, behavioural and motivational systems which are active during a clinical depression become organized over successive depressive episodes into a *depressive mode* which controls information processing and behaviour. With each episode the associations become stronger

and the mode is more easily triggered. Once it is activated it locks the person into a number of vicious maintaining cycles (Moorey 2010). Beck (2008) recently summarized the evolution of his model of depression and also suggested how neurobiological factors might interact with cognitive factors. Some individuals have a genetic predisposition for the amygdala to be hypersensitive and this is known to be associated with negative cognitive biases and dysfunctional beliefs: these biological and psychological factors all constitute risk factors for depression. Stressful life events and amygdala/cognitive reactivity lead to activation of the hypothalamic-pituitary-adrenal axis with associated dominance of limbic activity over prefrontal cortical activity. In effect, this means automatic thoughts or hot cognitions are believed and rational cognitive reappraisal of these negative cognitions becomes very difficult.

Cognitive model of personality disorders

In DSM-IV Axis I disorders, there are positive core beliefs which allow the person to function reasonably well between episodes. In Axis II disorders, the negative core beliefs are near the surface most of the time, and the associated maladaptive assumptions and interpersonal strategies give rise to what we term personality disorders (Fig. 38.1). For example, a woman had developed epilepsy in childhood and had been 'wrapped in cotton wool' by her parents. She believed that she was basically weak and unable to cope alone, but that if she had someone to rely on she could survive in life. She saw herself as incompetent, the world as a difficult place, and others as a source of support and rescue (*core beliefs*). Her *conditional assumption* was: 'If I have someone to look after me, I will be alright.' And the interpersonal strategy that flowed naturally from this was to attach herself to people stronger than herself (*compensatory strategy*).

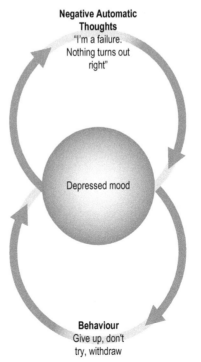

Negative Automatic Thoughts
"I'm a failure. Nothing turns out right"

Depressed mood

Behaviour
Give up, don't try, withdraw

Figure 38.1 • Vicious circles maintaining depression.

In psychiatric terms, she had a dependent personality. Beck et al (2007) have defined the relevant core beliefs and compensatory strategies for all the DSM personality disorders. A similar approach has been taken by Young who describes early maladaptive schemas, which are the equivalent of Beck's core beliefs. Young's schema-focused therapy (Young et al 2003) employs cognitive, behavioural, interpersonal and affective strategies to activate and restructure the schemas laid down in early childhood experience. Davidson (2007) has developed a cognitive therapy for personal disorders that incorporates aspects of Beck's and Young's approaches.

Characteristics of cognitive therapy

Cognitive therapy, like other behavioural and cognitive-behavioural approaches is a time-limited, structured therapy aimed at helping individuals cope with emotional problems and achieve symptom relief as well as reducing the chances of relapse. Like behaviour therapy it is structured, problem-focused and outcome oriented, placing great importance on the empirical testing of its theoretical and practical applications. In contrast to some forms of behaviour therapy, it always embeds its therapeutic techniques within a case conceptualization based on cognitive theory. The therapy takes place with weekly 50 min sessions (12–20 sessions in total), over 3–6 months. Because cognitive therapy seeks to change patients' longstanding beliefs about themselves and the world, it is necessary to establish a sound therapeutic alliance. Rather than tell patients their beliefs are unfounded, the therapist uses questioning and guided discovery to demonstrate that the beliefs are illogical or unhelpful. Beck coined the term 'collaborative empiricism' to describe the special nature of the relationship in cognitive therapy where patient and therapist test out the hypotheses of the cognitive model as applied to the patient's problems (Fig. 38.2). The therapy teaches a sceptical approach to cognitive events, encourages achieving distance from thoughts as a prelude to learning to modify them and thereby gain control over powerful negative feelings. While still requiring patients to engage actively in therapy, it has a set of techniques to work with patients who are sceptical, and so may be applicable to a wider range of less 'motivated' patients.

Conceptualization

Therapy is embedded in the cognitive model, and a conceptualization is developed for each patient to guide the treatment. For patients with clear diagnoses, the cognitive model for that particular disorder allows the therapist to plan a course of treatment and predict pitfalls. The assessment of the patient will therefore start with a cross-sectional problem-focused analysis of behaviour, cognition, emotion and physiological reactions. If a patient is depressed, the therapist will look at how the negative view of the self, the world and the future is operating in his or her life. He will assess the behavioural deficits which might be preventing the patient from engaging in activities to promote a sense of achievement, pleasure or control, and how negative automatic thoughts led to these behavioural deficits. He would

also be interested in the somatic symptoms of depression (e.g. is insomnia a problem? What are the patient's negative thoughts about their sleep disturbance?). Early experiences are important in shaping cognitive schemata (core beliefs and assumptions) and so developmental factors are also significant in a CBT assessment. How have early experiences led to certain core beliefs? What assumptions and compensatory strategies have arisen out of them? Have there been any critical incidents which have triggered the current episode? At the beginning of therapy various observer and self-report measures are used to establish a baseline so that the effectiveness of therapy can be assessed (e.g. Beck Depression Inventory, Beck Anxiety Inventory, Fear Questionnaire, Young's Schema Questionnaire). These instruments also give information about symptoms and cognitions which are of use in conceptualizing the case.

Case example

Philippa was a 35-year-old clerical worker with an 8-year history of panic and agoraphobia. She was unable to use public transport or to walk any distance alone. Her coping strategy was to ride everywhere on her bike, but she could only do this during daylight. She had 2–3 panics a week and felt pessimistic about the effectiveness of therapy: she had been treated for 5 years in analytic psychotherapy, and reported little or no improvement with her symptoms of panic and avoidance. Philippa was the daughter of an alcoholic. She had witnessed her father acting in an uncontrolled and sometimes aggressive fashion. She felt that the family pretended that her father did not have a problem, and kept it secret from the world. She was brought up in a strict religious family but was no longer religious.

By asking questions about her symptoms and inducing some of the panic feelings in the session through imagery, the therapist was able to map the interactions between her thoughts feelings and behaviours. During a panic, she started to feel out of control as she became more and more anxious. She feared that she would suddenly start crying in public, resulting in people rejecting her, or, even worse, taking pity and trying to help. At the height of the panic she would have an image of herself as a madwoman lying on the floor flailing about and moaning. As therapy progressed, she revealed that her sister had a bipolar affective disorder, and she feared that she too might be mad. She had not told her previous therapist this for fear of what they would think. She had been living with her sister some years before, when she had her first manic episode. Having seen her sister lose control and be admitted to hospital involuntarily, she thought the same might happen to her. Whenever she got panic symptoms she interpreted the anxiety as impending loss of control and catastrophized that she would go mad and be forcefully detained. The full conceptualization could not be developed until the seventh session, which illustrates how assessment in CBT is an ongoing process throughout treatment.

Initial phase of cognitive therapy

The initial phase of therapy concentrates on listening to the patient's account of their problems and forming a conceptualization, as described above. At the same time, the patient is

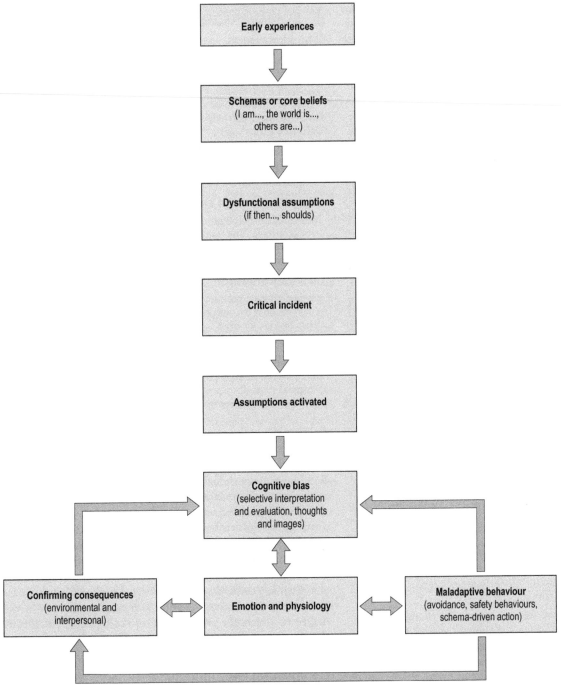

Figure 38.2 • The cognitive model.

introduced to the ideas and structure of the therapy, including the use of homework assignments. Self-help reading material can be used to aid the process of explanation (e.g. Fennell 1989). The conceptualization is shared with the patient as it is developed. This is helpful in building up an alternative picture of the problems. For instance, the depressive patient may attribute inactivity to laziness, while the cognitive conceptualization might reframe this inactivity as a symptom of depression associated with hopelessness. The basic idea to get across at this stage is that thoughts are not reality. Therapy is about clearing a space to examine thoughts and beliefs to see if they are realistic or helpful. In the first sessions problems are defined and the patient's goals for therapy established. Behavioural techniques are used to test out negative thoughts with a view to initial symptom management. In depression behavioural techniques include scheduling activities which give patients a sense of mastery or pleasure, graded tasks to help patients achieve success step by step, and specific experiments to test negative predictions. In anxiety, relaxation or distraction strategies might be taught to help the patient establish a sense of control. The aim in cognitive terms is to decrease the frequency of negative thinking and thus to improve symptoms. At all times

---

Box 38.5

CBT and medication

Depression

- CBT is as effective as antidepressant medication in outpatient depression
- The combination of CBT and antidepressants may be more effective than either alone in severe (inpatient) depression
- Combination of CBT and medication in mild – moderate (outpatient) depression is **not** more effective than either alone
- After ending treatment, relapse rates are lower with CBT than antidepressants

Anxiety

- Drug treatments have a higher relapse rate than CBT on discontinuation
- Antidepressants + exposure are the most effective treatment for panic and agoraphobia in the short term, but are not superior to CBT at long-term follow-up
- Combining exposure and medication (particularly high dose benzodiazepines) may decrease long term efficacy.

---

focused, e.g. identifying catastrophic beliefs in panic disorder and testing them with a specific behavioural experiment.

CBT (see Box 38.5) has been found to be effective for bulimia nervosa (Fairburn & Cooper 1989; Fairburn et al 1991), but insufficient evidence is available regarding anorexia. In bulimia, CBT is superior to antidepressants, waiting list controls and other psychotherapies, particularly for symptoms of the eating disorder and affective symptoms. NICE recommends CBT as the psychological treatment of choice for bulimia nervosa but it is more equivocal about recommending any particular therapy for anorexia, citing the possible helpfulness of cognitive analytic therapy, cognitive behaviour therapy, interpersonal therapy, focal psychodynamic therapy and family interventions (NICE 2004a).

There have been few trials of CBT for personality disorders. Dialectical behaviour therapy has been found to reduce parasuicidal behaviour in borderline personality disorder (Linehan et al 1991, 2006; Verheul et al 2003) and Young's schema therapy has been shown to improve a range of symptoms of borderline personality disorder (Giesen-Bloo et al 2006).

CBT in psychosis

One of the most exciting developments in CBT has been its application to psychosis. Two approaches have been demonstrated to be of benefit in schizophrenia.

Family interventions in schizophrenia

Following on from work which showed that high expressed emotion (EE), in a family with a schizophrenic member, was associated with higher relapse rates, Leff et al (1982) developed a family intervention to reduce high EE. Other behavioural interventions (e.g. Falloon 1988) do not focus purely on high EE. The various approaches share in common a focus on positive areas of family functioning and increasing family structure and stability (through problem-solving, goal-setting, cognitive restructuring, etc.). Family interventions have been extensively researched over the last 25 years and there is a very robust finding that they reduce relapse (e.g. meta-analysis of Pitschel-Waltz et al 2001).

CBT for hallucinations and delusions

Following the pioneering work of Kingdon and Turkington (1994), there has been a growing interest in the application of cognitive techniques in psychosis as an adjunct to antipsychotic medication. The therapy needs to be more flexible than standard cognitive therapy, and a great deal of emphasis is placed on establishing a good therapeutic relationship before any challenging of beliefs takes place. Kuipers et al (1997) describe the more flexible approach that was needed in their controlled trial:

> 'When necessary, treatment was arranged in locations convenient to the client, including home visits and proactive outreach following non-attendance. Within sessions the therapist was highly sensitive to changes in mental state and in particular the occurrence of paranoia. Active attempts were made to manage such problems so as to ensure that clients did not feel unduly pressured and to prevent treatment from becoming aversive. If necessary, sessions were cut short or rearranged. Difficult topics were discussed only when clients felt able to do so.'

As in all cognitive therapy, it is important to develop a shared model of the problems, gradually building up alternative explanations for symptoms the patient assumes are based on reality. The story of how the symptoms first appeared and what they meant to the patient is elaborated, and it is often possible to see that the first psychotic experiences occurred in states of altered consciousness through the impact of stress, sleep disturbance or drugs (Kingdon & Turkington 1994). If symptoms can be reconceptualized as stress reactions, the patient is then more willing to consider examining them and testing the validity of their beliefs. Delusional beliefs and beliefs about hallucinations are gently challenged and behavioural experiments devised. In addition, most of these treatment packages also teach coping strategies, challenge negative self-concepts and work on social disability and relapse. Evidence is beginning to emerge of the effectiveness of this therapy in improving symptoms. For instance, compared with treatment as usual, CBT showed a significant reduction in overall symptomatology (Kuipers et al 1997). Some 50% of the CBT group were treatment responders, compared with 31% of the control group. Comparisons with befriending or supportive therapy tend to show similar effects in the short term, but more benefit from CBT at follow-up. A meta-analysis (Pilling et al 2002) concluded CBT produced higher rates of 'important improvement' in mental state and demonstrated positive effects on continuous measures of mental state at follow-up. CBT also seems to be associated with low drop-out rates.

However, a note of caution has been sounded in recent years. A large and well-conducted randomized controlled trial failed to find an effect of CBT or family intervention on relapse rates in psychosis, but it did have some effect on depression, delusional distress and social functioning (Garety et al 2008). Wykes et al (2008) conducted a meta-analysis of CBT for psychosis: CBT plus treatment as usual demonstrated statistically significant effects on depression, anxiety, positive and negative symptoms and functioning, but not relapse rates.

CBT for bipolar disorder is in its infancy, but techniques now exist to help patients detect and attenuate hypomanic episodes. Lam et al (2003) demonstrated that CBT reduces bipolar episodes and admissions. However, Scott et al (2006) failed to find an effect on relapse rates. In their recent meta-analysis Lynch et al (2010) failed to find any effect of CBT for schizophrenia or bipolar disorder when compared to non-specific interventions. As has been found with medication, effectiveness trials in severe mental illness do not always support the initial enthusiasm generated by RCTs, but it is likely that, rather than expecting CBT to be a panacea, we should look more closely at the groups of patients who do respond and be clear about what the therapy can and cannot do. For psychosis this is probably the not inconsiderable number of stable patients who have chronic residual treatment resistant symptoms: reducing distressing symptoms and improving quality of life is surely a legitimate aim, even if therapy does not reduce the frequency of relapse.

Recent developments in CBT

Behaviour therapy was the first wave, cognitive the second wave, and now a resurgent form of behaviour therapy is on the scene. The term *third wave* therapy refers to a group of therapies including: dialectical behaviour therapy (DBT; Linehan 1993); acceptance and commitment therapy (ACT: Hayes et al 1999); behavioural activation (BA; Jacobson et al 2001); and functional analytic psychotherapy (FAP; Kohlenberg et al 2009). These therapies share a foundation in radical behaviourism and an interest in the *function* of problematic behaviours, thoughts, emotions and physical sensations rather than their *content* (Hayes 2004). According to Hayes they emphasize 'contextual and experiential change strategies rather than direct and didactic ones'. Their difference from traditional 'second wave' CBT is most obvious in their approach to cognition. Rather than challenge negative thoughts, patients are helped to acknowledge the thoughts without engaging with them. This is done through experiential exercises (ACT) or mindfulness practice (DBT). The behavioural component of therapy may involve a functional analysis of unhelpful behaviours (FAP) or identifying behaviours that help you work towards your life values (ACT). Another feature is an emphasis on directly experiencing negative emotions without engaging in ruminations or avoidance behaviour.

Evidence for these new therapies is limited, but studies suggest that behavioural activation for depression may be as effective or even more effective than traditional cognitive therapy (Cuijpers et al 2006). Mindfulness based cognitive therapy (MBCT; Segal et al 2002) is often included in this group, although it is not based on Skinnerian learning theory. MBCT has been developed to treat recurrent depression. It teaches mindfulness meditation, a secular application of Buddhist meditation practice. This develops the skill of being able to accept whatever we are experiencing in the moment without trying to fix or change it. By learning to be aware of what is happening to us here and now we can make skilful choices about how we act so that we do not get caught up in depressive ruminations or unhelpful behavioural patterns. MBCT is proving very popular and there is evidence that it can reduce relapse rates in recurrent depression (Teasdale et al 2000).

Conclusions

Cognitive behaviour therapy is a broad church, which embraces a variety of behavioural and cognitive theories and techniques. Its flexibility allows it to be applied to a wide range of conditions and there is strong evidence for its effectiveness (Butler et al 2006). Despite this empirical backing, CBT should not be considered a panacea. While statistical superiority over controls is well established the *clinical significance* of results is sometimes less dramatic, with many patients improved but still symptomatic. In severe mental illness the claims of CBT may have been overstated (Lynch et al 2010). Like all therapies CBT requires participation from the patient, and it may be less helpful with people who are unable or unwilling to engage in the self-help strategies required of them.

In Britain, the strength of the evidence base for CBT has significantly influenced the NICE guidelines and as a result it has become the dominant psychological therapy in the NHS. The Improving Access to Psychological Therapies (IAPT) programme will greatly increase the number of CBT therapists in primary care making it the largest naturalistic trial of CBT for anxiety and depression ever undertaken. One of the criticisms of CBT and the NICE guidelines approach has been that too much emphasis is placed on findings from randomized controlled trials which may not be applicable to the complexity, chronicity and co-morbidity seen in clinical services. IAPT will help to tell us how much these findings can be generalized. This move from efficacy studies, which show the treatment works in controlled settings, to effectiveness studies which assess its place in the 'real world' will be the next phase of CBT and promises to be a fascinating time.

Further reading

Beck, J.S., 1995. Cognitive therapy: basics and beyond. Guilford Press, New York.

Beck, A.T., Rush, A.J., Shaw, B.F., et al., 1979. Cognitive therapy of depression. Guilford Press, New York.

Clark, D.M., Beck, A.T., 2010. Cognitive therapy of anxiety disorders: science and practice. Guilford Press, New York.

Stern, R., Drummond, L., 1991. The practice of behavioural and cognitive

psychotherapy. Cambridge University Press, Cambridge.

Westbrook, D., Kennerley, H., Kirk, J., 2007. An introduction to cognitive behaviour therapy: skills and applications. Sage, London.

References

Adams, C.D., Dickinson, A., 1981. Instrumental responding following reinforcer devaluation. Q. J. Exp. Psychol. 33B, 109–121.

Bandura, A., 1971. Principles of behavior modification. Holt, Rhinehart & Winston, New York.

Beck, A.T., 1976. Cognitive therapy and the emotional disorders. International Universities Press, New York.

Beck, A.T., 1996. Beyond belief: a theory of modes, personality and psychopathology. In: Salkovskis, P.M. (Ed.), Frontiers of cognitive therapy. Guilford Press, New York.

Beck, A.T., 2008. The evolution of the cognitive model of depression and its neurobiological correlates. Am. J. Psychiatry 165, 969–977.

Beck, A.T., Clark, D.A., 1997. An information processing model of anxiety: automatic and strategic processes. Behav. Res. Ther. 35, 49–58.

Beck, A.T., Rush, A.J., Shaw, B.F., et al., 1979. Cognitive therapy of depression. Guilford Press, New York.

Beck, A.T., Emery, G., Greenberg, R.L., 1985. Anxiety disorders and phobias: a cognitive perspective. Basic Books, New York.

Beck, A.T., Freeman, A., Davis, D.D., 2007. Cognitive therapy of personality disorders, second ed. Guilford Press, New York.

Bell, A.C., D'Zurilla, T.J., 2009. Problem-solving therapy for depression: a meta-analysis. Clin. Psychol. Rev. 29, 348–353.

Bennet-Levy, J., Butler, G., Fennel, M., et al., (Eds.), 2004. Oxford guide to behavioural experiments in cognitive therapy. Oxford University Press, Oxford.

Blackburn, I.M., Moore, R.G., 1997. Controlled acute and follow-up trial of cognitive therapy and pharmacotherapy in out-patients with recurrent depression. Br. J. Psychiatry 171, 328–334.

Brewer, W., 1974. There is no convincing evidence for operant or classical conditioning in adult humans. In: Weimer, W., Palermo, D. (Eds.), Cognition and the symbolic processes1. Erlbaum, Hillsdale NJ, pp. 1–42.

Butler, A.C., Chapman, J.E., Forman, E.M., et al., 2006. The empirical status of cognitive-behavioral therapy: a review of meta-analyses. Clin. Psychol. Rev. 26, 17–31.

Chambless, D.L., Gillis, M.M., 1993. Cognitive therapy of anxiety disorders. J. Consult. Clin. Psychol. 61, 248–260.

Churchill, R., Hunot, V., Corney, R., et al., 2001. A systematic review of controlled trials of the effectiveness and cost-effectiveness of brief psychological treatments for depression. Health Technol. Assess. 5, 1–173.

Clark, D.A., Beck, A.T., 1999. Scientific foundations of cognitive theory and therapy of depression. Wiley, New York.

Clark, D.M., 1996. Panic disorder: from theory to therapy. In: Salkovskis, P.M. (Ed.), Frontiers of cognitive therapy. Guilford Press, New York, pp. 318–344.

Clark, D.M., Beck, A.T., 2010. Cognitive therapy of anxiety disorders: science and practice. Guilford Press, New York.

Clark, D.M., Wells, P.A., 1995. A cognitive model of social phobia. In: Heimberg, R.G., Liebowitz, M.R., Hope, D.A., et al., (Eds.), Social phobia: diagnosis, assessment and treatment. Guilford Press, New York, pp. 69–93.

Cuijpers, P., van Straten, A., Warmerdam, L., 2006. Behavioral activation treatments of depression: a meta-analysis. Clin. Psychol. Rev. 27, 318–326.

Davidson, K.M., 2007. Cognitive therapy for personality disorders: a guide for clinicians, second ed. Routledge, Hove.

Deckersbach, T., Gershuny, B.S., Otto, M.W., 2000. Cognitive behavioural therapy for depression: applications and outcome. Psychiatr. Clin. North Am. 23, 795–809.

De Rubeis, R.J., Crits Cristoph, P., 1998. Empirically supported individual and group treatments for adult mental disorders. J. Consult. Clin. Psychol. 66, 37–52.

D'Zurilla, T.J., Goldfried, M.R., 1971. Problem solving and behaviour modification. J. Abnorm. Psychol. 78, 107–126.

Ehlers, A., Clark, D.M., 2000. A cognitive model of posttraumatic stress disorder. Behav. Res. Ther. 38, 319–345.

Ellis, A., 1962. Reason and emotion in psychotherapy. Lyle Stuart, New York.

Emmelkamp, P.M.G., Wessels, H., 1975. Flooding in imagination versus flooding in vivo for agoraphobics. Behav. Res. Ther. 13, 7–15.

Evans, M.D., Hollon, S.D., DeRubeis, R.J., et al., 1992. Differential relapse following cognitive therapy and pharmacotherapy for depression. Arch. Gen. Psychiatry 49, 802–808.

Fairburn, C.G., Cooper, P.J., 1989. Eating disorders. In: Hawton, K., Salkovskis, P.M., Kirk, J. et al., (Eds.), Cognitive behaviour therapy for psychiatric problems. Oxford Medical, Oxford, pp. 277–314.

Fairburn, C.G., Jones, R., Peveler, R.C., et al., 1991. Three psychological treatments for bulimia nervosa. A comparative trial. Arch. Gen. Psychiatry 48, 463–469.

Falloon, I.R.H. (Ed.), 1988. Handbook of behavioural family therapy. Unwin Hyman, London.

Fennell, M.J., 1989. Depression. In: Hawton, K., Salkovskis, P.M., Kirk, J., et al., (Eds.), Cognitive behaviour therapy for psychiatric problems. Oxford Medical, Oxford, pp. 169–234.

Garety, P., Fowler, D.G., Freeman, D., et al., 2008. Cognitive–behavioural therapy and family intervention for relapse prevention and symptom reduction in psychosis: randomised controlled trial. Br. J. Psychiatry 192, 412–423.

Giesen-Bloo, J., van Dyck, R., Spinhoven, P., et al., 2006. Outpatient psychotherapy for borderline personality disorder: randomized trial of schema-focused therapy vs transference-focused psychotherapy. Arch. Gen. Psychiatry 63, 649–658.

Gould, R.A., Otto, M.W., Pollack, M.H., 1995. A meta-analysis of treatment outcome for panic disorders. Clin. Psychol. Rev. 15, 819–844.

Greenberger, D., Padesky, C.A., 1995. Mind over mood: a cognitive therapy treatment manual. Guilford Press, New York.

Hayes, S.C., 2004. Acceptance and commitment therapy and the new behavior therapies: mindfulness, acceptance and relationship. In: Hayes, S.C., Follette, V.M., Linehan, M. (Eds.), Mindfulness and acceptance: expanding the cognitive behavioral tradition. Guilford Press, New York, pp. 1–29.

Hayes, S.C., Strosahl, K.D., Wilson, K.G., 1999. Acceptance and commitment therapy: an experiential approach to behavior change. Guilford Press, New York.

Hollon, S.D., DeRubeis, R.J., Shelton, R.C., et al., 2005. Prevention of relapse following cognitive therapy vs medication in moderate to severe depression. Arch. Gen. Psychiatry 62, 417–422.

Jacobson, N.S., Martell, C.R., Dimidjian, S., 2001. Behavioral activation therapy for depression: returning to contextual roots. Clin. Psychol. 8, 255–270.

Kanfer, F.H., Karoly, P., 1972. Self control: a behavioristic excursion into the lion's den. Behav. Ther. 3, 398–416.

Kasvikis, Y., Marks, I.M., 1988. Clomipramine, self-exposure and therapist accompanied exposure in obsessive-compulsive ritualisers: two-year follow up. J. Anxiety Disord. 2, 291–298.

Kingdon, D.G., Turkington, D., 1994. Cognitive behaviour therapy of schizophrenia. Lawrence Erlbaum, Hove.

Kohlenberg, R.J., Tsai, M., Kanter, J.W., 2009. A guide to functional analytic psychotherapy: awareness, courage, love, and behaviorism. Springer, New York.

Kuipers, E., Garety, P., Fowler, D., et al., 1997. London-East Anglia randomised controlled trial of cognitive-behavioural therapy for psychosis. I: effects of the treatment phase. Br. J. Psychiatry 171, 319–327.

Kurtz, M.M., Mueser, K.T., 2008. A meta-analysis of controlled research on social skills training for schizophrenia. J. Consult. Clin. Psychol. 76, 491–504.

Lam, D.H., Watkins, E.R., Hayward, P., et al., 2003. A randomized controlled study of cognitive therapy for relapse prevention for bipolar affective disorder: outcome of the first year. Arch. Gen. Psychiatry 60, 145–152.

Leff, J., Kuipers, L., Berkowitz, R., Eberlein-Fries, R., et al., 1982. A controlled trial of intervention in the families of schizophrenic patients. Br. J. Psychiatry 141, 121–134.

Linehan, M., Bohus, M., Lynch, T., 2007. Dialectical behavior therapy for pervasive emotion dysregulation: theoretical and practical underpinnings. In: Gross, J. (Ed.), Handbook of emotion regulation. Guilford Press, New York.

Linehan, M.M., 1993. Cognitive-behavioural treatment of borderline personality disorder. Guilford Press, London.

Linehan, M.M., Armstrong, H.E., Suarez, A., et al., 1991. Cognitive-behavioral treatment of chronically parasuicidal borderline patients. Arch. Gen. Psychiatry 48, 1060–1064.

Linehan, M.M., Comtois, K.A., Murray, A.M., et al., 2006. Two-year randomized controlled trial and follow-up of dialectical behavior therapy vs therapy by experts for suicidal behaviors and borderline personality disorder. Arch. Gen. Psychiatry 63, 757–766.

Lynch, D., Laws, K.R., McKenna, P.J., 2010. Cognitive behavioural therapy for major psychiatric disorder: does it really work? A meta-analytical review of well-controlled trials. Psychol. Med. 40, 9–24.

Mahoney, M.J., 1974. Cognition and behavior modification. Ballinger, Cambridge MA.

Mahoney, M.J., 1995a. Theoretical developments in the cognitive psychotherapies. In: Mahoney, M.J. (Ed.), Cognitive and constructive psychotherapies: theory, research and practice. Springer, New York, pp. 3–19.

Mahoney, M.J. (Ed.), 1995b. Cognitive and constructive psychotherapies: theory, research and practice. Springer, New York.

Marks, I.M., 1987. Fears, phobias and rituals: panic anxiety and their disorders. Oxford University Press, New York.

Marks, I.M., O'Sullivan, G., 1988. Drugs and psychological treatments for agoraphobia/panic and obsessive compulsive disorders: a review. Br. J. Psychiatry 153, 650–658.

Marks, I.M., Swinson, R.P., Basoglu, M., et al., 1993. Alprazolam and exposure alone and combined in panic disorder with agoraphobia. J. Psychiatry 162, 776–787.

Marks, I.M., Kenwright, M., McDonough, M., et al., 2004. Saving clinicians' time by delegating routine aspects of therapy to a computer: a randomised controlled trial in phobia/panic disorder. Psychol. Med. 34, 9–17.

Mcdonald, R., Sartory, G., Grey, S.J., et al., 1978. Effects of self-exposure instructions on agoraphobic patients. Behav. Res. Ther. 17, 83–85.

McNally, R.J., Steketee, G.S., 1985. Etiology and maintenance of severe animal phobias. Behav. Res. Ther. 23, 431–435.

Meichenbaum, D., 1977. Cognitive behaviour modification: an integrative approach. Plenum Press, New York.

Meichenbaum, D., Cameron, R., 1973. Training schizophrenics to talk to themselves: a means of developing attentional controls. Behav. Ther. 4, 515–534.

Meichenbaum, D., Goodman, J., 1971. Training impulsive children to talk to themselves: a means of developing self-control. J. Abnorm. Psychol. 77, 115–126.

Monroe, S.M., Harkness, K.L., 2005. Life stress, the 'kindling' hypothesis and the recurrence of depression: considerations from a life stress perspective. Am. J. Psychiatry 112, 417–445.

Moorey, S., 1996. When bad things happen to rational people: cognitive therapy in adverse life situations. In: Salkovskis, P. (Ed.), Frontiers of cognitive therapy. Guilford Press, New York, pp. 450–470.

Moorey, S., 2010. The six cycles model: growing a 'vicious flower' for depression. Behav. Cogn. Psychother. 38, 173–184.

Moorey, S., Greer, S., 2002. Cognitive behaviour therapy for people with cancer. Oxford University Press, Oxford.

NICE, 2004a. CG9 Eating disorders: core interventions in the treatment and management of anorexia nervosa, bulimia nervosa and related eating disorders – NICE guideline. Online. Available: http://guidance.nice.uk/CG9.

NICE, 2004b. Anxiety: management of anxiety (panic disorder, with or without agoraphobia, and generalised anxiety disorder) in adults in primary, secondary and community care. Online. Available: http://guidance.nice.org.uk/CG22.

NICE, 2009a. Core interventions in the treatment and management of schizophrenia in primary and secondary care (update) NICE Guideline. Online. Available: http://guidance.nice.org.uk/CG82.

NICE, 2009b. Depression: management of depression in primary and secondary care (Update). NICE Guideline. Online. Available: http://guidance.nice.org.uk/CG90.

Padesky, C.A., 1994. Schema change processes in cognitive therapy. Clin. Psychol. Psychother. 1, 267–278.

Paykel, E.S., Scott, J., Teasdale, J.D., et al., 1999. Prevention of relapse in residual depression by cognitive therapy: a controlled trial. Arch. Gen. Psychiatry 56, 829–835.

Pilling, S., Bebbington, P., Kuipers, E., et al., 2002. Psychological treatments in schizophrenia: I. Meta-analysis of family intervention and cognitive behaviour therapy. Psychol. Med. 32, 763–782.

Pitschel-Waltz, G., Leucht, S., Bauml, J., et al., 2001. The effect of family interventions on relapse and rehospitalisation in schizophrenia – a meta-analysis. Schizophr. Bull. 27, 73–92.

Rachman, S.J., de Silva, P., 1978. Normal and abnormal obsessions. Behav. Res. Ther. 16, 233–238.

Rapee, R.M., 1991. The conceptual overlap between cognition and conditioning in clinical psychology. Clin. Psychol. Rev. 11, 193–203.

Roth, A., Fonagy, P., 2004. What works for whom? A critical review of psychotherapy research, second ed. Guilford Press, London.

Salkovskis, P.M., 1985. Obsessive-compulsive problems: a cognitive-behavioural analysis. Behav. Res. Ther. 23, 571–583.

Salkovskis, P.M., Harrison, J., 1984. Abnormal and normal obsessions: a replication. Behav. Res. Ther. 27, 549–552.

Sánchez-Meca, J., Rosa-Alcázar, A.I., Marín-Martínez, F., et al., 2010. Psychological treatment of panic disorder with or without agoraphobia: a meta-analysis. Clin. Psychol. Rev. 30, 37–50.

Scher, C., Ingram, R., Segal, Z.V., 2005. Cognitive reactivity and vulnerability: empirical evaluation of construct activation and cognitive diatheses in unipolar depression. Clin. Psychol. Rev. 25, 487–510.

Scott, J., Paykel, E., Morriss, R., et al., 2006. Cognitive–behavioural therapy for severe and recurrent bipolar disorders: randomised controlled trial. Br. J. Psychiatry 188, 313–320.

Segal, Z.V., Gemar, M., Williams, S., 1999. Differential cognitive response to a mood challenge following successful cognitive therapy or pharmacotherapy for unipolar depression. J. Abnorm. Psychol. 108, 3–10.

Segal, Z.V., Williams, J.M.G., Teasdale, J.D., 2002. Mindfulness-based cognitive therapy for depression: a new approach to preventing relapse. Guilford Press, New York.

Seligman, M.E.P., 1971. Phobias and preparedness. Behav. Ther. 2, 307–320.

Stern, R., Marks, I.M., 1973. Brief and prolonged flooding: a comparison in agoraphobic patients. Arch. Gen. Psychiatry 28, 270–276.

Stuart, S., Bowers, W.A., 1995. Cognitive therapy with inpatients: review and meta-analysis. J. Cogn. Psychother. 9, 85–92.

Teasdale, J.D., Segal, Z.V., Williams, J.M.G., et al., 2000. Prevention of relapse/recurrence in major depression by mindfulness-based cognitive therapy. J. Consult. Clin. Psychol. 68, 615–623.

Verheul, R., Van Den Bosch, L.M., Koeter, M.W., et al., 2003. Dialectical behaviour therapy for women with borderline personality disorder: 12-month, randomised clinical trial in the Netherlands. Br. J. Psychiatry 182, 135–140.

Warwick, H.M.C., Salkovskis, P.M., 1989. Hypochondriasis. In: Scott, J., Williams, J.M., Beck, A.T. (Eds.), Cognitive therapy in clinical practice. Croom Helm, London.

Watson, J.B., Rayner, R., 1920. Conditioned emotional reactions. J. Exp. Psychol. 3, 1–14.

Wells, A., 1997. Cognitive therapy of anxiety disorders. Wiley, Chichester.

Wells, A., 2000. Emotional disorders and metacognition: innovative cognitive therapy. Wiley, Chichester.

Wolitzky-Taylor, K.B., Horowitz, J.D., Powers, M.B., et al., 2008. Psychological approaches in the treatment of specific phobias: a meta-analysis. Clin. Psychol. Rev. 28, 1021–1037.

Wolpe, J., 1958. Psychotherapy by reciprocal inhibition. Standard University Press, Palo Alto CA.

Wykes, T., Steel, C., Everitt, B., et al., 2008. Cognitive behavior therapy for schizophrenia: effect sizes, clinical models, and methodological rigor. Schizophr. Bull. 34, 523–537.

Young, J.E., Klosko, J.S., Weishaar, M.E., 2003. Schema therapy: a practitioner's guide. Guilford Press, New York.

Psychopharmacology

Pádraig Wright   Michael F. O'Neill

CHAPTER CONTENTS

Introduction

This chapter provides an account of basic and clinical psychopharmacology, followed by an account of the main classes of psychotropic drugs.

Basic psychopharmacology

The human brain accounts for 2% of our bodyweight but utilizes 10% of the energy and 20% of the oxygen that we consume. Glucose is metabolized in the brain, as in all other tissues, by oxidative phosphorylation with the production of adenosine triphosphate. In addition, glucose is converted to glutamate, γ-amino butyric acid (GABA) and aspartate in the brain via the GABA shunt in which the enzyme glutamate decarboxylase catalyses the conversion of glutamate to GABA.

Every substance that enters the brain must cross the blood–brain barrier (BBB). The BBB maintains brain glucose levels at the expense of general blood glucose levels via a sodium-linked active transport system. The BBB prevents the passage of immunoglobulins, viruses and bacteria into the brain. Lipid-soluble substances, including lipid-soluble drugs, readily cross the BBB but lipid-insoluble drugs pass into the brain only very slowly.

Neurotransmitters and neuroreceptors

Neurotransmitters are substances that transfer signals across synapses between presynaptic and postsynaptic neurons. The neurotransmitters act on postsynaptic neurons via receptor molecules. Neurotransmitters (Fig. 39.1) may be defined as substances that:

- Are synthesized in the presynaptic neuron
- Are stored inactively in the presynaptic terminal
- Are released from the presynaptic terminal when the presynaptic neuron depolarizes
- Bind to a receptor at, and cause an effect (opening or closing of ion channels) in, the postsynaptic neuron
- Have a presynaptic reuptake mechanism and/or degrading enzymes in the synapse that inactivate them.

Neurotransmitters may be classified into families based upon their chemical structures. The most important neurotransmitter families are: (1) the monoamines dopamine (DA), histamine (H), noradrenaline or norepinephrine (NA) and serotonin (5HT); (2) the excitatory amino acids glutamate, glycine and aspartate; and (3) the neuropeptides (endorphins, somatostatin, cholecystokinin, vasoactive intestinal peptide, angiotensin, neurotensin and substance P). There are also inhibitory amino acids such as GABA. Other neurotransmitters include neurohormones (corticotrophin and thyrotrophin release hormones) and the neuronally synthesized gases, nitric oxide (see phosphodiesterase type 5 inhibitors below) and carbon monoxide.

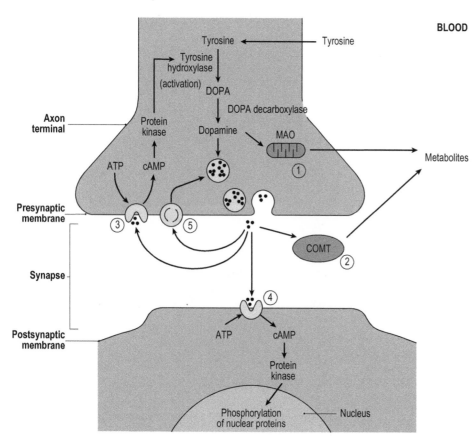

Figure 39.1 • Dopamine (and serotonin and noradrenaline) is: (1) degraded by monoamine oxidase (MAO) in presynaptic mitochondria, and (2) by synaptic catechol-O-methyltransferase (COMT) in the synapse. Dopamine binds to (3) presynaptic, as well as (4) postsynaptic membrane receptors, and is (5) actively transported back into the axon terminal.

Neurotransmitters bind to neuroreceptors which are classified into 'superfamilies' of which the two most important are the ligand gated ion channel receptors and the G-protein coupled (or gated) ion channel receptors. Ion channels are complex structures usually made up of several subunits, for example the nicotinic receptor is composed of five subunits. The pharmacological activity of ion channels may be altered significantly depending on their compositional subunits. Conformational changes in the structure of neurotransmitters allows them to adopt a range of forms and to bind to neuroreceptors with varying degrees of efficiency. This property bestows a range of activities at a large number of neuroreceptor subtypes on any single neurotransmitter. Dopamine has five receptor subtypes for example, while serotonin has 15.

Ligand gated ion channel receptors

Neuronal depolarization depends on the opening of ion channels in the neuronal membrane and the subsequent influx of sodium ions (Na^+) and efflux of potassium ions (K^+). The response of a neuron to ion channel receptor activation by either the natural ligand/neurotransmitter or a drug is rapid and brief. Examples of this mechanism include the action of ACh at the cholinergic nicotinic receptors of the neuromuscular junction, and GABA at $GABA_A$ receptors in the brain.

The ion channel of the cholinergic nicotinic receptor opens when Ach binds to it, allowing the influx of Na^+ ions and resulting in an excitatory postsynaptic potential. Glutamate receptors behave similarly.

$GABA_A$ receptors in the brain differ from nicotinic and glutamate receptors in that they open in response to GABA and allow the influx of both K^+ and chloride ions (Cl^-). This results in an inhibitory postsynaptic potential. BZD drugs such as diazepam have high affinity for, and are agonists at, the $GABA_A$ receptor. Binding of a BZD drug to the $GABA_A$ receptor enhances the effect of GABA and causes a greater influx of K^+ and Cl^- than binding of GABA alone.

G-protein coupled receptors

Some receptors are linked to ion channels and enzymes by guanine triphosphate binding, or G, proteins. The G-protein is embedded in the intracellular surface of the cell membrane and is activated when a ligand binds to the receptor. The activated G-protein then either stimulates or inhibits adenylate cyclase or other second messengers.

Examples of G-protein coupled receptors include adrenergic receptors that bind catecholamines (α_1 and α_2, β_{1-3}), serotonergic receptors ($5HT_{1A-1F}$, $5HT_2$), and dopaminergic receptors (D_1-like G_S coupled and D_2-like G_I coupled). Monoamine neurotransmitters bind exclusively to G-protein coupled receptors with the exception of the ligand gated ion channel $5-HT_3$ receptor.

The G-protein coupled receptors are of particular interest because all of the receptors important to psychiatry, with the exception of the ion channel glutamate and $GABA_A$ receptors, are G-protein coupled.

Mechanisms of action of psychotropic drugs

Psychotropic drugs may modify neuronal function through five mechanisms of action as follows:

* Increasing synthesis of neurotransmitter
* Promoting release of neurotransmitter into the synapse
* Mimicking the action of the endogenous neurotransmitter at the receptor (an agonist)
* Inhibiting the action of the endogenous neurotransmitter at the receptor (an antagonist)
* Prolonging the activity of the endogenous neurotransmitter by either preventing the action of degrading enzymes (e.g. acetylcholinesterase inhibitors) or preventing reuptake to the neurone (e.g. serotonin reuptake inhibitors).

Dopamine

Dopamine is described in some detail because of its role in the mechanism of action of antipsychotic drugs. The three dopaminergic systems of most importance to psychiatry originate in the midbrain and diencephalon and are depicted in Figure 39.2.

The mesocorticolimbic system

Dopaminergic neurons project from the ventral tegmental nucleus to the limbic, septal and frontocortical areas. The psychopharmacology of the mesocorticolimbic system may be summarized as follows:

* Drugs of abuse such as alcohol, cocaine and amphetamine release DA at the nucleus accumbens. It is therefore believed that this system is involved with reward and pleasure.
* All effective antipsychotic (AP) drugs are D_2 receptor antagonists. It is therefore believed that excess mesocorticolimbic dopaminergic function may underpin schizophrenia, especially its positive symptoms.
* Frontal D_1 receptors appear to play an important role in normal cognitive function, and deficient mesocorticolimbic dopaminergic function in the prefrontal and cingulate cortex has been implicated in the negative symptoms of schizophrenia.
* Mesocorticolimbic dopaminergic dysfunction has been implicated in mood disorders, particularly depression (prefrontal cortex/cingulate gyrus, nucleus accumbens), and in psychomotor retardation (dorsolateral prefrontal cortex, caudate nucleus).

The nigrostriatal system

Dopaminergic neurons project from the substantia nigra to the striatum. Degeneration of this system causes Parkinson disease, while blockade of D_2 receptors here by AP drugs causes extrapyramidal syndromes such as dystonia, akathisia and parkinsonism.

The tuberoinfundibular system

Dopaminergic neurons project from the arcuate nucleus of the hypothalamus to the pituitary gland. DA inhibits the release of prolactin and blockade of D_2 receptors here by AP drugs causes hyperprolactinaemia.

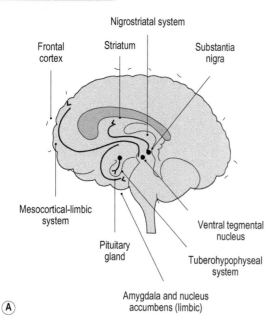

(A)

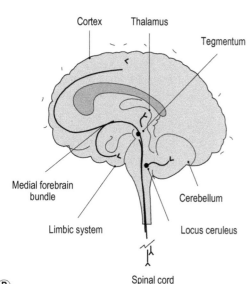

(B)

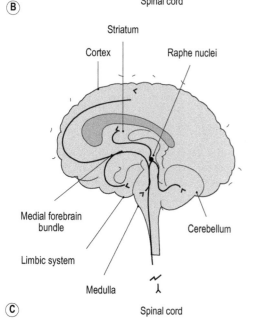

(C)

Biochemistry

DA is synthesized from phenylalanine via L-tyrosine and degraded by monoamine oxidase (MAO) and catechol-O-methyltransferase (COMT) to homovanillic acid (HVA) (Fig. 39.3). DA receptors are subdivided into the D_1-like GS coupled (D_1 and D_5) and the D_2-like G_I coupled (D_2, D_3 and D_4) classes (see below).

Clinical aspects

All AP drugs are potent D_2 receptor antagonists and many are also potent $5HT_{2A}$ receptor antagonists. Improvements in positive and negative symptoms are thought to result from altered dopaminergic function in the limbic and prefrontal cortex, respectively.

Tricyclic (TCA) antidepressant (AD) drugs inhibit the reuptake of DA to the presynaptic neuron by the DA transporter while monoamine type A oxidase inhibitor (MAOI) AD drugs increase synaptic DA by inhibiting MAO, its catalytic enzyme.

Amphetamines increase synaptic DA by causing its release into the synapse and both amphetamines and cocaine potently inhibit the DA reuptake transporter.

Noradrenaline (norepinephrine)

Noradrenergic neurons originate in the locus coeruleus in the floor of the fourth ventricle (Fig. 39.2). They project especially to the medulla and spinal cord, the cerebellum, the limbic system and thalamus, and the cortex. Noradrenergic systems are believed to be critical to arousal, attention, mood and pain because:

- Activity in noradrenergic neurons in the locus ceruleus increases in response to novel or aversive stimuli
- α_1- and α_2-receptor antagonists cause sedation
- Many antidepressant (AD) drugs increase noradrenergic neurotransmission
- Some AD drugs effectively alleviate pain.

Biochemistry

Noradrenaline (norepinephrine) is synthesized from phenylalanine (via dopamine) and degraded by MAO and COMT to 3-methoxy-4-hydroxy phenylglycol and 3-methoxy-4-hydroxy-mandelic acid respectively (Fig. 39.3). Noradrenergic receptor subtypes include α_1 and α_2 and β_{1-3} (see below).

Figure 39.2 • Schematic representation. (A) The mesocorticolimbic and nigrostriatal dopaminergic systems originate in the midbrain and project to the frontal cortex and limbic system, and to the striatum, respectively. The tuberohypophyseal dopaminergic system originates in the diencephalon and projects to the pituitary gland. (B) Noradrenergic neurons originating in the locus coeruleus project to the cortex, limbic system, thalamus, cerebellum and spinal cord. Tegmental noradrenergic neurons project to the brainstem and spinal cord. (C) Serotonergic neurons arise in the raphe nuclei and project to the cortex, limbic system, striatum, cerebellum, medulla and spinal cord.

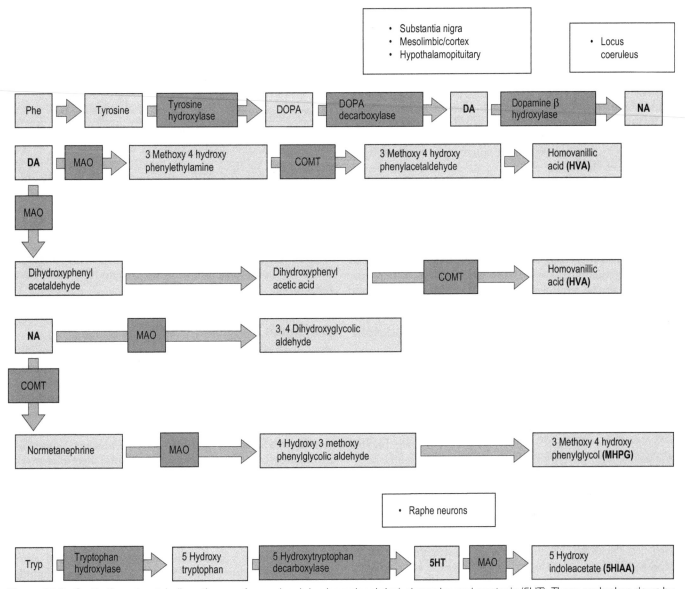

Figure 39.3 • Synthetic and metabolic pathways of: norepinephrine (norepinephrine), dopamine and serotonin (5HT). These are broken down by the monoamine oxidase (MAO) enzymes located in presynaptic mitochondria. Noradrenaline and dopamine are also broken down by the synaptic enzyme catechol-*O*-methyltransferase (COMT). Monoamines are all actively transported back into the neuron from the synaptic cleft by specific transporters.

Clinical aspects

Abnormalities of noradrenergic function are believed to play a role in depression and bipolar disorder. TCA AD drugs increase synaptic NA by inhibiting its reuptake to the presynaptic neuron by the NA transporter.

MAOI AD drugs increase synaptic NA by inhibiting MAO, its catalytic enzyme. There are two types of MAO, MAO-A and MAO-B. MAO-A is the most efficient in degrading NA (and 5HT) and its irreversible inhibition by MAOIs (especially phenelzine) may impair the metabolism of both dietary tyramine and sympathomimetic drugs such as phenyl-propanolamine and cause severe hypertension. Moclobemide, a reversible inhibitor of MAO-A, may pose less of a risk in this regard.

Amphetamines increase synaptic NA by promoting its rapid release into the synapse and both amphetamines and cocaine potently inhibit the NA reuptake transporter.

Serotonin

Serotonergic neurons originate in the dorsal and median raphe nucleii in the brainstem (Fig. 39.2). They project to the medulla and spinal cord, the cerebellum, the limbic system and striatum, and the cortex. Serotonergic systems are believed to be critical to sleep, appetite and mood because:

* Reduced serotonergic function may cause insomnia and depression

Despite the fact that psychotropic drugs are largely eliminated by renal excretion, there is no general restriction on the use of such drugs in patients with mild to moderate renal impairment. However, the dose of amisulpride should be reduced and chloral hydrate, lithium and acamprosate should be avoided in patients with moderate renal impairment, while clozapine is contraindicated in severe renal impairment.

Psychotropic drug development

Pharmaceutical companies wishing to license a new prescription psychotropic drug for clinical use must satisfy the requirements of regulatory authorities such as the European Medicines Agency in Europe as to the drug's quality, safety and efficacy. All drugs therefore undergo stringent preclinical and clinical evaluations before they are licensed for clinical use.

Preclinical evaluations precede clinical evaluations (e.g. 6-month primate toxicology studies must be undertaken before the drug may be administered chronically to humans) and include:

- Quality testing to ensure each tablet or parenteral formulation contains exactly the ingredients stated in its license and is stable under the storage conditions and for the period of time or shelf-life similarly stated
- Investigation of the mechanism of action of the drug including any transmitter, receptor, transporter or enzyme it affects either intentionally or unintentionally
- *In vitro* toxicological and pharmacodynamic testing in cultured cells and tissues
- *In vivo* toxicological, pharmacodynamic and behavioural testing in a range of animals (rodents, non-rodents and primates).

Clinical evaluations include:

- Phase I open-label clinical studies with single, escalating and multiple-doses in small numbers of healthy volunteers, the majority of whom are male because teratogenicity of the compound has not yet been investigated. These studies are primarily designed to determine the safety and pharmacokinetics of the new drug and to evaluate drug–drug interactions
- Phase II open-label and double-blind clinical studies with single, escalating and multiple-doses in relatively small numbers of patients suffering with the disease the new drug is designed to treat. These trials are designed to further evaluate safety, pharmacokinetics and pharmacodynamics, and to determine appropriate doses and dosing regimens
- Phase III clinical trials designed to provide statistical evidence that the drug is more effective than placebo and at least as effective and safe as a comparator drug (a drug that has already been licensed to treat the disease being investigated). Phase III trials usually involve large numbers (thousands) of patients treated double-blind with various doses of the drug being developed, a comparator and/or placebo.

The main classes of psychotropic drugs

There now follows an account of the pharmacokinetics and pharmacodynamics ('what the drug does to the body') of the main classes of psychotropic drugs. Our knowledge of drugs is changing constantly and the most up-to-date sources of information available should be consulted regularly. In the UK these include:

- The *Summary of Product Characteristics* or SPC, available online at: www.medicines.org.uk/EMC
- The *British National Formulary* (BNF, 2004), available online at: www.bnf.org
- The guidance available from the National Institute of Clinical Excellence (NICE), available online at: www.nice.org.uk
- The guidance available from the Committee on Safety of Medicines (CSM), available online at: www.mca.gov.uk/ aboutagency/regframework/csm/csmhome.htm.

The main groups of psychotropic drugs are now discussed in the following order:

- Antipsychotic drugs
- Antidepressant drugs
- Antimanic drugs
- Lithium and other mood-stabilizing drugs
- Drugs used in the treatment of anxiety disorders including sedative and hypnotic drugs
- Drugs used in the treatment of psychiatric disorders in children
- Antiepileptic drugs
- Drugs used in the treatment of erectile impotence, premature ejaculation and antisocial sexual behaviour
- Drugs used in the treatment of dementia
- Drugs used in the treatment of parkinsonism and related disorders
- Drugs used in the treatment of alcohol and drug dependency and cigarette smoking.

Antipsychotic drugs

Antipsychotic (AP) drugs are conventionally divided into the newer atypical and older typical groups although there is controversy about the significance of any differences between these groups. The atypical AP drugs include three dibenzazepines (clozapine, olanzapine and quetiapine), and several drugs with diverse structures (amisulpride, aripiprazole, paliperidone [a metabolite of risperidone], risperidone, sertindole, and ziprasidone). Clozapine may be regarded as the archetypal typical AP drug.

The typical AP drugs include the phenothiazines such as chlorpromazine, the thioxanthenes such as flupentixol and the butyrophenones such as haloperidol. Haloperidol may be regarded as the archetypal typical AP drug.

Pharmacokinetics and pharmacodynamics

The AP drugs have relatively similar pharmacokinetics and pharmacodynamics. Thus:

- They are rapidly and completely absorbed at the proximal small intestine, reaching C_{max} in 1–4 h
- They are subject to extensive first pass metabolism
- Their $t_{1/2}$ is generally of several days' duration (although the $t_{1/2}$ of depot preparations many extend over many weeks)

- Their plasma protein binding is in excess of 90%
- They are metabolized almost exclusively, and very extensively, in the liver, almost no parent drug being excreted.

Mechanism of action

Without exception, all effective AP drugs have a relatively high (and largely dose-dependent) affinity for mesolimbic (A10) postsynaptic D_2 receptors at which they are potent antagonists. Occupancy of at least 65% of D_2 receptors appears to be both necessary and sufficient for their antipsychotic efficacy.

The affinity of AP drugs for nigrostriatal (A9) postsynaptic D_2 receptors appears to determine their extrapyramidal safety. Atypical AP drugs differ from typical AP drugs in that they have relatively low affinity for nigrostriatal D_2 receptors. They also have relatively high $5HT_{2A}$ to D_2 receptor binding ratios. These properties, possibly combined with interactions with other receptor types, may be responsible for the improved extrapyramidal safety profile of atypical APs.

More recently, a fast dissociation hypothesis of AP efficacy and safety has been proposed (Kapur & Seeman 2001). This suggests that D_2 receptor occupancy produces the antipsychotic effect but that rapid dissociation from the D_2 receptor (rather than occupancy of $5HT_{2A}$ or other receptors), accounts for extrapyramidal safety.

Efficacy

AP drugs are effective in treating acute episodes of schizophrenia, mania and other psychoses, in preventing relapse in patients with schizophrenia and other psychoses, and in preventing relapse in patients with bipolar disease when mood-stabilizing drugs are ineffective or are not tolerated.

Schizophrenia

It is generally accepted that AP drugs are all equally effective in alleviating both the positive symptoms of schizophrenia and in treating other acute psychoses. There is some evidence that atypical AP drugs are more effective than typical AP drugs in alleviating negative symptoms and in reducing depressive symptoms, suicidal behaviour and completed suicide (Meltzer et al 2003, Wright & O'Flaherty 2003). More recent evidence suggests that atypical AP drugs such as olanzapine and possibly risperidone may improve cognitive function in patients with schizophrenia (Bilder et al 2002).

Atypical AP drugs have been recommended as the first-line treatment for almost all patients with schizophrenia by the National Institute for Health and Clinical Excellence, NICE (2002, 2009). It seems reasonable to extrapolate this recommendation to other patients who require AP drugs, for example those with acute mania (Box 39.1).

Treatment should commence with an adequate dose of a single atypical AP drug. If this is ineffective after 2–3 weeks the dose should be increased and treatment continued for a further 2–3 weeks. If treatment remains ineffective this drug should be discontinued, a second atypical AP drug should be prescribed and the same two-stage process should be repeated. If the second atypical AP drug proves ineffective, treatment with clozapine should be commenced. If the first atypical AP

Box 39.1

National Institute for Clinical Excellence (2002, 2009) Guidelines on atypical antipsychotics for schizophrenia

- The atypical antipsychotics (amisulpride, olanzapine, quetiapine, risperidone and zotepine) should be considered when choosing first-line treatment of newly diagnosed schizophrenia
- An atypical antipsychotic is considered the treatment option of choice for managing an acute schizophrenic episode when discussion with the individual is not possible
- An atypical antipsychotic should be considered for an individual who is suffering unacceptable side-effects from a conventional antipsychotic
- An atypical antipsychotic should be considered for an individual in relapse whose symptoms were previously inadequately controlled
- Changing to an atypical antipsychotic is not necessary if a conventional antipsychotic controls symptoms adequately and the individual does not suffer unacceptable side-effects
- Clozapine should be introduced if schizophrenia is inadequately controlled despite the sequential use of two or more antipsychotics (one of which should be an atypical antipsychotic) each for at least 6–8 weeks.

---

drug is not tolerated the patient should be switched to treatment with the second atypical AP drug. If this is not tolerated the patient should be switched to treatment with clozapine.

Clozapine is used as a second-line AP drug in patients with treatment resistant schizophrenia (inadequate efficacy of two different AP drugs prescribed in adequate doses for an adequate duration of time) and/or extrapyramidal side-effects caused by other AP drugs. Patients treated with clozapine require haematological monitoring because of the risk of agranulocytosis (see below).

Patients who refuse oral AP therapy or who are agitated may require a parenterally administered AP drug. Parenteral formulations of aripiprazole and olanzapine are available and are rapidly effective, for example i.m. olanzapine reduces agitation as effectively as, but more rapidly than i.m. haloperidol (Wright et al 2001).

The starting dose, dose range and available formulations of the atypical AP drugs that are currently licensed in the UK are presented in Table 39.1.

The relapse rate in untreated schizophrenia reaches almost 100% after 2 years. Long-term maintenance AP drug therapy is therefore essential for the majority of patients and should be continued indefinitely.

The majority of patients with schizophrenia do not realize that they are ill and they are therefore understandably reluctant to take AP drugs. This, and the adverse effects associated with these drugs, means that adherence to maintenance AP drug treatment is problematic. Injectable depot formulations of AP drugs reduce this problem to some extent in that patients may be more wiling to accept an i.m. injection every few weeks than tablets every day. Depot formulations of olanzapine and risperidone are available in the UK. The pharmacokinetics of depot AP drugs differ significantly from those of orally administered AP drugs in that $t_{1/2}$ may be of several weeks and steady state may not be reached for several months.

Table 39.1 The initial daily dose, daily dose range and available formulations of the atypical AP drugs currently licensed in the UK

	AP drug	Initial dose (mg)	Dose range (mg)	Available formulations
First-line AP drugs	Aripiprazole	10	10–30	Tablets, orodispersible tablets, oral solution, intramuscular injection
	Amisulpride	400–800	400–1200	Tablets, oral solution
	Olanzapine	10	5–20	Tablets, orodispersible tablets, oral solution, intramuscular injection, depot injection
	Paliperidone	6	3–12	Tablets
	Quetiapine	50	300–750	Tablets
	Risperidone	2	4–16	Tablets, orodispersible tablets, oral solution, depot injection
	Zotepine	75	75–300	Tablets
	Sertindole[a]	4	12–24	Tablets
Second-line AP drugs	Clozapine[b]	12.5–25	200–900	Tablets

[a]Sertindole has been reintroduced following an earlier suspension because of concerns about arrhythmias (QTc prolongation); its use is restricted to patients who are intolerant of at least one other AP drug and are enrolled in a clinical study.

[b]In order to use clozapine, both prescribers and patients must be registered with CPMS, the Clozaril Patient Monitoring Service.

Bipolar disorder

The relapse rate in untreated bipolar disorder is as high or higher than that in untreated schizophrenia. Bipolar patients are frequently treated with AP drugs when mood stabilizing drugs are ineffective or are not tolerated. Maintenance therapy should also be continued indefinitely in these patients because the risk of relapse never diminishes. Of the atypical AP drugs aripiprazole, olanzapine, quetiapine and risperidone are approved for the treatment of acute mania (see below) while olanzapine is approved for the prevention of manic and depressive relapse and quetiapine for the treatment of depressive relapse in patients with bipolar disease.

Safety

All effective AP drugs have a high affinity for, and are potent antagonists at, D_2 receptors but AP drugs also exert an effect at many other neuroreceptors. Antagonism at the $5HT_{2A}$ receptor may confer enhanced efficacy against negative symptoms but activity at other central receptors is, in the main, regarded as being responsible for adverse effects (Table 39.2).

The adverse effects listed in Table 39.2 occur to a great extent with all typical AP drugs. Atypical AP drugs also cause anticholinergic, antiserotonergic and antiadrenergic adverse effects but they are much less likely to cause antidopaminergic adverse effects such as extrapyramidal syndromes and, in some cases, hyperprolactinaemia.

AP drugs may also cause impaired temperature regulation, insomnia, dizziness, headache, confusion, gastrointestinal disturbance, blurred vision, contact sensitization, rashes, (cholestatic) jaundice and blood dyscrasias including leucopenia and agranulocytosis.

The most significant adverse effects associated with atypical AP drugs as weight gain, dizziness, postural hypotension (which may be associated with syncope or reflex tachycardia in some patients) and extrapyramidal symptoms occasionally including tardive dyskinesia on long-term administration. Hyperglycaemia and sometimes diabetes mellitus may also occur and neuroleptic malignant syndrome

Table 39.2 Adverse effects attributable to the antagonism of AP drugs at different types of neuroreceptors

Neuroreceptor effect	Adverse effect
Anticholinergic	Dry mouth, constipation (occasionally, paralytic ileus in older patients), dry eyes, blurred vision, closed angle glaucoma, urinary hesitancy, urinary retention (especially in males with prostatic hypertrophy), sexual dysfunction, mild tachycardia (because of reduced vagal tone), impaired memory and confusion
Antiserotonergic	Weight gain (antihistaminergic mechanisms also proposed)
Antiadrenergic	Dizziness, postural hypotension (may lead to falls and hip fractures in older patients), sexual dysfunction
Antidopaminergic	Extrapyramidal syndromes, hyperprolactinaemia

has been reported. More recently, it has been recognized that AP drugs increase the risk of cerebrovascular events and mortality in elderly patients with dementia. AP drugs should therefore not be used in elderly patients to treat mild to moderate psychotic symptoms and if used the dose should be reduced and treatment should be reviewed regularly.

Clozapine is associated with an increased risk of agranulocytosis and patients being treated with it require haematological monitoring. Reversible neutropenia occurs in 3% of clozapine treated patients while 0.8% of patients developed agranulocytosis prior to the introduction of haematological monitoring.

Their safety profile means that AP drugs should be prescribed cautiously in patients with hepatic and renal impairment, epilepsy, Parkinson disease, prostatism, blood dyscrasias and closed angle glaucoma. Some AP drugs cause photosensitivity. AP drugs are relatively contraindicated in patients with impaired consciousness and phaeochromocytoma.

Extrapyramidal adverse effects

Acute dystonia, parkinsonism, akathisia and tardive dyskinesia were described in patients with schizophrenia before the advent of AP drugs but typical AP drugs greatly increase the risk of these disorders. Acute dystonia occurs immediately or within a few days of treatment with an AP drug, especially in young male patients. Parkinsonism may only develop after many weeks of treatment and is commonest in older female patients. Akathisia occurs equally in both sexes and usually develops during the first few days or weeks of treatment.

Tardive dyskinesia is commonest in older female patients. Its incidence in patients treated with typical AP drugs is about 5% per year and the cumulative prevalence is between 20% and 25%. The incidence and cumulative prevalence in patients treated with atypical AP drugs is significantly lower.

Neuroleptic malignant syndrome

The neuroleptic malignant syndrome (NMS) consists of extrapyramidal symptoms (rigidity), fluctuating consciousness (delirium, stupor) and autonomic lability (hyperthermia, tachycardia, hypo- or hypertension, sweating, pallor, salivation and urinary incontinence). Marked elevation of creatinine phosphokinase occurs and thromboembolism and renal failure caused by myoglobinuria secondary to muscle necrosis are common. Untreated, death occurs in 10–20% of affected patients.

Neuroleptic malignant syndrome is a medical emergency that is best treated in an intensive care unit. Antipsychotic therapy must be discontinued, the patient's temperature normalized, fluid and electrolyte balance maintained and secondary infection treated. Diazepam, dantrolene or bromocriptine may be useful, as may amantadine and L-dopa. Recovered patients usually have no sequelae. Further antipsychotic treatment should be with a drug from a different chemical group and dosage should be increased extremely slowly and with careful monitoring.

Hyperprolactinaemia

Hyperprolactinaemia, a side-effect of all typical AP drugs, causes hypo-oestrogenaemia, and is associated with a number of different adverse effects in men and women:

* Men: gynaecomastia, impotence, loss of libido and impaired spermatogenesis

* Women: galactorrhoea, amenorrhoea, altered ovarian function, loss of libido and an increased long-term risk for osteoporosis.

Aripiprazole, olanzapine, quetiapine and clozapine do not appear to be associated with significant hyper-prolactinaemia, in contrast to both amisulpride and risperidone and to the typical AP drugs. Reducing risk for hyperprolactinemia is highly desirable given that impotence in men and loss of libido in both sexes may impair the quality of patients' lives and their adherence to treatment, while osteoporosis may present a longer-term personal and public health risk (Naidoo et al 2003).

Cardiovascular adverse effects

Sudden cardiac death has long been reported in otherwise healthy young people, especially men, treated with AP drugs. The causes of such deaths may include:

* Prolongation of the QTc interval on the electrocardiogram, which may lead to ventricular tachyarrhythmias and death. This is more likely to occur in patients who are hypokalaemic or have high sympathetic tone, both of which situations may prevail in agitated, overactive patients. The atypical AP drug sertindole has been reintroduced for use in the UK following an earlier suspension because of concerns about arrhythmias (see Table 39.1). Amisulpride, olanzapine, quetiapine and risperidone appear to have no clinically significant effect on the QTc interval. Of the typical AP drugs, droperidol is no longer available in the UK and thioridazine is restricted to second-line treatment of schizophrenia in adults under specialist supervision because of QTc prolongation

* NA α_1 blockade – some AP drugs, especially in high dosage, may cause marked NA α_1 blockade and lead to profound hypotension

* Concomitant treatment with drugs that act synergistically to cause cardiorespiratory collapse, for example BZD drugs.

Antidepressant drugs

The efficacy of AD drugs appears to depend on their ability to increase synaptic concentrations of some or all of the biogenic amines NA, 5HT and DA, which in turn enhances neurotransmission across the synapse. The mechanisms by which AD drugs increase synaptic concentrations of biogenic amines include:

* Inhibition of the transporter molecules responsible for the reuptake of NA, 5HT and DA from the synapse to the presynaptic neuron

* Inhibition of MAO, the catalytic enzyme for NA, 5HT and DA

* Blockade of presynaptic NA and 5HT neuroreceptors which prevents negative feedback by NA and 5HT at these receptors and thus permits the presynaptic neuron to continue secreting NA and 5HT.

The AD drugs may be pragmatically classified into the newer and older groups. The newer AD drugs include the following:

Table 39.3 The initial daily dose, daily dose range and available formulations of the AD drugs that are currently licensed in the UK

	AD drug	Initial dose (mg)	Dose range (mg)	Available formulations
Newer AD drugs	Citalopram	10–20	20–60	Tablets; liquid
	Duloxetine	60	120	Capsules
	Escitalopram	10	10–20	Tablets
	Fluoxetine	20	20	Capsules; liquid
	Fluvoxamine	50–100	100–300	Tablets
	Mirtazapine	15	15–45	Tablets
	Moclobemide	300	150–600	Tablets
	Paroxetine[a]	20	20	Tablets; liquid
	Reboxetine	8	8–12	Tablets
	Sertraline	50	50–200	Tablets
	Tryptophan[b]	3 g	3–6 g	Tablets
	Venlafaxine	75	75–375	Tablets; capsules
Older AD drugs	Amitriptyline	75	150–200	Tablets; liquid
	Amoxapine	100–150	150–300	Tablets
	Clomipramine	10	30–250	Tablets; capsules
	Dosulepin	75	150–225	Tablets; capsules
	Doxepin	75	75–300	Capsules
	Imipramine	75	150–20	Tablets
	Isocarboxazid	30	30–60	Tablets
	Lofepramine	140–210	140–210	Tablets; liquid
	Maprotiline	25–75	75–150	Tablets
	Mianserin	30–40	30–90	Tablets
	Nortriptyline	75–10	75–150	Tablets
	Phenelzine	45	45–90	Tablets
	Tranylcypromine	20	20–30	Tablets
	Trazodone	100–150	100–600	Tablets; capsules; liquid
	Trimipramine	50–75	150–300	Tablets; capules

The above dosing recommendations refer only to the treatment of depressive disorder and dosing recommendations may differ when the AD drugs listed are used in the treatment of anxiety or eating disorders (see below).

[a]The CSM recently recommended 20 mg as the daily dose of paroxetine in the treatment of depression and several anxiety disorders (see below).

[b]In order to use tryptophan both prescribers and patients must be registered with OPTICS, the OptiMax Information and Clinical Support unit.

Bipolar depression

AD monotherapy should be avoided in the management of depressive relapse in patients with bipolar disorder because of the risk of inducing rapid cycling or acute mania (SSRIs are probably safer than TCAs in this regard). Such patients should therefore be treated with an AD drug and a concomitantly administered mood-stabilizing drug such as lithium, valproate, olanzapine or quetiapine (see below).

Treatment-resistant depression

The following strategies may be useful in the management of treatment resistant depression:

- Consider misdiagnosis and/or co-morbidity
- Consider non-compliance, inadequate dosage or inadequate duration of treatment
- Prescribe a drug from a different AD class (including MAOI) or prescribe venlafaxine if not already tried

- Consider dual drug therapy with either an AD drug and lithium, an AD drug and an atypical AP drug or two AD drugs from two different classes (TCA with SSRI or TCA with MAOI)
- Consider the addition of thyroxine (as liothyronine) to one of the above strategies.

Safety

AD drugs primarily modify NA- and 5HT-mediated neurotransmission but they also exert an effect at many other central and peripheral receptors. These latter effects are, in the main, regarded as being responsible for the adverse effects of ADs.

AD drugs are associated with suicidal thinking and behaviour and children, young adults and patients with a history of suicidal behaviour are particularly at risk. The AD drug prescribed should reflect this risk and the possibility of overdosage (see below). Patients at risk should be monitored for suicidal behaviour, particularly at the beginning of treatment or following changes in dosage or AD drug.

Newer antidepressant drugs

SSRIs commonly cause nausea, dyspepsia, crampy abdominal pain and diarrhoea and all patients should be warned of this likelihood. These adverse effects will disappear in most patients after 7–10 days of treatment. In contrast, if headache occurs, it is likely to persist. Sexual dysfunction (diminished libido, erectile and ejaculatory impotence and anorgasmia) is much more common with SSRIs than TCAs and may affect as many as one in three patients. This is a major cause of treatment discontinuation in the later stages of recovery and during prophylaxis. Less common adverse effects associated with SSRIs include:

- Psychomotor arousal (which may be an advantage to some patients)
- Extrapyramidal syndromes
- Hyponatraemia (especially in older patients)
- Serotonin syndrome, characterized by confusion, fever, myoclonus, chorea, seizures and coma. This also occurs with venlafaxine. It is more likely to occur if SSRIs or SNRIs are administered with MAOIs.

Seizures may also occur. SSRIs have no effect on cardiac function and are therefore safe in overdosage (see below). They may cause mild anorexia and weight loss, although paroxetine may be associated with weight gain.

A discontinuation syndrome occurs in one in three patients within 24 h of abruptly discontinuing treatment with SSRIs or SNRIs. The symptoms may be moderate or severe and include anxiety, mood disturbance, gastrointestinal disturbance, dizziness, paraesthesia, sleep disturbance and an influenza-like syndrome. SSRI discontinuation syndrome is most common with paroxetine and venlafaxine, which have short $t_{1/2}$ and very uncommon with fluoxetine which has a long $t_{1/2}$ and an active major metabolite with a long $t_{1/2}$. SSRI and SNRI discontinuation syndrome may be avoided by gradual discontinuation of ADs over several weeks.

Older antidepressant drugs

TCAs are potent Ach, α_2-noradrenergic and H_1 neuroreceptor antagonists and some are also D_2 antagonists. These properties and as yet undefined central mechanisms are responsible for the adverse effects presented in Table 39.4. It is thought that the general increase in noradrenergic tone associated with TCAs is responsible for the anxiety, agitation, tremor and increased sweating experienced by some patients. TCAs also have class I or membrane stabilizing antiarrhythmic properties and may cause heart block in healthy individuals. TCAs, with the exception of lofepramine, are highly cardiotoxic in overdosage because:

- Their class I antiarrhythmic properties slow ventricular conduction and promote ventricular tachyarrhythmias
- A reservoir of potentially absorbable drug remains available in the proximal small intestine for a prolonged period following ingestion because their anticholinergic effects delay gastrointestinal motility
- They impair alveolar gas exchange and cause hypoxia, hypercapnia and acidosis. Acidosis in turn reduces protein binding and increases available free drug.

In contrast to TCAs apart from lofepramine, SSRIs have no appreciable effect on cardiac function and are relatively safe in overdosage. As is the case with many drugs, TCAs may cause rashes, hypersensitivity reactions, leukopenia, agranulocytosis,

Table 39.4 Adverse effects attributable to the antagonism of TCA AD drugs at different types of neuroreceptors

Neuroreceptor effect	Adverse effect
Anticholinergic	Dry mouth, constipation (occasionally, paralytic ileus in older patients), dry eyes, blurred vision, closed angle glaucoma, urinary hesitancy, urinary retention (especially in males with prostatic hypertrophy), sexual dysfunction, mild tachycardia (because of reduced vagal tone), impaired memory and confusion
Antiadrenergic (primarily α_1 antagonism)	Dizziness, postural hypotension (may lead to falls and hip fractures in older patients), sexual dysfunction, dry mouth, constipation
Antihistaminergic (primarily H_1 antagonism)	Sedation (impairs occupational and driving ability but may be a benefit for some patients), weight gain (antiserotonergic mechanisms also proposed)
Antidopaminergic	Extrapyramidal syndromes, hyperprolactinaemia (especially likely with amoxapine and clomipramine)
Complex central mechanisms	Lowered seizure threshold with increased risk of epileptic seizures, induction of manic episode (more likely in patients with recognized or unrecognized bipolar disorder)

eosinophilia, thrombocytopenia and hyponatraemia (especially in older patients and possibly due to inappropriate secretion of antidiuretic hormone). NMS occurs rarely. Mianserin and trazodone are associated with increased risks of white cell dyscrasias and priapism, respectively.

MAOIs may cause a potentially fatal hypertensive crisis because they inactivate MAO in the gut and prevent the neutralization of ingested sympathomimetic substances (dietary tyramine and histamine and drugs such as phenylpropanolamine and ephedrine). Patients being treated with MAOIs must be warned against eating certain foods (meat, soya or yeast extracts, mature cheeses, pickled herring, broad bean pods), drinking full bodied red wines or taking cough remedies containing phenylpropanolamine and ephedrine. These restrictions do not apply to patients treated with moclobemide.

The adverse effects associated with MAOIs include hypotension, insomnia and psychomotor arousal. MAOIs have no effect on cardiac function but they may cause dry mouth, constipation, urinary hesitancy and retention, sexual dysfunction and confusion. Phenelzine is a rare cause of peripheral neuropathy.

Antimanic drugs

The antimanic drugs include AP and BZD drugs along with lithium, carbamazepine and valproate (Keck 2003). These are all discussed in more detail elsewhere in this chapter.

Patients with acute mania (manic episode) almost always require hospitalization and treatment with antimanic drugs in order to rapidly control their behaviour and reduce risk, reduce their agitation and distress, alleviate their psychotic symptoms and prevent further episodes of mania. In general, AP drugs reduce manic symptoms in 1–2 days, lithium takes 1–2 weeks to be effective and carbamazepine and valproate have an intermediate onset of action.

Olanzapine, quetiapine and risperidone are approved for the treatment of acute mania and the vast majority of patients should be treated with one of these atypical AP drugs, either alone or in combination with BZD drugs (Goodwin & Young 2003). Parenteral administration of such drugs may be required, either because patients refuse oral therapy or in order to reduce risk. Patients with less severe mania may be treated with either lithium or carbamazepine alone, or with modest doses of atypical AP drugs.

Approximately half of all manic patients will not respond adequately to the treatments described above. Such patients will require combination therapy with an atypical AP drug and either lithium or carbamazepine. Clozapine has also been used successfully to treat patients with treatment resistant mania.

Lithium and other mood stabilizing drugs

Prophylactic mood-stabilizing drugs are recommended for patients who have experienced one of the following:

- Two manic episodes
- An episode of mania and an episode of depression or
- A single manic episode that caused very significant personal, domestic or occupational impact.

Some patients with recurrent depressive illness also benefit from mood-stabilizing drugs. The mood-stabilizing drugs that are currently available include:

- Lithium salts
- The antiepileptic drugs carbamazepine, lamotrigine and valproate
- The atypical AP drugs aripiprazole, olanzapine, quetiapine and risperidone.

NICE (2006) recommend lithium, olanzapine or valproate as first-line monotherapy agents for prophylaxis with any two of these agents in combination as second-line prophylaxis. Atypical AP drugs (including depot formulations of olanzapine and risperidone) represent third line prophylactic treatment in patients with bipolar disorder.

More recently, it has been suggested that the choice of prophylactic treatment should be guided by whether manic or depressive episodes dominate the illness. Thus, patients who experience predominantly manic episodes may be best treated with lithium, aripiprazole, quetiapine, valproate or olanzapine while those who experience predominantly depressive episodes may be best treated with quetiapine or lamotrigine (Goodwin et al 2009).

Lithium

Lithium salts will now be discussed (the antiepileptic and AP drugs are discussed below).

Pharmacokinetics and pharmacodynamics

Lithium is an alkali metal that may be administered as either its lithium carbonate or lithium citrate salt. The active component of both is the lithium cation (Li^+). Lithium:

- Is rapidly and completely absorbed at the proximal small intestine and, to a lesser extent, the stomach
- Reaches C_{max} in 1–2 h and has a $t_{1/2}$ of approximately 24 h (currently available tablets are coated so as to delay absorption and produce a non-toxic C_{max} approximately 4 hours after administration and effective blood levels throughout the day)
- Has a narrow therapeutic window, being largely ineffective at serum levels below 0.4 mmol/L and toxic at levels above 1.5 mmol/L
- Is not bound to plasma proteins and is eliminated unchanged via the kidney.

Mechanism of action

The mechanism of action of lithium is unknown. It may modify neuronal second messenger systems or stabilize neuronal membranes.

Efficacy

Lithium is indicated for the treatment of manic episode and the prevention of relapse in bipolar disorder. It is a second-line (after continuation of treatment with a newer type of AD drug) or adjuvant treatment (in combination with a newer type of AD) for the prevention of new depressive episodes in unipolar depressive disorder. Lithium may also be used to control aggressive or self-mutilating behaviour.

The daily dosage should be increased gradually until serum lithium measured 12 h after administration is maintained in the range 0.4–1.0 mmol/L (it was previously recommended to maintain serum lithium measured 12 h after administration in the range 0.6–1.2 mmol/L but this is now regarded as excessive for most patients). It is usual to measure serum lithium weekly while the dose is being titrated to the therapeutic range and every 3 months thereafter. Patients taking lithium require baseline and regular laboratory investigations in addition to serum lithium assays (see below).

Approximately 50% of patients in whom treatment with lithium is abruptly discontinued will develop mania within 1–2 weeks (Verdoux & Bourgeois 1993). Rebound mania may be avoided by gradual discontinuation of lithium over 6–8 weeks if treatment must cease.

Safety

The majority of patients taking lithium experience adverse effects even when their serum lithium levels are maintained within the therapeutic range. The body systems affected by these adverse effects include:

- Central nervous system – dysphoria, emotional and cognitive dulling (especially memory impairment) and tremor (this becomes more evident as serum lithium increases and may predict toxicity)
- Endocrine and reproductive systems – asymptomatic goitre, hypothyroidism (thyroid function should be evaluated every 6–12 months) and teratogenicity (there is an increased risk of cardiac malformations, especially Ebstein anomaly, if lithium is taken in the months before conception and/or during the first trimester). Lithium is secreted in breast milk and may cause neonatal hypothyroidism in breastfed babies
- Genitourinary system – polyuria, increased urinary output, diabetes insipidus and, very rarely, renal failure
- Gastrointestinal system – increased or decreased salivation, metallic taste (caused by secretion of lithium in saliva), polydipsia, nausea, vomiting, mild diarrhoea and weight gain
- Skin – rash, exacerbation of existing or development of *de novo* psoriasis and hair loss
- Cardiovascular system – clinically insignificant flattening or inverting of T waves on ECG and, rarely, symptomatic conduction defects.

Lithium toxicity is evident in some patients with serum lithium levels of 1.5 mmol/L and in almost all with levels >2.0 mmol/L. It usually develops over 1–2 days and may be precipitated by dehydration, impaired renal function, concomitant infection, treatment with diuretics or deliberate overdose. The adverse effects that may be present in the non-toxic state worsen during the initial stages of toxicity and patients experience severe vomiting and diarrhoea, marked thirst, polydipsia and polyuria and develop a coarse tremor. With increasing toxicity, the clinical picture progresses through hypertonicity, choreoathetoid movements, ataxia and dysarthria to delirium, seizures, renal failure and impaired consciousness. Untreated, cardiovascular collapse, coma and death soon follow.

There is no antidote to lithium toxicity and peritoneal dialysis or haemodialysis may be required. Toxicity may be prevented by advising patients of the importance of hydration and by temporarily discontinuing lithium and encouraging hydration at the first signs of toxicity.

Drugs used in the treatment of anxiety disorders including sedative and hypnotic drugs

The use of antidepressant, benzodiazepine and non-benzodiazepine drugs in the treatment of anxiety will now be discussed, as will sedative and hypnotic drugs.

Antidepressant drugs as anxiolytics

Older ADs are effective in treating anxiety disorders but their adverse effects militate against patients taking them. Newer ADs appear to be as effective in treating anxiety disorders as older ADs but cause fewer adverse effects and are therefore better tolerated by patients. The main difference between using newer ADs to treat anxiety and using them to treat depression is that somewhat different dosages are required (Table 39.5).

Benzodiazepine drugs

The risk of dependence is high with benzodiazepine (BZD) drugs and the last two decades have seen attempts to curb widespread prescribing. Nonetheless, the BZDs remain the most widely used anxiolytic and hypnotic drugs.

The BZDs available in the UK include alprazolam, chlordiazepoxide, clobazam, clonazepam, clorazepate, diazepam, flunitrazepam, flurazepam, loprazolam, lorazepam, lormetazepam, midazolam, nitrazepam, oxazepam and temazepam. Flurazepam, loprazolam, lormetazepam, nitrazepam and temazepam are usually prescribed as hypnotic drugs.

Pharmacokinetics and pharmacodynamics

Individual BZDs differ in the rate at which they are absorbed from the gastrointestinal tract. Diazepam is rapidly absorbed, for example, and reaches C_{max} in approximately 1 hour. In contrast, temazepam is absorbed slowly reaching C_{max} after 3 hours. Absorption of BZDs following i.m. administration is erratic. However, while the i.m. route has no therapeutic advantage over the oral route, it may be necessary to administer BZDs i.m. if it not possible to do so by the oral or i.v. route. Liquid formulations of BZDs are absorbed rapidly if administered rectally, C_{max} being reached in 15–30 min. Protein binding of BZDs is generally >90% but it is 75% for alprazolam.

Individual BZDs differ significantly in their lipid solubility. This is lowest for lorazepam and temazepam and highest for midazolam (which therefore rapidly crosses the BBB).

The $t_{1/2}$ of individual BZDs differ dramatically and this and the fact that many have active metabolites with long $t_{1/2}$ of their own complicates their clinical use. Flurazepam, for example, has a $t_{1/2}$ of 1–2 h but its active metabolite desalkylflurazepam has a $t_{1/2}$ of 75 h. Flurazepam therefore has a longer effective $t_{1/2}$ than the $t_{1/2}$ of the parent compound would suggest. Taking into account the $t_{1/2}$ of parent drug and the $t_{1/2}$ of any active metabolites, it is possible to divide BZDs into those

Non-benzodiazepine drugs

A number of non-BZD GABA$_A$ receptor agonists have become available in the last decade. These include the imidazopyridine zolpidem, the cyclopyrrolone zopiclone and the pyrazolopyrimidine zaleplon. These have very short (zaleplon) or short (zolpidem and zopiclone) durations of action and are licensed for the short-term treatment of insomnia. Their efficacy and safety is similar to that of BZDs. Tolerance and a withdrawal syndrome may occur and adherence to the prescribing guidelines applicable to BZDs is advised.

Pregabalin reaches C$_{max}$ in 1 hour and has a t$_{1/2}$ of 6 h. It is a GABA analogue that binds to the α_2-δ protein auxiliary subunit of voltage-gated calcium channels in the central nervous system. It is approved for the treatment of generalized anxiety disorder. The initial dose is 150 mg daily. This may be increased in weekly steps by 150 mg daily to a maximum of 600 mg daily. The commonest adverse effects associated with pregabalin include dizziness, somnolence, mood disturbance, visual disturbance, increased appetite and weight gain.

Sedative and hypnotic drugs

Chloral hydrate and triclofos sodium are safe, short-acting hypnotics with few adverse effects. They rarely cause hangover and are frequently used to treat insomnia in older patients. The prescribing guidelines applicable to BZDs should be followed when they are prescribed.

Barbiturates and paraldehyde are occasionally used to tranquillize patients who have not responded to other treatments or are in status epilepticus.

Antihistamines and low doses of older AP drugs are also widely used for their sedative or hypnotic properties.

Drugs used in the treatment of psychiatric disorders in children

Children differ from adults in their ability to absorb (usually faster), metabolize (usually faster) and eliminate drugs and psychotropic drugs are not tested extensively in children during clinical development. Great care is therefore required when treating children with such drugs and the manufacturer of the drug or the *British National Formulary* should always be consulted.

The disorders for which psychotropic drugs are widely prescribed during childhood include nocturnal enuresis, attention deficit hyperactivity disorder (ADHD), autism, sleep disorders, tic disorders and conduct disorder in children with learning disability. Children with anxiety disorders, depression and psychosis may also require medication.

Nocturnal enuresis

The first-line treatment of nocturnal enuresis is behavioural because this is generally effective. Drug therapy is appropriate after 7 years of age if behavioural treatment is ineffective or not possible and may be used alone or in combination with behavioural treatment. Short-term drug therapy in children under 7 years of age to cover periods away from home may be appropriate.

Imipramine (0.5–1.0 mg/kg) before going to bed is usually effective within 1–2 weeks. Amitriptyline is also used. The mechanism of action may involve direct anticholinergic effects on the bladder. Desmopressin (20–40 μg orally or by intranasal spray) before going to bed is also useful. Its adverse effects include fluid retention, hyponatraemia (which may cause seizures), headache, nausea, vomiting, nasal congestion and rhinitis. Treatment with imipramine or desmopressin should be reviewed every 3 months before a further 3 months of treatment is commenced. Treatment may need to continue for some years.

Oxybutynin is an anticholinergic drug that may be effective in children with treatment-resistant nocturnal enuresis caused by detrusor instability. Such treatment should only be initiated by a specialist following urodynamic studies.

Attention deficit hyperactivity disorder

The frequency with which attention deficit hyperactivity disorder (ADHD) is diagnosed and with which stimulant medication is prescribed to treat it is increasing. Concern that medication is being used to modify troublesome but appropriate childhood behaviour is probably unfounded and the response of children with ADHD to effective medication is among the most rapid and most dramatic in psychopharmacology.

The stimulant drugs licensed for the treatment of ADHD in the UK are methylphenidate, which is widely prescribed, and dexamphetamine, which is prescribed less frequently. Both are controlled drugs and subject to the prescription requirements of the Misuse of Drugs Regulations, 2001. Atomoxetine, a non-stimulant drug that has recently become available, is not a controlled drug and is licensed to treat ADHD in both children and adults.

NICE (2008a, b) recommend methylphenidate or atomoxetine as second-line treatment in moderate ADHD causing moderate impairment if non-pharmacological treatment is ineffective. Methylphenidate or atomoxetine are recommended as first line treatment in severe ADHD causing severe impairment.

Methylphenidate

Pharmacokinetics and pharmacodynamics
Methylphenidate is rapidly absorbed and protein binding is low. Hepatic metabolism and elimination are rapid, providing a t$_{1/2}$ of approximately 3 hours and clinical effects of approximately 5 hours duration. The drug must be administered 3–4 times per day (see below).

Methylphenidate causes the release of NA, DA and 5HT from, and blocks the reuptake of DA and NA to, presynaptic neurons, especially in the striatum.

Efficacy
Methylphenidate is administered in a dosage of 0.3–0.7 mg/kg per day. It is usually commenced at a dose of 5 mg twice daily and increased every 3–4 days until a beneficial effect is obtained or adverse effects prevent further dose increase. It is rarely necessary to dose above 60 mg/day. A long-acting formulation that is administered once daily in a dose range of 18–54 mg is available.

Most children with ADHD respond rapidly and significantly to methylphenidate or similar drugs. For example, Elia et al reported in 1991 that 96% of children showed behavioural improvement, while a recent review of clinical trials by Greenhill et al (1999) concluded that stimulants such as methylphenidate 'show robust short-term efficacy and a good safety profile'. Methylphenidate also remains effective in the long term. However, the effect of treating ADHD during childhood and adolescence with methylphenidate and other stimulants on eventual adult psychiatric morbidity is unclear.

Children whose ADHD has responded to methylphenidate will require prolonged treatment and may benefit from so-called drug holidays during which treatment is suspended, partly as a means of assessing the need for continuing medication.

Safety

The adverse effects commonly associated with methylphenidate include nervousness, insomnia, urticaria, fever, rash (which may progress to exfoliative dermatitis and erythema multiforme), anorexia, growth retardation (height should be monitored), nausea, dizziness, palpitations, headache, dyskinesia, drowsiness, hypertension, tachycardia, angina, abdominal pain and weight loss. Tics and organic psychosis may occur and abuse and diversion for recreational use are recognized. Greenhill et al (1999), on the basis of a literature review, reported no evidence of harmful effects from prolonged treatment.

Dexamphetamine

Pharmacokinetics and pharmacodynamics
The mechanism of action of dexamphetamine is similar to that of methylphenidate.

Efficacy
The efficacy of dexamphetamine is similar to that of methylphenidate. However, it should be regarded as a second-line treatment for children who do not respond to methylphenidate because of the risk of dependence and organic psychosis. Dexamphetamine is administered in a dosage of 5–20 mg/day with a maximum dosage of 40 mg/day in older children and adolescents.

Safety
The adverse effects commonly associated with dexamphetamine include insomnia, irritability, euphoria, tremor, headache, seizures, anorexia, growth retardation (height should be monitored), hypertension, dry mouth, tachycardia and sweating. Tics have been reported, organic psychosis may occur and dependence, tolerance and diversion for recreational use are recognized.

Atomoxetine

Pharmacokinetics and pharmacodynamics
Atomoxetine is rapidly absorbed and is 98% protein-bound. Hepatic metabolism is via the cytochrome P450 2D6 pathway and the $t_{1/2}$ of five hours in extensive metabolizers is increased to 24 h in poor metabolizers.

Atomoxetine is a highly selective inhibitor of the NA reuptake transporter. It increases synaptic concentrations of NA in the prefrontal cortex but has no effect on 5HT levels.

Efficacy
Atomoxetine may be administered to children and adolescents under 70 kg in body weight in an initial dose of 0.5 mg/kg per day. This may be increased after three days to 1.2 mg/kg per day. The total daily dose may be administered as a single dose or as two equal doses. Most children with ADHD respond significantly over 4–6 weeks to atomoxetine and its efficacy has also been established in adults with ADHD.

Atomoxetine may be administered to children and adolescents over 70 kg in body weight, and to adults, in an initial dose of 40 mg/day. This may be increased after 3 days to 80 mg/day and, if necessary, after 2 weeks to 100 mg/day.

Individuals whose ADHD has responded to atomoxetine will require prolonged treatment.

Safety
The adverse effects commonly associated with atomoxetine include dry mouth, insomnia, nausea, decreased appetite, constipation, dizziness, headache, sweating, sexual problems and palpitations. Modest increases in heart rate and blood pressure may occur. Hepatic disorders may occur (patients and parents should be advised to seek medical attention if abdominal pain, darkening of urine and/or jaundice occur) as may growth retardation (height should be monitored).

Autism

Psychotropic drugs play a modest but useful role in the alleviation of symptoms associated with autism:

- Atypical AP drugs, usually in low dosage, may help in the short-term treatment of agitation or aggression
- Stimulants and atomoxetine may help when ADHD symptoms are present, although they may worsen tic disorders
- AEDs should be prescribed for the control of seizures
- SSRIs may help in the management of anxiety, agitation and stereotypic behaviours.

Sleep disorders

Reassurance, education and behavioural treatment rather than psychotropic drugs are the mainstay of the management of sleep disorders in children. Sedating antihistamines, such as alimemazine (trimeprazine) 2 mg/kg daily, chloral hydrate 30–50 mg/kg daily or diazepam 0.1–0.3 mg/kg daily are occasionally prescribed for brief periods.

Diazepam 0.1–0.3 mg/kg daily or paroxetine 20–40 mg daily are very occasionally prescribed for night terrors.

Tic disorders

The motor and vocal tics of Gilles de la Tourette syndrome are commoner in children with autism, obsessive–compulsive disorder and ADHD than in otherwise healthy children. Clonidine (titrated to a maximum dose of 10 µg/kg per day), haloperidol (0.5–1.0 mg three times daily and slowly increased to a maximum of 10 mg daily or until a response is obtained) and pimozide are recognized treatments and atypical AP drugs and SSRIs are also used.

Conduct disorder

The use of psychotropic drugs for the primary purpose of controlling behaviour in children with learning disability is inappropriate because their adverse effects cause distress, impair cognition and may worsen the behaviour for which they were originally prescribed. Environmental management and psychological therapies are therefore the preferred treatments for such individuals. Psychotropic drugs should be prescribed for children with learning disability when the primary purpose is the short-term control of a crisis or the long-term treatment of a psychiatric disorder such as schizophrenia or depression.

AP drugs are widely prescribed for the control of agitation, self-harming and aggression in children with learning disability. Such individuals have brain damage by definition and are therefore at great risk of developing extrapyramidal adverse effects (which may exacerbate rather than reduce agitation and aggression) if treated with typical AP drugs. Atypical AP drugs in the lowest effective dose for the shortest duration of time necessary should therefore be the first choice if it is necessary to prescribe AP drugs for children with learning disability. Children with learning disability who have a psychotic disorder (e.g. at least 2% of such individuals have schizophrenia) may benefit from prolonged treatment.

Like AP drugs, antiepileptic drugs (AEDs) are also widely prescribed in children with learning disability, both in the treatment of epilepsy and recurrent mood disorders and in an attempt to reduce episodes of disturbed behaviour. Their use in the latter situation should only be commenced with recording of the target behaviour before and during treatment and with great attention to adverse effects. AEDs should be discontinued if the balance of benefits and risks proves unfavourable.

Newer AD drugs may help children with learning disability who have depression and may also reduce the frequency and severity of self-harming in some such individuals. Stimulant medications and atomoxetine may be beneficial if ADHD is present.

Anxiety disorders

SSRIs may be useful in the treatment of anxiety disorders, including obsessive–compulsive disorder, in childhood (see CSM advice, below). Psychotropic medication has no place in the management of school refusal unless there is an underlying psychiatric disorder.

Depression

The efficacy and safety of fluoxetine has been established in the treatment of depression in childhood (see CSM advice, below). Older AD drugs should be avoided.

Psychosis

Psychotic disorders are rare in childhood. Their treatment is with atypical AP drugs prescribed at low dosage, the dose being slowly titrated upwards until a response is obtained.

Antiepileptic drugs

Antiepileptic drugs (AEDs) are widely prescribed for the treatment of both epilepsy and bipolar disorder. The general pharmacological treatment of epilepsy will now be considered briefly. Following this, the AEDs available in the UK for the treatment of bipolar disorder – valproate, lamotrigine and carbamazepine, will be discussed.

General pharmacological treatment of epilepsy

NICE (2008a, b) recommend AED monotherapy with a combination of two or more AEDs being reserved for patients in whom several individual AEDs have proven ineffective or otherwise unsuitable. Newer AEDs (gabapentin, lamotrigine, levetiracetam, oxcarbazepine, tiagabine, topiramate, vigabatrin) are recommended when older AEDs (carbamazepine, valproate) are ineffective or otherwise unsuitable.

The plasma levels of AEDs should be monitored if clinically indicated (especially when prescribed in combination because of the risk of AED–AED interactions such as the induction of enzymes by carbamazepine). The patient, not the laboratory value, should be treated. Thus if seizures are controlled and the patient is not experiencing adverse effects, AED levels above the advised range may be acceptable. Conversely, if levels are within the advised range but seizures continue, dosage may be increased until efficacy is achieved or until adverse effects occur. Equally, the dosage should not be increased if it is effective, despite AED levels being below the advised range. Regular full blood counts and evaluations of thyroid, renal and hepatic function are advised with some AEDs.

The clinician is most often faced with the treatment of patients with either partial or focal epilepsy (which may or may not generalize) or with generalized epilepsy.

Partial or focal epilepsy

The recommended first-line monotherapy drugs for partial or focal epilepsy are carbamazepine, lamotrigine, phenytoin, valproate and topiramate. If none of these drugs are effective two of them may be prescribed in combination. Alternatively, a second-line AED such as clobazam, gabapentin, levetiracetam, phenytoin or tiagabine may be considered.

Generalized epilepsy

First-line monotherapy (and second-line AEDs) for generalized epilepsy depends on the type of seizure, as follows:

* Tonic/clonic seizures – carbamazepine, lamotrigine, valproate or topiramate (clobazam, levetiracetam or oxcarbazepine)
* Absence seizures – ethosuximide, lamotrigine or valproate, the latter also being effective in patients who experience both tonic/clonic and absence seizures (clobazam, clonazepam or phenytoin)
* Myoclonic seizures – valproate (clobazam, clonazepam, lamotrigine, levetiracetam, piracetam or topiramate).

Status epilepticus

Status epilepticus consists of recurrent seizures without recovery of consciousness between them. Treatment requires immediate intravenous lorazepam. Intravenous diazepam, midazolam and clonazepam may also be used. Paraldehyde or anaesthesia may occasionally be required.

If seizures are not controlled within 30 min, or if they recur, an intravenous loading dose of phenytoin and a subsequent phenytoin infusion should be administered. Patients with status epilepticus are best treated in an intensive care unit.

Contraception and reproduction

AEDs such as carbamazepine induce the metabolism of ethinylestradiol and either an alternative method of contraception or a contraceptive pill (or combination of pills) containing a dosage of 50 μg ethinylestradiol daily is necessary.

Women with epilepsy should plan their pregnancies and should consider withdrawing AEDs before conception and during pregnancy. However, it is almost certainly safer to take AEDs while pregnant than to have seizures. Carbamazepine is probably the least teratogenic AED. Folate supplements are advised for women taking AEDs (and are now advised for all women) before and during pregnancy and vitamin K supplements are advised for pregnant women taking carbamazepine or phenytoin.

Discontinuation of antiepileptic drugs

Patients who have not had seizures for a prolonged period may wish to discontinue their AEDs. Any decision to do so must be based upon:

* The length of time the patient has been free of seizures (a 2-year minimum is recommended)
* The normality of the electroencephalogram (EEG) with current AED treatment (it would be unwise to withdraw treatment from a patient whose EEG exhibits significant epileptic activity despite treatment with AEDs)
* The side-effects of current AEDs
* Social factors (occupation, need for a driving licence and hobbies).

A careful record of seizure type and frequency must be made and an EEG recorded before reducing dosage, when dosage is reduced to half the initial dosage and when AEDs are stopped. Any increase in seizure frequency or severity, or deterioration in the EEG, should lead to the planned withdrawal being reconsidered.

Alternative psychosis or forced normalization

Some epileptic patients who are being effectively treated with AEDs may experience depression, mania and/or psychotic symptoms in association with a reduction in seizures and normalization of their EEG. This alternative psychosis or forced normalization may be alleviated by a slight reduction in AED dosage, such that the EEG exhibits epileptic activity and/or occasional seizures occur.

Valproate

Pharmacokinetics and pharmacodynamics

Valproate is a branched chain fatty acid that is absorbed and metabolized (by oxidative enzymes) rapidly. Plasma protein binding is 90% while $t_{1/2}$ is 10–16 h. Valproate does not induce metabolic enzymes but it inhibits enzymes that metabolize carbamazepine, ethosuximide, lamotrigine and phenytoin and causes their plasma levels to increase. Semisodium valproate (or divalproex) is a dimer composed of two valproate molecules.

Mechanism of action

Valproate causes upregulation of $GABA_B$ receptors and also enhances 5HT neurotransmission.

Efficacy

In addition to use in patients with epilepsy, valproate may also be prescribed as an antimanic drug in the treatment of acute mania, or as a mood-stabilizer in the prophylaxis of bipolar disorder in patients unresponsive to or intolerant of lithium. In this case it may be prescribed alone or in combination with lithium.

Treatment with valproate should be commenced at 200 mg twice daily (250 mg twice daily for semisodium valproate) and increased by 200 mg/day (250 mg/day for semisodium valproate) every 2–3 days. Patients with mania may require doses of up to 2000 mg daily (2250 mg daily for semisodium valproate) while 1000–2000 mg daily (1250–2250 mg daily for semisodium valproate) are usually adequate for prophylaxis. Plasma valproate levels of 50–150 mg/L are recommended. However, clinical status is the best determinant of a patient's optimal dose.

Safety

Nausea, ataxia, tremor, weight gain and reversible hair loss (although regrown hair may be curly) are the commonest adverse effects of valproate. Less common but more serious adverse effects include:

* Hepatotoxicity, which may be fatal in children and in patients taking other AEDs in addition to valproate. Liver function should be evaluated before commencing and during the first 6 months of treatment with valproate
* Stevens–Johnson syndrome (the risk is increased if valproate and lamotrigine are prescribed in combination)
* Pancreatitis, hyperammonaemia with confusion and asterixis (clinical chemistry parameters should be monitored)
* Blood dyscrasias including leukopenia and pancytopenia (haematological parameters should be monitored).

Valproate is teratogenic and may cause congenital cardiac defects and neonatal seizures if taken during pregnancy.

Lamotrigine

Pharmacokinetics and pharmacodynamics

Lamotrigine is absorbed and metabolized (oxidative enzymes) rapidly. Plasma protein binding is 50% while $t_{1/2}$ is 24 h. Lamotrigine neither induces nor inhibits metabolic enzymes.

Box 39.4

National Institute for Clinical Excellence: Methadone and buprenorphine for the management of opioid dependence (2007) and Naltrexone for the management of opioid dependence (2007)

- Oral methadone and buprenorphine are recommended for maintenance therapy in the management of opioid dependence
- Patients should be committed to a supportive care programme including a flexible dosing regimen administered under supervision for at least 3 months, until compliance is assured
- Selection of methadone or buprenorphine should be made on a case-by-case basis, but methadone should be prescribed if both drugs are equally suitable
- Naltrexone is recommended for the prevention of relapse in formerly opioid dependent patients who are motivated to remain in a supportive care abstinence programme
- Naltrexone should be administered under supervision and its effectiveness in preventing opioid misuse reviewed regularly.

Methadone

Methadone is a long-acting opioid m receptor agonist that may be substituted for diamorphine and that will prevent withdrawal symptoms. It is less sedating and has a longer $t_{\frac{1}{2}}$ (24 h) than morphine. It is usually administered as a once daily oral solution in a concentration of 1 mg/mL but an injectable formulation is available. It is intrinsically addictive and should only be prescribed for individuals who are dependent upon opiates. The initial daily dose is 10–20 mg and this is increased by 10–20 mg/day until withdrawal symptoms have been controlled. The usual daily dose is then 40–60 mg (see Ch. 29). Withdrawal is accomplished by gradually reducing the daily dosage at a rate that is agreed between the patient and the psychiatrist. Alternatively, treatment with methadone may be continued indefinitely in order to provide 'harm reduction'.

The adverse effects of methadone include nausea, vomiting, constipation and drowsiness. Sweating, arrhythmias, hypothermia, hallucinations, dysphoria and rash may also occur. Respiratory depression and hypotension may occur at relatively high doses.

Buprenorphine

Buprenorphine is a partial antagonist at the opioid μ-receptor that will prevent withdrawal symptoms if substituted for diamorphine. However, it may precipitate withdrawal symptoms in patients dependent upon higher doses of opiates because of its partial antagonist properties.

Buprenorphine is subject to extensive first pass metabolism and must be administered sublingually. It is therefore important to instruct patients appropriately. Buprenorphine is initially prescribed at a dose of 0.8–4.0 mg daily. This may gradually be increased to a maximum of 32 mg daily. Withdrawal is accomplished by gradually reducing the daily dosage at a rate that is agreed between the patient and the psychiatrist.

The adverse effects of buprenorphine are similar to those of methadone.

Lofexidine

Lofexidine is an α_2 adrenergic agonist like clonidine (which is occasionally used for a similar purpose). It acts centrally to reduce NA secretion and thus reduce sympathetic tone. It will effectively prevent withdrawal symptoms in patients who are opiate dependent.

Lofexidine is usually prescribed in a dosage of 0.2 mg daily. This is gradually increased by 0.2–0.4 mg daily to a maximum dose of 2.4 mg daily.

The adverse effects of lofexidine include dry mouth, throat and nose, drowsiness, bradycardia and hypotension (it should not be administered if the pulse rate is below 50 b.p.m. and/or if systolic blood pressure is <90 mmHg). Sedation and coma may occur.

Naltrexone

Naltrexone is an orally administered opioid antagonist that neutralizes the euphoriant effects of opiates and alcohol. It may therefore trigger withdrawal symptoms in opiate dependent individuals. It my help formerly opiate dependent individuals maintain abstinence. Naltrexone may also be used for opiate withdrawal in hospitalized patients.

It is prescribed at a dose of 25–50 mg daily. Once an appropriate daily dose has been determined, the drug is usually administered on 3 days per week. Its adverse effects include nausea, vomiting, anorexia, diarrhoea, abdominal pain, anxiety, headache, insomnia, fatigue, sweating, lacrimation, hypothermia, rash and sexual dysfunction.

Cigarette smoking

Individuals who wish to discontinue cigarette smoking may benefit from nicotine replacement therapy, bupropion or varenicline. These should be prescribed in accordance with National Institute for Clinical Excellence (NICE) guidelines (Box 39.5).

Nicotine replacement therapy

Products are available that allow the administration of nicotine by sublingual (gum, lozenges), transdermal (patches) or transmucosal (nasal spray, inhaler) routes. The daily dosage of any

Box 39.5

NICE (2008a, b) guidelines on smoking cessation services

NICE has recommended (2008a, b) that nicotine replacement therapy, bupropion or varenicline should be prescribed as follows:
- To people who are planning to stop smoking as part of an abstinent-contingent treatment, in which the smoker makes a commitment to stop smoking on or before a particular date (target stop date)
- The prescription should be sufficient to last only until 2 weeks after the target stop date
- Subsequent prescriptions should be given only to people who have demonstrated, on re-assessment, that their quit attempt is continuing
- Varenicline or bupropion may be offered to people with unstable cardiovascular disorders, subject to clinical judgement
- A combination of nicotine patches and another form of nicotine replacement may be offered to people who show a high level of dependence on nicotine or who have found single forms of nicotine replacement inadequate in the past.

product should be titrated to the quantity of cigarettes smoked daily, maintained at this dosage for 3 months and then gradually reduced over a further period of 3 months.

Nicotine products may cause nausea, hiccups, dyspepsia, headache, palpitations, insomnia, abnormal dreams, myalgia, anxiety and somnolence. The combination of nicotine replacement therapy with bupropion or varenicline is not recommended.

Bupropion

Bupropion is a NA and DA reuptake inhibitor that has almost no antagonist effect at neuroreceptors. Most of its effects are mediated by its metabolite, hydroxybupropion.

Bupropion should be commenced 2 weeks before an agreed smoking cessation date at an initial dose of 150 mg daily. This dose is increased to 150 mg twice daily after 1 week and maintained at this for a further 9 weeks. Bupropion should then be gradually discontinued.

The adverse effects of bupropion include gastrointestinal disturbance, impaired concentration, anxiety and alterations in taste. Rarely, psoriasis may be exacerbated and Stevens–Johnson syndrome and psychosis may occur. The CSM has advised that bupropion is contraindicated in patients with a history of seizures or eating disorders, a CNS tumour or who are experiencing acute symptoms of alcohol or benzodiazepine withdrawal.

Varenicline

Varenicline is a selective partial agonist at the nicotine receptor. It should be commenced 2 weeks before an agreed smoking cessation date at an initial dose of 0.5 mg daily. This dose is increased to 0.5 mg twice daily after 3 days and to 1 mg twice daily after a further 4 days. It is then maintained at this dose (or at 0.5 mg twice daily if not tolerated) for a further 11 weeks. This 12-week course of treatment may be repeated if necessary.

The adverse effects of varenicline include gastrointestinal disturbances, appetite changes, dry mouth, taste disturbance, headache, drowsiness, dizziness and sleep disorders. It may be associated with an increased risk of suicidal behaviour and patients, particularly if they have a history of psychiatric disorder, should be monitored closely and advised to seek help if they become agitated, depressed or suicidal.

Special populations of patients

The treatment of children, women and elderly patients with psychoactive drugs merits special attention. Care must also be exercised when prescribing psychoactive drugs for motorists or individuals who operate machinery.

Children

Great care is required when treating children with psychoactive drugs because:

- Children generally absorb, metabolize and eliminate drugs more rapidly than adults
- Drugs are not extensively tested in children during clinical development, and

- Formulations may not be available to allow precise dosing based upon body weight.

Most psychotropic drugs used to treat children are prescribed off label, in that they are not specifically licensed for use in children. There are no psychoactive drugs that are specifically contraindicated in children but the manufacturer of the drug or a reference such as the *British National Formulary* should be consulted for dosing information and NICE guidance should be followed if available.

Women

Women receive twice as many prescriptions for psychoactive drugs as men but are largely excluded from clinical trials of new drugs because of the unknown potential for teratogenesis. The treatment of female patients with psychoactive drugs during their reproductive years therefore requires particular care (see Ch. 24).

Oral contraceptive pill

Psychotropic drugs that induce hepatic enzymes and increase the metabolism of both the combined and progesterone-only oral contraceptives include carbamazepine (see above), phenytoin, modafinil, phenobarbital and primidone. Women taking such drugs should either use an alternative method of contraception or take an oral contraceptive that provides 50 µg of ethinylestradiol per day.

Reproductive function

Psychoactive drugs should be avoided in women who are planning to become pregnant or who are already pregnant. However, this is not always possible and when a decision is taken to commence or continue a psychoactive drug during pregnancy because the potential benefit outweighs the potential risk, the following guidelines should be applied:

- Avoid treatment during the 1st trimester when the risk of teratogenicity is greatest if at all possible
- Use the lowest effective dose possible
- Ensure women taking antiepileptic drugs as mood-stabilizers or for epilepsy take appropriate doses of folate supplements before conception and during pregnancy in order to reduce the risk of neural tube defects (such advice is now applicable to all women contemplating pregnancy)
- Use established, rather than recently introduced drugs because more information on their use during pregnancy is available
- Consult the manufacturer of a drug for up-to-date information on its use in pregnancy.

Drugs of choice during pregnancy include carbamazepine and fluoxetine. Acamprosate, antiepileptic drugs other than carbamazepine, benzodiazepines, tricyclic ADs, lithium (see above) and quetiapine should be avoided.

Most psychoactive drugs are secreted in breast milk and although concentrations may be low, breast-feeding infants are at risk of the same adverse effects as adults taking such drugs. Guidelines similar to those applied to pregnant women should therefore be applied to women who are breast-feeding. Breast-feeding women may take AD drugs but should avoid

Electroconvulsive therapy and therapeutic neuromodulation

40

Ross A. Dunne   Declan M. McLoughlin

CHAPTER CONTENTS

Introduction

Italian psychiatrists Ugo Cerletti and Nicolas Bini developed electroconvulsive therapy (ECT) in Rome in 1938 and it was soon thereafter taken up all over the world as a treatment for major mental illness, especially depression and catatonia (Shorter & Healy 2007). In the last 70 years, clinicians and scientists have extensively refined the treatment which continues to be a vital alternative for patients with severe illnesses unresponsive to medications or psychotherapy, or indeed sometimes a treatment of first choice. Research is underway into its mode of action and understanding its antidepressant power may provide ways of elucidating the neurobiology of depression. However, both patients and psychiatrists have concerns about memory side-effects. So, today other methods of brain stimulation are in development with the aim of providing effective treatment but without associated cognitive side-effects. Up to 25% of people with depression do not respond to antidepressants and/or psychotherapy (Warden et al 2007). ECT represents an effective treatment for these people who then remit in 60–70% of cases.

Other neuromodulation techniques range from invasive therapies like deep brain stimulation (DBS) and, to a lesser extent, vagus nerve stimulation (VNS) to non-invasive therapies, such as repetitive transcranial magnetic stimulation (rTMS) and transcranial direct current stimulation (tDCS). DBS provides constant stimulation while rTMS intermittently stimulates the brain. Depending on the parameters used, these treatments can either activate or inhibit the stimulated region. The effectiveness of these therapies and their clinical utility varies widely.

Electroconvulsive therapy

Background

History

Use of deliberate seizure induction to treat severe mental illness has a peculiar, and somewhat serendipitous, history. In the 1920s, small doses of insulin were used in psychiatry to overcome anorexia and weight-loss in mood disordered patients (Kalinowsky & Hippius 1969). Manfred Sakel, an Austrian psychiatrist, subsequently used insulin to induce hypoglycaemia in patients withdrawing from alcohol and opiates. Some patients became comatose and Sakel noted 'a profound change in personality'. He went on to increase doses of insulin to deliberately induce coma and expanded its use to schizophrenia. This became known as 'insulin coma therapy' (ICT). Some patients reportedly had brief remissions following seizures during hypoglycaemic coma. The procedure had a high mortality rate and with the introduction of chlorpromazine in the 1950s, the use of ICT declined (Kalinowsky & Hippius 1969).

At approximately the same time as Sakel's introduction of ICT (1933), Ladislas Von Meduna, a Hungarian psychiatrist and neuropathologist, suggested that epilepsy and schizophrenia might be mutually exclusive because he observed low rates of seizure disorders in his psychotic patients and low rates of psychosis in epileptic patients (Shorter 2009; Fink 1984). He also noted that schizophrenia was associated with low numbers of glial cells in some brain areas, whereas epilepsy was associated with gliosis. Von Meduna suggested that seizures could be used therapeutically to relieve symptoms of schizophrenia and began using intravenous camphor, well known to induce seizures. However, such seizures took up to 3 h to develop and injections caused thrombophlebitis and other complications. So the faster-acting agent 'metrazol' (pentylenetetrazol) soon replaced camphor. Pharmacological convulsive therapy was reportedly successful for affective psychoses but serious complications were common, including vertebral fracture and aspiration pneumonia. Sympathetic discharge between injection and seizure caused a sense of 'impending doom' and there were unpredictable seizures due to increased cortical excitability (Shorter & Healy 2007). Later research has not supported Meduna's glial theories (Gaitatzis et al 2004). However, the glial abnormalities he noted are still a focus of much research in schizophrenia and depression (Cotter et al 2001).

Ugo Cerletti and Nicolas Bini were Roman psychiatrists studying epilepsy who realized they could safely apply an electrical charge to the scalp to stimulate the brain and produce convulsions, thereby producing an animal model of epilepsy (Shorter & Healy 2007). Following the success of pharmacological convulsive therapy, they began testing electroconvulsive therapy in humans and had some initial clinical success in treating psychosis. Soon afterwards, the German psychiatrist Lothar Kalinowsky took the treatment from Italy to the UK and USA through a series of seminars and demonstrations (Kalinowsky & Hippius 1969).

Refinement and development

Not surprisingly, and in the absence of any other reliable and effective intervention, ECT was soon used throughout the world for the treatment of all major mental illnesses. It was effective in severe affective psychosis and offered new hope to those who had previously been considered 'untreatable'. Patients had a series of electrically induced grand-mal seizures and often recovered from their mental illness but, because of the intensity of the uncontrolled seizure, they were prone to fractures and soft tissue injuries. In 1940, the British anaesthetist A.E. Bennett

introduced curare, the first neuromuscular blocking agent, specifically for use in convulsive therapies. This successfully reduced physical movements but was replaced in 1951 by the more reliable agent suxamethonium, now widely used in many anaesthetic settings (Bennett 1994). Barbiturate anaesthetics were introduced soon afterwards, heralding modern 'modified' ECT.

Efforts to further refine ECT began with unilateral stimulation to reduce physical side-effects. The electrodes were placed on one side of the head only, beginning with very low levels of current in order to gradually induce a seizure (Pacella & Impastato 1954). Unilateral ECT caused less memory impairment (Lancaster et al 1958) but was initially shown to be less effective. Later studies showed its effectiveness depended on higher doses of charge. By 1960, the widespread introduction of tricyclic antidepressants had reduced the need for ECT. ECT was further refined by using brief pulses of square-wave stimulation rather than sine-wave stimulation. This aimed to decrease transmitted charge and stimulate neurons more efficiently and thereby possibly reduce cognitive side-effects (Sackeim et al 2007). In the late 1970s and early 1980s, several UK hospitals produced randomized controlled trials to examine ECT vs sham ECT (in which anaesthetic is given without any electrical stimulus or seizure). Meta-analysis of these trials shows clearly that ECT is an effective treatment (UK ECT Review Group 2003). More recently, efforts to minimize the cognitive side-effects of ECT, while maintaining its undoubted clinical effectiveness have focused on modifying electrode placement and narrowing stimulus pulse width in order to stimulate neurons more efficiently (Sackeim et al 1993). These modifications are currently under evaluation in clinical trials.

Stimulus dosing

The seizure threshold (ST) is conventionally defined as the minimum charge required to induce a 25 s EEG seizure (Scott 2005). This can theoretically vary up to 40-fold between individuals (Sackeim et al 1987), although in routine practice there is usually a three- to five-fold difference between patients. A key factor in successful ECT is that the charge used should be appropriately supra-threshold, e.g. at least $1.5 \times$ ST for bilateral ECT. Indeed, it is possible to induce seizures using just a threshold charge but such seizures have less therapeutic value (Thirthalli et al 2009). Seizure threshold should be measured at the first treatment by repeated administration of gradually increasing stimuli, so that the minimum amount of charge is delivered. This is best done by increasing the charge according to a set protocol (Scott 2005). Both psychiatrist and anaesthetist should be aware at the patient's first treatment that they may require re-stimulation. Consequences of not using a stimulus-dosing protocol are over-estimation of the seizure threshold, unnecessary use of too much charge and increased risk of cognitive side-effects. The seizure threshold is higher with bilateral ECT than unilateral ECT. ST often rises during a course of ECT and the duration of seizures may fall in parallel. However, it is clear that seizure duration itself does not correlate well with seizure threshold or antidepressant efficacy of ECT, except that sub-convulsive stimulation appears to be ineffective (Chung 2002; Kales et al 1997).

Electrode placement and treatment frequency

Electrode placement may be either bitemporal (BT), bifrontal (BF) or unilateral (UL) (Fig. 40.1). At seizure threshold, bilateral electroconvulsive therapy (ECT) is more effective than unilateral ECT. As the dose (in millicoulombs, mC) above seizure threshold increases, the efficacy of UL ECT increases. A 1.5 × ST bilateral ECT may have similar efficacy to UL ECT at ~6 times the seizure threshold, but UL ECT may have fewer cognitive side-effects even at this dose. It is believed that unilateral ECT should be given on the language non-dominant side (the right side in the majority of both right and left-handed patients) to avoid structures important for verbal memory. As the dose of UL ECT is increased above 6 × ST, more cognitive impairment becomes evident (Tew et al 2002). Currently, the Royal College of Psychiatrists recommends 4 × ST UL ECT for patients where there is a concern regarding cognitive impairment (Scott 2005). For bitemporal ECT, electrodes are placed 4 cm above the midpoint of a line between the tragus of the ear and the external canthus (Fig. 40.1). For UL ECT, one electrode is placed in this position, the other on the same side, approximately 4 cm inferolateral to the midpoint of a line joining the right and left tragi in a coronal plane. Patients are treated twice weekly in the UK and Ireland and three times per week in the USA. Thrice weekly treatment is not associated with a faster remission but may provoke more memory problems (UK ECT Review Group 2003).

ECT and the media

Attitudes to ECT have changed many times over the last 70 years, varying from positive to negative and from realistic to melodramatic (Pirsig 1974; Ward 1947; Manning 1994). Many

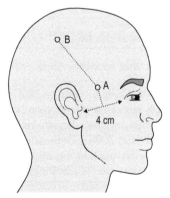

Figure 40.1 • Electrode placements. The figure demonstrates the d'Elia (1970) placement for right unilateral treatment, with one electrode (A) placed 4 cm above the midpoint of a line joining the lateral canthus of the eye and the tragus of the ear. The other electrode (B) is placed approximately 3–4 cm from the vertex. For bitemporal stimulation, both electrodes are placed at point (A) on either side of the head. In bifrontal stimulation both electrodes are placed more anteriorly over the superior orbital ridge on both sides of the forehead (not shown).

portrayals have entered the public consciousness. Ken Kesey's description of the treatment in his novel 'One Flew Over The Cuckoo's Nest' (Kesey 1962) was made more famous by the 1975 film. Indeed, those who have written about ECT have often used the artistic image rather than evidence or experience in order to evoke an emotional response in their audience rather than reasoned deliberation (Healy & Charlton 2009). Many of the most forthright opponents of ECT have based their ideology on artistic and media portrayals of the treatment rather than scientific evidence.

Physical principles of ECT

In ECT, a small electrical current is passed through the brain of an anaesthetized patient given a muscle relaxant. An electrical field is generated between two hand-held electrodes on the scalp separated by several centimetres (Fig. 40.1). This creates a potential difference (voltage), across which an electrical current may flow. An electrolyte gel may be used to aid conduction. Much of the current will flow through the skin and subcutaneous fascia (shunting). Some of the current will pass into the brain inducing widespread stimulation of neurons. This causes a chain-reaction and neuronal firing becomes recurrent and synchronous. There are paroxysmal discharges of large groups of neurons with synchronous electrical discharges involving many areas of the cortex and subcortical structures.

For the patient, this initially results in a facial grimace due to direct stimulation of temporalis muscles. With adequate (above seizure threshold) stimulation, there is an initial tonic phase with extension of the limbs followed by the clonic phase with rhythmic physical movements at roughly 3 beats per second. In some patients, these movements are barely detectable, while for others movement can be stronger. The typical fronto-mastoid EEG recording of 3 Hz spike-wave complexes is most likely generated by thalamocortical circuitry (Destexhe et al 1999; Niedermeyer & Lopes da Silva 2005). Because of the neuromuscular blockade induced by suxamethonium, the most accurate measure of seizure length is duration of EEG seizure activity. Typically, after 30–40 s of ictal activity, there is a flattening of the EEG, with less activity than at baseline and this is referred to as 'EEG suppression' (Fig. 40.2).

Charge in millicoulombs (mC) is the unit of electrical measurement used. The majority of contemporary ECT machines deliver a fixed current of approximately 800 milliamperes (mA) and automatically alter their voltage. Therefore, a higher charge can be delivered only by a longer train of brief pulses. In this way, the patient is exposed to the minimum of energy.

Neurobiology of ECT

Molecular mechanism of action

Short-term changes in synaptic levels of monoamine neurotransmitters, such as serotonin (5HT), noradrenaline (norepinephrine) (NA) and dopamine (DA), are no longer considered the sole biological basis of depression. Increasingly, the focus has moved to cerebral plasticity and its role in mood and cognition.

has been traditionally indicated for postpartum psychosis. Puerperal psychoses show both familial and individual risk-associations with bipolar disorder and mania and therefore may be considered on the spectrum of affective psychoses (Spinelli 2009).

Catatonia

Catatonia is a final common pathway for many severe mental illnesses (Fink et al 2009). Currently, most catatonia occurs in the context of the severe psychomotor retardation of depression. It is now less frequently seen in patients with schizophrenia than in the early twentieth century. Catatonia may also occur in the context of neuroleptic malignant syndrome. ECT and benzodiazepines are the most effective treatments for catatonia. A recent Cochrane systematic review and meta-analysis (Tharyan & Adams 2005) did not support the use of ECT in other presentations of schizophrenia, and a 2005 meta-analytic assessment of the utility and cost-effectiveness of ECT in schizophrenia suggested 'ECT either combined with antipsychotic medication or as a monotherapy is not more effective than antipsychotic medication in people with schizophrenia' (Greenhalgh et al 2005). Clozapine was more clinically effective and cost-effective. The literature on concurrent use of clozapine with ECT in those refractory to clozapine alone is limited to open trials and retrospective studies. There is little evidence to support the combination and there are reports of both prolonged seizures and cardiac arrhythmias during treatment (Tharyan & Adams 2005). However, for schizophrenic patients with catatonia, ECT remains an effective treatment. Due to ethical concerns, it is unlikely such severely ill patients will be included in large-scale randomized controlled trials.

Neurological disorders

Since 1975, many case reports describe that patients with Parkinson disease who had ECT for depression had dramatic, short-term improvements in their tremor and bradykinesia. However, there is little randomized controlled trial evidence for treating psychiatrically well patients with Parkinson's and a recent meta-analysis found only modest effects (Fregni et al 2005). Only case series support the use of maintenance ECT in treatment refractory Parkinson disease.

There are reports that patients with intractable neuropathic pain, or pain associated with thalamic lesions, may benefit from ECT (Abdi et al 2004). Epilepsy is not an absolute contraindication to ECT (although it requires expert neurological assessment and supervision), and case reports even support ECT as an adjunct in those with intractable epilepsy or status epilepticus in expert settings (Kamel et al 2009).

Consent and capacity

To have ECT, patients must have the capacity to give sustained informed consent. Documenting capacity includes assessing the ability to communicate a choice, to understand relevant information, to appreciate the consequences of a decision and to reason about treatment choices. The essential information to communicate to a patient are: the reasons for treatment (Why?, Why now?); the nature of ECT (the deliberate induction of a seizure using a small amount of electricity); its side-effects (physical and cognitive); the use of a general anaesthetic; the nature of the desired outcome and the reasonably expected consequences of not having treatment. Patients should have time to evaluate and weigh their choices before making the decision to have ECT. Patients who are in hospital involuntarily may sometimes be treated without their consent, according to the jurisdiction's guidelines. The UK has a separate Mental Capacity Act (2005) to inform practice. Similar legislation is under consideration in the Republic of Ireland.

Pre-anaesthetic assessment

Before treatment, a complete medical history should be taken and all patients should have a full medical examination. A history of stroke, cardiac ischaemia, gastro-oesophageal reflux disease, hypertension, increased intracranial pressure or respiratory disease is particularly salient. 12-Lead ECG and blood tests, including full blood count and electrolyte levels, are routine. Further tests are performed as indicated according to the medical history and examination. Heavy smokers, the elderly and those with a history of acute respiratory illness should have a chest X-ray (Tess & Smetana 2009). On the morning of ECT, patients should take antihypertensive or antiarrhythmic therapy as normal. As no definitive airway is used and there is a theoretical risk of aspiration of stomach contents, all patients are fasting prior to ECT.

Anaesthesia

ECT should be administered in a dedicated suite if in a psychiatric hospital, preferably with separate waiting, treatment and recovery areas. In a general hospital, it has been successfully used in the theatre recovery area. Any such area should have facilities for continuous monitoring of ECG, blood pressure, pulse-oximetry and end-tidal CO_2. Patients should be medically fit for anaesthesia. The short-acting barbiturate anaesthetic methohexitone sodium is commonly given. Other anaesthetics which may be used include propofol, etomidate and thiopental. Propofol is associated with shorter seizures (Eranti et al 2009). Suxamethonium is the most commonly used muscle relaxant. Immediately after the seizure is induced there is a parasympathetic discharge which causes bradycardia. A short asystole sometime occurs, but rarely needs intervention. Occasionally patients are given atropine or glycopyrrolate to reduce secretions and stop the vagally-mediated bradycardia. However, routine atropine pre-medication is no longer recommended because it may precipitate arrhythmias. Parasympathetic vagal discharge is followed by sympathetic discharge during the seizure accompanied by tachycardia and hypertension. It is important that all patients are oxygenated with 100% oxygen via face-mask prior to the ECT stimulus. Beta adrenoreceptor antagonists are sometimes used in tolerant patients to reduce hypertension. This hypertension usually lasts only minutes, but should be monitored in the recovery area.

Safety

Preoperative anaesthetic evaluation and the facilities required for the safe treatment of patients are described by the Royal College of Psychiatrists (Scott 2005). The mortality for ECT is estimated at <2/100 000 treatments (Munk-Olsen et al 2007; Nuttall et al 2004; Scarano et al 2000), which is similar to that expected with other elective interventions involving anaesthesia. ECT rapidly reduces suicidal ideation; however, demonstrating 'anti-suicidal' properties would require prospective evaluation on an impractically large scale due to the low baseline probability of completed suicide (Kellner et al 2005).

Groups who oppose ECT on ideological grounds often allege that ECT causes 'brain damage'. If this is taken to mean prolonged or permanent loss of brain tissue then there is no evidence in support of this allegation (Dwork et al 2004; Devanand et al 1994). Indeed, ECT in animals fails to mimic the neurotoxic effects of repeated epileptic seizures unless ECT seizures are produced a mere 2 h apart (Cardoso et al 2008). Most of the evidence from animal models suggests that histological change due to ECT is limited to increasing the formation of synapses and neuronal precursors in the hippocampus and possibly mossy fibre sprouting. These changes may correlate with memory impairment, memory improvement relative to baseline depression or mood improvement, but this remains to be investigated.

Cardiac complications are rare, but are still the most common serious adverse effect. Reported incidences for cardiac complications vary. Dec et al (1985) found ECT to be well tolerated using serial ECG and cardiac enzyme monitoring, while Huuhka et al. (2003) used a 24 h Holter recording before and after 26 elderly patients had their first ECT treatment. Bigeminy and supraventricular tachycardia were increased but the presence of arrhythmias before ECT largely predicted their presence after ECT (Huuhka et al 2003). There is no evidence of a cumulative negative effect of ECT treatments on cardiovascular measures (Prudic et al 1987). Aspiration pneumonitis, dental fracture and other serious side-effects are rare in modified ECT but more common in unmodified ECT (Tecoult & Nathan 2001). Modified ECT is thus a medically safe procedure. So when patients are treated by experienced staff in an appropriately equipped setting they can be assured that the minimum of risk applies.

Psychotropic medications and ECT

In the UK and Ireland, most patients continue to receive medications during treatment. In practical terms, this usually causes few concerns. There is a theoretical risk of prolonged seizures with some SSRIs and neuroleptics which may reduce the seizure threshold (Scott 2005). This may only be of practical importance in young people on high dosages. On the other hand, ECT providers should liaise with clinical teams in order to minimize the amount of medications that might raise the seizure threshold, e.g. benzodiazepines or anticonvulsant mood-stabilizers. One recent trial showed some evidence of slightly improved outcomes for patients maintained on SSRI medications during ECT, although this has yet to be replicated (Sackeim et al 2009). After ECT, medications are routinely continued. This reduces the relapse rate after finishing ECT by up to half (Scott 2005; Sackeim et al 2001).

Side-effects

Physical side-effects

Headache affects nearly half of patients after ECT and may be caused by muscle contraction, serotonin release or blood-flow changes. Treatment with non-steroidal anti-inflammatory medications or paracetamol is usually sufficient to manage post-ECT headache (Leung et al 2003). Rarely, some patients may require opioid analgesics. Intranasal sumatriptan given pre-ECT may prevent severe headaches in those with a history of migraine (White et al 2006). Nausea and vomiting occur in 5% of patients after intravenous general anaesthesia for any indication, and rates are similar after ECT (Hofer et al 2003; Gomez 1975). This may be managed during a course of ECT using antiemetic pre-medication. Changing anaesthetic agent from methohexitone to propofol can reduce nausea at the expense of a higher seizure threshold and shorter seizures, though not necessarily less effective treatment (Tramèr et al 1997; Eranti et al 2009).

Cognitive side-effects

Concerns about memory side-effects of ECT have existed since the early 1940s. Psychiatrists often did not take patients' reports of memory impairment seriously, or attributed such impairments solely to depression. This has resulted in a lack of longitudinal research and a paucity of knowledge about ECT-induced memory impairments, especially retrograde amnesia. It has also resulted in much mistrust among those who oppose the use of ECT on ideological grounds. A systematic review of surveys of subjective side-effects found patients more likely to report side-effects to lay organizations than their doctor (Rose et al 2003). Discussing memory impairment freely and openly is a vital part of the informed consent procedure. Patients' concerns should not be minimized and all available facts should be used to help the patient make informed decisions.

Both retrograde and anterograde memory can be affected. Retrograde amnesia involves forgetting already learned facts or events. Anterograde amnesia describes difficulties in encoding new memories. While anterograde amnesia is common during a course of electroconvulsive therapy, it passes on average 14 days after the last treatment and anterograde memory function improves beyond pre-treatment levels (Semkovska & Mcloughlin 2009). Retrograde amnesia is much more difficult to assess as it involves each person's singular memories. In particular, autobiographical memory (memory for personal events) is thought to be affected. Questionnaires designed to test this differ in their sensitivity and validity (Kopelman et al 1989). One such questionnaire used in a large ($n=260$) New York population found autobiographical memory deficits in some patients at 6 months. These deficits were associated with older sine-wave stimulation and the use of bilateral ECT. No data were published to estimate memory impairment in depressed patients who had not received ECT or in a control population (Sackeim et al 2007).

Contraindications

There are few absolute contraindications to ECT. However, certain illnesses increase the risk of complications and therefore must be evaluated before ECT. For patients in whom there is a suspicion of raised intracranial pressure (ICP), space occupying lesion or vascular malformation, there should be appropriate neurological and neurosurgical consultation. During ECT there is a loss of auto-regulatory control of cerebral blood flow, resulting in transiently increased cerebral blood pressure and ICP. Such patients have been treated but may be at increased risk of complications, including death. Recent myocardial infarction and/or cerebrovascular accident are contraindications to ECT as are physical morbidities which would prevent the use of anaesthetic agents, such as severe COPD or congestive heart failure. Congestive heart failure represents a particular risk due to transiently increased blood pressure and associated sympathetic vasoconstriction and tachycardia, resulting in increased afterload and potential decompensation. Treating patients during pregnancy is possible, but should be undertaken in an obstetric environment with expert support.

ECT and the multidisciplinary team

Modern treatment for mental illness is delivered by teams of professionals working together to provide a broad biopsychosocial approach. Patients having ECT are often the most severely ill, but ECT can provide remission from depression within six to eight treatments. However, full recovery from a depressive episode involves more than mere improvement in mood and cognition. People may be returning to stressful life situations or family conflict. Some people choose to share their experience of ECT while others feel that this adds to the stigma of illness. It is easy for medical personnel to focus on the biological power of ECT but miss the maintenance of social and psychological wellbeing that requires input from occupational therapists, psychologists and social workers. Such professionals might not be familiar with ECT and may share many widespread and stereotyped misconceptions. Education of the multidisciplinary team towards realistic expectations of ECT is therefore vital to provide effective care and follow-up.

Therapeutic neuromodulation

Vagus nerve stimulation (VNS)

Vagus nerve stimulation has been used for epilepsy refractory to medication since 1988. Soon after its introduction, some patients with co-morbid depression displayed improvements in mood symptoms independent of reduction in seizures, so clinical trials in treatment-resistant depression began. A pacemaker-like stimulator in the chest wall transmits a pulse to the left cervical vagus nerve via a bipolar electrode for approximately 30 s every 5 min. Vocal hoarseness during stimulation is the main side-effect and complicates treatment blinding in clinical trials (McLoughlin 2008). Other transient side-effects include headache, neck pain, dyspnoea and cough. Rare cardiac side-effects have been reported. Unfortunately, the effectiveness of VNS apparently declines with increasing pre-treatment resistance to established therapies and with severity of depression. The only randomized, sham-controlled trial found VNS not to be effective vs sham treatment (Rush et al 2005). Despite this negative finding, the treatment has been licensed in several countries solely on the basis of longer term open studies demonstrating some, if limited, efficacy (Nahas et al 2005).

Repetitive transcranial magnetic stimulation (rTMS)

rTMS uses a high-powered hand-held electromagnetic coil positioned on the head to create a strong oscillating magnetic field in the brain and therefore an electrical field in underlying brain tissue according to Lenz's law (Feynman et al 2006). The relationship between resulting blood-flow changes and behaviour can then be studied and compared with neurocognitive observations from fMRI studies. Thus, rTMS has had its greatest success as an experimental tool. Initially, it might have represented an alternative to ECT by altering blood-flow in brain areas controlling mood. Although the first clinical trials were encouraging, later trials have shown progressively decreasing effect-sizes and one trial vs ECT showed limited relative efficacy for rTMS (Ebmeier et al 2006; McLoughlin et al 2007) and found ECT to be more cost-effective (Knapp et al 2008). rTMS has failed to demonstrate antidepressant efficacy in treatment-resistant depression in multi-centre sham-controlled trials (Herwig et al 2007; O'Reardon et al 2007; Mogg et al 2008). Recent meta-analyses show that some statistically significant effects can be detected vs sham, but the clinical usefulness of this treatment is very limited, with only 25% of patients responding vs 9% of sham-treated patients (Lam et al 2008). Despite disappointing clinical trial results, several international governing bodies have licensed rTMS for clinical use. It remains to be seen whether future refinements or trials will enhance its clinical utility. Notably, sham control in trials is difficult due to scalp sensations associated with a strong magnetic field.

Transcranial direct current stimulation (tDCS)

Transcranial direct current stimulation (tDCS) is not a new treatment, but remains highly experimental, with little good quality clinical evidence to support its use. It was first evaluated in the late nineteenth century and then again in the middle of the twentieth century (Bindman et al 1964; Lippold & Redfearn 1964). Pre-clinical evidence of an effect on cerebral blood flow has been equivocal and the treatment needs much further pre-clinical and clinical evaluation.

Neurosurgery for mental illness

Antonio Egas Moniz was a Portuguese neurologist who won the 1949 Nobel Prize for Medicine or Physiology for his introduction of prefrontal leucotomy, the crude ablation of prefrontal white matter tracts. In an era when mental illness was regarded as a process of inevitable decline in mental functioning which would always involve institutional care, Egas Moniz aimed to reduce the suffering of those he saw as incurably mentally ill. However, the technique was mimicked and altered by unskilled practitioners with often disastrous consequences. During these latter procedures, techniques were often unsterile or performed without patients' consent. Now, stereotactic neurosurgery for mental illness bears more resemblance to modern neurosurgical techniques used to relieve chronic physical pain or dystonia. However, its controversial history means that it is subject to the strictest controls of any medical treatment (Matthews et al. 2006).

Stereotactic neurosurgery for mental illness is now used only for selected patients with chronic, treatment-resistant depression or obsessive compulsive disorder. In the UK, Europe and the USA, patients are referred to national tertiary care centres. Referral to these services results in further assessment and intervention with psychological, pharmacological and physical interventions including occasionally VNS and DBS. Of patients referred, approximately 10% finally undergo ablative surgery. Patients continue their pharmacological and psychotherapeutic management after surgical treatment. Therefore surgery is not a 'last resort', but an additional treatment for patients who remain pervasively disabled by their mental illness after multiple therapies. Techniques have developed considerably in the past 50 years and bilateral anterior cingulotomy and bilateral anterior capsulotomy are the two techniques commonly used to thermally ablate ventral and medial prefrontal cortical areas. Modern functional and anatomical studies confirm the importance of these structures in depression and OCD. Neurosurgery for mental illness is not performed without the patient's consent and contraindications include the inability to provide sustained informed consent, substance misuse, organic pathology or the presence of primary personality disorder (Matthews et al. 2006).

Deep brain stimulation (DBS)

Deep brain stimulation has had success in the treatment of dystonia, chronic pain and Parkinson disease (PD). Fine electrodes are placed neurosurgically under local anaesthesia in areas of the brain involved in the particular pathology. Tremor in PD can be alleviated by stimulation of the subthalamic nucleus or globus pallidus. Treatment of depression has focused on similar areas as ablative surgery, i.e. subgenual cingulate gyrus (Brodmann area 25). Complications can include infection, involuntary laughter and hypomania. As yet, DBS for depression is an experimental non-ablative treatment in depression and OCD but small case series and open trials have suggested some utility (Mayberg et al 2005; Greenberg et al 2006).

Summary

- ECT is a medically safe procedure, giving 60–70% of those with treatment-resistant depression remission after 6–8 treatments, and has been the most acutely effective treatment for depression for over 70 years. It is now used primarily for severe or treatment-resistant depression and is a first-line treatment for catatonia.

- Current trials are underway to further refine ECT, reducing cognitive side-effects while maintaining its undoubted efficacy.

- DBS, VNS, rTMS and tDCS are experimental treatments awaiting large-scale clinical trials showing robust evidence of clinical utility. They show promise in developing treatments using burgeoning neuroscientific knowledge.

- Neurosurgery for mental illness is practised in a few specialized centres worldwide. It provides additional therapeutic options for those with treatment-resistant, disabling depression or OCD. It bears little resemblance to older procedures.

References

Abdi, S., Haruo, A., Bloomstone, J., 2004. Electroconvulsive therapy for neuropathic pain: a case report and literature review. Pain Physician 7, 261–263.

Bennett, A.E., 1994. Curare: a preventive of traumatic complications in convulsive shock therapy (including a preliminary report on a synthetic curare-like drug). Am. J. Psychiatry 151, 248–258.

Bindman, L.J., Lippold, O.C., Redfearn, J.W., 1964. The action of brief polarizing currents on the cerebral cortex of the rat (1) during current flow and (2) in the production of long-lasting after-effects. J. Physiol. 172, 369–382.

Campbell, S., Marriott, M., Nahmias, C., et al., 2004. Lower hippocampal volume in patients suffering from depression: a meta-analysis. Am. J. Psychiatry 161, 598–607.

Cardoso, A., Assunção, M., Andrade, J.P., et al., 2008. Loss of synapses in the entorhinal-dentate gyrus pathway following repeated induction of electroshock seizures in the rat. J. Neurosci. Res. 86, 71–83.

Chung, K.F., 2002. Relationships between seizure duration and seizure threshold and stimulus dosage at electroconvulsive therapy: implications for electroconvulsive therapy practice. Psychiatry Clin. Neurosci. 56, 521–526.

Cotter, D., Mackay, D., Landau, S., et al., 2001. Reduced glial cell density and neuronal size in the anterior cingulate cortex in major depressive disorder. Arch. Gen. Psychiatry 58, 545–553.

Czeh, B., Lucassen, P.J., 2007. What causes the hippocampal volume decrease in depression? Are neurogenesis, glial changes and apoptosis implicated? Eur. Arch. Psychiatry Clin. Neurosci. 257, 250–260.

Dec Jr., G.W., Stern, T.A., Welch, C., 1985. The effects of electroconvulsive therapy on serial electrocardiograms and serum cardiac enzyme values. A prospective study of depressed hospitalized inpatients. J. Am. Med. Assoc. 253, 2525–2529.

Destexhe, A., McCormick, D.A., Sejnowski, T.J., 1999. Thalamic and thalamocortical mechanisms underlying 3 Hz spike-and-wave discharges. Prog. Brain Res. 121, 289–307.

Devanand, D.P., Dwork, A.J., Hutchinson, E.R., et al., 1994. Does ECT alter brain structure? Am. J. Psychiatry 151, 957–970.

Dwork, A.J., Arango, V., Underwood, M., et al., 2004. Absence of histological lesions in primate models of ECT and magnetic seizure therapy. Am. J. Psychiatry 161, 576–578.

Index

Note: Page numbers followed by *b* indicate boxes, *f* indicate figures and *t* indicate tables.